Seventh Edition

Shortell and Kaluzny's
Health Care Management
Organization Design and Behavior

Seventh Edition

Shortell and Kaluzny's
Health Care Management
Organization Design and Behavior

Lawton Robert Burns | Elizabeth Howe Bradley | Bryan Jeffrey Weiner

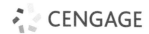

CENGAGE

Australia • Brazil • Mexico • Singapore • United Kingdom • United States

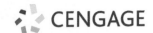

Shortell and Kaluzny's Health Care Management: Organization Design and Behavior, Seventh Edition
Lawton Robert Burns, Elizabeth Howe Bradley, and Bryan Jeffrey Weiner

SVP, GM Skills & Global Product Management: Jonathan Lau

Product Director: Matthew Seeley

Product Team Manager: Stephen Smith

Associate Product Manager: Lauren Whalen

Product Assistant: Jessica Molesky

Executive Director, Content Design: Marah Bellegarde

Director, Learning Design: Juliet Steiner

Learning Designer: Deborah Bordeaux

Vice President, Marketing Services: Jennifer Ann Baker

Marketing Director: Sean Chamberland

Marketing Manager: Jonathan Sheehan

Senior Director, Content Delivery: Wendy Troeger

Senior Content Manager: Thomas Heffernan

Digital Delivery Lead: Derek Allison

Managing Art Director: Jack Pendleton

Senior Designer: Angela Sheehan

Cover Image: Excellent backgrounds/ ShutterStock.com

Compositor: Lumina Datamatics, Inc.

For product information and technology assistance, contact us at **Cengage Learning Customer & Sales Support, 1-800-354-9706**

For permission to use material from this text or product, submit all requests online at **www.cengage.com/permissions.** Further permissions questions can be e-mailed to **permissionrequest@cengage.com**

Library of Congress Control Number: 2018964616

Student edition:
ISBN: 978-1-305-95117-4

Loose-leaf edition:
ISBN: 978-1-337-90554-1

Cengage
20 Channel Center Street
Boston, MA 02210
USA

Cengage is a leading provider of customized learning solutions with employees residing in nearly 40 different countries and sales in more than 125 countries around the world. Find your local representative at: **www.cengage.com**

Cengage Learning products are represented in Canada by Nelson Education, Ltd.

To learn more about Cengage platforms and services, register or access your online learning solution, or purchase materials for your course, visit: **www.cengage.com**

Notice to the Reader

Printed in Mexico
Print Number: 01   Print Year: 2018

Contents

Contributors

Jane Banaszak-Holl, PhD

Professor of Public Health
School of Public Health and Preventive Medicine
Monash University
Melbourne, Australia

Elizabeth Howe Bradley, PhD, MBA

President
Vassar College
Poughkeepsie, New York

Amanda Brewster, PhD

Assistant Professor of Health Policy & Management
School of Public Health
University of California
Berkeley, California

Lawton Robert Burns, PhD, MBA

The James Joo-Jin Kim Professor, Professor of Health
Care Management, and Director of the Wharton
Center for Health Management and Economics
The Wharton School, University of Pennsylvania
Philadelphia, Pennsylvania

Martin P. Charns, MBA, DBA

Professor of Health Policy and Management
School of Public Health, Boston University
Investigator and Director Emeritus
Center for Healthcare Organization &
Implementation Research
VA Boston Healthcare System
Boston, Massachusetts

Jon A. Chilingerian, PhD

Professor of Management
Heller School, Brandeis University
Adjunct Professor of Public Health & Community
Medicine
Tufts School of Medicine
Waltham, Massachusetts

Ann F. Chou, PhD, MPH, MA

Associate Professor of Family and Preventive Medicine
College of Medicine
University of Oklahoma Health Sciences Center
Oklahoma City, Oklahoma

Ann Leslie Claesson-Vert, PhD, MSN, PSP

Associate Clinical Professor
Lead Faculty Personalized Learning MSN Program
Northern Arizona University, North Valley Campus
Phoenix, Arizona

Thomas D'Aunno, PhD

Professor of Management
Robert F. Wagner Graduate School of
Public Service
New York University
New York, New York

Mark L. Diana, MBA, MSIS, PhD

Drs. W.C. Tsai and P.T. Kung Professor in Health
Systems Management
Associate Professor and Chair, Department of Health
Policy and Management
Tulane University
New Orleans, Louisiana

Amy C. Edmondson, PhD

Novartis Professor of Leadership and Management
Harvard Business School
Boston, Massachusetts

Bruce Fried, PhD

Associate Professor
Department of Health Policy and Management
University of North Carolina at Chapel Hill
Chapel Hill, North Carolina

Mattia J. Gilmartin RN, PhD, FAAN

Executive Director
NICHE I Nurses Improving Care for Healthsystem
Elders
Rory Meyers College of Nursing
New York University
New York, New York

Jennifer L. Hefner, PhD, MPH

Assistant Professor
Division of Health Services Management and Policy
College of Public Health
The Ohio State University
Columbus, Ohio

Christian D. Helfrich, PhD, MPH

Core Investigator, VA Puget Sound Health Services
Research and Development
Research Associate Professor, Health Services
School of Public Health
University of Washington
Seattle, Washington

Timothy Hoff, PhD

Professor of Management, Healthcare Systems,
and Health Policy
D'Amore-McKim School of Business
School of Public Policy and Urban Affairs
Northeastern University
Boston, Massachusetts

Peter D. Jacobson, JD, MPH

Professor Emeritus of Health Law and Policy
Director, Center for Law, Ethics, and Health
University of Michigan School of Public Health
Ann Arbor, Michigan

John R. Kimberly, PhD

Henry Bower Professor of Entrepreneurial Studies
Professor of Management
Professor of Health Care Management
The Wharton School, University of Pennsylvania
Philadelphia, Pennsylvania

Sumit R. Kumar, MD, MPA

Resident Physician, Yale New Haven Hospital
Department of Internal Medicine
Yale School of Medicine
New Haven, Connecticut

Kristin Madison, JD, PhD

Professor of Law and Health Sciences
Northeastern University
Boston, Massachusetts

Ann Scheck McAlearney, ScD, MS

Executive Director, Professor of Family Medicine
CATALYST, The Center for the Advancement of Team
Science, Analytics, and Systems Thinking
College of Medicine, Ohio State University
Columbus, Ohio

Eilish McAuliffe, PhD, MSc, MBA

Professor of Health Systems
School of Nursing, Midwifery, and Health Systems
College of Health and Agricultural Sciences
University College Dublin
Dublin, Ireland

Mario Moussa, PhD, MBA

Adjunct Instructor
Division of Programs in Business
School of Professional Studies
New York University
New York, New York

Ingrid M. Nembhard, PhD, MS

Fishman Family President's Distinguished Associate
Professor of Health Care Management
The Wharton School, University of Pennsylvania
Philadelphia, Pennsylvania

Derek Newberry

Adjunct Professor
Organizational Dynamics and Anthropology
University of Pennsylvania

Ann Nguyen, PhD, MPH

Postdoctoral Fellow
Department of Population Health
School of Medicine
New York University
New York, New York

Laurel E. Radwin, PhD, RN

Research Health Scientist (formerly)
Center for Healthcare Organization and
Implementation Research
Boston VA Healthcare System
Boston, Massachusetts

Kevin W. Rockmann, PhD

Professor, School of Management
George Mason University
Fairfax, Virginia

Aditi Sen, PhD

Assistant Professor of Health Policy and
Management
Bloomberg School of Public Health
Johns Hopkins University
Baltimore, Maryland

Lauren Taylor, MPH

Doctoral Candidate
Harvard Business School
Harvard University

Gregory L. Vert

Assistant Professor
College of Security and Intelligence
Embry Riddle Aeronautical University
Prescott, Arizona

Karen A. Wager, DBA

Professor and Associate Dean for
Student Affairs
Department of Healthcare Leadership
and Management
College of Health Professions
Medical University of South Carolina
Charleston, South Carolina

Stephen L. Walston, PhD

Professor
Director, MHA Program
David Eccles School of Business
University of Utah
Salt Lake City, Utah

Bryan Jeffrey Weiner, PhD
Professor, Departments of Global Health
and Health Services
University of Washington
Seattle, Washington

Gary J. Young, JD, PhD
Director, Northeastern University Center for
Health Policy and Healthcare Research
Professor of Strategic Management
and Healthcare Systems
Northeastern University
Boston, Massachusetts

Edward J. Zajac, PhD
James F. Beré Professor of Organization Behavior
J. L. Kellogg Graduate School of Management
Northwestern University
Evanston, Illinois

Foreword

For twenty-five years and six editions, we have attempted to provide an integrative perspective to the organization and management of health services, presenting the major management theories, concepts, and practices of the day. We have also provided practical illustrations and guidelines to assist managers and prospective managers in the provision of health services in a variety of settings.

As we go to press, we have entered the era of health care reform, presenting new and perhaps not so new challenges and opportunities. Under the leadership of Rob Burns, Elizabeth Bradley, and Bryan Weiner, the invited chapter authors have provided a thoughtful and in-depth analysis of the theories, concepts, and approaches that managers and prospective managers need to address the critical issues in the provision of health services as well as meet the challenges and opportunities resulting from health care reform.

The passage of health care reform brings a great deal of uncertainty as it attempts to address the long-standing problems of access, quality, cost containment, and significant disparities under unprecedented economic conditions. Much has changed as reflected in the mandates regarding access to coverage, coverage itself, the role of public and private programs, and health insurance exchanges as well as the role of comparative effective studies, payment reforms, accountable care organizations, and patient-centered medical homes.

While these represent significant changes in the operation of the delivery system, the fundamental managerial challenges remain and will continue to require skillful attention if health care and the various delivery organizations are to realize their potential. Issues of maintaining a motivated workforce, assuring state-of-the-art practice patterns, coordinating various disciplines and specialties to the benefit of patient care, and accommodating an ever-expanding technology within a market economy that would benefit the patient and the larger community have been and will continue to be the major responsibility of management.

This seventh edition provides readers with the relevant theories, concepts, tools, and applications to address operational issues that managers face on a daily basis. As described in the lead chapter, the key challenge facing organizations and their managers is to deliver "value"— the ratio of quality to cost. While this has always been a concern, the reality of present-day economics and the developing science has made this imperative.

The book is divided into three sections. The first section provides two insightful introductory chapters presenting the challenges of providing health services and some of the conceptual maps necessary to help guide managers in the decision-making process and providing a framework for understanding the role and contributions of management and leadership within a variety of health care settings.

The next section focuses on the Micro Perspective— Managing the Internal Environment. This perspective addresses the classic issues of organization design, motivation, communications, power, organizational learning, performance/quality improvement, and managing groups and teams. Each chapter provides an "In Practice" scenario that sets the scene for the concepts and tools for effective management.

The last section, the Macro Perspective—Managing the External Environment, focuses on the organizational context and addresses the challenge of achieving competitive advantage and managing alliances. Four new chapters will help prepare managers for the uncertainty of the years ahead. These include the challenges of managing an ever-expanding information technology, consumerism, an increasingly complex regulatory environment, and finally the recognition that we live in a globalized world.

Health services management has come of age, and Burns, Bradley, Weiner, and their colleagues have presented the theories, concepts, and guidelines that future managers will need to succeed in the years ahead.

Stephen M. Shortell, PhD
Blue Cross of California Distinguished
Professor of Health Policy & Management
Professor of Organizational Behavior,
Haas School of Business and Dean,
    School of Public Health
University of California, Berkeley
Berkeley, California

Arnold D. Kaluzny, PhD
Professor Emeritus of Health and Policy
    & Management,
Gillings School of Global Public Health, and Senior
    Research Fellow
Cecil G. Sheps Center for Health Services Research,
University of North Carolina at Chapel Hill,
Chapel Hill, North Carolina

Preface

INTRODUCTION

This book is intended for those interested in a systemic understanding of organizational principles, practices, and insights pertinent to the management of health services organizations. The book is based on state-of-the-art organization theory and research with an emphasis on application. Although the primary audience is graduate students in health services administration, management, and policy programs, the book will also be of interest to undergraduate programs, extended degree programs, executive education programs, and practicing health sector executives interested in the latest developments in organizational and managerial thinking. It is also intended for students of business, public administration, medicine, nursing, pharmacy, social work, and other health professions who will assume managerial responsibilities in health sector organizations or who want to learn more about the organizations in which they will spend the major portion of their professional lives. Previous editions have been translated into Polish, Korean, Ukrainian, and Hungarian, and we look forward to the book's continued use by our international colleagues.

TEXT APPROACH

The seventh edition broadens the view of the health care sector beyond the traditional focus on hospitals and other provider organizations to include suppliers, buyers, regulators, and public health and financing organizations. It offers a comparative, global perspective on how the United States and other countries address issues of health and health care. Additionally, the book discusses managerial implications of emerging issues in health care such as public reporting, pay for performance, information technology, retail medicine, ethics, and medical tourism. Finally, this seventh edition expands upon a major theme of prior editions: health care leaders must effectively design and manage health care organizations while simultaneously influencing and adapting to changes in environmental context. Managing the boundary between the internal organization and its external environment is therefore a central task of health care leadership.

ORGANIZATION

The organization of the book reflects this expanded theme. Part 1 provides an overall perspective on the health care sector, discusses the distinctive challenges facing health care organizations, and examines the roles of leaders and managers in influencing organizational culture, performance, and change. Part 2 focuses on core leadership and managerial tasks within organizations. These include motivating people, guiding teams, designing structure, coordinating work, communicating effectively, exerting influence, resolving conflict, negotiating agreements, improving performance, and managing innovation and change. Part 3 describes the broader context in which health care organizations operate and discusses the managerial implications of several emerging trends and issues. These include the pursuit of strategies to achieve the organization's mission, the growth of strategic alliances in the health sector, the expansion and complexity of health law and regulation, the uses and challenges of health information technology, the rise of consumerism in health care, and the global interconnectedness of health systems.

FEATURES

The Seventh edition continues several popular features from the sixth edition. These include the following:

- An explicit list of topics provided at the beginning of each chapter.
- Specific behaviorally oriented Learning Objectives highlighted at the beginning of each chapter.
- A list of Key Terms that readers should be able to define and apply as a result of reading each chapter.
- An "In Practice" column describing a practical situation facing a health services organization.
- A section in several chapters called "Debate Time," which poses a controversial issue or presents divergent perspectives to stimulate the reader's thinking.
- Comprehensive Managerial Guidelines and Summary points at the conclusion of each chapter.
- Discussion Questions that help reinforce chapter concepts.

NEW TO THIS EDITION

The seventh edition updates the case studies included in the sixth edition along with the case discussion questions. It also updates the ongoing developments in health policy and regulation, as well as the research evidence in each chapter's subject matter. It also includes several new authors, expanding the community of healthcare management scholars contributing to this volume.

MINDTAP

MindTap is a personalized teaching experience with relevant assignments that guide students to analyze, apply, and improve thinking, allowing you to measure skills and outcomes with ease.

- MindTap features a complete integrated course combining additional quizzing and assignments, and application activities along with the enhanced ebook to further facilitate learning.

- **Personalized Teaching:** Becomes yours with a Learning Path that is built with key student objectives. Control what students see and when they see it. Use it as-is or match to your syllabus exactly–hide, rearrange, add and create your own content.

- **Guide Students:** A unique learning path of relevant readings and activities that move students up the learning taxonomy from basic knowledge and comprehension to analysis and application.

- **Promote Better Outcomes:** Empower instructors and motivate students with analytics and reports that provide a snapshot of class progress, time in course, engagement and completion rates.

INSTRUCTOR RESOURCES

Instructor Companion Site

The Instructor Companion site for this text offers many valuable support materials. To access the Instructor Companion site, go to http://login.cengage.com.

If you have a Cengage SSO account: Sign in with your e-mail address and password.

If you do not have a Cengage SSO account: Click Create My Account and follow the prompts.

The following support materials are included:

- **Electronic Instructor's Manual**—The Instructor's Manual that accompanies this book includes an overview of the In Practice and Debate Time material from the text, suggested solutions to the end-of-chapter discussion questions and case studies, teaching tips and exercises, complimentary reading lists, suggested solutions to the Vignette material in the study guide, and an overview of additional Debate Time material from the study guide.

- **PowerPoint presentations**—This book comes with Microsoft PowerPoint slides for each chapter. They're included as a teaching aid for classroom presentation, to make available to students on the network for chapter review, or to be printed for classroom distribution. Instructors, please feel free to add your own slides for additional topics you introduce to the class.

- **ExamView®**—ExamView®, the ultimate tool for objective-based testing needs, is a powerful test generator that enables instructors to create paper, LAN, or Web-based tests from test banks designed specifically for their Cengage Course Technology text. Instructors can utilize the ultraefficient QuickTest Wizard to create tests in less than five minutes by taking advantage of Cengage Course Technology's questions banks or customize their own exams from scratch.

- **Sample Course Syllabus**—The Sample Syllabus was developed to help instructors customize specific course titles.

ABOUT THE AUTHORS

Lawton Robert Burns is the James Joo-Jin Kim Professor and Professor of Health Care Management in the Health Care Management Department at the Wharton School, University of Pennsylvania. He is also Director of the Wharton Center for Health Management and Economics, and Co-Director of the Roy & Diana Vagelos Program in Life Sciences and Management. His research focuses on hospital–physician relationships, strategic change, integrated health care, supply chain management, health care management, formal organizations, physician networks, and physician practice management firms. Dr. Burns is the author of several books, including *Managing Discovery: Harnessing Creativity to Drive Biomedical Innovation* (2018), *China's Healthcare System and Reform* (2017), *India's Healthcare Industry* (2014), *The Business of Healthcare Innovation* (2012), *Health Care History and Policy in the United States* (2006), *and The Health Care Value Chain* (2002). He is the recipient of numerous grants, fellowships, and awards, including the 2015 Keith Provan Distinguished Scholar Award from the Academy of Management and its Health Care Administration Division. Dr. Burns has also provided expert witness testimony for the federal government as well as for the private sector. He is a member of the Academy of Management and the American Hospital Association. Lawton R. Burns has a Bachelor of Arts Degree in Sociology and Anthropology, a Master's Degree in Sociology, a Masters in Business Administration, and a Doctor of Philosophy Degree in Sociology.

Elizabeth Howe Bradley, PhD, is the President of Vassar College in Poughkeepsie, New York. She was previously a Professor of Public Health at the Yale School of Public Health, where she directed the Health Management Program for a decade and subsequently the Global Health Leadership Institute. Bradley is renowned internationally for her work on quality of hospital care and large-scale health system strengthening efforts within the US and abroad. Bradley is the author of *The American Healthcare Paradox: Why Spending More Is Getting Us Less* and the 2018 recipient of the William B. Graham Prize for Health Services Research, the highest distinction that researchers in the health services field can achieve. Bradley was elected to the National Academy of Medicine in 2017. President Bradley has a Bachelor of Arts Degree in Economics, a Master of Business Administration, and a Doctor of Philosophy Degree in Health Policy and Health Economics.

Bryan Jeffrey Weiner, PhD, is Professor in the Departments of Global Health and Health Services at the University of Washington. Dr. Weiner directs the Implementation Science Program in the Department of Global Health and serves as the Strategic Hire in Implementation Science for the School of Public Health. His research focuses on the adoption, implementation, and sustainment of innovations and evidence-based practices in health care organizations. He is member of the Academy of Management, Academy Health, and the American Public Health Association. Dr. Weiner has a Bachelor of Arts Degree in Psychology, a Master of Arts Degree in Organizational Psychology, and a Doctor of Philosophy Degree in Organizational Psychology.

ACKNOWLEDGMENTS

We believe that the major strength of this text is the diversity of the talented authors, who contributed multiple perspectives, experiences, skills, and expertise to each chapter. The new and substantially revised chapters reflect the breadth and depth of the authors' expertise as well as their fresh perspectives. We wish to acknowledge with gratitude the immeasurable contribution that Stephen Shortell and Arnold Kaluzny have made in the fields of health care management research and education. As scholars, advisors, mentors, and colleagues, they have deeply influenced our work and our professional lives. Through the six editions of this book, over the past twenty-five years, they have helped educate a generation of health services researchers, policy makers, managers, and health professionals. We hope that the seventh edition sustains the tradition of excellence that these gentlemen have established.

Finally, we wish to acknowledge Lauren Taylor and Rachelle Alpern for their excellent editorial assistance.

Lawton Robert Burns
University of Pennsylvania
Elizabeth Howe Bradley
Vassar College
Bryan Jeffrey Weiner
University of Washington

1

PART ONE
Introduction

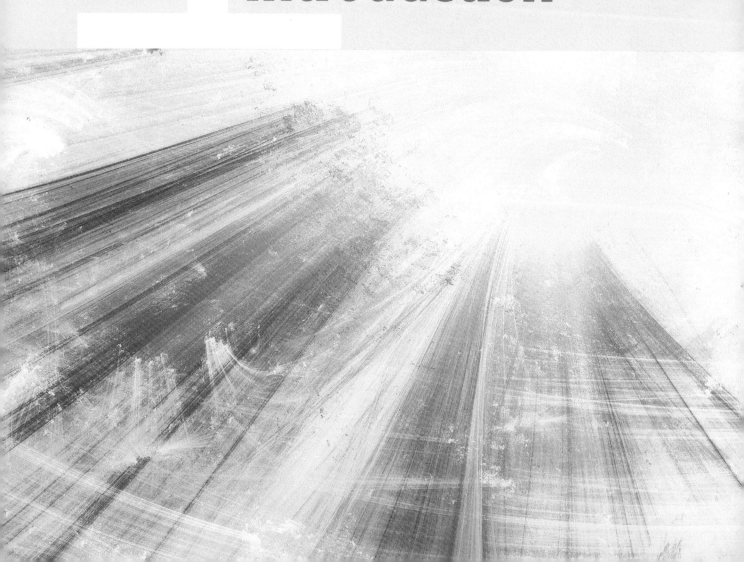

Chapter 1

Delivering Value: The Global Challenge in Health Care Management

Lawton Robert Burns, Elizabeth H. Bradley, and Bryan J. Weiner

CHAPTER OUTLINE

- The Challenge: Deliver Value
- Challenge of Rising Health Care Costs: Supply- and Demand-Side Price and Volume Drivers
- Other Challenges Exacerbating the Value Challenge
- The Challenges are Global
- Complexity of the U.S. Health Care System
- Why Changing the Health Care System Is So Difficult
- Systemic Views of Health and U.S. Health Care
- Organization and Management Theory
- Summative Views of Organization Theory
- Organization Theory and Behavior: A Guide to This Text

LEARNING OBJECTIVES

After completing this chapter, the reader should be able to:

1. Discuss the challenge of delivering value in health care
2. Identify the major forces affecting the delivery of health services
3. Distinguish the similarities and differences in the forces shaping health services globally
4. Discuss why it is difficult to change the health care industry
5. Develop a system view of health care delivery
6. Discuss the different types of firms operating in a health care system
7. Identify, discuss and apply the major perspectives and theories on organizations to real problems facing health care organizations
8. Analyze in analyzing problems from multiple theoretical lenses

KEY TERMS

Ambidexterity	Evidence-Based Medicine
Bending the Cost Curve	External Environment
Bounded Rationality	Health Systems
Bureaucracy	Hospital–Physician Relationships
Classical School of Administration	Human Relations School
Complex Adaptive System	Institutional Theory
Contingency Theory	Iron Triangle
Decision-Making School	Macro Perspective

Micro Perspective	Social Network Approach
Moral Hazard	Strategic Management Perspective
Open Systems Theory	System Perspectives
Population Ecology	Triple Aim
Resource Dependence Theory	Value
Scientific Management School	Value Chain

• • • IN PRACTICE: The GAVI Alliance

The Global Alliance for Vaccines and Immunization (GAVI) is one of the largest global health initiatives (GHIs) that targets specific diseases/conditions to help meet Millennium Development Goals. GAVI was launched at the World Economic Forum on January 31, 2000, to improve the distribution of new and underused vaccines to low-income countries and thereby reduce childhood mortality and morbidity, and increase the health status of these populations (GAVI Alliance, 2010; Martin and Marshall, 2003; Milstien et al., 2008).

GAVI was a partnership of developing countries, organizations involved in international development and finance (e.g., United Nations Children's Fund, the World Health Organization, the World Bank), the pharmaceutical industry, and philanthropic organizations (e.g., the Bill and Melinda Gates Foundation provided seed funding of $750 million). GAVI lacked presence at the local level, and thus relied on its partners for planning and implementation in each country.

A number of managerial challenges faced the GAVI Alliance in achieving its goals. First, the vision of the GAVI Alliance had to motivate local countries to participate in this vaccination program and gradually increase their own funding for it. Second, local countries needed to accept the responsibility to deliver the vaccine programs and the attendant results. Third, these countries had to help develop and manage local infrastructure to deliver the vaccines to rural populations—often referred to as the last hundred yards or miles of the supply chain. This meant the countries needed not only transportation and distribution networks but also a cadre of local health care workers with training in vaccine storage and administration. Fourth, the GAVI Alliance had to manage diverse stakeholders, including its core founding members such as the World Bank, WHO, UNICEF, and the Gates Foundation. Fifth, the GAVI Alliance had to operate with a lean structure such that bureaucracy did not slow its progress. Sixth, the alliance had to develop leverage over pharmaceutical firms to purchase the needed drugs at a lower cost, which local countries could afford. Last, the GAVI Alliance needed a clear governance structure with defined responsibilities for partners.

Since its inception in 2000 through 2013, GAVI directly supported the immunization of 440 million children (e.g., for Hepatitis B, Haemophilus influenzae type B (Hib), and yellow fever), with an increase in global immunization coverage rates from 70 percent to 83 percent. Such efforts have helped to decrease the global under-five mortality rate. In addition to speeding up population access to underused vaccines, GAVI has also pursued efforts in strengthening health systems, improving vaccine storage and delivery, getting immunization onto national health agendas, and stimulating research and development for vaccines (World Bank Group, 2012).

Despite its success, GAVI has not been without its problems. Although the alliance necessarily focused heavily on developing partnerships and initiating vaccine coverage, less attention was paid to implementation of plans and mobilization of resources for ongoing treatment (in-country follow-up). One reason may be that vaccine costs have risen both absolutely and as a percentage of the total health expenditures, and vaccinations may not be the top priority of developing-country governments (Milstien et al., 2008; Muraskin, 2004). Moreover, the alliance partners needed to grapple with the large supply chain "system costs" required to handle, transport, and store the drugs (Lydon et al., 2008) and the issue of securing long-term financial commitments from its partners. An additional problem is that GAVI's single-minded focus on vertical programs such as vaccination may have diverted countries from broader efforts to develop and finance their health systems. The "Gates Foundation approach" to global health, focused on targeted technical solutions with clear and measurable outcomes, did not fit easily with broader investments needed in the social determinants of health (e.g., social and economic development) (Storeng, 2014). GAVI acknowledged this issue by adopting "health system strengthening" (HSS) as a core principle, but such support was still heavily concentrated on procuring drugs, equipment, and supplies (Tsai, Lee, and Fan, 2016). Finally, in 2008, GAVI reorganized its informal alliance model to become an independent legal entity that diluted the influence of its founding partners. World Bank interactions with and financing of GAVI immunization efforts subsequently declined.

CHAPTER PURPOSE

A central challenge in delivering health care services in the new millennium is the challenge of delivering value. *Value* is created when (a) additional features of quality or customer service desired by a customer can be provided at the same cost or price, (b) a given set of features of quality or customer service can be delivered at a lower cost or price relative to other producers, or (c) additional features of quality can be provided at a lower cost. At a societal level, health and wealth exert beneficial effects on one another. Investments in health care delivery that improve quality and/or reduce cost can improve health status, which in turn can support economic growth and political stability (Burns, D'Aunno, and Kimberly, 2003; Esty et al., 1999; Sachs, 2001). Conversely, economic development that raises the standard of living and socioeconomic conditions improves the population's health (Cutler, Deaton, and Lleras-Muney, 2006; Liu, Yao, and Du, 2015).

Nevertheless, health investments that enhance value are not always made. For instance, despite evidence of the benefits of immunization coverage (Martin and Marshall, 2003; World Health Organization, 1996) and a steady increase globally during the 1970s and 1980s, immunization coverage declined sharply in the 1990s due to curtailed government funding in low-income countries. For example, Mao's agenda to increase public health investments in China, which led to rapidly increasing life expectancy, was reversed and subordinated to economic growth under Deng Xiaoping as a part of the country's economic liberalization reforms.

The GAVI Alliance entered in 2000 and, during its first 13 years, raised over $8.4 billion, disbursed over $6 billion to 76 countries, improved the quality and safety of vaccines administered in poor countries, reduced the procurement cost of these drugs through centralized purchasing, and immunized nearly half a billion children against deadly or disabling diseases.

Why was this approach not already taken? To effect major changes in health care delivery and increase value, as the GAVI Alliance has, organizations require extraordinary approaches. Such approaches critically hinge on several management competencies. These include assembling (global) alliances, clarifying the governance structure of the alliance, developing the local health care infrastructure to deliver the needed services, balancing global and local commitments, and developing local ownership of health initiatives. Managerial skills (including but not limited to developing alliances, negotiating governance and roles, conflict management, managing change, forging strategic plans and leadership) are critical components of the manager's "tool kit" in any health care system. These skills are described in subsequent chapters in this volume.

THE CHALLENGE: DELIVER VALUE

The key challenge facing health care firms is to deliver **value**, defined as the quotient of quality divided by cost (Porter and Teisberg, 2006). That is, firms are asked to deliver a higher level of quality at the same cost, the same level of quality at a lower cost, or higher quality at a lower cost (Institute for Health Care Improvement, 2009). More expansive definitions include patient access and convenience along with quality features (Lee, 2015). In the United States, this challenge has been proposed to (a) providers, in the form of accountable care organizations (ACOs), pay-for-performance (P4P), and other types of value-based contracting; (b) insurers, in the form of value-based insurance design (VBID); and (c) suppliers, in the form of outcomes-based contracts with insurers (Barlas, 2016).

Value-based health care has recently become a global concern. In 2016, the World Economic Forum launched its "Value in Healthcare" project to stimulate national health system reforms around value. That same year, The Economist Intelligence Unit (2016) issued its global assessment of value-based health care across 25 countries. Common components of value-based health care include an ecosystem of supporting institutional and policy structures, coalitional support from broad stakeholders, support of professionals who are trained in value-based health care, quality measurement and standardization, cost measurement, integrated and patient-focused care, and payment based on outcomes.

In order to create and deliver value, health care organizations must find a way to address three health policy goals of our health care system since the late 1920s: improve the quality of care, improve access to care, and reduce cost and cost acceleration—for example, **bending the cost curve**, or the reducing of health spending relative to projected trends (Commonwealth Fund, 2007a). In past decades, providers have been asked to demonstrate a similar value (quality/cost) proposition using a series of management techniques, such as total quality management (e.g., reducing process variation and simultaneously raising the level of process performance), supply chain management (e.g., standardizing products to achieve consistency in use and lower unit cost), and clinical integration (standardizing care paths and protocols to reduce clinical practice variations and improve quality of care).

Numerous health services researchers have questioned whether all three goals are simultaneously attainable (Chen et al., 2010; Katz, 2010) or require a balancing act (Berwick, Nolan, and Whittington, 2008). The achievement of these three goals is sometimes referred to as the **iron triangle** of health care (Kissick, 1994). Picture an equilateral triangle, with three equal angles of

60 degrees, and assume that each angle is one of these three policy goals. Any effort to address one policy angle widens that angle (e.g., access) at the expense of one or both of the other two angles (e.g., quality or cost). For example, the Patient Protection and Affordable Care Act (PPACA) expanded insurance coverage to 24 million citizens but at a cost of roughly $1 trillion that needed to be recouped via taxes, lower provider reimbursements, and other programmatic savings (CMS, 2010).

Provider organizations in the health care industry have nevertheless been required to accomplish the quality and cost goals at the same time. Since the 1990s, employers have monitored health plans (and thus their provider networks) in terms of four domains of measures known as the Healthcare Effectiveness Data and Information Set (HEDIS), which resemble the iron triangle: effectiveness of care, access/availability of care, utilization and relative resource use, and experience of care. The Institute of Medicine (IOM, 2001)—now known as the National Academy of Medicine—articulated six "aims for improvement" in a high-performing health care system: care should be safe, effective, patient-centered, timely, efficient, and equitable. Most recently, providers in the United States have been encouraged to pursue "the triple aim" that builds upon the IOM's six aims: improving the patient's experience of care, improving the health of the population, and reducing the per capita cost of care (Berwick, Nolan, and Whittington, 2008). These three aims have been baked into the quality scorecard used to measure ACO performance in the Medicare program.

The balancing of broad health policy goals is apparent on a global scale as well. The World Health Organization (WHO, 2000) uses three criteria to rank national **health systems**: health status (similar to quality), responsiveness to the expectations of the population (similar to access), and social and financial risk protection (similar to cost).

CHALLENGE OF RISING HEALTH CARE COSTS: SUPPLY- AND DEMAND-SIDE PRICE AND VOLUME DRIVERS

One reason why the health system is challenged to deliver value is that the denominator—health costs—has risen steadily over time and proven difficult to restrain. National health expenditures in the United States have been rising at roughly 2.3 percent annually above the growth in gross domestic product for the past five decades (Altman, 2010; Blumenthal, Stremikis, and Cutler, 2013). Some have argued that public and private sector efforts work to temporarily rein in this rate of increase, only to see the cost escalation return (Altman

and Levitt, 2002; Jost, 2012). Such rising costs make health care increasingly unaffordable to the individual and crowd out other public spending.

Why do costs rise inexorably? Many experts argue that the underlying driver of rising costs is technology and its broad application to new patients and patient indications (Aaron and Ginsburg, 2009; Commonwealth Fund, 2007b; Congressional Budget Office, 2008a, b). Following Weisbrod (1991), technological improvements spur higher prices, higher demand, and higher costs—all of which call for greater insurance coverage for the new technology, which then drives further technological innovation. Technology contributes to rising costs in other ways. In contrast to other industries, health care technology is often a complement rather than a substitute for labor—for example, requiring many technicians to utilize the new equipment. Moreover, providers often compete for patients based on the sophistication of the services and equipment they offer, leading to expensive excess capacity and duplication in a local market ("technology wars"). Insurance is another driver of rising costs, as broader coverage (e.g., for more people or more benefits) increases demand and thus health spending, as well as the attendant problem of **moral hazard** (Arrow, 1963) whereby the insured utilize more health care than they would if they paid for services out of pocket (i.e., from their own resources without insurance).

There are several supply- and demand-side drivers of rising health costs. On the supply side, costs are driven by imperfect information markets whereby purchasers and consumers of health care are not able to discern quality differences perfectly among health care providers, make few repeat purchases, and enjoy less transparency of pricing, which allows great variation in the economic rents earned by providers of the same product or service. Such rents also result from provider market power. Costs are also driven in part by providers' practice of defensive medicine, providers' focus on acute rather than chronic care or prevention, and poor coordination of services among providers (Studdert et al., 2005; Towers Perrin, 2008). Finally, costs are driven by geographic variations in the supply of hospital beds and specialist physicians, which may induce demand (Roemer, 1961).

On the demand side, costs are driven by the tax-free treatment of health care benefits (which contributes to richer health benefit packages and induces moral hazard), as well as public and private sector financing of health care through a third-party payment system of insurers and other fiscal intermediaries outside the patient–provider relationship. Favorable tax treatment and a third-party payer system combine to insulate the consumer/patient from the true cost of the health care services they demand. In addition, demand is driven by a country's national wealth, the expectations of its population, the highly technological nature of health care

GEOGRAPHIC VARIATION IN HEALTH CARE SPENDING: A CLOSER LOOK

Health care expenditures in the United States have been rising for decades (Jost, 2012), but per capita spending on health care varies widely across the country. There are well-known variations in spending across states, hospitals, and even physicians to treat the same condition. Earlier, the Dartmouth Atlas suggested that the cost and quality of the services rendered to the Medicare population were either negatively correlated or not correlated at all, suggesting that Medicare spending could be reduced by decreasing such variations without harming quality (Wennberg, Fisher, and Skinner, 2002).

Why does health care spending vary so much across the country? The reasons are complex and difficult to tease apart. Differences in prices of health care services and severity of illness play an important role, but together these factors account for only half of the geographic variation in spending. Regional differences in the supply of specialist physicians and health care facilities are also thought to play a role. Regional differences in provider willingness to adopt new technologies or provide costly treatments that might or might not improve health care outcomes are also thought to increase costs. Most recently, research has identified variations in the cost and utilization of post-acute care services (e.g., nursing homes) as a major driver (Newhouse and Garber, 2013). Researchers have also challenged the Dartmouth Atlas research findings noted above by showing that across all funding sources (e.g., Medicare, commercial payers, etc.) higher levels of spending in wealthier states may translate into higher quality of care (Cooper, 2008).

Scholars and policy makers looking to slow the rate of growth in health care expenditures ("bend the cost curve") point to organized delivery systems that focus on coordinated care and prevention as a promising way to reduce the costs associated with the efficiencies, misaligned incentives, and poor quality attributed to the highly fragmented nature of the health care system that currently exists in the United States. In his efforts to promote health reform, for example, President Barack Obama praised the Mayo Clinic in Minnesota and the Cleveland Clinic in Ohio as examples of hospitals providing the highest-quality care at costs well below the national norm and suggested that all providers in the country practice their type of medicine.

DEBATE TIME: Overuse, Underuse, and Misuse of Health Care

Researchers at the Rand Corporation suggest that the health care system suffers from three process problems in delivering quality: overuse of services, underuse of other services, and misuse of still other services (Schuster, McGlynn, and Brook, 1997). Overuse characterizes those services and procedures that are expensive and where the potential for harm to patient's health exceeds the possible benefit, such as the excessive use of antibiotics for viral infections. Underuse characterizes those services that are likewise costly to perform but increase the quality of care and produce favorable patient outcomes, such as vaccinations, preventive visits, and taking medications as prescribed. Misuse, finally, characterizes those services that add costs without necessarily harming the patient, such as extra lab tests, unnecessary screening (PSA), or avoidable complications. In early 2017, *The Lancet* devoted an entire issue to the global nature of these three problems.

What do you think?

- Which of these three problems do you think is most prevalent?
- Which of these three problems do you think is most important to address?
- What managerial strategies might you employ to address each one?

services, and the health behaviors of its population. These supply and demand drivers are listed in Table 1.1.

There are many price and volume drivers of rising costs as well. Price drivers include provider consolidation and the resulting lack of competition, development of new technologies, rising labor costs, provider cost-shifting, and consumer preferences for care in higher-cost settings. Volume drivers include fee-for-service payment,

rise of chronic diseases, consumer demand, defensive medicine, lack of care coordination, and fraud and abuse.

A handful of axioms govern the demand side of this vast system that may be peculiar to health care. The first is that technological innovations and their application are desired by providers, desired by patients, and drivers of rising health care costs ("the technological imperative")

(Fuchs, 1986; Gelijns and Rosenberg, 1994). A second axiom is that technology drives specialization in the medical (and nursing) field, which further drives up health care costs. A third axiom is that every citizen deserves the finest health care now made available by these technological developments (often defined as the product or service offered by my firm) as long as someone else pays for it. Another axiom following from the technological imperative is that cost and price are the key issues germane to all parties. Indeed, the one issue that currently unites the entire value chain in health care is reimbursement; many analysts anticipate that it will be the patient/consumer who unites the chain in the future. Last, technological innovation and its attendant costs spur the spread of insurance coverage for such innovation, which increases spending on innovation, which fuels yet more innovation (Weisbrod, 1991).

OTHER CHALLENGES EXACERBATING THE VALUE CHALLENGE

Complicating the difficulty of providing value, health care systems face a number of other challenges. One key problem involves measuring and managing quality of care. Providers are confronted by multiple payers with different quality performance scorecards; moreover, many of the quality metrics are not highly correlated with one another (cf. Smith et al., 2017). Another key

problem is the growing burden of chronic illness in the population (both in the United States and globally), which requires more clinician time and resources to treat. Other challenges include increasing patient demand and expectations, increasing payer and societal demands for accountability, unexpected epidemiological shifts, calls for greater patient safety, increasing complexity, strains on federal and state government budgets, inadequate supply of primary care practitioners, reported shortages of specialists and other health personnel, erosion of the public's trust in physicians and hospitals, growing concerns over privacy of personal health information, lack of transparency in prices and information, conflicts of interest and incentives, lack of consumerism, lack of efficient and effective use of information technology, and provider resistance to change (Dranove, 2008; Herzlinger, 2006; Porter and Teisberg, 2006).

On top of these challenges one can lay a series of delicate balancing acts that health care firms (and society as a whole) must deal with beyond the value equation. These include meeting rising demand and expectations with finite resources (both capital and labor), addressing chronic care needs with an acute care–based delivery system, fostering population-based models of care amidst a system based on physicians in small groups or solo practice, sharing information while respecting patient privacy, incorporating modern therapeutic and technological advances while restraining the rate of growth in cost, and promoting wellness behaviors in a system that finances acute care seeking.

Table 1.1 Supply- and Demand-Side Drivers of Health Costs

Supply-Side Drivers	Demand-Side Drivers
Imperfect information regarding price and quality	Tax treatment of health care benefits
Provider market power	Third-party payment system
Nonprice competition (e.g., technology wars)	Breadth and depth of insurance coverage
Technology and its diffusion	Moral hazard
Geographic variations	Rising national income
Poor coordination among providers	Poor healthy behaviors
Fee-for-service payment systems	Private sector financing of care, which supplements public spending, encourages greater coverage, and may promote cost-shifting
Excess capacity	
Acute care focus of delivery system	
Limited primary care	
Malpractice fears and pressures	

THE CHALLENGES ARE GLOBAL

The problems, issues, and challenges facing the health care industry are global, confronting health care systems in many countries (Burns, 2014; Burns and Liu, 2017; see also Chapter 15). As an illustration, Table 1.2 identifies some of the common issues and problems facing the health care systems of India, China, and the United States. These countries have populations that are quickly aging—true especially of China, and increasingly so for both India and the United States. All three countries face a huge epidemiologic transition from acute care to chronic illness, with underdeveloped systems for dealing with chronic care (especially true in the East). Populations in all three countries have developed more sedentary lifestyles, with increasing incidence of diabetes, obesity, and hypertension. All three countries have populations with substantial national wealth that are now demanding more health care services and thereby increasing health care costs rapidly. Not surprisingly, all three countries also report that health care costs are a major source of personal and family bankruptcy. Finally, all three countries face the common issue of how to balance the demand for technological innovation by providers and patients with its high cost.

At the same time, there are several major divergences between these health care systems (see Table 1.3). The U.S. health care system compared with India or China spends a much higher proportion of its gross domestic product on health care and provides a higher level of insurance coverage to its population. While health insurance programs are now spreading across India (increasingly private sector) and China (mostly public sector), they provide coverage for a limited range of services (e.g., focused until recently on hospital inpatient care). Hospital ownership patterns also diverge widely. China's hospital system is almost entirely public sector (although the country recently announced its intention to allow more entry by private hospitals), while India's formerly public sector hospital system has seen the emergence of a thriving private sector comprised of multihospital systems (e.g., Apollo, Fortis, Wockhardt, and MaxHealthcare). By contrast, much of the U.S. hospital market is voluntary and nonprofit in character. Such differences and commonalities suggest that management strategies to meet the value challenge must consider the local context, but may nevertheless share many similar elements. As Chapter 15 notes, these strategies may encompass prospective payment systems, enhanced provider reimbursement rates, patient marketing and recruitment, etc.

Table 1.2 Parallel Concerns in the United States, India, and China

- Concern with iron triangle
- Concern with high hospital costs as cause of impoverishment/bankruptcy
- Concern with the high costs of technology
- Concern with geographic disparities in health status
- Concern with conflicts of interest and supplier-induced demand
- Concern with prices as driver of rising health care costs
- Concern with lifestyle issues and behaviors
- High number of specialists
- Hospital waste and inefficiency
- Lack of a primary care system
- Fee-for-service payment system
- Mixture of financing mechanisms: government, employer, individual
- Fragmentation in government ministries/bureaucracy
- Low consumer information
- Competing spending priorities (education, social services, health) at the local government level

Table 1.3 Areas of Divergence: United States versus India and China

- Health care spending per capita
- Percentage of national health expenditures (NHE) accounted for by patient out-of-pocket spend
- Development of private health insurance
- Depth and breadth of insurance coverage
- Presence of centralized purchasers
- Percentage of NHE spent on drugs
- Tradition of private sector ownership of hospitals
- Development of the central government's role in health care
- Development of governance mechanisms to monitor providers

COMPLEXITY OF THE U.S. HEALTH CARE SYSTEM

The United States lacks a single national health insurance program (other than the Medicare program for the elderly) to pay for health care. Thus, one confronts a variety of mechanisms to finance health care by federal, state, and local governments, as well as employers, individuals, and philanthropic organizations. Over time, the financing system has shifted from private payers to public payers, and from out-of-pocket payment to third-party payment using insurers.

The U.S. system also has a fully developed **value chain** (i.e., interlinked activities among a set of firms whereby suppliers provide raw material inputs to manufacturers who process them and produce outputs for downstream markets) (Burns, 2002; Porter, 1985). For example, the United States has thousands of product manufacturers (pharmaceuticals, biotechnology, medical-surgical supplies, capital equipment, medical devices, and information technology), wholesalers and distributors, hospitals,

physicians, nursing homes, pharmacies, home health agencies, insurers and insurance brokers, and employers offering health insurance coverage to their employees. It also has hundreds of group purchasing organizations (GPOs) and public health agencies; 50 State Medicaid programs; a vast federal **bureaucracy** (literally, government by bureaus or offices), which finances care, delivers health care services, regulates providers, approves new innovation, funds basic and applied research, and provides public health; and lots of niche firms offering pharmacy benefit management and disease management services (see Figure 1.1). This is a huge industry with lots of stakeholders, divergent interests and perspectives, and entrenched positions.

Effective management of any one sector of this system requires not only an understanding of the competitive developments within that sector but also an understanding of the other sectors, what is taking place within them, and how they interact with one another (Burns, 2005). Some of the health care managerial approaches and actions over the last decade reflect cross-sector understanding

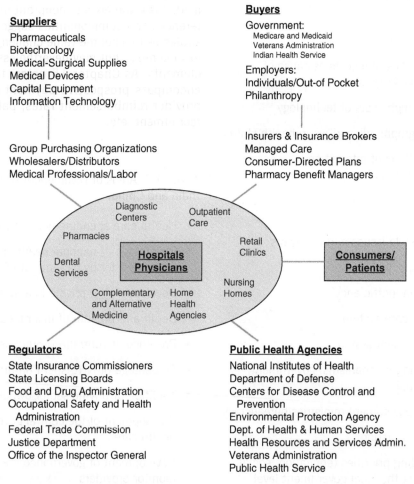

Figure 1.1 System View of the U.S. Health Care Industry.

and efforts. Such efforts include but are not limited to: managing under new P4P systems developed by both public and private sector payers; working with outside vendors (e.g., hotel chains, consulting firms, General Electric) to improve customer service, patient flow, and revenue cycle management; working with information technology companies to develop and implement electronic medical records (EMRs) systems (see Chapter 13); hospitals partnering with physicians to improve quality of care or develop new ambulatory care sites; and hospitals working with GPOs to lower supply costs.

WHY CHANGING THE HEALTH CARE SYSTEM IS SO DIFFICULT

In addition to being complex, the health care system is slow to change. There are several reasons for this. First, the industry is heavily regulated at both the state and federal levels by myriad agencies and professional associations. The federal government is also the dominant payer, reimbursing health care via administered prices. Market forces have thus given way to more regulation and piecemeal legislative action (due to legislative gridlock) at the federal level (Altman and Rodwin, 1988; Field, 2007).

Second, consumerism is a newcomer to health care. Until recently, consumerism was stifled by the prevalence of third-party payment and first-dollar coverage, the old

sociological view of the patient playing the "sick role" (Parsons, 1951), the prevalence of customized transactions, infrequent (and few repeat) purchases, uncertainty over product quality, and the fact that roughly three-quarters of all monies spent were on products and services previously unseen by the patient. Today, consumerism can be found in a number of areas: high-deductible health plans (HDHPs) and health savings accounts (HSAs), boutique/concierge medicine offered by physicians seeking to avoid managed care organizations (MCOs), complementary and alternative medicine (CAM), personal health records (PHRs), direct-to-consumer (DTC) advertising by pharmaceutical and medical device firms, health care financial services (smart cards), employer wellness programs, and consumer cost-sharing programs (see Chapter 14). However, in most of these areas, consumer engagement is not widespread. Studies suggest that perhaps as many as 40 percent of all patients are not "activated" in taking care of themselves. Moreover, there is a fair degree of "health illiteracy" among the U.S. population, preventing them from making wise choices about providers, health plans, and their own health (Parker, Regan, and Petroski, 2014; Schlesinger and Grob, 2017; Thorpe, 2007).

Third, health care delivery is heavily influenced by the medical profession, which controls (directly or indirectly) up to 85 percent of all spending (Sager and Socolar, 2005). While physicians do compete with one another, they nevertheless enjoy a monopoly or near monopoly over most important decisions governing resource allocation, including prescribing an ethical pharmaceutical,

• • • IN PRACTICE: Does Pay-for-Performance Work? The Case of the Premier Hospital Quality Incentive Demonstration

In 2003, the Centers for Medicare and Medicaid Services (CMS) and Premier Inc., a large national GPO, launched the Premier Hospital Quality Incentive Demonstration (PHQID) to determine if economic incentives are effective at improving the quality of inpatient care. Hospitals participating in the PHQID collected and submitted data on 33 quality measures for five clinical conditions. For each condition, hospitals performing in the top decile (i.e., 10 percent) received a 2 percent bonus in addition to their usual Medicare payment. Hospitals in the second decile received a 1 percent bonus. Hospitals that underperformed on quality indicators were liable for a 1–2 percent financial penalty in the third year.

Initial results suggested P4P was value-enhancing. Between 2003 and 2007, CMS awarded more than $36.5 million to high-performing hospitals; bonuses averaged $71,960 per year, and ranged from $914 to $847,227 (Premier, 2009). According to Premier, participating hospitals raised their overall quality by an average of 17.2 percent over four years and outperformed nonparticipating hospitals by an average of 6.9 percentage points on 19 quality measures.

Academic research tells a more mixed story. Lindenauer et al. (2007) compared 207 PHQID hospitals with 406 hospitals that did not participate in the demonstration and found modest differences in quality (about 3 percent) after statistically adjusting for other factors. Conversely, Ryan (2009) found no evidence that PHQID had a significant effect on risk-adjusted 30-day mortality or risk-adjusted 60-day cost for four of the conditions, suggesting no value effect. Another evaluation found no impact on outcome measures of quality in hospitals (Jha et al., 2012). A meta-analysis of P4P programs reported no positive impact on patient outcomes in any care setting but did find positive effects on process measures in ambulatory care (Mendelson et al., 2017).

performing a surgical procedure, scheduling a laboratory or imaging test, and admitting a patient to a hospital bed. Freidson (1970) long ago discussed the professional dominance of physicians. Physicians are largely autonomous, community-based entrepreneurs with (until recently) little employment relationship with hospitals in which many of these decisions are made (Burns, Goldsmith, and Sen, 2013). Due to professional training and the legal distinction between the hospital and its medical staff, hospitals have historically been challenged to alter the practice patterns and behaviors of their physicians. Moreover, while provider organizations are increasingly being reimbursed using "alternative payment methods" (APMs) such as P4P and shared risk, the organizations do not pass these incentives down to their physician members. The most recent effort to push APMs (MACRA, 2015) will reportedly impact not more than 800,000 physicians in 2017 by giving them a reprieve from reporting requirements.

Fourth, most of the nongovernmental sectors in health care have consolidated over the past two to three decades, thereby reducing competition, conferring market power and fostering higher prices. Consolidation has occurred in the following sectors (time periods): pharmaceuticals (late 1980s to the present), pharmaceutical wholesalers (1980s–1990s), medical devices (1990s), hospitals (1990s), insurers (1990s), GPOs (1990s), pharmacy benefit managers (1990s–2000s), and hospitals again (2010s to the present). These trends have fostered the emergence of several bilateral monopolies (e.g., big insurers negotiating with large hospital systems) in local markets.

Fifth, the delivery of hospital care (which accounts for roughly 30 percent of national health expenditures) is heavily dominated by nonprofit institutions, such as non-profit community hospitals and municipal/state-owned facilities. Investor-owned facilities comprise only about 15–20 percent of the hospital sector—a percentage that has remained relatively flat for decades. Nonprofit hospital ownership and accountability to local boards and communities (rather than shareholders) may mitigate against pressures to alter their missions, strategies, and operating practices. Theory suggests that nonprofits exhibit relatively poor supply response to changes in demand, more limited entrepreneurship owing to constraints on the distribution of earnings, and choice of optimization of various outcomes (e.g., quantity of services provided, focus on physician convenience and returns) rather than profits (Hansmann, 1987). The empirical evidence here is generally equivocal outside of the nursing home industry (Sloan et al., 2001).

Sixth, like politics, health care delivery is largely local. Physicians are licensed to practice in a given state and, like most hospitals, generally draw their patients from the local geographic area. Insurance companies are likewise licensed and regulated at the state level, and credential

and contract with provider networks in local markets. The United States has 389 metropolitan statistical areas that act as local markets with different configurations of power among key stakeholders (e.g., employers, insurers, hospitals, local government, etc.). Such differences necessitate tailored strategies by manufacturers in order to sell their products. While there has been much talk about medical tourism, more domestic tourism (e.g., to regional centers of excellence) than foreign tourism (e.g., to Thailand or India) seems to take place (Deloitte, 2009). Similar barriers have inhibited the utilization of telemedicine to span across markets. The largely local character of health care certainly complicates (and perhaps mitigates against) any concerted efforts to try to change the system from above.

Seventh, there is a widespread lack of valid data about quality and cost in health care. Until recently, most patient–provider transactions were captured and stored in paper-based systems (e.g., physician notes, patient charts, and medical records). This made it nearly impossible to analyze practice patterns to improve care quality and efficiency. To the extent that good patient care data existed, it rested in the hands of insurers who reimbursed providers for the care but did not share the granular information with them. This information asymmetry benefited insurers at the bargaining table with providers. In 2009, President Obama's stimulus package included funding for the diffusion of EMRs across physician offices to begin to address problems of data capture, although the issues of data validity and complexity of interpretation remain.

Eighth, and finally, efforts to change the health care system using business practices imported from the outside have repeatedly come up short (Arndt and Bigelow, 2000a; Burns and Pauly, 2002; Westphal, Gulati, and Shortell, 1997). One reason is that these practices have been adopted for normative reasons (e.g., to look efficient, to satisfy boards they are improving efficiency, and/or to imitate what other forward-looking organizations in the market are doing) as well as, or sometimes rather than, rational reasons (e.g., to remedy their operating problems). This would explain, for example, why hospitals have not invested more time and capital in the implementation of any given practice, or the coordination and integration among multiple practices, but rather pursued a series of discrete practice solutions over time (see Table 1.4) as they have come into vogue (flavor-of-the-month management) (Pfeffer and Sutton, 2006). Another reason is that such practices may not fully consider the institutional differences noted above and thus are not customized to health care settings.

Given the managerial problems that need to be confronted in health care, and given the complexity of the health care system and its peculiarities, what approaches seem fruitful for addressing them? One approach is to

Table 1.4 Business Practices Adopted by Hospitals, 1985–2010

- Corporate restructuring/holding companies
- Corporate diversification into new businesses
- Theory Z management
- Total quality management/continuous quality improvement (TQM/CQI)
- Horizontal integration (e.g., mergers and acquisitions)
- Vertical integration (physician acquisition, continuum of care, insurance)
- Strategic alliances with physicians and hospital networks
- Reengineering/work restructuring
- Product line management/service line management
- Customer focus/patient-centered care
- Focused factories
- Lean manufacturing and the Toyota Production System

apply system analysis to glean insights into the behavior of complex settings. Another approach is to apply organization and management theory. The next two sections sketch out some of these perspectives and how they might be usefully applied.

SYSTEMIC VIEWS OF HEALTH AND U.S. HEALTH CARE

A major source of complexity is the multifactorial nature of the determinants of health including social and environmental determinants (e.g., housing, occupation, income, access to parks and recreation), behavioral determinants (e.g., smoking, drug use, exercise), and medical determinants (e.g., blood pressure, cholesterol, mental health). Decades of research in public health has suggested that the vast majority of a population's health is determined by social, environmental, and economic factors and less by medical factors, including the use of biomedical care. Nevertheless, the United States spends far more on medical care than on social services that may greatly influence health (Bradley and Taylor, 2013; Bradley et al., 2016). Research has indicated that among high-income countries, those that spend relatively more on social services and relatively less on medical care, have subsequently better health outcomes, adjusted for gross domestic product (Bradley and Taylor, 2013);

similar patterns of spending and health outcomes are also apparent within the United States (Bradley et al., 2016).

Descriptions of the health care industry in the United States often begin with a discussion of whether it is a "system." Webster's dictionary defines a system as a complex unity formed of many, often diverse, parts subject to a common plan or serving a common purpose. Clearly, the U.S. health care industry does not meet this standard. As noted above, the multiple players have different goals (**triple aim**) and divergent interests ("patients need my product/service, you should pay for it," consolidation versus competition, integrated versus niche models).

Is a system view important? We think so, for many reasons. First, from a **macro perspective**, health outcomes are determined by an array of forces and factors that spans much more than a nation's health care infrastructure. There are multiple systems frameworks that describe these forces and factors (Shakarishvili, 2009). Hsiao (2003), World Health Organization (2000), and Roberts et al. (2003) have each developed a generic framework for the overall structure of any country's health care system. These frameworks describe several background forces (environment, nutrition, sanitation, professional training, and others) that affect the policy levers available to a system. These levers ("control knobs") include financing, payment, organization, regulation, and behavior. These control knobs are modeled to impact intermediate health system outcomes (efficiency, quality, and access—similar to the iron triangle), which in turn produce the ultimate health outcomes of health status, financial risk protection, and satisfaction (see Figure 1.2).

Second, as noted earlier, there are so many interdependent players that a systemic view helps to organize them and their interactions. Figure 1.1 provides such a framework for the U.S. context. Providers of health care services occupy the middle of the diagram for a specific reason: they are the main focus of everyone else. Buyers reimburse them for services rendered to their employees/beneficiaries, suppliers seek to sell them their products, regulators spend much of their time overseeing their quality/safety environment and their competitive conduct, and public health agencies seek to enhance population health by financing research and educational activities undertaken by providers as well as exercising oversight generally outside the direct provision of health care services. For the two parties in the upper-left and upper-right portions of the diagram (suppliers and buyers, respectively), two sets of intermediaries channel their services to providers.

This suggests a third reason for the importance of system views. The concept of a value chain (Porter, 1985)—that is, a firm or industry's input, throughput, and output activities that are served by a host of support functions—suggests that value is created along this collection of activities and requires effective partnerships. Value can be created by making the appropriate

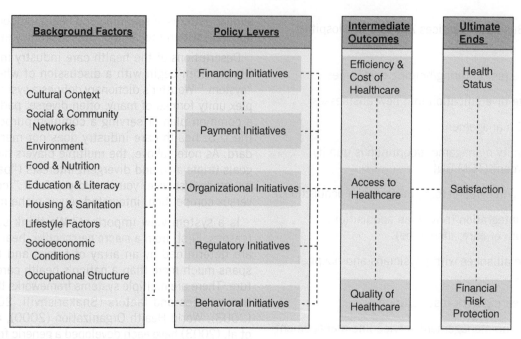

Figure 1.2 The Health Care System.

make-versus-buy decisions on how much of the value chain to occupy. For example, should providers operate their own insurance vehicles or contract with payers in the local market? Much of health care today is undertaking an analysis of make-buy decisions with this system view in mind. Pharmaceutical firms are now considering whether or not they should shed their research and development arms, allow such functions to be performed by smaller and more nimble actors like biotechnology firms, and concentrate their efforts on the sales and marketing functions. Conversely, hospitals are now considering whether they should assume more of the functions of the GPOs they have historically contracted with and do their own in-house contracting. Historically, suppliers have deliberated whether or not they should serve as their own wholesalers/distributors, while employers/buyers have experimented with operating their own provider networks.

A system view is important for a fourth reason. Management theory teaches that successful innovation requires concomitant changes among the system's components (sectors) to achieve congruence or "fit" (Senge, 2006; Tushman and O'Reilly, 1997). Similar thinking has been applied to the U.S. health care system: payment reforms in the buyer sector must be accompanied by corresponding reforms in the provider delivery system. Thus, for proposed payment changes—P4P, gainsharing, or bundled payment—to work, provider organizations require new models of physician–hospital collaboration (Burns, Goldsmith, and Muller, 2010). This perspective is at the center of current calls for "transformation from volume to value" in the U.S. system (Miller, 2008).

More broadly, efforts to reform one sector of the health care system must consider their impacts on the others to assess congruence with their interests and resources.

Fifth, as noted above, organizations within the health care industry have increasingly consolidated into systems over the past two decades with the stated objective of being more efficient, but may not operate as such. While mergers and acquisitions (M&A) have received a lot of attention (both by the merging firms and the media), postmerger integration activities have not. It is not clear that large multiunit systems can operate in a systemic fashion; extract scale economies from their operations; increase their productivity; add value; and address the multiple goals of access, quality, and acceptable cost. Systemic views of newly consolidated health care organizations and their potential (if any) to add value may thus be in society's interest. Indeed, between 2002 and 2004, the Federal Trade Commission (FTC) and Department of Justice (DOJ) conducted a series of workshops to assess the competitive and efficiency benefits of horizontal and vertical forms of consolidation (FTC/DOJ, 2004).

Thus, for example, despite the continuation of larger mergers (Pfizer and Wyeth, Merck and Schering Plough), research suggests that pharmaceutical M&A does not improve research productivity or profitability over the long term (Burns, Nicholson, and Evans, 2005). Instead, there are now suggestions that "big pharma" needs to "get small," perhaps by de-verticalizing their value chains, shedding their R&D activities, and focusing on a smaller set of activities. Similarly, the hospital systems that developed during the 1990s have devolved into more decentralized collections of autonomous operating units rather than centralized operations acting in concert (Burns et al., 2012). Indeed, the systems lens of federalism (the appropriate division of federal and state powers) suggests alternative ways for these hospital systems to organize themselves.

ORGANIZATION AND MANAGEMENT THEORY

Schools of management thought have evolved over the past century to provide conceptual maps of how to deal with internal and external challenges. These conceptual maps include theories of how things work, what causes what, and how to act. The theories are not mutually exclusive and can serve as multidimensional or multilayered models to guide managerial action. Executives benefit from being familiar with, and adept at using, many of these conceptual maps. This is no easy task; it is akin to being ambidextrous, both left-brain and right-brain, and more a fox than a hedgehog (Berlin, 1953).

Early Writings on Bureaucracy and Organization

Western management theory received its early impetus in the writings of Max Weber (1964), a German sociologist writing about the Prussian civil service in the late nineteenth century. Weber described the prominent features of this "bureaucracy" (literally, government by bureaus or offices) in terms of offices and officeholders, a vertical hierarchical ordering of these offices into organizational pyramids, a horizontal division of labor that separated offices and their functions, the use of explicit procedures to govern activities, the presence of records and files, and the selection of officeholders based on achievement rather than ascription. For Weber, bureaucracy was that form of administrative organization that operated under legal authority and was capable of the highest level of efficiency.

Research suggests that the bureaucratic model of organization is technically efficient and even superior to other forms under certain environmental, technological, and task conditions (Lawrence and Lorsch, 1967; Woodward, 1965). There is also considerable research on how to apply this model to the six common pathologies of the bureaucratic division of labor (Bacharach, Bamberger, and Conley, 1990):

- Role overlap (duplication): two roles perform the same task
- Role gap (accountability): neither role performs the needed task
- Role underuse (boredom): role not assigned enough tasks

- Role overload (burnout): role assigned too many tasks
- Role ambiguity (anxiety): role not clear what the tasks are
- Role conflict (stress): role's tasks are at cross-purposes

Bureaucracies are endemic to all organizations, including those in the health care industry. The degree of bureaucracy tends to be associated with both the firm's size and age. Thus, bureaucracy is less pronounced in small work groups and entrepreneurial start-ups (e.g., biotechnology firms) and more pronounced in hospitals and large consolidated firms (e.g., pharmaceuticals). Hospitals are peculiar bureaucracies in that they feature a "dual hierarchy"—a centralized system governing the nonmedical activities and a decentralized, collegial one governing the medical staff (Begun, Luke, and Pointer, 1990; Pool, 1991). Physician group practices, the majority of which are quite small, are peculiar in that they feature consensual governance rather than a bureaucracy. As many researchers have noted, physicians dislike and distrust authority (Burns and Wholey, 2000).

Organization size has been a staple of management research. This is due to ease of measurement as well as a range of hypotheses regarding its impact on survival, efficiency and performance, innovation, change (or inertia), entrepreneurship and risk-taking, firm legitimacy and influence, top management cohesion, political activity (both internal and external), employee commitment and human resource practices, internal coordination of market exchanges, internal coordination of different specialties, and (more recently) social responsibility practices and market power. Across all of these impacts, size has both positive and negative effects. There is nothing inherently evil in large size. To be sure, there is a managerial bias to pursue growth and larger scale (Josefy et al., 2015).

Bureaucracy has also become a staple of management research. There is nothing inherently evil in bureaucracy, given that it is needed to help coordinate the efforts of interdependent departments and personnel, control decision making to yield more standardized decisions, and develop routines for efficient functioning (e.g., delegation and decentralization). However, in modern parlance bureaucracy has taken on a negative connotation of poor service, lack of responsiveness, lack of consensus and change, and inscrutable, byzantine operation.

At its essence, management and bureaucracy are all about "control." The word "manage" derives from the French word *manege*, used in dressage, meaning to put a horse through its paces (Braverman, 1974). Control is not necessarily evil either. Control involves mechanisms to orient workers' attention toward firm goals, as well as motivate and encourage them to act in ways that support these objectives (Cardinal, Kreutzer, and Miller, 2017). To be sure, these goals may conflict with the goals of

• • • IN PRACTICE: Efforts to Deal with Bureaucratic Dysfunctions

Considerable research has highlighted the dysfunctional consequences of bureaucracy including its inward focus (rather than focus on the client or the environment), its tendency to rigidity and inertia, and its stultifying effects on individual creativity and thus organizational change. Nothing has changed here; as late as the 1980s and 1990s, major firms such as General Electric (GE) used change programs like "Work-Out" to attack their bureaucracies (Ulrich, Kerr, and Ashkenas, 2002). After downsizing its workforce, GE found that the remaining managers and employees had more work and responsibilities to handle. To reduce the load, they gathered employee suggestions for how to get non-value-adding work out of GE's processes (hence, the title of the program). The company discovered that Work-Out was more than just trimming excess work, however. It was also an "exercise" work-out for employees to study and diagram their work processes, as well as a mechanism for conflict resolution as different departments worked out their differences in how processes overlapping their areas might be simplified.

the employees. The challenge for the modern manager is to utilize the clarifying elements of bureaucracy (e.g., to resolve the six pathologies above) while at the same time avoiding the classic bureaucratic pitfalls of too many hierarchical levels that separate executives at the top from frontline workers down below, or too many horizontal divisions or units that effectively create boundaries inside and outside the firm, which impede interaction and the flow of information, or too many rules and regulations, which stifle creative problem-solving. Chapters 3, 4, and 8 in this book consider these issues.

Frederick Taylor and Scientific Management

The **scientific management school** (Taylor, 1911) extended the Weberian model by explicitly emphasizing the "control" element of bureaucracy. Scientific management was an attempt to apply the methods of science to increasingly complex problems of controlling work in rapidly growing firms (Braverman, 1974). For example, Frederick Taylor employed time–motion studies to analyze a steelworker's task into its simplest components and then systematically improve the worker's performance of each component to maximize productivity and ensure conformity to the one best way of production. Such thinking became embedded in assembly-line technologies like auto making by industrialists like Henry Ford.

Scientific management had an enormous impact on management practice and theory for decades to come. Of particular importance to us are three assumptions. First, Taylor assumed that workers were guided by intuition and variable training and thus were unable to perform their tasks in the best way. Instead, armed with scientific techniques (e.g., time–motion studies), management must control every aspect of the labor process and dictate precisely how it should be done. Workers were left with no discretion in their jobs, while managers were vested with all decision making regarding task

design. This separation of decision making at the top from execution/implementation down below in the firm came to pervade all management and strategy thinking (Mintzberg, 1994). A second related assumption was that management needed to closely supervise workers to ensure adherence to standardized tasks and prevent any "soldiering" (deliberate restriction of output); rather than being intrinsically motivated, workers responded primarily to monetary incentives and external control. Third, due to the large variability in how to do one's job (e.g., which methods, which tools), scientific management focused on reducing the variations and finding the one best way to perform the work in order to maximize productivity.

This school presaged several recent movements in management thinking. The emphasis on decomposing tasks into their constituent elements and worker training anticipated the early work on job design; later efforts to amend this approach included the job redesign approach (Hackman et al., 1975; Hackman, 1981), human factors engineering (Herzberg, Mausner, and Snyderman, 1959), and the quality of work life movement. These topics are taken up in Chapters 3 and 5. The emphasis on reducing variations in work anticipated the later work of W. Edwards Deming and total quality management movement in the United States of the 1980s—a topic taken up in Chapter 9. And the emphasis on specialized tasks and productivity anticipated the focused factories of the 1980s and 1990s (Herzlinger, 1997).

Classical School of Administration

The writings of Gulick (1937), Gulick and Urwick (1937), and Fayol (1949) collectively known as the **Classical School of Administration** took many of the concepts developed by Weber and Taylor and formulated them into general principles of management—essentially continuing Taylor's view of "one best way" to manage. These principles included unity of command (i.e., one boss), unity of direction (one objective, one plan, one boss), subordination of individual interest to general interest, centralization, authority, span of control (optimal number of people to supervise), and departmentalization (Fayol, 1949). Much attention was also paid to the construction of "organizational charts" depicting these principles on paper. Such principles directed managerial practice for much of the twentieth century.

Departmentalization has been one of the most enduring principles articulated by this school. These writers identified two principal models for the firm's division of labor: process departmentalization and purpose departmentalization. These have since been relabeled functional and divisional organization: organizing by functional area versus organizing by product line, customer, or geographic area. Alfred Chandler (1962) depicted the large-scale shift in the organization of American enterprise from the former to the latter. Twenty years later, Goldsmith (1981) described a similar transformation taking place among U.S. hospitals. Efforts to commingle the two forms of management gave rise to matrix structures utilized both in industry and in health care (Burns, 1989; Galbraith, 1973). Alternative forms of departmentalization comprise the core of thinking on organization design and coordination, the topic of Chapter 3.

Human Relations School

The human relations school developed a model of worker motivation that sharply differed from the Taylorist approach and thus suggested a different way of management. Work conducted by Elton Mayo (1945) and Roethlisberger and Dickson (1947) at the Hawthorne plant of the Western Electric Company ironically began as a Taylorism project to assess the impact of lighting changes on worker productivity. In contrast to Taylor's focus on individual workers and their jobs, their research anticipated Kurt Lewin's (1951) insight about the primacy of the group in structuring individual behavior. The findings implied that to improve productivity, management must attend to a new set of considerations beyond monetary incentives and top-down control of work. Managers must instead understand the informal organization of workers (groups, group sentiments, team work), the need of workers to be listened to and participate in the design of their work (participation, self-governance), and the importance of morale and satisfaction as motivators of worker effort. This view also anticipated later research on social networks of relationships and informal social structures (that emerged as employees pursued their own interests and needs), which supplanted earlier research on the organizational charts for which the Classical School was so famous (McEvily, Soda, and Tortoriello, 2014). Group structure and process are considered in Chapter 5; communication skills are discussed in Chapter 6.

Mayo's work suggested that workers are less rational than Taylor believed, guided less by financial incentives and more by human sentiments. Workers were also motivated to be accepted by their peer groups and achieve social solidarity. Finally, workers had an array of goals and needs that did not necessarily coincide with, or were subordinated to, the firm's interests. This insight led to an entirely new managerial approach called "organization development," which recognized the interdependence of the organization and groups of employees and sought ways to simultaneously achieve both the firm's goals and those of its workers. By extension, this school paved the way for later recognition of the employee as the firm's key asset.

Subsequent research and writing expanded the human relations school's approach. Douglas McGregor (1960) contrasted this school and its emphasis on managing human resources (Theory Y) with scientific management and its emphasis on control and coercion (Theory X). For McGregor, human relations management sought ways to integrate the firm and the worker, as well as ways to harness the worker's creativity and imagination. Taking account of Maslow's (1943) hierarchy of needs, McGregor argued that satisfying the worker's higher-order needs of belongingness, esteem, and self-actualization was critical. Herzberg refined Maslow's approach and suggested that such intrinsic motivation was inherently satisfying, while extrinsic factors were merely dissatisfying if not met. These approaches led to the entire field of job-redesign (Hackman, 1981) and self-managing work teams. The topics of motivating people and developing teams are considered in Chapters 4 and 5.

Contingency Theory of Leadership

By the mid-twentieth century, two schools of management thought had been established. One argued for greater structure, control, top-down decision making, and reliance on extrinsic rewards (Theory X); the other argued for more participative management, self-governance, bottom-up decision making, and reliance on intrinsic rewards (Theory Y). For decades, these schools were often (but erroneously) viewed as polar opposites. Subsequent research conducted during the 1960s and 1970s (summarized in Bass, 1981) suggested the choice of leadership style is not either-or. Instead, the effectiveness of specific management approaches depends on key situational factors (see Chapter 2), now known as Contingency Theory.

Decision-Making School

The decision-making school of management—also labeled the "Neo-Weberian" model (Perrow, 1986)—developed during the 1950s and 1960s, spearheaded by researchers at Carnegie Mellon University (Cyert and March, 1963; March and Simon, 1958; Simon, 1947). This school focused as much on how decisions were made and goals were set as on the structure of the firm—but all within a context with which Weber and scientific managers were comfortable: control of the work process and the worker.

In contrast to both scientific management and human relations, the decision-making school focused neither on top executives nor on lower-level workers, but rather on the large cadre of middle managers that had developed inside the large firms of the mid-twentieth century. Such managers and their decisions needed to be controlled. Because of limits on managers' cognition—known as **bounded rationality**—decision making needed to be guided by "satisficing" behavior (limited search among alternative options and selection of first acceptable solution) and the use of "programs" and "routines" (e.g., solutions or problem-solving paths used before) (cf. March and Simon, 1958; Simon, 1947). Such approaches served as points of stability and biases against innovation by narrowing the strategic choices available to managers. Decision making was also organized and controlled through means-ends hierarchies, in which the goal (ends) of one layer of management (e.g., increase profits) became translated into subgoals (means) pursued by the subordinate layer of management (e.g., raise revenues, decrease costs). They also presaged the "garbage can model" of decision making, in which solutions have a life of their own distinct from the problems they are called on to solve and may behave as answers looking for questions to solve (March, 1994).

The decision-making school had entirely different views of worker motivation as well. Rather than viewing workers as extrinsically or intrinsically motivated, or having goals that were shared or divergent from the firm, researchers described "inducements-contributions contracts" through which the firm and the worker engaged in exchange (Barnard, 1938). This had implications for the goals pursued by the firm. There was no necessary harmony or consistency in the goals pursued. Instead, firms could have multiple coalitions, each in pursuit of their own subgoals. Conflict could thus exist internally, and conflict resolution was never complete. Agreement on firm goals was thus accomplished through bargaining and negotiation. This school of thought thus presaged more political theories of the firm, which viewed organizations not as unified hierarchies but as competing coalitions pursuing self-interests (see Chapter 7). Such theories recognized the role of interest groups and factions that make goal attainment and unified action more difficult, as well as the importance of bargaining and negotiation among internal stakeholders that can affect how well the firm can respond to its environment and competitors. To the extent that firms "make decisions," these decisions do not flow from any formal rationality or structure but instead from a struggle between interest groups for power and control. Moreover, some internal

interest groups (such as professionals) can have stronger ties to their external counterparts than to their internal colleagues (Weber and Waeger, 2017).

Finally, the decision-making school introduced several new themes in organization theory and analysis. Rather than overt supervision and control espoused in Taylorism and scientific management, this school emphasized more unobtrusive controls over managerial decisions and behaviors. These controls included the following: standard operating procedures (SOPs), decision-making routines, socialization and training, organizational vocabularies and communication, and uncertainty absorption strategies (e.g., techniques to filter, process, edit, classify, and restrict the flow of information inside the firm). Its focus on politics and internal struggles for control also paved the way for research on professionals working within organizational bureaucracies. In health care, much of the early work here was conducted by Freidson's (1970) study of physicians, Scott's (1982) models for managing professionals, and Abbott's (1988) study of contests among professions for jurisdictional control over a set of tasks (Anteby, Chan, and Dibenigno, 2016).

Institutional Theory

In contrast to the scientific management and classical administration schools, which viewed organizations as rational tools for achieving purposive goals, **institutional theory** viewed organizations as organisms that adapt to pressures from without and within. What are these pressures? Similar to the decision-making school, firms here are limited in their degree of rationality by both the environment (which can deflect the firm's purposes) and internal members (who bring their own goals and interests that may vary from those of the firm's).

According to Selznick (1957), the early proponent of this perspective, firms develop a distinctive character through a process of institutionalization: they take on a distinctive set of values, structures, and capacities as part of a natural history of development. Selznick's (1949) history of the Tennessee Valley Authority (TVA) illustrates its strategy of co-optation of local leaders to ensure the agency's survival long after its initial goals were met, but at the expense of some of the agency's own goals. In this manner, the firm becomes endued with values and goals from its environment as well as its initial charter. The history of hospitals shows how board members initially endowed and financed many facilities in the late nineteenth century to support charity care. They then broadened the medical staff in the early twentieth century to include many community practitioners to attract paying patients. However, by virtue of their control over patient access and medical knowledge, the medical staff came to dominate decision making within the institution and broadened its goals from charity care to provision of quality care to the middle class and supporting the physician's private practice (Perrow, 1963). Indeed, Pauly and Redisch (1973) argued that hospitals became the de facto workshop of physicians during much of the twentieth century.

The institutional view received further impetus from the work of Meyer and Rowan (1977) and DiMaggio and Powell (1983). They outlined the normative pressures in the environment that constrained the choice of organizational form and other structural elements adopted by the firm, leading to similarities across firms. Such structural similarities were not enacted for efficiency reasons but rather for the sake of conformity with prevailing norms and values of what represented appropriate modes of organizing. Burns and Wholey (1993) documented the impact of local networks of influence in promoting the diffusion of matrix management among hospitals; Arndt and Bigelow (2000b) documented the impact of such normative ideologies and pressures on hospital management during the past century; D'Aunno, Sutton, and Price (1991) described the impact of such forces on the organization of drug abuse treatment centers; and Ruef and Scott (1998) examined the characteristics affecting hospital legitimacy over a 55-year period.

Open Systems and Resource Dependence Theories

The idea that organizations exist within an environmental context, from which it must secure resources, support, and legitimacy in order to survive and operate, received a more complete explication in **open systems theory** (Katz and Kahn, 1966). The institutional theorists described one set of (normative) constraints on the firm's structures and behaviors imposed by environmental forces. Thompson (1967) extended the decision-making view and its attempt to deal with bounded rationality by describing organizations as "open systems, hence indeterminate and faced with uncertainty, but at the same time as subject to criteria of rationality and hence needing determinateness and certainty." At lower levels in the organization, managers would seek to seal off the firm from its environment through a host of "uncertainty absorption" techniques. At higher levels, the firm embraced and actively sought to manage its interdependence with the environment.

Additional research conducted during the 1960s suggested that the effectiveness of specific management and structural approaches depended on the firm's environment, technology, and critical tasks. Thus, a more bureaucratic or "mechanistic" approach is suitable when the environment is stable and the tasks are routine and well understood, while a less bureaucratic or "organic" approach is more suitable when the environment is turbulent and the tasks are complex and less well understood

(Burns and Stalker, 1961; Woodward, 1965). Thus emerged a "contingency theory" of organization structure, which suggested the effectiveness of organizational action rested on the "fit" between the degree of uncertainty in environmental demands and two dimensions of its internal arrangements, differentiation and integration (Lawrence and Lorsch, 1967). Extensions of this approach also emphasized the need for "fit" between the firm's key components of formal organization, informal organization, people, and tasks (Nadler and Tushman, 1997; Van de Ven, Ganco, and Hinings, 2013).

Later researchers went further to suggest the bureaucratic and participative structures are neither opposites nor a one-dimensional linear continuum, but rather two different dimensions on which firms and their management approaches may rest. That is, the most effective approaches are not "either or" but "both and" (Blake and Mouton, 1964; Collins and Porras, 1994; Johnson, 1996; Misumi and Peterson, 1985). Indeed, recent research emphasizes the importance of **ambidexterity** in organizational performance: for example, firms that are both centralized and decentralized, firms that have units that are both mechanistic and organic in structure, etc. (Beer and Nohria, 2000; Quinn, 1988; Tushman and O'Reilly, 1997).

The open-system view of organizations (Katz and Kahn, 1966; Thompson, 1967) contained within it the seeds of **resource dependence theory**. In this model, organizations depend on other firms for critical resources and engage in strategies to protect themselves. Thompson described four elements in the firm's task environment (customers, suppliers, competitors, and regulators) and the firm's interdependence with its task environment and technology. Subsequent scholars (Pfeffer and Salancik, 1978) described the firm's effort to manage or strategically adapt to this task environment. This research suggested that organizations were not passive recipients of environmental change but actively sought to change their environments. Interorganizational relationships (IORs) constitute one key adaptive strategy for managing this interdependence. IORs have become a major focus of corporate activity and can take many forms, including horizontal mergers and vertical integration (see Chapter 10), strategic alliances (see Chapter 11), lobbying and managing regulatory demands (see Chapter 12), and managing community physicians (see Chapters 4 and 11). In this manner, organization theory began to confront the emerging field of corporate strategy and the strategic management perspective.

Another key insight of the resource dependence school is that the firm's environment contains other firms with competing interests and agendas, not just resources the firm needs (Wry, Cobb, and Aldrich, 2013). The firm's efforts to not only transact with external organizations but also to compete with them helped to focus attention on a new perspective—strategic management.

Strategic Management Perspective

The **Strategic Management Perspective** has evolved considerably since the 1960s, when it was dominated by the logic of top-down decision making, deliberate corporate rationality, and environmental stability. The field now encompasses at least three main schools of thought, many of which have their precursors in the schools discussed above. One school of thought emphasizes industry structure and competitive forces (Porter, 1980), similar to Thompson's articulation of the task environment. A second school of thought emphasizes the firm's distinctive capabilities and resources, building upon the decision-making school's discussion of organization programs and routines (Barney, 1991; March and Simon, 1958). A third school emphasizes the firm's relational capabilities and collaboration with upstream suppliers and downstream distributors and customers (Dyer and Singh, 1998). Such relationships can be developed with other constituents as well, including competitors, regulators, or other firms in the task environment. These schools are covered in depth in Chapter 10.

More recent perspectives include "sensemaking" and "organizational learning." Sensemaking is the process by which managers come to understand (i.e., make sense of) unexpected or confusing events in their environments and then craft strategic responses to them (Weick, 1995). This perspective clearly links to other schools of thought like decision-making and open-systems theory. In contrast to those schools, however, it points toward a new perspective on how corporate strategy is "enacted" rather than planned and is more emergent than deliberate (Maitlis and Christianson, 2014). Organizational learning has both internal and external referents. Internally, the firm learns how to perform its tasks more efficiently or at a higher quality (e.g., move down the learning curve, practice makes perfect); externally, firms learn how to identify potential partners for strategic alliances and develop skills in managing those partners (Inkpen and Tsang, 2007).

Organizational Ecology

The school of organizational ecology, or **population ecology**, is typically associated with the work of Hannan and Freeman (1977) and Aldrich (1979) but developed out of early sociological work conducted by Amos Hawley (1950) and his mentor Roderick McKenzie (1968) on organizational forms, competition among forms for resource space, and organization–environment covariation. Borrowing from a biological metaphor, organizational ecology principles suggest that the environment selects out and retains the most appropriate organizational form from an existing population of various forms (Baum and Amburgey, 2005). Such forms are selected out due to their superior ability to compete for and acquire scarce resources. In this school, the emphasis is on (a) the population of firms rather than the individual firm, and (b) changes in organizational populations due to variation, selection, retention, and competitive forces. In contrast to the institutional school, organizational ecology focuses on diversity rather than isomorphism. It also suggests that environmental forces make managerial choice and discretion very important for organizational survival and growth.

Research on organizational ecology has tended to focus on the economic and social conditions that affect the number and diversity of organizations, and their changing composition over time (Baum and Amburgey, 2005). Thus, some common themes studied include conditions that explain organization foundings (entries) and failures (exits), organizational inertia versus momentum, and changes to organizational niches (generalist versus specialist firms).

This perspective has been quite helpful in understanding the transition among competing organizational forms in certain sectors of the health care industry. Researchers have identified the environmental conditions under which generalist and specialist hospitals will survive (Alexander, Kaluzny, and Middleton, 1986), the environmental selection pressures in the hospital industry (Alexander and Amburgey, 1987), the impact of size on the failure rates of health maintenance organizations (HMOs) (Wholey, Christianson, and Sanchez, 1992), the transition from the original group-model and staff-model HMOs to the more prevalent IPA model (Wholey and Burns, 1993), and the transition of the hospital industry from a cottage industry to a more organized industry of 600 systems and networks (Bazzoli et al., 1999).

Social Network Perspective

Sociologists have long taken the **social network approach** in describing the embeddedness of human behavior in social relationships (Granovetter, 1985). As noted by the human relations school, these social networks can operate within formal and informal work groups to shape and constrain individual behavior. As noted by the institutional theorists, they can also operate at the interfirm level to exert normative pressures on managerial choice and organizational structure.

Social network structure can be analyzed in two ways: in terms of interaction patterns and in terms of structural similarity (Knoke, 1990). The interaction approach emphasizes the consequences of interaction and the ability to control interactions because of a central role in the network. Actors who have relationships with one another are grouped together in a network. This network has certain dimensions. "Network centrality" refers to the actor's linkage to others within the network who themselves are connected. "Strength of ties" refers to the frequency and intensity of interaction with others in the network; such ties can be direct or indirect (mediated by another). "Network density" refers to the number of different linkages between two or more actors (Uzzi, 1999); the greater the number of linkages, the more dense the network, and the more embedded the network's actors. Such networks may have a greater capacity for transferring knowledge and facilitating learning across network members (Gulati, 1995; Uzzi, 1997). For example, opinion leaders on the medical staff have often been utilized by hospitals to influence adoption of new practices by their colleagues, just as manufacturers have used them to sway adoption of new products.

The structural approach, on the other hand, groups actors by the similarity in their relations with others. "Structural equivalence" refers to two actors who have no direct connection but have similar ties with others. "Structural holes" refer to networks of actors who are interdependent but are not interacting; the presence of such holes has been shown to retard innovation (Ahuja, 2000). Structural holes can become filled by a third party who mediates their exchange (Burt, 1992). For example, foundation grants established "community care networks" during the late 1990s to bring a variety of local health agencies and providers together to promote primary care and health promotion activities (Bogue et al., 1997; Bazzoli et al., 1997). Similarly, integrated delivery networks (IDNs) can fill the structural hole between independent physician groups who can jointly develop and implement care management practices (Shortell and Rundall, 2003).

Social networks are also important for understanding team functioning and performance. Medical clinics exhibit varying levels of information provision among their professionals depending on network centrality, density, and homophily (Wholey et al., 2009). Similarly, strength of ties with academic researchers and centrality in research and development collaboratives furthers the access of biotechnology companies to labor expertise and capital as well as to promising projects and future collaborations (Powell, Koput, and Smith-Doerr, 1996). Finally, research on innovation within medical device firms suggests that new ideas are more likely to emerge from heterophilous networks with weak ties (to generate variations) but are more likely to be widely adopted in homophilous networks with strong ties (Van de Ven et al., 1999).

System Perspectives

In recent years, management theory and health care professionals have developed a host of new **system perspectives**, focused on the broader system in which individual and organizational behavior occurs. Some of these perspectives have focused on health systems broadly conceived. Hsiao and the World Health Organization have both developed models linking the major inputs, throughputs, and outputs of health care (see Figure 1.2). The Centers for Disease Control (CDC) has likewise developed its "Health Run" model of the determinants of health outcomes (Figure 1.3). Other models have been developed to

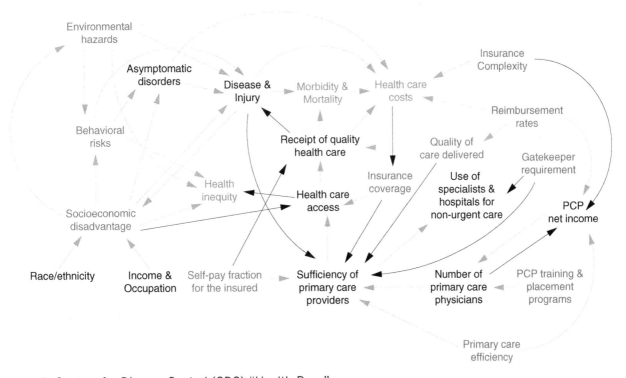

Figure 1.3 Centers for Disease Control (CDC) "Health Run."

SOURCE: Adapted from the Centers for Disease Control.

encapsulate the delivery system portion of the health care industry. During the 1990s and the rise of IDNs, Shortell and colleagues described a conceptual model of system integration based on functional, physician-system, and clinical integration. Nelson et al. (2008) described the embeddedness of patients and clinical microsystems that treat them within a larger network of mesosystems (collection of clinical microsystems treating a shared patient population) and the larger macrosystem.

Other system analogies rest on biological metaphors. For example, interactions of insects (e.g., termites or ants) can result in self-organized, coordinated teamwork characterized as "swarm intelligence" (Bonabeau and Meyer, 2001). Such interactions promote robustness, flexibility, and adaptability without the need for central control or local supervision. More broadly, firms can employ the "wisdom of crowds" (Surowiecki, 2004) via social networks with customers and innovators, collaborative software, wikis, and other information markets to develop collective intelligence and make better decisions (Bonabeau, 2009).

Such approaches are referred to as **complex adaptive systems** (or, alternatively, complexity science). They are complex in that they are composed of multiple, diverse, interconnected elements; they are adaptive in that they have the capability to change and learn from their experience (see Chapter 9). Thinking on complex adaptive systems has been applied to health care in the study of clinical pathway development (Priesmeyer et al., 1996), the nursing profession's resistance to change (Begun and White, 1999), medication errors in hospitals (Dooley and Plsek, 2001), and innovations in health care delivery such as HIV/AIDS prevention and treatment and the structure and performance of IDNs (Begun, Zimmerman, and Dooley, 2003). In the broader management literature, thinking on complex adaptive systems has been widely applied to strategic change and implementation.

SUMMATIVE VIEWS OF ORGANIZATION THEORY

The various theoretical schools reviewed above should be viewed not as competing but rather as complementary approaches for understanding and managing organizational behavior. Collectively, they provide the practitioner as well as the researcher with a rich, diverse set of lenses or frames. Some schools clearly operate at distinct *levels* of analysis: for example, Taylorism focuses on structuring the tasks of individual workers; the human relations and social networks schools focus on groups; the decision-making school focuses on middle managers; the Weberian and classical administration schools focus on top executives who structure the firm and its activities; while the resource dependence, population

ecology, and institutional schools focus heavily on the external environment.

In addition to the different levels of analysis, the schools also suggest different *strategies* for changing organizations and different *competencies* that managers need to develop. Thus, Weber, the neo-Weberians, and the classical administration theorists focus on how to design organization structures and control (worker and managerial) behavior. Researchers in the human relations school focus heavily on motivating workers, satisfying employee needs, promoting quality of life at work, and managing conflict. Resource dependence focuses on the development of interorganizational relationships and market strategies the firm can use to control its environment, while the population ecologists and institutional theorists highlight the environmental forces (both ecological and normative) that constrain such use. Finally, the network and complex adaptive system perspectives highlight the importance of social networks—especially network structure and interactions—for generating and diffusing new ideas, forming bonds of solidarity, and promoting adaptability.

Applying Organizational Theory to Practice: Hospital–Physician Relationships

How might the perspectives and insights of these different schools be used together? We can illustrate this with a concrete example: executives' efforts to foster improved **hospital–physician relationships** (HPRs). In what ways are these relationships tied to the delivery of value in health care? Studies from the 1990s suggest that excellent HPRs are tied to hospital profitability under the Medicare program (Bray et al., 1994; ProPAC, 1992). The Health Systems Integration Study suggests that economic integration of hospitals and physicians forms part of the bedrock for improving clinical integration (Shortell et al., 1996). Empirical evidence suggests that a handful of models of economic integration help to control cost and improve quality (Bazzoli et al., 2000; Burns and Muller, 2008; Shortell, Gillies, and Anderson, 1994). Most recently, researchers have suggested that a key driver of ACO performance is physician motivation and engagement by hospitals (D'Aunno et al., 2016; Phipps-Taylor and Shortell, 2016; Skillman, Cross-Barnet, and Singer, 2017).

We should note that researchers have devoted considerable attention to the application of management theory to the HPR. Long ago, Scott (1982) described three models for organizing the work of professionals (like physicians) inside organizations: autonomous, heteronomous, and conjoint. The autonomous model delegates control over work to the professionals, the heteronomous

• • • IN PRACTICE: Physician Employment in China

The United States and China have taken entirely opposite approaches to the hospital–physician relationship. In the United States, the two parties have historically been independent of one another and paid by different sources (Blue Cross and Medicare Part A for hospitals, Blue Shield and Medicare Part B for physicians). Physician–hospital arrangements in general and hospital employment in particular have developed in the past three decades to combat this lack of alignment. By contrast, China outlawed private medical practice and turned physicians into hospital employees starting in the 1950s. Physicians were not allowed to leave hospital practice without the permission of their hospitals. Only recently has the Chinese central government begun to loosen the close dependency of the physician on the hospital.

Health care systems in both countries are shifting the relationships in search of better performance. In the United States, policy makers and system executives hope that closer alignment breeds greater cooperation on quality improvement, cost reduction, revenue enhancement, and market share growth. In China, policy makers hope that looser ties foster greater mobility in the physician labor market and development of an ambulatory care system. The fact that the United States and China are moving in totally opposite directions suggests that neither a hierarchical approach nor a market approach is inherently superior to managing the hospital–physician relationship.

model imposed some administrative controls and routine supervision, and the conjoint model is characterized by more power-sharing between the administrative and professional hierarchies. Begun, Luke, and Pointer (1990) developed a different, fourfold typology to describe this relationship along the two strategic dimensions of "tightness of coupling" and "degree of strategic purpose": conjoint firm (high, high), latent conjoint firm (high, low), quasi firm (low, high), and network (low, low). Shortell and Rundall (2003) investigated this relationship from the perspective of social network theory and strategic adaptation theory to derive hypotheses regarding the likelihood of success in forming successful partnerships. Casalino and Robinson (2003) also examined three different models for organizing HPRs that parallel use of the market (traditional hospital medical staff), strategic alliances (PHOs, IPAs), and hierarchies (hospital employment). Most recently, Alexander and Young (2017) explained that efforts to move physicians from autonomous to heteronomous arrangements have not been successful, while other professional occupations in hospitals (e.g., nurses) have long operated under such structures. They then explored conjoint models that recognize the value of both professional ("micro care") and administrative ("macro care") hierarchies and the necessary infrastructure to be successful.

From the Weberian perspective, executives might seek to resolve the dual hierarchy in hospitals that has long divided the medical staff from administration, perhaps by creating a more unified organization. For example, in many academic medical centers, the two lines of authority over (a) the medical school and its faculty and (b) the hospital and its professional and ancillary departments have been consolidated under one individual—the medical school dean. Alternatively, there are calls today to reorganize the hospital medical staff and improve its

governing structure to promote greater accountability for quality of care.

From a scientific management perspective, hospitals might more vigorously pursue efforts at clinical integration, such as developing and disseminating clinical guidelines, and monitoring their physicians' adherence to them. Such efforts are believed to promote higher quality of care. They also serve to reduce unwanted variations in clinical practice, and to promote **evidence-based medicine**, in which health care professionals identify and apply scientific information in order to make clinical decisions.

Classical administration's focus on organization design orients hospital executives to develop the most appropriate structures within which their clinicians work. As an illustration, during the 1990s executives erected multiple vehicles for partnering with physicians and contracting with managed care organizations. These included the physician-hospital organization (PHO), the independent practitioner association (IPA), the management services organization (MSO), and the integrated salary model (ISM). Each model offered a different level of professional autonomy and hospital financial support that catered to the individual physician's needs and desires. More recently, hospitals have shifted away from their process/functional structures and developed new organizational designs based on purpose departmentalization. These are alternatively called service line management models, hospitals within hospitals, and centers of excellence. Following the dictates of the classical school, they decentralize authority for a clinical area, along with supporting personnel and/or ancillary functions, to physicians in that specialty area.

Following the human relations approach, hospitals have long engaged in efforts to include physician representatives on their board and give them the opportunity to express their voice in governing the institution. In addition, they have long conducted surveys of the medical staff to understand trends in physician morale, to identify sources of physician satisfaction and dissatisfaction with the hospital, and to elicit physician suggestions for change. More recently, some medical schools have begun training future physicians in areas such as teamwork and analysis of the health care system, partly to satisfy new requirements from the AMA's Committee on Graduate Medical Education (COGME).

The decision-making school emphasizes the importance of unobtrusive controls to reduce discretion and shape the premises of decisions made by managers. Leading IDNs in the United States, such as the Mayo Clinic and the Kaiser Permanente Medical Groups, have long utilized an internally developed and inculcated corporate culture of teamwork to promote collaborative medicine. During the 1990s, some community-based hospital systems sought to emulate this approach by developing questionnaires to evaluate prospective new members of the medical staff in terms of their orientation to quality and efficient health care delivery. Other hospitals utilized clinical databases to develop practice profiles of their physicians; such profiles were then disseminated to the practitioners with the aim of steering them to more cost-effective practice patterns. Some went so far as to perform "economic credentialing" for prospective or current members of the medical staff.

HPRs are a domain in which strong professional forces (e.g., the logics, values, norms, and beliefs of the medical profession) confront a host of institutional and market forces (Alexander and D'Aunno, 2003). At one extreme, medical profession desires for open medical staffs have long competed with hospitals' financial interests to exclusively contract with one group to cover hospital ancillary services (Burns, Goldsmith, and Muller, 2010). HPRs have also been shaped by strong institutional forces such as government reimbursement systems (e.g., diagnosis-related groups or DRGs, bundled payment) that have led hospitals to engage their medical staffs in more cooperative decision making. Since the 1990s, the physicians' professional interests have been subsumed under a series of market-based arrangements—in effect, reducing the traditional loose-coupling between the hospital and medical staff. These reflect heteronomous professional organizations (Scott, 1982) such as the PHO, IPA, and ISM models.

Open systems theory has been applied to HPRs in several ways. During the 1990s, hospitals located in markets subject to intense managed care pressures (or the anticipation of managed care) were encouraged by consultants and academics to develop vertically integrated delivery networks; these could include the acquisition of primary care physician practices, medical groups, or specialist practices. Conversely, hospitals in markets characterized by low managed-care penetration were

encouraged to focus on more traditional activities to work with their medical staffs (APM/University HealthSystem Consortium, 1995). Later thinking suggested that hospitals develop ambidextrous approaches for dealing with their medical staffs—in effect, being both hospital-centric and physician-centric at the same time. Some IDNs in the 1990s aspired to hospital systems that were organizations of physicians, or to promote clinical autonomy through the collectivization of physicians (Burns, 1999).

Following resource dependence theory, HPRs can be characterized as external strategies engaged in by hospitals to control inputs critical to their survival. Hospitals have traditionally depended on community physicians to refer patients to their specialists, to admit patients to their inpatient areas, and to provide specialty coverage in the emergency room. More recently, they have depended on physicians to assist in the provision of efficient care (to manage under DRGs or bundled payments) and quality care (e.g., under P4P programs). HPRs can be viewed as efforts to partner with community physicians in strategic alliances—in effect, developing IORs—and co-opt the desired behaviors in a variety of economic exchanges. Alexander et al. (1996) described a host of physician-organization arrangements developed by hospital systems in the 1990s to ensure these critical physician inputs.

From the strategic management perspective, some types of HPRs reflect not only a strategy of securing critical inputs (similar to resource dependence) but also a deliberate effort to foreclose competitors' access to those inputs. Thus, during the 1990s, hospitals engaged in a bidding war with one another and with physician practice management companies to acquire the primary care physicians in the local area. This acquisition strategy was viewed as a zero-sum gain: that is, the physicians my hospital acquired would be loyal to my institution and direct all of their referrals and admissions to my institution (rather than yours). HPRs thus represented a classic vertical integration strategy (Porter, 1980). A smaller number of hospitals and IDNs viewed HPRs as a platform for developing strategic capabilities and resources (e.g., cooperation with the medical staff, physician teamwork, physician leadership, etc.) that could be applied to solving other business problems or pursuing other economic ventures.

Ecological analysis has not been widely applied to the analysis of HPRs. Nevertheless, the health care reform debates of 1993 and 2009 pointed to particular models of delivery as being the most efficient mode of organizing. In 1993, the Clinton health plan called for accountable care plans (consortiums of providers) to contract with state-based health insurance purchasing cooperatives in risk-bearing contracts. The 2010 health reform encourages pilot demonstration projects for ACOs (again, consortiums of local providers—this time, community hospitals and the physicians that utilize them) to deliver on both cost and quality metrics in contractual, risk-based agreements with the Medicare program. Tightly coupled HPRs—such as the Cleveland Clinic, the Mayo Clinic, Kaiser Permanente Medical Groups, and the Geisinger Clinic—have been touted as the model for other providers to emulate (Whitley, 2009).

Research applying social network analysis to HPRs has developed several important hypotheses (Shortell and Rundall, 2003). The "strength of strong ties" among physician organizations is associated with the success of HPRs in developing economic exchange and altruism. Moreover, as social linkages (both direct and indirect) increase in a network, the network becomes more embedded, thus facilitating more weak ties and the spread of information and cost-effective opportunities for learning. Centrality in HPR networks, the presence of organizations that can fill structural holes in the network, and the strength of ties linking the physician organization to the network will facilitate adoption and implementation of clinical process innovations.

Finally, Begun, Zimmerman, and Dooley (2003) utilize the complex adaptive perspective to analyze the Minneapolis-based merger of HealthSpan and Medica into the Allina Health System in 1994. Rather than focus on the explicit merger strategy and intent, the researchers analyze how the merger actually unfolded and how Allina's strategy and structure coevolved over time. They suggest that integration of entities would be more effective if they were allowed to "e-merge" rather than "be-merged."

In a similar vein, Cappelli et al. (2010) attribute the ascendance of Indian firms in a number of industries, including health care, to managerial practices of improvisation and adaptability. Emergent business practices and models, rather than explicit strategies or even Western theories, have enabled Indian firms to develop solutions such as micro-insurance and low-cost hospital care for the poor to address the needs of the "bottom of the pyramid." The researchers characterize these practices and models as "the Indian way" of learning by doing and suggest they may serve as sources of learning and reverse innovation for Western organizations.

ORGANIZATION THEORY AND BEHAVIOR: A GUIDE TO THIS TEXT

The challenge for managers is to understand the complexity of the health care system (e.g., Figures 1.1 and 1.2), and the interests and roles of the different actors within it, and then determine which managerial perspectives discussed above can be usefully applied, at what level of analysis, and using what levers to address the value equation. Table 1.5 attempts to summarize this and describe where the book's chapters tackle these issues.

The book is divided into three parts. This chapter and the next introduce the reader to the issues of leadership and management in health care. The next part considers the **micro perspective**: the internal environment of organizations. Topics taken up here include organization design, motivation, groups and teams, communication, power/politics/conflict, organization learning and innovation, and organizational performance, improvement, and change management. The last part of the book considers the *macro perspective*: the external environment of organizations. Topics here include strategy, strategic alliances, policy and regulation, information technology, consumerism, and forces shaping health care throughout the rest of the world.

Table 1.5 Organization Theory and Behavior: A Guide to the Text

Health Care Organizations and Their Managers Organization Theory and Management of Health Care Firms (Chapter 1) Leadership, Management, and Culture in Health Care Firms (Chapter 2)	
Micro Perspective: Manage the Internal Environment	**Macro Perspective: Manage the External Environment**
Organization Design (Chapter 3)	Achieving Competitive Advantage (Chapter 10)
Motivating People (Chapter 4)	Managing Strategic Alliances (Chapter 11)
Managing Groups and Teams (Chapter 5)	Health Care Policy and Regulation (Chapter 12)
Communication (Chapter 6)	Managing Information Technology (Chapter 13)
Managing Power, Politics, and Conflict (Chapter 7)	Consumerism (Chapter 14)
Organization Learning and Innovation (Chapter 8)	Globalization and Health Management (Chapter 15)
Organization Performance, Improvement, and Change Management (Chapter 9)	

CASE

Can Organization Theory Inform Efforts to Improve Health Care Quality?

Improving the quality of health care has proven to be an elusive and difficult task (Nembhard et al., 2009). Health care organizations have experienced considerable difficulty in grasping all of the individual-level, team-level, organization-level, and system-level factors that shape quality. They have also been challenged to measure quality, to motivate providers to change their practices, and to implement quality improvement projects. The problems have been manifest in high rates of hospital readmission, high rates of preventable deaths and medical errors, uneven quality of care for people with inadequate insurance, and the introduction of new and expensive medical technologies without concomitant gains in life expectancy.

Questions

1. Does theory and research in management offer *any* guidance for practitioners seeking to improve quality of care?
2. What does *each* school of thought reviewed in this chapter suggest about what to do?
3. Which of the schools of thought seem to offer the *most* useful advice?

REFERENCES

Aaron, H., & Ginsburg, P. (2009). Is health spending excessive? If so, what can we do about it? *Health Affairs, 28,* 1260–1275.

Abbott, A. (1988). *The system of professions.* Chicago, IL: University of Chicago Press.

Ahuja, G. (2000). Collaboration networks, structural holes, and innovation: A longitudinal study. *Administrative Science Quarterly, 45*(3), 425–455.

Aldrich, H. E. (1979). *Organizations and environments.* Englewood Cliffs, NJ: Prentice-Hall.

Alexander, J. A., Kaluzny, A. D., & Middleton, S. C. (1986). Organizational growth, survival and death in the U.S. hospital industry: A population ecology perspective. *Social Science and Medicine, 22*(3), 303–308.

Alexander, J. A., & Amburgey, T. (1987). The dynamics of change in the American hospital industry: Transformation or selection? *Medical Care Research and Review, 44*(2), 279–321.

Alexander, J. A., Burns, L. R., Zuckerman, et al. (1996). An exploratory analysis of market-based physician-organization arrangements. *Hospitals and Health Services Administration, 41*(3), 311–329.

Alexander, J. A., & D'Aunno, T. A. (2003). Alternative perspectives on institutional and market relationships in the U.S. health care sector. In S. Mick & M. Wyttenbach (Eds.), *Advances in health care organization theory* (pp. 45–77). San Francisco, CA: Jossey-Bass.

Alexander, J. A., & Young, G. (2017). Health professionals and organizations – Moving toward true symbiosis. In T. Hoff, K. Sutcliffe, & G. Young (Eds.), *The healthcare professional workforce* (pp. 77–102). New York: Oxford University Press.

Altman, S., & Rodwin, M. (1988). Halfway competitive markets and ineffective regulation: The American health care system. *Journal of Health Politics, Policy and Law, 13*(2), 323–339.

Altman, D., & Levitt, L. (2002). The sad history of health care cost containment as told in one chart. *Health Affairs, 23,* W83–W84.

Altman, S. (2010). Is it possible for the U.S. to control health care costs? Presentation to the Leonard Davis Institute, University of Pennsylvania. January 29, Philadelphia.

APM/University HealthSystem Consortium. (1995). How markets evolve. *Hospitals and Health Networks, 69,* 60.

Anteby, M., Chan, C., & Dibenigno, J. (2016). Three lenses on occupations and professions in organizations. *Academy of Management Annals, 10*(1), 183–244.

Arndt, M., & Bigelow, B. (2000a). The transfer of business practices into hospitals: History and implications. In L. Friedman, J. Goes, & G. Savage (Eds.), *Advances in health care management* (Vol. 1, pp. 339–368). New York: Elsevier.

Arndt, M., & Bigelow, B. (2000b). Presenting structural innovation in an institutional environment: Hospitals' use of impression management. *Administrative Science Quarterly, 45,* 494–552.

Arrow, K. (1963). Uncertainty and the welfare economics of medical care. *American Economic Review, 53*(5), 941–973.

Bacharach, S., Bamberger, P., & Conley, S. (1990). Work processes, role conflict, and role overload. *Work and Occupations, 17*(2), 199–228.

Barlas, S. (2016). Health plans and drug companies dip their toes into value-based pricing. *Pharmacy & Therapeutics, 41*(1), 39–41, 53.

Barnard, C. (1938). *The functions of the executive.* New York: Oxford University Press.

Barney, J. (1991). Firm resources and sustained competitive advantage. *Journal of Management, 17,* 99–120.

Bass, B. (1981). *Stogdill's handbook of leadership.* New York: Free Press.

Baum, J., & Amburgey, T. (2005). Organizational ecology. In J. Baum (Ed.), *The Blackwell companion to organizations* (pp. 304–326). Oxford, UK; Malden, MA: Blackwell Business.

Bazzoli, G. J., Stein, R., Alexander, J. A., et al. (1997). Public-private collaboration in health and human services delivery: Evidence from community partnerships. *Milbank Quarterly, 75*(4), 533–561.

Bazzoli, G. J., Shortell, S. M., Dubbs, N., et al. (1999). A taxonomy of health networks and systems: Bringing order out of chaos. *Health Services Research, 33*(6), 1683–1717.

Bazzoli, G. J., Chan, B., Shortell, S. M., et al. T. (2000). The financial performance of hospitals belonging to health networks and systems. *Inquiry, 37*, 234–252.

Beer, M., & Nohria, N. (2000). *Breaking the code of change.* Cambridge, MA: Harvard Business School Press.

Begun, J. W., & White, K. R. (1999). The profession of nursing as a complex adaptive system: Strategies for change. In J. J. Kronenfeld (Ed.), *Research in the sociology of health care* (pp. 189–203). Greenwich, CT: JAI Press.

Begun, J. W., Luke, R. D., & Pointer, D. D. (1990). Structure and strategy in hospital–physician relationships. In S. Mick (Ed.), *Innovations in health care delivery: Insights from organization theory.* San Francisco, CA: Jossey-Bass.

Begun, J. W., Zimmerman, B., & Dooley, K. J. (2003). Health care organizations as complex adaptive systems. In S. Mick & M. Wyttenbach (Eds.), *Advances in health care organization theory* (pp. 253–288). San Francisco, CA: Jossey-Bass.

Berlin, I. S. (1953). *The hedgehog and the fox: An essay on Tolstoy's view of history.* New York: Simon & Schuster.

Berwick, D. M., Nolan, T. W., & Whittington, J. (2008). The triple aim: Care, health, and cost. *Health Affairs, 27*, 759–769.

Blake, R., & Mouton, J. (1964). *The managerial grid.* Houston, TX: Gulf Publishing Co.

Blumenthal, D., Stremikis, K, & Cutler, D. (2013). Health care spending – a giant slain or sleeping? *New England Journal of Medicine, 369*, 2551–2557.

Bogue, R., Antia, M., Harmata, R., & Hall, C. (1997). Community experiments in action: Developing community-defined models for reconfiguring health care delivery. *Journal of Health Politics, Policy and Law, 22*, 1051–1076.

Bonabeau, E. (2009). Decisions 2.0: The power of collective intelligence. *Sloan Management Review, 50*, 45–52.

Bonabeau, E., & Meyer, C. (2001). Swarm intelligence: A whole new way to think about business. *Harvard Business Review, 79*(5), 107–114.

Bradley E. H., & Taylor L. A. (2013). *The American health care paradox: Why spending more is getting us less.* New York: Public Affairs, 2013.

Bradley, E., Canavan, M., Rogan, E., et al. (2016). Variation in health outcomes: The role of spending on social services, public health, and health care, 2000–09. *Health Affairs, 35*(5), 760–768.

Braverman, H. (1974). *Labor and monopoly capital.* New York and London: Monthly Review Press.

Bray, N., Carter, C., Dobson, A., et al. (1994). An examination of winners and losers under Medicare's prospective payment system. *Health Care Management Review, 19*, 44–55.

Burns, T., & Stalker, G. M. (1961). *The management of innovation.* London: Tavistock.

Burns, L. R. (1989). Matrix management in hospitals: Testing theories of matrix structure and development. *Administrative Science Quarterly, 34*, 349–368.

Burns, L. R. (1999). Polarity management: The key challenge for integrated health systems. *Journal of Healthcare Management, 44*, 14–33.

Burns, L. R. (2002). *The health care value chain.* San Francisco, CA: Jossey-Bass.

Burns, L. R. (2005). *The business of healthcare innovation.* Cambridge, UK: Cambridge University Press.

Burns, L. R. (2014). *India's healthcare industry: Innovation in delivery, financing, and manufacturing.* Cambridge, UK: Cambridge University Press.

Burns, L. R., & Liu, G. (2017). *China's healthcare system and reform.* Cambridge, UK: Cambridge University Press.

Burns, L. R., & Wholey, D. (1993). Adoption and abandonment of matrix management programs: Effects of organizational characteristics and interorganizational networks. *Academy of Management Journal, 36*, 106–138.

Burns, L. R., & Wholey, D. R. (2000). Responding to a consolidating healthcare system: Options for physician organizations. In L. Friedman, J. Goes, & G. Savage (Eds.), *Advances in health care management* (Vol. 1, pp. 273–335). New York: Elsevier.

Burns, L. R., & Pauly, M. V. (2002). Integrated delivery networks: A detour on the road to integrated health care? *Health Affairs, 21*(4), 128–143.

Burns, L. R., D'Aunno, T. D., & Kimberly, J. R. (2003). Globalization and its many faces: The case of the health care sector. In H. Gatignon and J. R. Kimberly (Eds.), *The INSEAD-Wharton alliance on globalizing: Strategies for building successful global businesses* (pp. 395–421). Cambridge, UK: Cambridge University Press.

Burns, L. R., Nicholson, S., & Evans, J. (2005). Mergers, acquisitions, and the advantages of scale in the pharmaceutical sector. In L. R. Burns (Ed.), *The business of health care innovation* (pp. 223–268). Cambridge, UK: Cambridge University Press.

Burns, L. R., & Muller. R. (2008). Hospital-physician collaboration: Landscape of economic integration and impact on clinical integration. *Milbank Quarterly, 86*, 375–434.

Burns, L. R., Goldsmith, J. C., & Muller, R. (2010). History of physician-hospital collaboration: Obstacles and opportunities. In J. Crosson and L. Tollen (Eds.), *Partners in health: How physicians and hospitals can be accountable together (pp. 18–45).* Oakland, CA: Kaiser Institute for Health Policy.

Burns, L. R., Wholey, D., McCullough, J., et al. (2012). The changing configuration of hospital systems: Centralization, federalization, or fragmentation? In L. Friedman, G. Savage, and J. Goes (Eds.), *Annual review of health care management: Strategy and policy perspectives on reforming health systems* (Vol. 13, pp. 189–232). Bingley, UK: Emerald Group Publishing.

Burns, L. R., Goldsmith, J., & Sen, A. (2013). Horizontal and vertical integration of physicians: A tale of two tails. In L. Friedman, G. Savage, & J. Goes (Eds.), *Annual review of health care management: Revisiting the evolution of health system organization* (Vol. 15, pp. 39–117). Bingley, UK: Emerald Group Publishing.

Burt, R. S. (1992). *Structural holes: The social structure of competition.* Cambridge, MA: Harvard University Press.

Cappelli, P., Singh, H., Singh, J., & Useem, M. (2010). *The India way.* Cambridge, MA: Harvard Business School Press.

Cardinal, L., Kreutzer, M., & Miller, C. (2017). An aspirational view of organizational control research: Re-invigorating empirical work to better meet the challenges of 21st century organizations. *Academy of Management Annals, 11*(3), 559–592.

Casalino, L., & Robinson, J. (2003). Alternative models of hospital-physician affiliation as the United States moves away from tight managed care. *Milbank Quarterly, 81*(2), 331–351.

Chandler, A. D. (1962). *Strategy and structure*. Cambridge, MA: MIT Press.

Chen, L., Jha, A., Guterman, S., et al. (2010). Hospital cost of care, quality of care, and readmission rates: Penny wise and pound foolish? *Archives of Internal Medicine, 170*(4), 340–346.

Centers for Medicare and Medicaid Services (CMS). (2010, April 22). *Estimated financial effects of the "Patient Protection and Affordable Care Act" as amended*. Washington, DC: CMS.

Collins, J. C., & Porras, J. (1994). *Built to last: Successful habits of visionary companies*. New York: Harper Business.

Commonwealth Fund. (2007a, December). *Bending the curve: Options for achieving savings and improving value in U.S. health spending*. New York: The Commonwealth Fund.

Commonwealth Fund. (2007b, January). *Slowing the growth of U.S. health care expenditures: What are the options?* New York: The Commonwealth Fund.

Congressional Budget Office. (2008a, January). *Technological change and the growth of health care spending*. Washington, DC: CBO.

Congressional Budget Office. (2008b, February). *Geographic variation in health care spending*. Washington, DC: CBO.

Cooper, R. (2008). States with more health care spending have better-quality health care: Lessons about Medicare. *Health Affairs, 28*(1), w103–w115.

Cutler, D., Deaton, A., & Lleras-Muney, A. (2006). The determinants of mortality. *Journal of Economic Perspectives, 20*(3), 97–120.

Cyert, R. M., & March, J. G. (1963). *A behavioral theory of the firm*. Englewood Cliffs, NJ: Prentice-Hall.

D'Aunno, T. D., Sutton, R., & Price, R. (1991). Isomorphism and external support in conflicting institutional environments: A study of drug abuse treatment units. *Academy of Management Journal, 34*, 636–661.

D'Aunno, T., Broffman, L., Sparer, M., et al. (2016). Factors that distinguish high-performing accountable care organizations in the Medicare shared savings program. *Health Services Research, 53*(1), 1–18. Epub: doi: 10.1111/1475-6773.12642.

Deloitte. (2009). *2009 survey of health care consumers: Key findings, strategic implications*. Washington, DC: Deloitte Center for Health Solutions.

DiMaggio, P. J., & Powell, W. W. (1983). The iron cage revisited: Institutional isomorphism and collective rationality in organizational fields. *American Sociological Review, 48*, 147–160.

Dooley, K., & Plsek, P. (2001). A complex systems perspective on medication errors. Working paper, Arizona State University.

Dranove, D. (2008). *Code red*. Princeton, NJ: Princeton University Press.

Dyer, J. H., & Singh, H. (1998). The relational view: Cooperative strategies and sources of interorganizational competitive advantage. *Academy of Management Review, 23*, 660–679.

Economist Intelligence Unit. (2016). *Value-based healthcare: A global assessment*. Retrieved June 1, 2017, from http://vbhcglobalassessment.eiu.com/wp-content/uploads/sites/27/2016/09/EIU_Medtronic_Findings-and-Methodology.pdf.

Esty, D. C., Goldstone, J., Gurr, T.R., et al. (1999, Summer). State failure task force report: Phase II findings. *Environmental change and security project report*. No. 5 (pp. 49–72). Washington, DC: Woodrow Wilson Center.

Fayol, H. (1949). *General and industrial management*. London: Sir Isaac Pitman & Sons.

Federal Trade Commission and Department of Justice (FTC/DOJ). (2004). *Improving health care: A dose of competition*. Washington, DC: FTC and DOJ.

Field, R. (2007). *Health care regulation in America: Complexity, confrontation, and compromise*. New York: Oxford University Press.

Freidson, E. (1970). *Professional dominance*. Chicago, IL: Aldine.

Fuchs, V. (1986). *The health economy*. Cambridge, MA: Harvard University Press.

Galbraith, J. (1973, February). Matrix organization designs. *Business Horizons, 14*(1), 29–40.

GAVI Alliance. (2010). *Saving lives and protecting health: Results and opportunities*. Geneva, Switzerland: The GAVI Alliance.

Gelijns, A., & Rosenberg, N. (1994). The dynamics of technological change in medicine. *Health Affairs, 13*(3), 28–46.

Goldsmith, J. C. (1981). *Can hospitals survive?* Homewood, IL: Dow Jones-Irwin.

Granovetter, M. (1985). Economic action and social structure: The problem of embeddedness. *American Journal of Sociology, 91*, 481–510.

Gulati, R. (1995). Does familiarity breed trust? The implications of repeated ties for contractual choice in alliances. *Academy of Management Journal, 38*, 85–112.

Gulick, L. (1937). *Notes on the theory of organization*. Memorandum prepared for the President's Committee on Administrative Management.

Gulick, L., & Urwick, L. (1937). *Papers on science of administration*. New York: Columbia University Press.

Hackman, J. R., Oldham, G. R., Janson, R., et al. (1975). A new strategy for job enrichment. *California Management Review, 17*(4), 57–71.

Hackman, J. R. (1981). Work redesign for organization development. In H. Meltzer (Ed.), *Making organizations humane and productive* (pp. 373–387). New York: John Wiley & Sons.

Hannan, M. T., & Freeman, J. H. (1977). The population ecology of organizations. *American Journal of Sociology, 82*, 929–964.

Hansmann, H. (1987). Economic theories of nonprofit organizations. In W. W. Powell (Ed.), *The nonprofit sector: A research handbook* (pp. 27–42). New Haven, CT: Yale University Press.

Hawley, A. (1950). *Human ecology*. New York: Ronald Press.

Herzberg, F., Mausner, B., & Snyderman, B. (1959). *The motivation to work* (2nd ed.). New York: John Wiley & Sons.

Herzlinger, R. E. (1997). *Market-driven health care.* Reading, MA: Addison-Wesley.

Herzlinger, R. E. (2006). Why innovation in health care is so hard. *Harvard Business Review, 84*(5), 58–66.

Hsiao, W. C. (2003). What is a health system? Why should we care? In M. Roberts, W. Hsiao, P. Berman, & M. Reich (Eds.), *Getting health reform right: A guide to improving performance and equity.* New York: Oxford University Press.

Inkpen, A., & Tsang, E. (2007). Learning and strategic alliances. *Academy of Management Annals, 1*(1), 479–511.

Institute for Health Care Improvement. (2009). How do they do that? Low-cost, high-quality health care in America. Retrieved February 12, 2010, from http://www.IHI.org/IHI/Programs/StrategicInitiatives/HowDoTheyDoThat.htm?TabId=4.

Institute of Medicine (2001). *Crossing the quality chasm: A new health system for the 21st century.* Washington, DC: National Academy Press.

Jha, A., Joynt, K., Orav, E., et al. (2012). The long-term effect of Premier pay for performance on patient outcomes. *New England Journal of Medicine, 366*(17), 1606–1615.

Johnson, B. (1996). *Polarity management: Identifying and managing unsolvable problems.* Amherst, MA: HRD Press.

Josefy, M., Kuban, S., Ireland, R., et al. (2015). All things great and small. *Academy of Management Annals, 9*(1), 715–802.

Jost, T. (2012). Eight decades of discouragement: The history of health care cost containment in the USA. *Forum for Health Economics & Policy, 15*(3), 53–82.

Katz, M. (2010). Decreasing hospital costs while maintaining quality: Can it be done? *Archives of Internal Medicine, 170*(4), 317–318.

Katz, D., & Kahn, R. L. (1966). *The social psychology of organizations.* New York: Wiley.

Kissick, W. L. (1994). *Medicine's dilemmas.* New Haven, CT: Yale University Press.

Knoke, D. (1990). *Political networks: The structural perspective.* Cambridge, UK: Cambridge University Press.

Lawrence, P., & Lorsch, J. (1967). *Organization and environment.* Cambridge, MA: Harvard University Press.

Lee, V. (2015). The journey to value. Retrieved June 1, 2017, from http://healthsciences.utah.edu/notes/021015_journey.value.php#.WTAZFWWwM7c.

Lewin, K. (1951). *Field theory in social science.* New York: Harper.

Lindenauer, P. K., Remus, D., Roman, S., Rothberg, M. B., Benjamin, E. M., Ma, A., & Bratzler, D. W. (2007, February 1). Public reporting and pay for performance in hospital quality improvement. *New England Journal of Medicine, 356*(5), 486–496.

Liu, G., Yao, Y., Du, N., et al. (2015). *Health and economic prosperity.* Beijing: Peking University National School of Development.

Lydon, P., Levine, R., Makinen, M., et al. (2008). Introducing new vaccines in the poorest countries: What did we learn from the GAVI experience with financial sustainability? *Vaccine, 26,* 6706–6716.

MACRA. (2015). Medicare Access and CHIP Reauthorization Act. Retrieved from https://www.cms.gov/Medicare/Quality-Initiatives-Patient-Assessment-Instruments/Value-Based-Programs/MACRA-MIPS-and-APMs/MACRA-MIPS-and-APMs.html.

Maitlis, S., & Christianson, M. (2014). Sensemaking in organizations: Taking stock and moving forward. *Academy of Management Annals, 8*(1), 57–125.

March, J. G. (1994). *A primer on decision making: How decisions happen.* New York: Free Press.

March, J., & Simon, H. A. (1958). *Organizations.* New York: John Wiley & Sons.

Martin, J. F., & Marshall, J. (2003). New tendencies and strategies in international immunization: GAVI and the vaccine fund. *Vaccine, 21,* 587–592.

McEvily, B., Soda, G., & Tortoriello, M. (2014). More formally: Rediscovering the missing link between formal organization and informal social structure. *Academy of Management Annals, 8*(1), 299–345.

Maslow, A. (1943). A theory of human motivation. *Psychological Review, 50,* 370–396.

Mayo, E. (1945). *The social problems of an industrial civilization.* Boston, MA: Harvard University Press.

McGregor, D. (1960). *The human side of enterprise.* New York: McGraw-Hill.

McKenzie, R. (1968). The scope of human ecology. In A. Hawley (Ed.), *Roderick D. McKenzie: On human ecology* (pp. 19–32). Chicago, IL: University of Chicago Press.

Mendelson, A., Kondo, K., Damberg, C., et al. (2017). The effects of pay-for-performance programs on health, health care use, and processes of care. *Annals of Internal Medicine, 166*(5), 341–353.

Meyer, J., and Rowan, B. (1977). Institutionalized organizations: Formal structure as myth ceremony. *American Journal of Sociology, 83,* 340–363.

Miller, H. D. (2008). *From volume to value: Transforming health care payment and delivery systems to improve quality and reduce costs.* Recommendations of the 2008 NRHI Healthcare Payment Reform Summit (Pittsburgh, PA). Network for Regional Healthcare Improvement.

Milstien, J., Kamara, L., Lydon, P., et al. (2008). The GAVI financing task force: One model of partner collaboration. *Vaccine, 26,* 6699–6705.

Mintzberg, H. (1994). *The rise and fall of strategic planning.* New York: Free Press.

Misumi, J., & Peterson, M. (1985). The performance-maintenance (PM) theory of leadership: Review of a Japanese research program. *Administrative Science Quarterly, 30,* 198–223.

Muraskin, W. (2004). The global alliance for vaccines and immunization: Is it a new model for effective public-private cooperation in international public health? *American Journal of Public Health, 94*(11), 1922–1925.

Nadler, D., & Tushman, M. (1997). *Competing by design: The power of organizational architecture.* Oxford, UK: Oxford University Press.

Nelson, E. C., Godfrey, M. M., Batalden, P. B., et al. (2008). Clinical microsystems, part I: The building blocks of health systems. *Joint Commission Journal on Quality and Patient Safety, 34,* 367–378.

Nembhard, I., Alexander, J., Hoff, T., et al. (2009). Why does quality of health care continue to lag? Insights from management research. *Academy of Management Perspectives, 23*(1), 24–42.

Newhouse, J. P., & Garber, A. (2013). Geographic variation in Medicare services. *New England Journal of Medicine, 368,* 1465–1468.

Parker, J., Regan, J., & Petroski, J. (2014). Beneficiary activation in the Medicare population. *Medicare and Medicaid Research Review, 4*(4), E1–E14.

Parsons, T. (1951). *The social system.* Glencoe, IL: Free Press.

Pauly, M. V., & Redisch, M. (1973). The not-for-profit hospital as a physicians' cooperative. *American Economic Review, 63,* 87–99.

Perrow, C. (1963). Goals and authority structures: A historical case study. In E. Freidson (Ed.), *The hospital in modern society* (pp. 112–146). New York: Free Press.

Perrow, C. (1986). *Complex organizations: A critical essay* (3rd ed.). Glenview, IL: Scott Foresman & Co.

Pfeffer, J., & Salancik, G. R. (1978). *The external control of organizations.* New York: Harper & Row.

Pfeffer, J., & Sutton, R. (2006). *Hard facts, dangerous half-truths and total nonsense; Profiting from evidence-based management.* Cambridge, MA: Harvard Business School Press.

Phipps-Taylor, M., & Shortell, S. M. (2016). More than money: Motivating physician behavior change in accountable care organizations. *Milbank Quarterly, 94*(4), 832–861.

Pool, J. (1991). Hospital management: Integrating the dual hierarchy. *International Journal of Health Planning and Management, 6*(3), 193–207.

Porter, M. E. (1980). *Competitive strategy: Techniques for analyzing industries and competitors.* New York: Free Press.

Porter, M. E. (1985). *Competitive advantage: Creating and sustaining superior performance.* New York: Free Press.

Porter, M. E., & Teisberg, E. O. (2006). *Redefining health care.* Boston, MA: Harvard Business School Press.

Powell, W. W., Koput, K., & Smith-Doerr, A. (1996). Interorganizational collaboration and the locus of innovation: Networks of learning in biotechnology. *Administrative Science Quarterly, 41,* 116–145.

Premier. (2009). Model hospital value-based purchasing program continues to improve patient outcomes. Retrieved October 1, 2018, from https://www.businesswire.com/news/home/20090817005609/en/Model-Hospital-Value-Based-Purchasing-Program-Continues-Improve/.

Priesmeyer, H. R., Sharp, L. F., Wammack, L., et al. (1996). Chaos theory and clinical pathways: A practical application. *Quality Management in Health Care, 4,* 63–72.

ProPAC. (1992). *Evaluation of winners and losers under Medicare's prospective payment system.* Washington, DC: Prospective Payment Assessment Commission.

Quinn, R. (1988). *Beyond rational management: Mastering the paradoxes and competing demands of high performance.* San Francisco, CA: Jossey-Bass.

Roberts, M. J., Hsiao, W., Berman, P., & Reich, M. R. (2003). *Getting health reform right.* New York: Oxford University Press.

Roemer, M. (1961, November 1). Bed supply and hospital utilization: A natural experiment. *Hospitals,* 36–42.

Roethlisberger, F. G., & Dickson, W. (1947). *Management and the worker.* Cambridge, MA: Harvard University Press.

Ruef, M., & Scott, W. R. (1998). A multidimensional model of organizational legitimacy: Hospital survival in changing institutional markets. *Administrative Science Quarterly, 43*(4), 877–904.

Ryan, A. M. (2009). Effects of the Premier hospital quality incentive demonstration on Medicare patient mortality and cost. *Health Services Research, 44*(3), 821–842.

Sachs, J. (2001). *Macroeconomics and health: Investing in health for economic development.* Geneva, Switzerland: World Health Organization.

Sager, A., and Socolar, D. (2005). *Health costs absorb one-quarter of economic growth, 2000–2005.* Data Brief No. 8. Health Reform Program. Boston University School of Public Health. Boston, MA.

Schlesinger, M., & Grob, R. (2017). Treating, fast and slow: Americans' understanding of and responses to low-value care. *Milbank Quarterly, 95*(1), 70–116.

Schuster, M., McGlynn, E., & Brook, R. H. (1997). *Why the quality of U.S. health care must be improved.* Santa Monica, CA: Rand Corporation.

Scott, W. R. (1982). Managing professional work: Three models of control for health organizations. *Health Services Research, 17,* 213–240.

Selznick, P. (1949). *TVA and the grass roots.* New York: Harper & Row.

Selznick, P. (1957). *Leadership in administration.* New York: Harper & Row.

Senge, P. (2006). *The fifth discipline.* New York: Doubleday.

Shakarishvili, G. (2009). Building on health systems frameworks for developing a common approach to health systems strengthening. Paper prepared for the World Bank, the Global Fund, and the GAVI Alliance Technical Workshop on Health Systems Strengthening. Washington, DC, June 25–27.

Shortell, S. M., Gillies, R. R., & Anderson, D. (1994). The new world of managed care: Creating organized delivery systems. *Health Affairs, 13,* 46–64.

Shortell, S. M., Gillies, R. R., Anderson, D. A., et al. (1996). *Remaking health care in America: Building organized delivery systems.* San Francisco, CA: Jossey-Bass.

Shortell, S. M., & Rundall, T. G. (2003). Physician-organization relationships: Social networks and strategic intent. In S. Mick & M. Wyttenbach (Eds.), *Advances in health care organization theory* (pp. 141–173). San Francisco, CA: Jossey-Bass.

Simon, H. A. (1947). *Administrative behavior.* New York: MacMillan.

Skillman, M., Cross-Barnet, C., Singer, R., et al. (2017). Physician engagement strategies in care coordination: Findings from the Centers for Medicare and Medicaid Services Health Care Innovation Awards Program. *Health Services Research, 52*(1), 291–312.

Sloan, F., Picone, G., Taylor, D., et al. (2001). Hospital ownership and cost and quality of care: Is there a dime's worth of difference? *Journal of Health Economics, 20*(1), 1–21.

Smith, S., Reichert, H., Ameling, J., et al. (2017). Dissecting Leapfrog: How well do Leapfrog practice scores correlate with Hospital Compare ratings and penalties, and how much do they matter? *Medical Care, 55*(6), 606–614.

Storeng, K. (2014). The GAVI Alliance and the "Gates approach" to health system strengthening. *Global Public Health, 9*(8), 865–879.

Studdert, D. M., Mello, M. M., Sage, W. M., et al. (2005). Defensive medicine among high-risk specialist physicians in a volatile malpractice environment. *Journal of American Medical Association, 293*(21), 2609–2617.

Surowiecki, J. (2004). *The wisdom of crowds*. New York: Doubleday.

Taylor, F. W. (1911). *The principles of scientific management*. New York: W. W. Norton.

Thompson, J. D. (1967). *Organizations in action*. New York: McGraw-Hill.

Thorpe, K. (2007). *An unhealthy truth: Rising rates of chronic disease and the future of health in America*. Partnership to Fight Chronic Disease. Retrieved May 16, 2017, from http://www.prevent.org/data/files/initiatives/thorpeslides11-30-07.pdf.

Towers Perrin. (2008). 2008 update on U.S. tort cost trends. Retrieved July 31, 2010, from http://www.towersperrin.com/tp/getwebcachedoc?webc=USA/2008/200811/2008_tort_costs_trends.pdf.

Tsai, F-J., Lee, H., & Fan, V. (2016). Perspective and investments in health system strengthening of Gavi, the Vaccine Alliance: A content analysis of health system strengthening-specific funding. *International Health, 8*, 246–252.

Tushman, M. L., & O'Reilly, C. (1997). *Winning through innovation: A practical guide to leading organizational change and renewal*. Cambridge, MA: Harvard Business School Press.

Ulrich, D., Kerr, S., and Ashkenas, R. (2002). *GE Work-Out*. New York: McGraw-Hill.

Uzzi, B. (1997). Social structure and competition in interfirm networks: The paradox of embeddedness. *Administrative Science Quarterly, 42,* 35–67.

Uzzi, B. (1999). Embeddedness in the making of financial capital: How social relations and networks benefit firms seeking financing. *American Sociological Review, 64*, 481–505.

Van de Ven, A., Polley, D. E., Garud, R., & Venkataraman, S. (1999). *The innovation journey*. New York: Oxford University Press.

Van de Ven, A., Ganco, M., & Hinings, C. R. (2013). Returning to the frontier of contingency theory of organizational and institutional designs. *Academy of Management Annals, 7*(1), 393–440.

Weber, M. (1964). *The theory of social and economic organization*. Glencoe, IL: Free Press.

Weber, K., & Waeger, D. (2017). Organizations as polities: An open systems perspective. *Academy of Management Annals, 11*(1), 886–918.

Weick, K. (1995). *Sensemaking in organizations*. Thousand Oaks, CA: Sage Publications.

Weisbrod, B. A. (1991). The health care quadrilemma: An essay on technological change, insurance, quality of care, and cost containment. *Journal of Economic Literature, 29*, 523–552.

Wennberg, J. E., Fisher, E. S., & Skinner, J. S. (2002). Geography and the debate over Medicare reform. *Health Affairs,* Web Exclusive, W96–W114.

Westphal, J. D., Gulati, R., & Shortell, S. M. (1997). Customization or conformity: An institutional and network perspective on the content and consequences of TQM adoption. *Administrative science quarterly, 42*(2), 366–394.

Whitley, M. A. (2009, June 4). Cleveland Clinic praised by President Barack Obama for efficiency, control of costs. *The Plain Dealer* (Cleveland, OH). Retrieved July 31, 2010, from http://www.cleveland.com/medical/index.ssf/2009/06/cleveland_clinic_praised_by_pr.html.

Wholey, D. R., Christianson, J. C., & Sanchez, S. (1992). Organization size and failure among health maintenance organizations. *American Sociological Review, 57*, 829–842.

Wholey, D. R., & Burns, L. R. (1993). Organizational transitions: Form changes by health maintenance organizations. In S. Bacharach (Ed.), *Research in the sociology of organizations* (pp. 257–293). Greenwich, CT: JAI Press.

Wholey, D. R., Wilson, A. R., Riley, W., & Knoke, D. (2009). Work and talk: Information provision in informal consulting in medical clinics. Unpublished manuscript.

Woodward, J. (1965). *Industrial organization: Theory and practice*. London: Oxford University Press.

World Bank Group. (2012). *Global Program review: The GAVI Alliance*. Washington, DC: World Bank.

World Health Organization. (1996). *The world health report 1996: Fighting disease, fostering development*. Geneva, Switzerland: WHO.

World Health Organization. (2000). *The world health report 2000: Health systems: Improving performance*. Geneva, Switzerland: WHO.

Wry, T., Cobb, J. A., & Aldrich, H. (2013). More than a metaphor: Assessing the historical legacy of resource dependence and its contemporary promise as a theory of environmental complexity. *Academy of Management Annals, 7*(1), 441–488.

Chapter 2

Leadership and Management: A Framework for Action

Elizabeth H. Bradley, Ingrid M. Nembhard, Lauren Taylor, Amanda Brewster, and Jane Banaszak-Holl

CHAPTER OUTLINE

- Introduction
- Concepts of Leadership and Management
- Theories of Leadership
- Leadership Internal and External Roles
- Challenges for Leadership in Health Care
- An Approach to Address the Challenges: Strategic Problem Solving
- Relationship of Leadership to Organizational Performance
- Sustaining Leadership

LEARNING OBJECTIVES

After completing this chapter, the reader should be able to:

1. Differentiate between leadership and management
2. Describe the evolution of leadership theory
3. Comprehend internal and external challenges for leadership and management
4. Apply a strategic problem-solving method to health care challenges
5. Appreciate current research findings in leadership literature
6. Discuss how to sustain successful leadership

KEY TERMS

Adaptive Leadership	Governing Board
Administrative Leadership	Inclusive Leadership
Behavioral Theories	Instrumental Support
Clinical Leadership	Interpersonal Support
Competencies	Leadership
Contingency Theories	Leader-Member Exchange (LMX)
Donors	Management
Followership	Middle Managers
Front-Line Managers	Objectives
Goals	Organizational Culture

Path-Goal Model

Relational Theories

Senior Management

SMART

Strategic Problem Solving

Technical Leadership

Trait Theories

Transactional Leadership

Transformational Leadership

• • • IN PRACTICE: The Case of Paul Levy, CEO of Beth Israel Deaconess Medical Center[1]

Paul Levy is an unusual leader in health care because his first job in health services was as CEO of Beth Israel Deaconess Medical Center (BIDMC). Immediately prior to taking the job at BIDMC, Mr. Levy was executive dean for administration at Harvard Medical School, and prior to that, he directed the Massachusetts Water Resources Authority (1987–1992) and worked in public utilities. Mr. Levy became the CEO at BIDMC as it struggled to become financially stable, and he successfully turned the health system around. His success illustrates how individuals can succeed as leaders across multiple situations and that the challenges at BIDMC required a leader with new ideas about how to meet the medical center's challenges.

BIDMC is a large medical center associated with Harvard University. In 2001, the year Paul Levy became CEO of BIDMC, the medical center had 1,200 physicians on its staff, 4,500 full-time employees, and 513 licensed beds.[2] It also experienced total losses of $28 million and losses in the operating budget were as high as $58 million.[3] These losses were attributed to limited integration of duplicative and costly operations after BIDMC was created from the merger of two large hospitals and a number of other smaller community hospitals in the extremely competitive Boston area. Mr. Levy forced change to happen quickly after taking office; within a year of becoming CEO, BIDMC experienced several months of positive financial status relative to budget and subsequently experienced steady improvement in financial health.

How did he implement change so quickly? Both he and others argue that it came not from making quick decisions about how to make cuts within the health system but from empowering others to make these decisions more efficiently. He changed the culture to emphasize staff-driven change. Partly, this was and still is done by more clearly outlining both the positive and negative consequences of the situation, setting expectations for what should come from organizational change, and repeatedly communicating how change is going and whether expectations are met, which includes being transparent about the organization's operations, successes, and failures. Today, Paul Levy blogs regularly on the Internet and you will find on his blog forthright discussions of both positive aspects of BIDMC's health care and the financial troubles the institution now faces again.

The mechanisms of Paul Levy's leadership are visible today as BIDMC again confronts financial trouble. In 2009, BIDMC had the worst financial year since 2001, and these problems are expected to continue at least through 2010 as the economic downturn persists and the health care environment in Boston changes. Indeed, all the hospitals in Boston have been facing a similar situation. Levy though has insisted that his staff will contribute to the solution. In his communication to staff, Mr. Levy writes, "Our task, it seems to me, and the one with which you have been so helpful in your comments [via e-mail and other mechanisms], has been to come up with alternatives that dramatically reduce this number of layoffs [set at 600]"[4] while achieving our cost-cutting goals. Mr. Levy received these suggestions after asking employees for help in identifying options. Now, his challenge is to determine which suggestions to use and to convey to staff the value of all the recommendations received. How would you weigh the multitude of options employees suggest? Who should contribute ultimately to decisions about where the biggest cuts in hospital operations occur? What values would you commit to maintaining through periods of cost cutting and economic downturn? All these questions reflect hard decisions about the process by which a leader both inspires followers and maintains the organization's culture and mission.

---

[1] The topic and historical timeline in this case are based roughly on the Harvard Business School Case # 9-303-008, "Paul Levy: Taking Charge of the Beth Israel Deaconess Medical Center (A)," written by Professors David A. Garvin and Michael A. Roberto, 2002.

[2] These data are taken from the Harvard Business School Case # 9-303-008, "Paul Levy: Taking Charge of the Beth Israel Deaconess Medical Center (A)," written by Professors David A. Garvin and Michael A. Roberto, 2002.

[3] Ibid.

[4] Retrieved from: http://www.bidmc.org/GivetoBIDMC/NewsRoom/CommunicationFromPaulLevy.aspx, retrieved January 24, 2010.

CHAPTER PURPOSE

The purpose of this chapter is to provide an understanding of and distinctions between leadership and management functions within organizations facing complex and changing environments. We describe the historical evolution in leadership theories up to contemporary models and explore leadership and management challenges the stewards of modern health care organizations may face. The chapter seeks to help those in leadership and management roles anticipate challenges, perform more effectively, and sustain themselves and their organizations in the dynamic environment of health care.

INTRODUCTION

The chapter is organized in seven sections. The first section distinguishes the concepts of leadership and management and explains that both of these functions occur at many levels of the organizational hierarchy. The second section reviews prominent theories of leadership. The third section describes two roles of effective organizational leadership: improving the execution of the primary task of the organization (internal leadership) and creating effective relationships with external stakeholders (external leadership). The fourth section describes contemporary challenges faced by leadership of health care organizations. The fifth section introduces a strategic problem-solving framework that can be used to address these challenges at different levels of the organization. The sixth section summarizes recent research findings concerning the influence of leadership on health care organizational performance. The chapter ends with the seventh section, which addresses issues of succession planning for organizations to sustain effective leadership over time as well as sustaining oneself in leadership roles.

CONCEPTS OF LEADERSHIP AND MANAGEMENT

Leadership can be defined as the process in which one engages with others to set and achieve group objectives, often an organizationally defined goal (Robbins and Judge, 2010). In contrast, **management** can be defined as the process of accomplishing predetermined objectives through the effective use of human, financial, and technical resources (Longest, Rakich, and Darr, 2000). Although the same person may execute leadership in some circumstances and management in others, the two activities are conceptually distinct. Importantly, both leadership and management activities may be undertaken by managers at all levels of the organizational hierarchy, although the scope of the goals, strategies, and tactics will vary with position in the organization.

Modern health care organizations are often large bureaucracies requiring management at multiple levels.

In many health organizations, it is possible to distinguish three levels of managers, many of whom both lead and manage as part of their positions: (1) **front-line managers** provide direct supervision for clinical, technical, and administrative staff involved directly in patient care and support services; (2) **middle managers** have responsibility for specific departments or units within the health care organization; and (3) **senior managers** are responsible for managing the entire organization, overseeing all units within it, and managing relationships with the governing board of the organization.

Front-line managers assign tasks and hold supervisees accountable for performing job responsibilities. Effective performance often involves implementing strategies through teams and coordinating cross-functional groups. The leadership activities of front-line managers have direct and immediate effects on how the work of the organization is performed, as the relationship between employees and their immediate supervisors strongly influences perceptions of the work climate and what is expected (Purcell and Hutchinson, 2007).

Middle managers have been called the "linking pins" within organizations because of their fundamental roles in communication and coordination (Floyd and Wooldridge, 1992; Likert, 1961). Middle managers implement strategies developed at the senior management level but can also play important roles in shaping strategy; in fact, involvement of middle management in setting strategy has been associated with better organizational performance (Floyd and Wooldridge, 1992). Middle managers are often the ones who act as organizational champions for innovation, bringing ideas developed on the front lines to the attention of senior managers (Floyd and Wooldridge, 1992) and ushering idea implementation (Birken, Lee, and Weiner, 2012; Birken et al., 2013; Birken et al., 2016). Operating in the middle of the organization, they manage the front-line managers but report to senior managers.

Senior managers are often referred to as the "C-suite" because their job titles include chief executive officer, chief financial officer, chief information officer, chief nursing officer, and chief medical officer, among others. Senior management sets strategic direction for the organization, with input from the governing board where applicable, and is responsible for defining and communicating the mission and values of the organization as well as managing middle managers.

Although many metaphors have been used to characterize organizations (Morgan, 2006), conceptualizing organizations as living systems is particularly helpful for understanding leadership and management functions. In this conceptualization, organizations are seen as open systems, receiving inputs (e.g., financing, information, raw materials) from their environments, processing these inputs, and releasing outputs back to the environment (Katz and Kahn, 1978). A key function of leadership in open system theory is the managing of the boundary

DEBATE TIME: Leadership and Management: Any Differences?

1. Many leadership experts argue that leadership is a role rather than a personal or professional trait. Is this a distinction worth making?
2. Many people, even those well acquainted with the two concepts, confuse management and leadership. Some argue that management is simply one skill that a leader may or may not possess. Others depict leadership as enlightened management, saying, "Management is doing things right. Leadership is doing the right things." Are they really two separate ideas?
3. Many professional development courses are available for building leadership skills and competencies. Courses differ substantially, but most presuppose that leadership can be taught or developed within a person. Is this presupposition valid? Based on what you know of your peers and the leaders you consider to be great, can anyone demonstrate leadership?

between the internal functioning of the organization and its external environment, including the market, community, and political realities of the day. This boundary management function seeks to maintain an optimally permeable boundary, which involves engagement with external stakeholders and market forces while also protecting the organization from external threats and using internal resources (e.g., human, financial, and technical staff and materials) to execute the primary tasks of the organization.

THEORIES OF LEADERSHIP

The popular images of people who are successful in leadership roles evoke charismatic, larger-than-life personalities. Take, for example, Paul Levy, whom we described at the start of this chapter and who is seen as largely responsible for the turnaround of Beth Israel Deaconess Medical Center. Early in his tenure at Beth Israel Deaconess, the *Boston Globe* reported, "The turnaround of Beth Israel Deaconess is as much about management as health care. By most accounts Levy's predecessor, Dr. James Reinertsen, understood well the hospital's problems. But every time he pushed, the institution pushed back and little got done. Levy, best known for running the Massachusetts Water Resources Authority got things done, big and small" (Bailey, 2002).

Theories about what makes effective leadership are many; however, they can be categorized as follows: (1) trait theory, which posits that individuals are effective in leadership roles based on innate traits; (2) behavioral theory, which suggests that people are effective in leadership roles based a set of behaviors that are learned over time with training and experience, instead of their traits; (3) contingency theory, which argues that no singular set of traits and behaviors are adequate for explaining who will be effective in leadership roles; rather, the needed behaviors depend on the circumstance or environment in which one is leading; and (4) relational theory, which emphasizes the importance of relationships between those in leadership and followership roles. We review each in turn to chart the development of the field.

Trait Theory

In the late nineteenth century and early twentieth century, experts believed that innate physical and personality traits were strongly linked to leadership capacity. In other words, people are born leaders or not. Research on critical traits reached its peak during the early twentieth century and has since declined as other determinants of leadership performance have become better understood and more widely endorsed. It is now accepted that people with a wide range of personal traits can be successful in leadership roles, although certain personal characteristics such as personality and gender have been shown to influence leadership approaches.

Trait researchers have evaluated the influence of more than 40 individual traits and personality characteristics on leadership performance (Landy and Conte, 2004), but only a handful of traits have been empirically linked to leadership performance. Gender, which was long thought to be an innate trait, has been found to be associated with leadership performance in many instances, although the literature is mixed on the magnitude and direction of this influence. Some evidence suggests that women and men use different behaviors in leadership roles. A review of meta-analyses found that women were more likely than men to use transformational leadership styles and demonstrate greater support for subordinates (Eagly and Carli, 2007). Gender-based differences in leadership effectiveness appear to depend on the context, and particularly the degree to which a woman's leadership role is seen to conflict with gender-based cultural norms. For example, women have been rated as less effective than men in positions that have been usually filled by men, such as the military, but have been rated more positively than men in leadership roles in education, government, and social service organizations (Eagly, 2007).

Researchers have also examined the link between personality and leadership, finding that extraversion, emotional stability, and openness to experience are associated with leadership effectiveness (Judge, Bono, and Locke, 2000); nevertheless, some evidence indicates that the influence of personality differs markedly across settings, with personality exerting more influence on the perceived effectiveness of leadership in unstructured settings (e.g., among student groups) than in work organizations (Judge, Bono, and Locke, 2000). The literature has also suggested that the relationship between personality and leadership performance is likely mediated by the behaviors that people with different personalities are likely to choose (Judge, Bono, and Locke, 2000).

Behavioral Theory

In the 1930s, the behavioral school of thought about leadership evolved to argue that individuals' behaviors, rather than their traits, explained the difference between effective and ineffective leadership. The behavioral approach to leadership emphasized the actions that the person in the leadership role takes on the job. Such behaviors were readily observable by another party and could be developed through education and work experience. The popularization of behavioral theory in leadership coincided with the growth of business schools within which behaviors could be taught.

Some of the earliest studies to map leadership behaviors, conducted by researchers at the Ohio State University and the University of Michigan in the late 1940s (Stogdill and Coons, 1957), identified two dimensions along which leadership behavior could vary. The first, consideration for the satisfaction of employees, focused on the use of behaviors that build trust with employees by, for example, demonstrating interest in their ideas and regard for their feelings (Bass, 1990). The second, initiation of structure, focused on setting reasonable objectives and defining employee roles (Bass, 1990). This distinction is similar to the distinction made between relationship- and task-oriented approaches to leadership, where relationship-oriented leadership concentrates on maintaining supportive interactions with employees and task-oriented leadership concentrates on achievement of work results. Although different individuals may emphasize one or the other domain, effective performance typically requires both (Bass, 1990).

The effective use of emotional intelligence (Goleman, 2006), or the ability to understand and manage emotions in oneself and others, has also been associated with leadership effectiveness. In its most classic formulation, emotional intelligence includes (1) being self-aware (to recognize one's own emotions), (2) controlling one's emotions to use them effectively for decision making and action, (3) detecting others' emotions, and (4) managing others' emotions in work interactions (Salovey and Meyer, 1990). Emotional intelligence is thought to facilitate skill with a number of effective leadership behaviors (George, 2000).

Models of leadership behavior have become more complex in order to fit the reality that those in leadership roles usually respond to a situation with a set of behaviors rather than a single behavior. **Transformational leadership** refers to a set of behaviors used by leaders to influence (or transform) the attitudes, values, and behaviors of staff in ways that inspire staff to go beyond minimum job requirements and strive to contribute to the achievement of the larger organizational mission. Transformational leadership can enable the accomplishment of immediate goals while also anticipating and better meeting the needs of a changing environment and has been associated with organizational performance (Lowe, Kroeck, and Sivasubramaniam, 1996). Table 2.1 lists the four key behaviors that characterize transformational leadership (Bass, 1990).

Transformational leadership is often contrasted with **transactional leadership**, which uses explicit reward structures (e.g., recognition, compensation, and promotions) to influence performance of staff. Classically, the transactional leadership literature discusses four behaviors: (1) making rewards contingent on performance, (2) correcting problems actively when performance goes wrong, (3) refraining from interruptions of performance if it meets standards (i.e., passive management of exceptions), and (4) a laissez-faire approach to organizational change. Transactional leadership accomplishes the required tasks on time and completely but does not seek to move the organization and its staff to a new value system or way of working together. It is worth noting that transactional and transactional leadership may be appropriate separately or together, depending on the context. While the initial conceptualization of transformational and transactional leadership argued that leadership within a specific situation could be defined as one or the

Table 2.1 Defining Characteristics in Transactional and Transformational Leadership

Transactional Leadership	Transformational Leadership
Reward contingent on performance	Employ idealized role model
Correct performance problems actively	Motivate through inspiration
Refrain from interrupting performance if acceptable	Stimulate the intellect of subordinates
Use laissez-faire approach	Use individualized consideration

other, a review of many studies on the topic concluded that transactional approaches—particularly contingent rewards—are important complements to transformational approaches (Lowe, Kroeck, and Sivasubramaniam, 1996; Gilmartin and D'Aunno, 2007).

Contingency Theory

Contingency theory, which first emerged in the 1960s, expands previous behavioral frameworks to suggest that the effectiveness of specific leadership behaviors and actions depends on the context in which one is leading. Behaviors that may be very effective in one situation can be ineffective in another, adding a premium to being able to not only understand the context but also adapt one's behaviors and actions to it. Contingency theory elevates leadership from a property of a single individual and makes it a property of a system.

One of the first extensive descriptions of contingency factors in leadership came from Fred Fiedler in 1967 who argued that an individual's success in leadership positions depends not just on one's behaviors but also on one's relationship to people in followership roles and the tasks these people are expected to undertake (Berg, 1998). Even greater elaboration of how the work environment affects success in leadership is explored in the **path-goal model**, which argues that effective leadership requires a supervisor who provides the information, support, and resources that staff need to achieve the objectives in a particular situation (House, 1996). Victor Vroom and colleagues focused on how the effectiveness of decision-making processes between leadership and subordinates varies by the type of decisions being made, differentiating situations in which effective decisions can be made by leadership alone from situations in which effective decision making requires varying degrees of consultation with subordinates (Vroom and Yetton, 1973).

Another contingency model, which has been central in theories of leadership, is the **leader-member exchange (LMX)** theory, which recognizes distinctive relationships between people in leadership roles and each of their staff in followership roles (Graen and Uhl-Bien, 1995). LMX theories argue that those in the leadership role react differently to their trusted and limited "in group," who are given more autonomy and flexibility in tasks than the "out group," who may also report to the person in the leadership role, but among whom clearly defined roles and greater formality is the norm. LMX theories have also considered the potential movement of individuals from "out group" to "in group" as individuals gradually become trusted and tasked with the in-group activities. Some researchers have suggested that people in leadership roles need to evolve their behavior as subordinates gain experience and ability over time (Hersey and Blanchard, 1969).

A final prominent model within the contingency theory of leadership is **adaptive** versus **technical leadership** (Heifetz, 1994), which describes how effective leadership techniques vary according to the amount of uncertainty in the environment. Adaptive leadership, required in uncertain environments characterized by complex problems and dynamic contexts and risk, involves mobilizing people to confront changed circumstances (Heifetz, 1994). Technical leadership, appropriate for situations with less uncertainty, involves motivating the execution of established problem-solving processes. For instance, adaptive leadership asks questions to allow staff to unearth the problems whereas technical leadership would define the problem for staff. Faced with threats to the organization, adaptive leadership would disclose the threat to the organization whereas technical leadership would seek to protect the organization from the threat. Concerning roles and norm setting, adaptive leadership challenges traditional roles and social norms, as new roles and norms must evolve to meet a changing environment, while technical leadership defines roles more clearly and reinforces existing social norms. Consistent with contingency theory, alternative approaches are thought to be effective for varying environments.

Relational Theory of Leadership

Building on contingency theories, relational theories of leadership suggest that the relationship between people in leadership and followership roles is essential to any conception of leadership (Berg, 1998). Attention to followership has developed in recent decades, following social movements of the 1960s and 1970s that encouraged the questioning of authority and broadened the concept of leadership beyond getting subordinates to go along with decisions made by the person in the leadership (Kellerman, 2008). Like leadership, followership is a critical role in an organization. Effective **followership** has been defined as "enthusiastic, intelligent, and self-reliant participation in the pursuit of an organizational goal" (Kelley, 1988). Most people in an organization play both leadership and followership roles at varying times and in varying assignments within their position responsibilities (Kellerman, 2008).

The effectiveness of people in leadership roles may be measured by the extent to which they are able to leverage the capacities of those in followership roles. Five types of followership have been identified (Kelley, 1988): "sheep" are passive and uncritical; "yes people" are more active but never question the leader. "Alienated followers" are independent thinkers but cynical and passive about performing their roles. "Survivors" are hesitant to commit to new ideas until most colleagues do. Last, "effective followers" think for themselves and are proactive in carrying out their work. People who are effective in followership roles are adept at managing themselves and readily share dissenting views with people in the leadership roles. The degree to which one can exhibit effective followership depends on one's relationship with those in leadership roles, reinforcing both leadership and followership not as individual traits or capacities but rather relational concepts.

Despite the centrality of the leadership-followership relationship, people in leadership roles may not always manage subordinates in a way that fosters genuine, participatory followership. People in leadership roles can fail to fully incorporate people in followership roles in agenda- and priority-setting processes and decision making. Such failures come with enormous opportunity costs, as the participation of energetic people in the followership role has been consistently shown to strengthen group performance (Kellerman, 2008). Similarly, people in followership roles may find it uncomfortable to manage people in leadership roles. People in followership roles may fear "overstepping" their professional boundaries or being seen as either overly eager or overly critical of their supervisor's plans or actions. Nevertheless, willingness to actively engage with the person in the leadership role in an enthusiastic, intelligent, and self-reliant manner is what distinguishes effective followership.

The relationship between the people in leadership roles and people in followership roles can provide the organization with a greater range of capacities to draw upon in pursuit of organizational goals. When this relationship is weak or nonexistent, the person in the leadership role is apt to overtax themselves, resort to rigid role boundaries or hierarchical structures, and be unreceptive to the input of followers (Kelley, 1988). Those in followership roles in these cases are apt to participate in a more limited, dogmatic fashion and to keep potentially useful perspectives to themselves. This leaves the organization limited in the scope of its functioning and less able to react strategically and on a timely basis. In contrast, when the relationship between those in leadership and those in followership roles is strong—that is, built on a history of trust and mutual appreciation—people can fearlessly contribute their unique skills and perspectives as needed to the accomplishment of the goal (Berg, 1998; Weick, 1993). Strong relationships between those in the leadership and followership roles thus provide organizational durability, allowing it to have collaborative connections across the hierarchy (Berg, 1998) and to adapt and respond to changing circumstances and challenges.

LEADERSHIP INTERNAL AND EXTERNAL ROLES

People in leadership positions will inevitably face a multitude of constantly evolving challenges based on shifting internal capacities and external conditions—including new market conditions, emerging regulatory and legal standards, and shifting norms about what communities want from their health care organizations. In this section, we identify two primary roles of leadership: (1) facilitating effective and efficient execution of the primary task of the organization (internal leadership) and (2) creating effective relationships with stakeholders in the external environment (external leadership). Both roles present challenges for organizational leadership.

Facilitating Execution of the Primary Tasks of the Organization

The primary tasks of the organization are the set of activities that enable the organization to achieve its objectives, goals, and overall mission. For instance, delivering high-quality acute patient care at reasonable cost might be a primary task of a hospital, providing health education may be a primary task of a school-based clinic, and improving residential quality of life for adults with functional impairments might be a primary task of a nursing home. Many additional tasks are in service to the primary tasks and keenly important such as finance, marketing, human resources, materials management, and many others. A set of management and quality improvement tools are typically deployed to ensure the accomplishment and sustaining of these primary tasks. In addition to technical, financial, strategic, and material inputs to executing the primary task, research has shown that organizational culture is fundamental for executing the tasks of organizations (Bradley et al., 2012; Curry et al., 2011; Schneider, Erhart, and Macey, 2013).

Effective leadership entails not just attending to technical, financial, strategic, and material inputs but also diagnosing, cultivating, and altering organizational culture as needed to support task accomplishment (Kotter, 2007; Longest, Rakich, and Darr, 2000; Schein, 2006; Senge, 1990). According to Schein (2006), organizational culture is the deepest level of assumptions and beliefs that are shared by members of an organization. These assumptions and beliefs are learned responses to organizations' efforts to survive within the external environment. The culture survives because it solves problems for the organization, and hence it is de facto considered valid. Additionally, the organizational culture is thought to operate unconsciously and defines the "way we do things around here." Schein (2006) proposed the following definition:

> A pattern of basic assumptions—invented, discovered, or developed by a given group as it learns to cope with its problems of external adaptation and internal integration—that has worked well enough to be considered valid and, therefore, to be taught to new members as the correct way to perceive, think and feel in relation to those problems.

Although the essence of organizational culture is basic assumptions and beliefs shared in the organization, culture is nonetheless manifest in more visible levels of organizational life, including tangible artifacts and expressed values that operate at more superficial levels of the organization. Although the more surface levels of artifacts and values may not be the essence of culture, they do signal the essence of culture and are therefore important to understand, interpret, and use as part of the leadership role of influencing organizational culture. The relationships among basic assumptions and beliefs, values, and artifacts are illustrated in Table 2.2.

Artifacts are signs of the physical, psychological, or social environment. These might include the physical space, modes of communication both written and verbal, signage in the organization, language used, and other overt behaviors. In the health care setting, artifacts might include the terms used to describe the people served by the organization. Consider the difference between, for example, "diabetic patients" and "patients with diabetes." This simple wording change shifts the focus from the disease to the person, who happens to have a disease. In another example, consider the artifact of referring to "mental health patients" to "clients with mental health issues." Other artifacts might include the way in which an organization uses e-mail, the approach to staff meetings, physical layout of offices or patient care areas, the use or nonuse of uniforms for staff, and so on.

Values are the organization's stated values and rules of behavior. For instance, patient-centeredness is an example of an organizational value. In reality, some activities may suffer from inadequate patient-centeredness, but the organization might still hold the value, and its value would be a sign of the culture. Such a value is often semi-visible to the degree that it is expressed in communication of all kinds. People seeking to influence organizational culture, therefore, can start with discussions of values in forums where they can be debated and challenged, and gradually, if successful, integrated into the basic beliefs and assumptions of members of the organization. This visibility distinguishes values from shared basic assumptions, which are deeply embedded, taken-for-granted behaviors that operate at an unconscious level but usually constitute the essence of the organizational culture.

Table 2.2 Elements of Organizational Culture: Assumptions and Beliefs, Values, and Artifacts

Basic Assumptions and Beliefs	Values	Artifacts
The organization has patients' best interests at heart	Patient safety and patient-centeredness	Employee orientation includes patient safety Board reporting on patient safety indicators Reading library for patients and families Satisfaction surveys reviewed by senior management Customer relations programs
Health is multifaceted	Interdisciplinary care	Interdisciplinary care teams and rounds Matrix reporting relationships Interdisciplinary quality teams Green programs to sustain environment Social support groups with patients and families
High-quality care is essential	Quality of care	Quality metrics defined, measured, and reported Incentive systems (monetary and nonmonetary) for quality Performance reviews include quality-of-care goals Public reporting of quality outcomes Quality improvement committee structure
Health care is a human right	Equity and ethics	Free clinic partnerships Outreach to low-income communities Staff voluntarism in community Ethical review boards Medical ethics training for staff of all levels
Health care resources are limited	Efficiency	Process improvement efforts to reduce redundancy Pay scales within range Physical plant is cost-efficient Limit staffing to what is necessary Clear travel and conference rules

Creating Effective Relationships with External Stakeholders

According to an open systems view of organizations (Katz and Kahn, 1978), leadership can be understood as centrally concerned with the management of boundaries (Gilmore, 1982; Lawrence and Lorsch, 1967). Managing boundaries entails protecting the distinctive competence to which the organization lays claim (Selznick, 1957). This management of the boundary may require defending the perimeter to maintain an inner environment that is conducive to achieving the primary tasks of the organization but also may require opening a perimeter in order to allow new information, personnel, or capital to be incorporated into organizational workflows. In the latter case, it is useful to keep in mind that each boundary crossing carries with it not only the potential for learning but also the risk of subversion by outsider's values and practices (Gilmore, 1982).

This boundary-management aspect of leadership has been brought into sharp relief in an age of specialization and resource scarcity within the health care landscape. Together, these environmental characteristics increase the degree of interdependence among actors (Gilmore, 1982). If we consider a health care organization as the focal organization, key external stakeholders include the governing board and donors (who are not immersed in the daily activities of the organization), potential collaborators and competitors in the marketplace, regulators and politicians, and communities or populations served by the organization. Each has its own interests that may or may not be able to be aligned with those of the focal organizations.

The **governing board** (sometimes called trustees or the board of directors) typically plays a critical role both in setting the overall mission of the organization and in establishing organizational accountability. **Donors** (in the case of nonprofit health care organizations) are also not involved in the day-to-day operation but nonetheless can have substantial influence on the mission and activities of the organization. Yet, board members and donors may be active not only because of their business expertise or knowledge of the organization's services but also because they are community opinion leaders or representatives of community interests. Communicating with board members and donors can be challenging as a consequence of these dual roles.

In the past, experts have provided simple rules for making communication with the board and donors go more smoothly (Letts, Ryan, and Grossman, 1999). First, organizational leadership must make clear to stakeholders that nonprofit performance cannot be reduced to financial profits. Particularly in the nonprofit sector, the organization's overall performance depends on a balanced scorecard of outcome measures, and that must be communicated effectively to external stakeholders. Second, external stakeholders do not always have strong incentives to contribute to the organization's performance, and hence, people in leadership positions must strive to motivate external stakeholders to contribute positively to performance. Last, in effective organizations, leadership recognizes external stakeholders as champions of the organization within the community.

Managing Partnerships

For many years in U.S. health care, it has been expected that people in leadership positions would think strategically about how their organizations could compete with others. Increasingly, to manage change in health care is to analyze the potential for health care organizations to coordinate, partner, or merge in an effort to lower costs, enhance market share, or improve quality and reach care. Against this backdrop, people in leadership positions must identify not only key competitors who pose a threat to the core business but also potential allies and partners—including government agencies, community groups, and other provider or payer organizations—who may provide a comparative advantage in the marketplace.

Notable alliances in health care have occurred between insurers and providers (e.g., Kaiser Permanente, traditional HMOs) and among groups of providers (e.g., physician groups). Increasingly, alliances are taking new forms based on the need to create accountable care organizations (ACOs), patient-centered medical homes, and other types of integrated delivery systems. Such organizational forms link a range of provider and payer types, including not only primary and specialty care but also long-term care and community-based care.

Relationships between health care providers and community-based social service organizations are also becoming more popular in response to increasing focus on population health. Through these kinds of relationships, the scope of traditional health care providers can be enlarged to attend to not only medical but also social determinants of health through coordinated services to address housing, legal, nutrition, or other needs. As payment systems, such as ACOs and accountable health communities (Centers for Medicare & Medicaid Services, 2016), expand incentives to improve the population's health outcomes, health care providers and payers may direct attention toward the social determinants of health and, hence, social service providers. The literature on the degree to which social service investments can offset health care costs and improve outcomes is still developing (Bradley and Taylor, 2013; Taylor et al., 2015); however, partnerships between health care and social service providers are likely to expand in complexity and prevalence in the decades ahead.

CHALLENGES FOR LEADERSHIP IN HEALTH CARE

Focusing both internally and externally is critical for effective leadership in the context of the contemporary challenges in health care. The American College of Healthcare Executives' 2017 survey of top issues confronting hospital CEOs indicates that CEOs view their top three challenges as relating to financing, governmental mandates, and personnel shortages in that order. See Table 2.3 for their top 10 challenges. From 2015 to 2017, the top challenges have largely remained the same, with financial challenges unequivocally cited as the top challenge year after year since at least 2006. The rankings indicate that, although patient safety and quality as well as patient satisfaction are top priorities, health care leadership is conscious that they must lead their organizations to deliver quality care within the context of changing payment systems, government mandates, and personnel shortages. The rankings for 2017 also indicate noticeable shifts in concern from prior years. Personnel shortages have leaped forward as a concern (from eighth to ninth place in prior years to third place in 2017). In contrast, leaders no longer report health care reform implementation and care for the uninsured/underinsured among their top 10 concerns. These concerns have been replaced by related issues: reorganization and access to care.

Existing evidence suggests that hospital board members share CEOs' perceptions of the challenges facing people in hospital leadership roles. Survey results show that board members rate financial performance, quality of care, operations, and business strategy among the top priorities for hospital board oversight (Jha and Epstein, 2009). Thus, there appears to be some consensus about the challenges facing people in senior leadership roles in hospitals. More research is needed to understand whether the perceived leadership challenges are the same for those in other positions and those in other types of health care organizations such as medical groups, health insurance companies, long-term facilities, and biopharmaceutical firms.

Irrespective of individual perception, a seminal analysis of the U.S. health system conducted by the Institute of Medicine (IOM, 2001) indicates that all individuals in leadership roles are responsible for

Table 2.3. Top 10 Challenges Confronting Hospital Leadership (2013–2017)

Issue	2017	2016	2015	2014	2013
Financial challenges	1 (2.0)	1 (2.7)	1 (3.2)	1 (2.5)	1 (2.4)
Governmental mandates	2 (4.2)	2 (4.2)	3 (4.5)	2 (4.6)	3 (4.9)
Personnel shortages	3 (4.5)	4 (4.8)	4 (5.1)	8 (7.4)	9 (8.0)
Patient safety and quality	4 (4.9)	3 (4.6)	2 (4.2)	3 (4.7)	3 (4.9)
Patient satisfaction	5 (5.5)	5 (5.5)	5 (5.3)	5 (5.9)	5 (5.9)
Physician-hospital relations	6 (5.9)	7 (5.9)	6 (5.7)	5 (5.9)	6 (6.0)
Access to care	7 (5.9)	6 (5.8)	7 (6.2)		
Technology	8 (7.0)	9 (7.1)	9 (7.1)	7 (7.3)	8 (7.9)
Population health management	9 (7.3)	8 (6.6)	8 (6.3)	6 (6.8)	7 (7.6)
Reorganization (e.g., mergers, acquisitions, restructuring, partnerships)	10 (7.5)	10 (7.8)	10 (7.4)		
Health care reform implementation				2 (4.6)	2 (4.3)
Care for the uninsured/underinsured				4 (5.5)	4 (5.6)

SOURCE: American College of Healthcare Executives. Survey: Healthcare Finance, Safety and Quality Cited by CEOs as Top Issues Confronting Hospitals in 2015, 2016, and 2017. https://www.ache.org/pubs/research/ceoissues.cfm.

NOTE: The first number is the absolute rank and the second number is the average rank. Issues are listed by the average rank, with the lower numbers indicating the higher concerns. CEO were asked to rank 10 issues affecting their hospitals in order of importance and to identify specific areas of concern within each of those issues. The survey was limited to CEOs of community hospitals (nonfederal, short-term, and nonspecialty hospitals).

helping their organizations to achieve six aims for the health system. According to the IOM, leadership should develop, implement, and maintain systems, cultures, and relationships that improve the (1) safety, (2) timeliness, (3) efficiency, (4) cost-effectiveness, (5) equity, and (6) patient-centeredness of care. The IOM explained that these six aims need to be met for the health system to "cross the chasm" between current practice, which often results in patient harm and waste, and best practice, which would provide the best known care for patients. Subsequent work further summarizes that leadership must attend to the broader "triple aim" of "improving the experience of care, improving the health of populations, and reducing per capita costs of health care" (Berwick, Nolan, and Whittington, 2008).

AN APPROACH TO ADDRESS THE CHALLENGES: STRATEGIC PROBLEM SOLVING

In many instances, addressing the challenges confronting leadership—both those that relate to the internal functioning required to accomplish primary organizational tasks as well as those that involve external stakeholders—requires problem solving to make the shift from current state to desired state. One useful approach for leaders at multiple levels of organization is **strategic problem solving**. Strategic problem solving is a management approach that integrates the strategic function of leadership involving goal and objective setting with the subsequent organizational action required to achieve the set objectives. Strategic problem solving uses an eight-step approach, outlined in Figure 2.1. The steps, while sequenced in the description, are more realistically completed in an iterative fashion with feedback loops and

adjustments throughout the process. The approach can be applied to narrowly defined operational problems or expansive strategic challenges faced at the highest levels of the organization or community.

The eight steps in the strategic problem-solving model are designed to help an organization (or organizational unit) move from a current state to a desired future state, where strategy is viewed as the road map for the trip between where the organization presently is and where the organization would like to be. The eight steps are the following: define the problem, set the overall objective, conduct a root cause analysis, generate alternative strategies that could be used to address the problem given the root causes identified, perform a comparative analysis of the alternative strategies, select the strategy, develop an implementation plan and implement, and develop an evaluation plan and evaluate.

Step 1: Define the Problem.

The first step to strategic problem solving is to define the problem in a way that allows the identification of solutions. Writing down the problem in a clear "problem statement" is one way to clearly define what one is trying to fix. Critical to this is conducting a valid landscape analysis by examining as much of the current environment, resources available, demands from stakeholders including staff, and current performance in meeting those demands. Consistent with the principles of achievability and realism, it is helpful to define a single problem. While people in leadership roles face complex circumstances with multiple facets, strategic problem solving identifies an important but single problem in order to focus attention. Ideally, many strategic problem-solving efforts are ongoing throughout organizations; however, in each, the problem is clearly articulated and can be realistically addressed with the potential resources available. The best problem statements are short, widely shared by key constituents, and do not include a solution to the problem. Table 2.4 shows weak problem statements and how they may be strengthened to foster more effective strategic problem solving.

Step 2: Set the Overall Objective.

Once the problem is clearly defined, the problem statement can be translated into an overall objective. Goal setting is a critical function of leadership, conducted most effectively in ways that engage affected groups within the organization as well as key external stakeholders. The terms goals and objectives have different, although related, uses. **Goals** refer to the larger aspirations of the organization, whereas **objectives** refer to the subordinate goals that must be accomplished to meet the larger aspirations. Research suggests that goal achievement is most likely when the goals are broadly shared in the organization, perceived to be challenging but feasible, include a time element, and are aligned with reward

1. Define the problem,

2. Set the overall objective,

3. Conduct a root cause analysis,

4. Generate alternative strategies to interventions,

5. Perform a comparative analysis of alternatives,

6. Select the best strategy and address its limitations,

7. Develop an implementation plan and implement, and

8. Develop an evaluation plan and evaluate

Figure 2.1 The Eight-Step Strategic Problem-Solving Process.

Table 2.4 Writing Problem Statements

Weak Problem Statements	Suggestions for Improvement	Strong Problem Statements
"We need more regular delivery of supplies."	Focus on a problem, rather than the solution. In this case, why is more regular delivery important?	"Stock-outs of essential supplies are common in our organization."
"Due to understaffing, nurses are overworked."	Focus on a single problem, rather than the cause of the problem.	"Nurses are overworked."
"Our budgets are too small; we have a rundown building, and our medical director is leaving the organization soon, along with several key nurses and paraprofessionals."	Focus on a single problem; keep the problem statement short.	"There is not sufficient revenue to cover costs."

systems (Bogardus, Bradley, and Tinetti, 1998; Locke and Latham, 1990; March and Simon, 1958).

The approach to organizational leadership termed "Management by Objectives" (MBO) (Drucker, 1954) is the most commonly discussed method of using goals and objectives to align organizational action toward achieving organizational goals. The MBO school of thought argued that objectives should be designed to be what is termed **SMART** (Doran, 1981). The acronym stands for specific, measurable, assignable, realistic, and time bounded. Specific means that the objective is concrete and well defined with adequate detail. Measurable means that there are metrics that can be assessed that will determine if the objective has been met. Assignable means the person or team that will be responsible for achieving the objective can be identified. Realistic mean that the objective has been defined in a way that can be accomplished if prioritized with the resources available and time given. Time bound means that target times are specified for when the objective will be achieved. Theoretically, managing by SMART objectives makes explicit

the process of goal setting and facilitates shared expectations about what is to be accomplished, how, and by when. Such a process can enhance motivation and, with clear metrics, organizational units can be held accountable for progress toward the shared objectives and goals.

Effective objectives address the problem defined in the problem statement and are SMART objectives as shown in Figure 2.2. For instance, an organization with a poor inventory control system might define the problem statement as "Supply stock-outs are common." An overall SMART objective that addresses that problem might be "Reduce supply stock-out events by 25 percent by the end of the quarter."

Step 3: Conduct a Root Cause Analysis.

In order to design strategies, a root cause analysis can help identify the causal factors associated with the problem. With clarity about the problem causes, a more effective set of alternative strategies to address the problem can be designed. Finding the root cause requires careful analysis. Several management tools can help people in leadership

Specific—What exactly are we going to do, with or for whom? The program states a precise outcome to be accomplished. This outcome is often stated in numbers, percentages, or frequencies.

Measurable—Is the target of the objective measureable? How will it be measured, including the metrics to be tracked and the methods for data collection and analysis?

Achievable—Can the objective be accomplished in the proposed time frame given the economic and political environment?

Realistic—Will this objective realistically bring the organization closer to accomplishing our goal or overall objective?

Time bound—Is a time frame for achieving the objective provided?

Figure 2.2 Is Your Objective Statement SMART?

roles find the root causes of the problem, including but not limited to Ishikawa (fishbone) diagramming, flow charting, Pareto charts, histograms, scatter plots, and regression analyses. Analyzing data and patterns of action is key.

Step 4: Generate List of Possible Strategies.

Based on the results of the root cause analysis, a list of possible strategies to address the root causes and hence reduce the problem and fulfill the objective can be designed. The list should be tractable in number, and each strategy can include multiple interventions, although as a full strategy, each should be mutually exclusive with the other strategies listed. For instance, one strategy might include doing A and not B. An alternative might be to do B and not A, and a third alternative might be to do both A and B. In addition, each strategy should be reasonable for addressing the problem; hence potential strategies that are known to be unrealistic or ineffective should not be considered in the alternative strategy list. Because it cannot address the problem, typically, the strategy to do nothing is not included in such an exercise. An effective set of alternative strategies then are clearly described, comprehensive but not overwhelming in number (try to identify three to four strategies), feasible to implement, and mutually exclusive so they can be compared as alternatives.

Step 5: Perform Comparative Analysis of Alternative Strategies.

Once several alternative strategies have been generated, it is important to perform a side-by-side comparison of the options using evaluative criteria to rate and choose among the strategies. Evaluative criteria are characteristics that are important to the organization and by which the potential merit of each alternative can be judged. Illustrative evaluative criteria are the degree to which the strategy under consideration is (1) effective to addressing the problem, (2) cost-effective, (3) consistent with the organization's overall strategy, (4) timely in effect, or (5) politically feasible. Alternative strategies can then be rated either with quantitative measures (using a single scoring system or natural units) or with qualitative scales using a matrix as shown in Tables 2.5 and 2.6. If the matrix is quantitative, scores can be summed or weighted and summed to identify the most desired strategy. If the matrix is qualitative, ratings can be integrated to discuss the merits and disadvantages overall of each alternative strategy. Sensitivity analysis, taking into account the riskiness of alternative outcomes from a single strategy, can be conducted as desired to understand the impact of alternative scoring or weighted on the choice of alternatives to pursue. This type of analysis is shown in Table 2.7. Such matrices are merely guides to frame collective discussions and arguments; they cannot provide a definitive answer that will always be a right answer, as strategy has substantial flexibility and judgment involved. However, the approach is useful for organizing much information and communicating about the decision-making criteria and process.

To get the weighted value, multiply the raw score by the percentage (as a decimal). Then add the weighted values across the row to get the total weighted score.

Example: Increasing staff has a raw score of 5 in "impact on productivity," and the criterion, impact on productivity,

Table 2.5 Qualitative Rating Matrix for Comparative Analysis

Options	Evaluative Criteria			
	Impact on Productivity	Annual Expense	Political Feasibility	Time Required
1: Increase Staff	Very Good	High	Low	3 Months
2: Increase Pay	Unclear	High	Very Low	1 Year
3: Improve Supervision	Fairly Good	Low	High	1 Month

Table 2.6 Quantitative Rating Matrix for Comparative Analysis

Options	Evaluative Criteria				
	Impact on Productivity	Annual Expense	Political Feasibility	Time to Effect	Total Score
1: Increase Staff	5	1	2	4	12
2: Increase Pay	3	1	1	1	6
3: Improve Supervision	3	4	4	4	15

Table 2.7 Quantitative Rating Matrix with Weighting for Comparative Analysis

Implementation Options		Evaluative Criteria				
	Impact on Productivity	Annual Expense	Political Feasibility	Time to Effect	Total	
Weighting:	50%	20%	15%	15%	100%	
1: Increase Staff	5 (2.5)	1 (.2)	2 (.3)	4 (.6)	12 (3.6 weighted)	
2: Increase Pay	3 (1.5)	1 (.2)	1 (.15)	1 (.15)	6 (2 weighted)	
3: Improve Supervision	3 (1.5)	4 (.8)	4 (.6)	3 (.45)	14 (3.35 weighted)	

is weighted by 50 percent. The weighted value is therefore the raw score (5) multiplied by the weighting percent as a decimal ($5 \times 0.50 = 2.5$; the weighted value is 2.5). Summing the weighted values across the row provides the total weighted score for the strategy listing in that row (i.e., the total weighted score for the strategy "increasing staff" is 3.6). Based on the raw score (without weighting), the strategy "improve supervision" has the highest total score; based on the total weighted score, the strategy "increase staff" has the highest score.

Step 6: Select the Best Intervention and Explain Your Decision.

Based on the results of the comparative analysis, select the best intervention. As part of this, it is critical to describe the potential limitations to the selected alternative and, ideally, address these limitations, recognizing that managerial problem solving involves trade-offs and nearly all management decisions have limitations. The strongest approach to problem solving identifies and refutes the limitations of the managerial choices. The ability to foster support for a strategic direction, despite its recognized drawbacks, is an important skill for leadership.

Step 7: Develop Implementation Plan and Implement.

Implementation plans identify the steps to take in order to put the selected strategy into action. A strong implementation plan specifies major tasks to be completed, timelines for each task, and the people or groups accountable to complete each task. Implementation plans often include a work plan organizing the various tasks, timelines, and resources involved in the implementation. To be complete, implementation plans might include early tasks related to fostering key stakeholder support for subsequent strategies and tasks. An example work plan, also known as a Gantt chart, is included in Figure 2.3. An implementation plan is critical to strategic problem solving as it provides a clear timeline for

the overall project, a sequencing of steps to complete a larger strategy, a method of assigning responsibility to individuals and groups for accomplishing tasks, and a vehicle for communicating expectations and monitoring progress toward meeting objectives.

Step 8: Develop Evaluation Plan and Evaluate.

Although evaluation is listed as the last step of strategic problem solving, the conceptualization of the evaluation should begin at the start of the problem-solving process. Often, evaluation includes both monitoring of progress as well as final evaluation of the degree to which the objective was met. A strong monitoring and evaluation plan creates a transparent process for understanding how a project's progress and outcomes will be assessed and can motivate staff to work toward a common target.

Central to evaluation is the selection of performance indicators. Indicators, sometimes termed metrics, are the items measured to determine performance (e.g., profit, mortality rates, adherence to medications). Many evaluation plans also include targets, or the level one wants to reach in the indicator. For instance, the indicator might be "reduce mortality rates after acute myocardial infarction," and the target might be "reduce mortality rates after acute myocardial infarction by 1 percent in the next year."

Indicators may be process or outcome indicators. Process indicators measure whether specific activities needed to achieve the objective have been accomplished (e.g., number of staff trained, whether or not a workshop was held, amount of new equipment purchased). Outcome indicators, in contrast, measure whether or not the overall objective was achieved. To make sure that your indicators are meaningful and realistic, be sure to consider who will use the data, how it will be collected and verified, how it will be analyzed, and how it will be reported. As a cautionary note, data collection, analysis, and reporting can be expensive and overwhelming for organizations. It is important, therefore, to select a modest number of indicators that

PLAN FOR IMPROVED MANAGEMENT AND LEADERSHIP CAPACITY AT HOSPITAL LEVEL

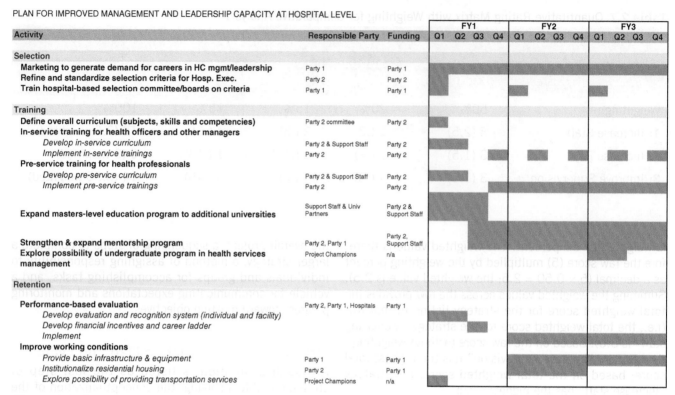

Figure 2.3 Example of a Gantt Chart.

are viewed as most meaningful. Tracking a few indicators consistently and accurately is more useful than tracking many indicators that are measured or analyzed imperfectly.

RELATIONSHIP OF LEADERSHIP TO ORGANIZATIONAL PERFORMANCE

Because leadership is a process that touches various aspects of organizations, many have been interested in the link between leadership and organizational performance in health care. Empirical researchers in health services and general management have pursued this subject with fervor. Most of the resulting articles in PubMed, the electronic bibliographic database of health care–related articles, have focused on reviewing theories of leadership in relation to performance, providing anecdotes of successful individual leaders, or conjecturing on how performance results may be explained by leadership behaviors, without testing their hypotheses. A relatively small number of the articles have reported on data-driven, original research studies. These studies suggest that leadership can contribute substantially to organizational performance.

Organizational performance in health care is classified into three major categories: (1) patient-related, (2) staff-related, and (3) management-related (Schofield and Amodeo, 1999). Patient-related outcomes are those that indicate quality of patient care, such as prevalence of adverse events, patient mortality, and patient satisfaction. Staff-related outcomes are those that indicate staff satisfaction with the organization, such as reported job satisfaction, retention rates, and staff commitment to the organization. Last, management-related outcomes are the remaining indicators of organizational performance for which management is responsible, such as productivity, effectiveness (i.e., goal achievement), and financial performance. Researchers have found links between leadership and performance outcomes in each of the three categories. They have also found that leadership effectiveness is associated with a core set of leadership competencies. We review key findings from these streams of work in this section, drawing from a set of extensive and systematic reviews (Altieri and Elgin, 1994; Cummings et al., 2008, 2010; Gilmartin and D'Aunno, 2007; McCloskey and Molen, 1987; Wong, Cummings, and Ducharme, 2013).

Leadership and Patient-Related Outcomes.

A growing body of research documents a significant relationship between leadership and a variety of patient-related outcomes. A systematic review of research on nursing leadership, surveying literature from 1985 to 2012, found that leadership was correlated with patient satisfaction, patient mortality, adverse events (e.g., medication errors, hospital-acquired infections), complications for patients, and patient health care utilization (e.g., length of stay) (Wong, Cummings, and Ducharme, 2013). Of the 43 relationships between leadership and patient outcomes examined, 26 (60 percent) were found to be significant and positive, one was found to be significant and negative, and the remainder were not significant. The evidence of relationship was strongest for patient mortality and satisfaction. Overall, the research, including subsequent studies (McKinney et al., 2016), indicates that patient outcomes are more favorable when individuals in leadership roles employ relational leadership styles. The use of these styles has also been correlated with the achievement of clinical goals for patients (e.g., appropriate hemoglobin A1c levels for diabetic patients and prenatal care [Xirasagar, Samuels, and Stoskopf, 2005]).

Additionally, the literature indicates that task-oriented leadership contributes positively to patient satisfaction and clinical quality of care. McCutcheon et al. (2009) found that hospital nurse managers' use of a transactional leadership style was positively associated with patient satisfaction, particularly for leadership with larger spans of control. Likewise, Havig et al. (2011) found that task-oriented leadership by nursing home managers was positively associated with family satisfaction with residents' care. Data collected from surveys of nationally representative groups of hospitals in the United States and England have also documented a positive link between hospital leaderships' use of management practices focused on tasks such as operations, monitoring, human resources management, and quality of care delivered to patients with respect to 19 evidence-based practices across three clinical conditions (acute myocardial infarction, congestive heart failure, and pneumonia) (Tsai et al., 2015).

Together, the findings related to relational and task-oriented leadership suggest that both types of leadership can contribute to processes that enhance patient satisfaction and result in high-quality clinical care. It may be necessary to have both for effectiveness: task-oriented leadership to clarify standards and roles in a way that facilitates good care and relational leadership to foster intergroup collaboration (Wong, Cummings, and Ducharme, 2013) and effective knowledge management (Gowen, Henagan, and McFadden, 2009).

Leadership and Staff-Related Outcomes.

One of the most robust findings in health care leadership research is a significant link between leadership style and staff-related outcomes. Studies of nurses,

physicians, and other health professionals have consistently shown that the use of relational leadership styles (transformational, LMX, empowering, supportive, etc.) is positively associated with staff job satisfaction, satisfaction with the leadership, reduced burnout, staff motivation to perform, improved work environment, retention, staff commitment to the organization, engagement, and reduction in staff absences (Bobbio, Bellan, and Manganelli, 2012; Brady Germain and Cummings, 2010; Chullen et al., 2010; Cowden, Cummings, and Profetto-McGrath, 2011; Cummings et al., 2010; Lavoie-Tremblay et al., 2016; Lewis and Cunningham, 2016; Nembhard and Edmondson, 2006; Schreuder et al., 2011; Shanafelt et al., 2015; Wong, Cummings, and Ducharme, 2013). Even emotionally exhausted staff members reported job satisfaction if their managers used emotionally intelligent leadership (Cummings, Hayduk, and Estabrooks, 2005). Conversely, task-oriented leadership styles were negatively associated with staff-related outcomes, according to this body of work.

The data suggest that the positive effect of relational leadership styles stems from their effect on intermediate staff outcomes such as workgroup cohesion, reduced stress, empowerment over decisions, and self-efficacy—all of which have been associated with increased job satisfaction and retention (Gilmartin and D'Aunno, 2007). Furthermore, when staff work with managers who used relational leadership styles, staff health, anxiety, and well-being were improved (Cummings et al., 2010). Research suggests that the effects of leadership on staff experience are part of the reason why leadership is correlated with patient-related outcomes. In addition to the aforementioned staff-related consequences, relational leadership has been shown to influence staff development of expertise, communication, and collaboration, which were, in turn, associated with patient-related outcomes (Hu et al., 2016; Wong, Cummings, and Ducharme, 2013).

Leadership and Management-Related Outcomes.

Relational leadership has also been associated with several management-related outcomes, including productivity, effectiveness, and staff effort to meet organizational goals involving innovation and change. A systematic review of 18 studies of nursing leadership found individual, team, and workgroup effectiveness and productivity were higher in association with relational leadership styles in 13 of the studies (Cummings et al., 2010). Six of the eighteen studies also found significantly reduced effectiveness and productivity associated with task-oriented styles. Relational leadership has been positively associated with interdisciplinary teamwork, role clarity, innovation, and the use of evidence-based practices (Aarons and Sommerfeld, 2012; Cummings et al., 2010)—all of which contribute to management-related outcomes. Additionally, this leadership approach has been associated with the development of organizational climates supportive of organizational goals. For example, studies have shown that transformational leadership is associated with safety climate, which is associated with process quality (McFadden, Stock, and Gowen, 2015). Researchers have also reported that leadership that is able to shift from a focus on inclusive decision making to task achievement over time is able to increase the perceived value of organizational goals such as participation in multistakeholder alliances, which bring together diverse organizations to work on health-related issues, an increasingly common goal (D'Aunno, Alexander, and Jiang, 2015).

Limited work exists to examine the relationship between leadership and financial performance that does not focus on the governing board. Such studies are often self-reported case studies that describe positive effects of proactive leadership on financial performance (Goetz, Janney, Ramsey, 2011; Zwingman-Bagley, 1999). Work on boards, however, has indicated that board involvement and composition can have mixed effects. Some work, for example, has found that board involvement in strategic planning, a leadership activity, was associated with higher net income (Kaissi and Begun, 2008), as was having a board with a culture of inclusivity and a strong relationship between board and the CEO (Kane, Clark, and Rivenson, 2009). Other work has found that involving the CEO has no effect, while involving more managers in governing boards was associated with lower total margin and return on assets, potentially because greater manager involvement interferes with the board's ability to monitor management behavior effectively (Kuntz, Pulm, and Wittland, 2016).

The management outcome that has received substantial attention is successful organizational change. Researchers have found that transformational leadership is correlated with more innovative work climate (Aarons and Sommerfeld, 2012), and staff less likely to view implementation as a burden (Brimhal et al., 2015), contributing to HCOs' success implementing change. Such leadership, however, may be insufficient for success in some cases. One study showed that managers who received high scores for transformational leadership, received low scores from peers and subordinates for effectiveness in leading organizational change (Kan and Parry, 2004). This finding has led scholars to conclude that additional factors—beyond transformational leadership—are required for successful change in health care (Gilmartin and D'Aunno, 2007).

Much work theorizes and shows that leadership support for change efforts greatly impacts the success of such efforts (Bradley et al., 2003, 2006; Greenhalgh et al., 2004; Lukas et al., 2007; Nembhard, Morrow, and Bradley, 2015). Additionally, this work has identified two types of support that those in leadership roles must provide for successful change: **instrumental support** and **interpersonal support** (Yukl, 2006). Instrumental support refers to various forms of tangible assistance such as providing resources, removing organizational barriers such as existing institutional policies, developing structures to facilitate change efforts, and information sharing. Interpersonal support refers to intangible actions that often contribute to individuals' feeling valued and appreciated, such as providing encouragement, offering feedback, and being inclusive. **Inclusive leadership** invites and appreciates others' words and deeds, collaborates with others across the professional hierarchy, shares power with others, frames tasks as a team effort, and facilitates a positive work climate for all staff members, regardless of profession and position (Nembhard and Edmondson, 2006). In theory, the combination of instrumental and interpersonal support fosters intrinsic motivation within staff, which increases staff commitment and effort in support of change. In turn, staff commitment and effort—in conjunction with a compelling vision and staff accountability—contribute to successful organizational change.

Studies have shown that the support of administrative leadership and clinical leadership is needed for successful organizational change (Bradley et al., 2001; Greenhalgh et al., 2004). **Administrative leadership** support refers to the instrumental and interpersonal support provided by those who hold senior positions in the organization, such as chief executive officer, chief operating officer, and vice president for performance improvement. **Clinical leadership** support refers to instrumental and interpersonal support provided by those who hold clinical positions, such as physicians and nurses. Research on organizational change efforts has consistently shown that the support of physicians, and in particular a respected physician champion (of change), is critical to the success of change efforts (Greenhalgh et al., 2004).

Leadership and Competencies.

The complexity and difficulty of leading health care organizations in a changing world has spurred interest in identifying the **competencies**—defined as knowledge, skills, and abilities—needed for effective leadership. Consortia of major professional organizations such as the Healthcare Leadership Alliance (HLA), leadership development organizations such as National Center for Healthcare Leadership (NHCL), accrediting organizations such as the Commission on the Accreditation of Healthcare Management Education (CAHME), and other researchers have conducted studies to identify core competencies for those in leadership positions in HCOs. These studies

(American College of Healthcare Executives [ACHE], 2014; Bradley et al., 2008; Calhoun et al., 2008; CAHME, 2017; Stefl, 2008) consistently point to four competency areas for effective leadership: (1) knowledge of the health care industry, (2) technical skills, (3) analytic/conceptual skills, and (4) interpersonal/communication skills. Studies on the effectiveness of educational programs designed to increase competencies for leadership, which generally evaluate programs based on participants' self-ratings of learning, ability, or behavior, provide support for the notion that such programs enhance leadership capability for students in health care management degree programs (Bradley et al., 2008), physicians (Frich et al., 2015), nurses (Cummings et al., 2008), and other health professionals (Baer et al., 2015; Pecukonis et al., 2013).

Summary of the Literature on Leadership and Performance.

Existing research offers a number of insights. It shows that relational leadership styles have been positively correlated with patient-, staff-, and management-related performance outcomes, and task-oriented styles have been associated with improved patient outcomes as well. The extent to which causal inferences can be made based on existing research is limited due to study design issues—e.g., sample selection, variable measurement, and data analytic choices. Nevertheless, the descriptive and statistical findings support the notion that leadership plays a critical role in influencing performance of health care organizations (Wells and Hejna, 2009).

SUSTAINING LEADERSHIP

Organizations are successful in achieving their goals because even when individuals come and go, organizational structure provides a way for activities to continue through personnel changes. Well-designed organizational structures are important in the health care sector, in which approximately 18 percent of hospital CEOs have left their positions each year since 2014, and where rates of turnover have been persistently high across years and across states (ACHE, 2017). Costs of leadership turnover can be reduced by clearly defining the needed competencies for succession planning for leadership positions, which requires leadership to lay out explicitly the strategic and cultural plans for the organization.

Succession planning is not only limited to planning for who moves into leadership roles but also includes review and codification where possible of organizational cultural elements, work practices, and job design. These additional activities prepare the organization for the cyclical nature of succession planning, which involves (1) first, that individuals with the potential for greater responsibility are identified; (2) next, these individuals are prepared to take on those greater responsibilities through mentoring and training; and (3) finally, after they are moved to higher-level positions, new individuals with potential must be identified and the cycle starts again (Garman and Tyler, 2004).

A key element of preparing new people for leadership positions includes giving them the opportunity to take on critical assignments that provide the opportunity to develop leadership skills. This must include providing such individuals with decision-making roles. McCall, Lombardo, and Morrison (1988) asked CEOs to identify developmental experiences critical to their own success and from their experiences identified five critical abilities necessary in early leadership experiences: (1) the ability to set and implement agendas, (2) to handle complex relationships, (3) to promote basic organizational values, (4) to manage the personal demands of top management positions, and (5) to maintain a critical self-awareness, especially in terms of performance. Succession planning should include ways to provide individuals with opportunities to develop these abilities.

Given the substantial personal stress that accompanies leadership roles and the negative organizational impact of poorly managed stress among those in leadership roles (Heifetz and Linsky, 2002), caring for oneself is fundamental to sustaining leadership. Key approaches to managing oneself involve the recognition, analysis, and processing of stressful situations regardless of what changes in the situation. Recognition begins with developing a perspective on the larger picture of what might be occurring in one's environment while still engaging in daily core tasks. Holding both perspectives, that of the larger picture and that of the more immediate situation, has been suggested as fundamental to sustained leadership (Bradley, 2006; Heifetz, 1994; Johnson, 1992). Additionally, successfully managing stress requires distinguishing one's role from oneself. The approach of viewing the failures, conflicts, and setbacks as attributed to the role rather than one's personal actions can help address undue stress of leadership.

Analysis of the situation can also be helpful in addressing personal stress and allowing for sustained leadership despite challenges. Analysis might include focused efforts to understand the origins of conflict and to avoid internalizing conflicts as one's own problem when such conflicts may be among or between others (Heifetz, 1994). Such analysis is only possible with adequate listening to the evidence around oneself. Therefore, the ability to listen, hear, and absorb potentially difficult or ambiguous information as part of analyzing sources and solutions to stress is a critical skill for people in leadership roles to practice in order to sustain their personal balance.

Finally, leadership roles in health care remain highly stressful as the health care environment remains highly turbulent. The president of the ACHE, Deborah Bowen, articulated this in her 2013 statement: "Elevated turnover among hospital CEOs seems to be a feature of the current health care environment . . . The continuing trend of consolidation among organizations, the increasing demands on chief executives to lead in a complex and rapidly changing environment, and retirement of leaders from the baby boomer era may all be contributing to this continuing higher level of change in the senior leadership of hospitals" (ACHE, 2015). Health system leadership can benefit from a proactive approach in supporting leadership succession with structured coaching and mentoring directed at preserving oneself and one's sense of purpose (ACHE, 2015).

SUMMARY AND MANAGERIAL GUIDELINES

1. Leadership and management are complementary, but distinct fields of study. Leadership can be defined as the process in which one engages others to set and achieve a common goal, often an organizationally defined goal. In contrast, management can be defined as the process of accomplishing predetermined objectives through the effective use of human, financial, natural, and technical resources.

2. Management and leadership are neither exhaustive not mutually inclusive. A person may occupy a management role but not a leadership role, a leadership role but not a management role, or both roles at the same time.

3. The effectiveness of specific leadership behaviors and actions depends on the context in which one is leading. Behaviors that may be very effective in one situation can be ineffective in another, adding a premium to being able to not only understand the context but also adapt one's behaviors and actions to it.

4. Leadership is born of the relationship between the person(s) in the leadership role and the person(s) in the followership role. The effectiveness of people in leadership roles may be measured by the extent to which they are able to leverage the capacities of those in followership roles.

5. Transformational leadership can create changes in organizational culture, but it is important to consider the reasons why a given organization gave rise to the culture. Organizational culture survives because in one way or another, it solves problems for the organization.

6. Research suggests a host of leadership approaches that have been linked to improved organizational performance across a range of health care organizations and services.

7. Strategic problem solving is a useful approach by which those in leadership and management positions may integrate the strategic functions of their roles with the subsequent organizational action required to achieve the set objectives.

8. Succession planning is a crucial part of leadership, particularly in the turbulent health care environment.

DISCUSSION QUESTIONS

1. Where do leadership and management overlap in definition and responsibilities? Where do they diverge?

2. How have theories of leadership evolved over the course of the twentieth century and into the twenty-first century? When compared with the trait theories of the early 1900s, have modern theories of leadership been simplified, or grown more complex?

3. What is the relationship between emotional intelligence and leadership?

4. How do transformational and transactional leadership differ? Give an example of each type of leadership and when it might be preferable to the other.

5. What is organizational culture?

6. What are artifacts, and how might they play a role in organizational change?

7. What is a "SMART" objective? Give an example that lays out how the objective meets each of the "SMART" requirements.

8. How might one compare a series of alternative strategies? What are the concerns in using a purely quantitative scale of evaluation?

9. What are the responsibilities of a person who is effective in the followership role? How does leadership foster effective followership?

10. What kind of actions might an organization take in order to ensure sustained leadership?

CASE

The New Department Director

As a new director of ambulatory care at the Kennedy Medical Center, Dr. Grant started to review issues in the hospital; it was clear that something was wrong. Every day, a large crowd of patients and families waited for hours in the emergency department. Although the outpatient ambulatory practices seemed to be running smoothly, the emergency department, which was within Dr. Grant's responsibility, seemed to be a mess. The hospital was typically going "on divert," meaning they would divert ambulances from the emergency room, sending them to another hospital in the city because Kennedy Medical Center did not have the beds and staff to accept more patients. Dr. Grant was embarrassed by the situation and was surprised that no one higher up in the administration had noted this as a concern. When he asked about it, his boss, the chief operating officer of the hospital, said it had been this way for a while.

Dr. Grant approached Ms. Downs, the nurse manager of the emergency department and a nurse with 25 years of experience at the hospital, about the issue. She also reported that the situation was no worse than usual and, while it was not ideal, Kennedy Medical Center did better than other hospitals in the area. Still, the situation bothered Dr. Grant, and he made a promise to himself that he would fix it, setting a goal of having 90 percent of the emergency department outpatients in and out of the emergency department in four hours and having the emergency department be on divert no more than once per month. He was not sure what the current percentage meeting this goal was, but given his previous experience at other hospitals, he aimed to accomplish these objectives in six months.

With his problem identified and clear objectives set, Dr. Grant set out to implement a new strategy, which involved (1) teaching the staff about root cause analysis, (2) reengineering the triage work flow to speed access to a clinician, and (3) making what he viewed as a minor fix to the current electronic registration system to improve team communication. This approach had worked well in his former hospital, reducing wait times by more than 30 percent within six months.

After much planning, Dr. Grant held a staff meeting of the nurse manager and the three emergency department supervisors who reported to her to discuss the new strategy. He described the new processes, which were supposed to smooth out redundancies and save time. The staff seemed to like the reengineering process ideas best, so Dr. Grant decided to start with those. He suggested that they could begin the new workflow in two weeks, after staff education and training. The staff meeting was friendly, and no one said much. Ms. Downs had to leave slightly early to pick up her son from school, but the supervisors said that training should be no problem and that two weeks gave them plenty of time. They agreed as a group to start two weeks from Monday.

On the "go live" Monday, Dr. Grant had a morning of meetings outside the hospital but was comforted that Ms. Downs was there and in charge. Unfortunately, two clerks had days off requested months earlier, and the charge nurse for the day had a family emergency over the weekend and was late to work. The staff members remaining were thankfully the most efficient.

When Dr. Grant returned to the hospital after his outside meeting, Ms. Downs was waiting in his office and upset. She said that the new workflow process had fallen apart and that the crowds were worse than ever. She raised her voice and then turned quickly away to go back to her work area, saying, "You have not fixed anything. You have made it worse here. Look at the mess we have today. And it will be just as bad tomorrow. We need to go back to the way it used to be."

Dr. Grant was surprised at how angry Ms. Downs seemed to be. He looked in at the emergency department triage area, and it did look very crowded. The efficient registration clerks were there working, but they could not keep up with the crowds. The beds in the emergency department were already full, and the medical director was suggesting it was time to divert ambulances already even though it was only Monday at noon. Dr. Grant went back to his office and wondered what he should do.

Questions

1. What problem(s) does Dr. Grant face?
2. Consider individual-level, team-level, and system-level problems. For each, set an objective that is SMART.
3. Could Dr. Grant have avoided the current situation? How?
4. Use concepts of leadership and management from this chapter to recommend what Dr. Grant should do going forward.

REFERENCES

Aarons, G. A., & Sommerfeld, D. H. (2012). Leadership, innovation climate, and attitudes toward evidence-based practice during a statewide implementation. *Journal of the American Academy of Child and Adolescent Psychiatry, 51*(4), 423–431.

Altieri, L. B., & Elgin, P. A. (1994). A decade of nursing leadership research. *Holistic Nursing Practice, 9*(1), 75–82.

American College of Healthcare Executives (ACHE). (2014). Professional Development Task Force 2014–2015 Annual Report. Retrieved September 27, 2018, from http://www. ache.org/professionaldevelopmenttaskforce/FINAL-REPORT-RECOMMENDATIONS.pdf.

American College of Healthcare Executives (ACHE). (2015). Hospital CEO turnover rate remains elevated. Retrieved September 27, 2018, from http://www.ache.org/pubs/Releases/2015/hospital-ceo-turnover-rate15.cfm.

American College of Healthcare Executives (ACHE). (2017). Hospital CEO turnover rate remains steady. Retrieved September 27, 2018, from http://www.ache.org/pubs/research/ceoturnover_2017.cfm.

Baer, M. T., Harris, A. B., Stanton, R. W., et al. (2015). The future of MCH Nutrition Services: A commentary on the importance of supporting leadership training to strengthen the nutrition workforce. *Maternal and Child Health Journal, 2*(19), 229–235.

Bailey, S. (2002). A hospital heals itself. *Boston Globe*. Boston. Reprinted in Paul Levy, Taking charge of the Beth Israel Deaconess Medical Center (B). Harvard Business School Case 9-303-080 by Professors David A. Garvin and Michael A. Roberto (December 10, 2002).

Bass, B. (1990). *Bass & Stogdill's handbook of leadership: Theory, research & managerial applications*. New York: Free Press.

Berg, D. (1998). Resurrecting the muse: Followership in organizations. In E. Klein, F. Gabelnick, & P. Herr (Eds.), *The psychodynamics of leadership.* Madison, CT: Psychosocial Press.

Berwick, D. M., Nolan T. W., & Whittington, J. (2008). The triple aim: Care, health, and cost. *Health Affairs, 27*(3), 759–769.

Birken, S. A., DiMartino, L. D., Kirk, M. A., et al. (2016). Elaborating on theory with middle managers' experience implementing healthcare innovations in practice. *Implementation Science, 11*(1), 2.

Birken, S. A., Lee, S. Y., & Weiner, B. J. (2012). Uncovering middle managers' role in healthcare innovation implementation. *Implementation Science, 7*, 28.

Birken, S. A., Lee, S.-Y. D., Weiner, B. J., et al. (2013). Improving the effectiveness of health care innovation implementation: Middle managers as change agents. *Medical Care Research and Review, 70*(1), 29–45.

Bobbio, A., Bellan, M., & Manganelli, A. M. (2012). Empowering leadership, perceived organizational support, trust, and job burnout for nurses: A study in an Italian general hospital. *Health Care Management Review, 37*(1), 77–87.

Bogardus, S. T., Bradley, E. H., & Tinetti, M. E. (1998). A taxonomy for goal setting in the care of persons with dementia. *Journal of General Internal Medicine, 13*(10), 675–680.

Bradley, E. H. (2006). Achieving rapid door-to-balloon times: How top hospitals improve complex clinical systems. *Circulation, 113*(8), 1079–1085.

Bradley, E. H., Cherlin, E. J., Busch, S. H., Epstein, A., Helfand, B., & White, W. D. (2008). Adopting a competency-based model: Mapping curricula and assessing student progress. *Journal of Health Administration Education, 25*, 37–51.

Bradley, E. H., Curry, L. A., Spatz, E. S., et al. (2012). Hospital strategies for reducing risk-standardized mortality rates in acute myocardial infarction. *Annals of Internal Medicine, 156*(9), 618–626.

Bradley, E. H., Holmboe, E. S., Mattera, J. A., et al. (2001). A qualitative study of increasing beta-blocker use after myocardial infarction: Why do some hospitals succeed? *Journal of American Medical Association, 285*(20), 2604–2611.

Bradley, E. H., Holmboe, E. S., Mattera, J. A., et al. (2003). The roles of senior management in quality improvement efforts: What are the key components? *Journal of Healthcare Management, 48*(1), 15–28.

Bradley, E. H., & Taylor, L. A. (2013). *The American health care paradox: Why spending more is getting us less.* New York: Public Affairs Press.

Bradley, E. H., Webster, T. R., Schlesinger, M., Baker, D. W., & Inouye, S. K. (2006). The roles of senior management in improving hospital experiences for frail older adults. *Journal of Healthcare Management, 51*, 323–337.

Brady Germain, P., & Cummings, G. G. (2010). The influence of nursing leadership on nurse performance: A systematic literature review. *Journal of Nursing Management, 18*(4), 425–439.

Brimhall, K. C., Fenwick, K., Farahnak, L. R., et al. (2015). Leadership, organizational climate, and perceived burden of evidence-based practice in mental health services. *Administration and Policy in Mental Health, 43*(5), 629–639.

Calhoun, J. G., Dollett, L., Sinioris, M. E., et al. (2008). Development of an interprofessional competency model for healthcare leadership. *Journal of Healthcare Management, 53*(6), 375–390.

Centers for Medicare & Medicaid Services. (2016). Accountable health communities model. Retrieved September 27, 2018, from https://innovation.cms.gov/initiatives/AHCM.

Chullen, C. L., Dunford, B. B., Angermeier, I., et al. (2010). Minimizing deviant behavior in healthcare organizations: The effects of supportive leadership and job design. *Journal of Healthcare Management, 55*(6), 381–397; discussion 397–398.

Commission on Accreditation of Healthcare Management Education (CAHME). (2017). Criteria Program Review Worksheet. Retrieved September 27, 2018, from https://cahme.org/healthcare-management-education-accreditation/resources/.

Cowden, T., Cummings, G., & Profetto-McGrath, J. (2011). Leadership practices and staff nurses' intent to stay: A systematic review. *Journal of Nursing Management, 19*(4), 461–477.

Cummings, G., Hayduk, L., & Estabrooks, C. (2005). Mitigating the impact of hospital restructuring on nurses: The responsibility of emotionally intelligent leadership. *Nursing Research, 54*(1), 2–12.

Cummings, G., MacGregor, T., Davey, M., et al. (2008). Factors contributing to nursing leadership: A systematic review. *Journal of Health Services Research & Policy, 13*(4), 240–248.

Cummings, G. G., MacGregor, T., Davey, M., et al. (2010). Leadership styles and outcome patterns for the nursing workforce and work environment: A systematic review. *International Journal of Nursing Studies, 47*(3), 363–385.

Curry, L. A., Spatz, E., Cherlin, E., et al. (2011). What distinguishes top-performing hospitals in acute myocardial infarction mortality rates? *Annals of Internal Medicine, 154*(6), 384–390.

D'Aunno, T., Alexander, J. A., & Jiang, L. (2015). Creating value for participants in multistakeholder alliances: The shifting importance of leadership and collaborative decision-making over time. *Health Care Management Review, 42*(2), 100–111.

Doran, G. T. (1981). There's a S.M.A.R.T. way to write management's goals and objectives. *Management Review, 70*(11), 35–36.

Drucker, P. F. (1954). *The practice of management.* New York: Harper.

Eagly, A. H. (2007). Female leadership advantage and disadvantage: Resolving the contradictions. *Psychology of Women Quarterly, 31*, 1–12.

Eagly, A. H., & Carli, L. L. (2007). *Through the labyrinth: The truth about how women become leaders.* Boston, MA: Harvard Business School Press.

Floyd, S. W., & Wooldridge, B. (1992). Middle management involvement in strategy and its association with strategic type: A research note. *Strategic Management Journal, 13*(S1), 153–167.

Frich, J. C., Brewster, A. L., Cherlin, E. J., & Bradley, E. H. (2015). Leadership development programs for physicians: A systematic review. *Journal of General Internal Medicine, 30*(5), 656–674.

Garman, A. N., & Tyler, J. L. (2004). Strategic planning: What kind of CEO will your hospital need next? A model for succession planning. *Trustee, 57*(9), 38–40.

George, J. (2000). Emotions and leadership: The role of emotional intelligence. *Human Relations, 53*, 1027–1055.

Gilmartin, M. J., & D'Aunno, T. A. (2007). 8 leadership research in healthcare: A review and roadmap. *The Academy of Management Annals, 1*(1), 387–438.

Gilmore, T. (1982). Leadership and boundary management. *Journal of Applied Behavioral Science, 18*(2), 343–356.

Goetz, K., Janney, M., & Ramsey, K. (2011). When nursing takes ownership of financial outcomes: Achieving exceptional financial performance through leadership, strategy, and execution. *Nursing Economics, 29*(4), 173–182.

Goleman, D. (2006). *Emotional intelligence.* New York: Bantam Dell.

Gowen, C. R., 3rd, Henagan, S. C., & McFadden, K. L. (2009). Knowledge management as a mediator for the efficacy of transformational leadership and quality management initiatives in U.S. health care. *Health Care Management Review, 34*(2), 129–140.

Graen, G., & Uhl-Bien, M. (1995). Relationship-based approach to leadership: Development of leader-member exchange (LMX) theory of leadership over 25 year: Applying a multi-level multi-domain perspective. *The Leadership Quarterly, 6*, 219–247.

Greenhalgh, T., Robert, G., Macfarlane, F., et al. (2004). Diffusion of innovations in service organizations: Systematic review and recommendations. *Milbank Quarterly, 82*(4), 581–629.

Havig, A. K., Skogstad, A., Kjekshus, L. E., et al. (2011). Leadership, staffing and quality of care in nursing homes. *BMC Health Services Research, 11*, 327.

Heifetz, R. (1994). *Leadership without easy answers.* Cambridge, MA, Belknap Press of Harvard University Press.

Heifetz, R., & Linsky, M. (2002). *Leadership on the line: Staying alive through the dangers of leading.* Boston, MA: Harvard Business School Press.

Hersey, P., & Blanchard, K. (1969). Life cycle theory of leadership. *Training and Development Journal, 23*, 26–34.

House, R. J. (1996). Path-goal theory of leadership: Lessons, legacy and a reformulated theory. *The Leadership Quarterly, 7*, 323–352.

Hu, Y. Y., Parker, S. H., Lipsitz, S. R., et al. (2016). Surgeons' leadership styles and team behavior in the operating room. *Journal of American College of Surgeons, 222*(1), 41–51.

Institute of Medicine (2001). *Crossing the quality chasm: A new system for the 21st century.* Washington, DC: National Academy Press.

Jha, A. K., & Epstein, A. M. (2009). Hospital governance and the quality of care. *Health Affairs, 29*(1), 182–187.

Johnson, B. (1992). *Polarity management: Identifying and managing unsolvable problems.* Amherst, MA: HRD Press.

Judge, T. A., Bono, J. E., & Locke, E. A. (2000). Personality and job satisfaction: The mediating role of job characteristics. *Journal of Applied Psychology, 85*(2), 237–249.

Kaissi, A. A., & Begun, J. W. (2008). Strategic planning processes and hospital financial performance. *Journal of Healthcare Management, 53*(3), 197–208; discussion 208–209.

Kan, M. M., & Parry, K. W. (2004). Identifying paradox: A grounded theory of leadership in overcoming resistance to change. *The Leadership Quarterly, 15*(4), 467–491.

Kane, N. M., Clark, J. R., & Rivenson, H. L. (2009). The internal processes and behavioral dynamics of hospital boards: An exploration of differences between high- and low-performing hospitals. *Health Care Management Review, 34*(1), 80–91.

Katz, D., & Kahn, R. L. (1978). *The social psychology of organizations*. New York: Wiley.

Kellerman, B. (2008). *Followership: How followers are creating change and changing leaders*. Boston, MA: Harvard Business School Press.

Kelley, R.E. (1988). In praise of followers. *Harvard Business Review, 66*(6), 142–148.

Kotter, J. (2007). Leading change: Why transformation efforts fail. *Harvard Business Review, 85*(1), 96–103.

Kuntz, L., Pulm, J., & Wittland, M. (2016). Hospital ownership, decisions on supervisory board characteristics, and financial performance. *Health Care Management Review, 41*(2), 165–176.

Landy, F. G., & Conte, J. M. (2004). *Work in the 21st century: An introduction to industrial and organizational psychology*. Boston, MA: McGraw-Hill.

Lavoie-Tremblay, M., Fernet, C., Lavigne, G. L., et al. (2016). Transformational and abusive leadership practices: Impacts on novice nurses, quality of care and intention to leave. *Journal of Advances Nursing, 72*(3), 582–592.

Lawrence, P. R., & Lorsch, J. W. (1967). Differentiation and integration in complex organizations. *Administrative Science Quarterly, 12*(1), 1–47.

Letts, C., Ryan, W., & Grossman, A. (1999). *High performance nonprofit organizations: Managing upstream for greater impact*. New York: John Wiley.

Lewis, H. S., & Cunningham, C. J. (2016). Linking nurse leadership and work characteristics to nurse burnout and engagement. *Nursing Research, 65*(1), 13–23.

Likert, R. (1961). *New patterns of management*. New York: McGraw-Hill.

Locke, E. A., & Latham, G. P. (1990). *The theory of goal setting and task performance*. Englewood Cliffs, NJ: Prentice Hall.

Longest, B. B., Rakich, J. S., & Darr, K. (2000). *Managing health services organizations and systems*. Baltimore, MD: Health Professions.

Lowe, K. B., Kroeck, K. G., & Sivasubramaniam, N. (1996). Effectiveness correlates of transformational and transactional leadership: A meta-analytic review of the MLQ literature. *The Leadership Quarterly, 7*(3), 385–425.

Lukas, C. V., Holmes, S. K., Cohen, A. B., et al. (2007). Transformational change in health care systems: An organizational model. *Health Care Management Review, 32*(4), 309–320.

March, J. G., & Simon, H. A. (1958). *Organizations*. New York: John Wiley.

McCall, M., Lombardo, M., & Morrison, A. (1988). *The lessons of experience: How successful executives develop on the job*. New York: Free Press.

McCloskey, J. C., & Molen, M. T. (1987). Leadership in nursing. *Annual review of nursing research, 5*, 177.

McCutcheon, A. S., Doran, D., Evans, M., et al. (2009). Effects of leadership and span of control on nurses' job satisfaction and patient satisfaction. *Nursing Leadership (Toronto, Ont.), 22*(3), 48–67.

McFadden, K. L., Stock, G. N., & Gowen, C. R., 3rd. (2015). Leadership, safety climate, and continuous quality improvement: Impact on process quality and patient safety. *Health Care Management Review, 40*(1), 24–34.

McKinney, S. H., Corazzini, K., Anderson, R. A., et al. (2016). Nursing home director of nursing leadership style and director of nursing-sensitive survey deficiencies. *Health Care Management Review*.

Morgan, G. (2006). *Images of organization*. Thousand Oaks, CA: Sage Publications, *41*(3), 224–32.

Nembhard, I. M., & Edmondson, A. C. (2006). Making it safe: The effects of leader inclusiveness and professional status on psychological safety and improvement efforts in health care teams. *Journal of Organizational Behavior, 27*(7), 941–966.

Nembhard, I. M., Morrow, C. T., & Bradley, E. H. (2015). Implementing role-changing versus time-changing innovations in health care: Differences in helpfulness of staff improvement teams, management, and network for learning. *Medical Care Research and Review, 72*(6), 707–735.

Pecukonis, E., Doyle, O., Acquavita, S., et al. (2013). Interprofessional leadership training in MCH social work. *Social Work in Health Care, 52*(7), 625–641.

Purcell, J., & Hutchinson, S. (2007). Front line managers as agents in the HRM-performance causal chain: Theory, analysis and evidence. *Human Resource Management Journal, 17*, 3–20.

Robbins, S. P., & Judge, T. A. (2010). *Essentials of organizational behavior* (10th ed.). Upper Saddle River, NJ: Pearson Prentice Hall.

Salovey, P., & Meyer, J. D. (1990). Emotional intelligence. *Imagination, Cognition and Personality, 9*(3), 185–211.

Schein, E. H. (2006). *Organizational culture and leadership*. San Francisco, CA: John Wiley & Sons.

Schneider, B., Erhart, M., & Macey, W. (2013). Organizational climate and culture. *Annual Review of Psychology, 64*, 361–388.

Schofield, R. F., & Amodeo, M. (1999). Interdisciplinary teams in health care and human services settings: Are they effective? *Health & Social Work, 24*(3), 210–219.

Schreuder, J. A., Roelen, C. A., van Zweeden, N. F., et al. (2011). Leadership styles of nurse managers and registered sickness absence among their nursing staff. *Health Care Management Review, 36*(1), 58–66.

Selznick, P. (1957). *Leadership in administration: A sociological interpretation*. Evanston, IL: Row, Peterson.

Senge, P. (1990). The leader's new work: Building learning organizations. *Sloan Management Review, 31*(1), 7–23.

Shanafelt, T. D., Hasan, O., Dyrbye, L. N., et al. (2015). Changes in burnout and satisfaction with work-life balance in physicians and the general US working population between 2011 and 2014. *Mayo Clinic Proceedings, 90*(12), 1600–1613.

Stefl, M. (2008). Common competencies for all healthcare managers: The healthcare leadership alliance model. *Journal of Healthcare Management, 53*(6), 360–373.

Stogdill, R., & Coons, A. (1957). *Leader behavior: Its description and measurement*. Columbus: Bureau of Business Research, College of Commerce and Administration, Ohio State University.

Taylor, L. A., Coyle, C. E., Ndumele, C. D., et al. (2015). *The social determinants of health: What works?* Boston: Blue Cross Blue Shield of Massachusetts Foundation.

Tsai, T. C., Jha, A. K., Gawande, A. A., et al. (2015). Hospital board and management practices are strongly related to hospital performance on clinical quality metrics. *Health Affairs (Millwood), 34*(8), 1304–1311.

Vroom, V., & Yetton, P. (1973). *Leadership and decision-making.* Pittsburgh, PA: University of Pittsburgh Press.

Weick, K. E. (1993). The collapse of sensemaking in organizations: The Mann Gulch disaster. *Administrative Science Quarterly, 38*(4), 628.

Wells, W., & Hejna, W. (2009). Developing leadership talent in healthcare organizations: There are five key areas in which healthcare organizations can better foster the development of strong leaders among their employees. *Healthcare Financial Management, 63*(1), 66–70.

Wong, C. A., Cummings, G. G., & Ducharme, L. (2013). The relationship between nursing leadership and patient outcomes: A systematic review update. *Journal of Nursing Management, 21*(5), 709–724.

Xirasagar, S., Samuels, M. E., & Stoskopf, C. H. (2005). Physician leadership styles and effectiveness: An empirical study. *Medical Care Research and Review, 62*, 720–740.

Yukl, G. A. (2006). *Leadership in organizations.* Upper Saddle River, NJ: Pearson Prentice Hall.

Zwingman-Bagley, C. (1999). Transformational management style positively affects financial outcomes. *Nursing Administration Quarterly, 23*(4), 29–34.

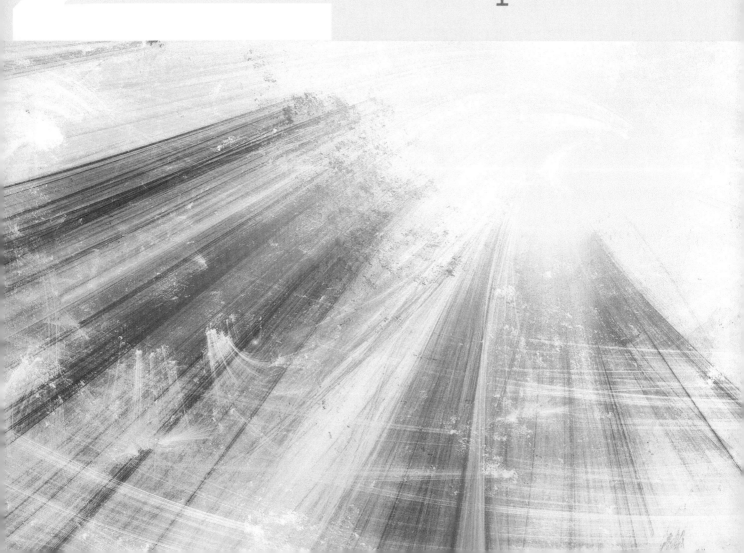

2

PART TWO
Micro Perspective

Chapter 3

Organization Design and Coordination

Martin P. Charns, Gary J. Young, and Laurel E. Radwin

CHAPTER OUTLINE

- Why Is Organization Design Important?
- Twin Structural Issues: Differentiation and Integration
- Coordination at the Macro Level
- Service Lines
- Line and Staff Positions
- Integrated Delivery Systems
- Centralization and Decentralization
- Parallel Organization
- Hybrid Structures
- Organizations with Multiple Goals
- Governance and the Three-Legged Stool of Administration, Medical Staff, and the Board
- Micro-Level Coordination

LEARNING OBJECTIVES

After completing this chapter, the reader should be able to:

1. Describe the variants of organization structure found in health care organizations
2. Describe the facilitating and hindering effects of organization structure on coordination
3. Provide a framework for determining what organization design is most appropriate for a given health care organization
4. Describe the mechanisms and processes of coordination at the micro level and their effects on quality of care

KEY TERMS

Accountable Care Organization

Centralization

Communication

Coordination

Decentralization

Differentiation

Direct Contact

Feedback

Functional Structure

Governance

Group Coordination

Hierarchy of Authority

Hybrid Organization

Integrated Delivery Networks

Integration

Integrators

Interdependence

Liaison Roles

<table>
<tr><td>Matrix Organizations</td><td>Rules and Procedures</td></tr>
<tr><td>Mutual Adjustment</td><td>Sequential Interdependence</td></tr>
<tr><td>Organization Design</td><td>Service Line</td></tr>
<tr><td>Organization Structure</td><td>Simultaneous Interdependence (Team Interdependence)</td></tr>
<tr><td>Parallel Organization</td><td>Specialization</td></tr>
<tr><td>Planning and Goal Setting</td><td>Standardization of Output</td></tr>
<tr><td>Pooled Interdependence</td><td>Standardization of Skill</td></tr>
<tr><td>Program Organization Structure</td><td>Standardization of Work</td></tr>
<tr><td>Programming</td><td>Supervision</td></tr>
<tr><td>Reciprocal Interdependence</td><td>Task Force</td></tr>
<tr><td>Relational Coordination</td><td>Task Uncertainty</td></tr>
<tr><td>Relationships</td><td>Team</td></tr>
</table>

• • • IN PRACTICE: A Tale of Two Units

Unit A, a general medical unit in a major Eastern teaching hospital, is characterized by high dissatisfaction among the nursing staff and is the target of frequent complaints from residents and attending physicians. Communication among the nurses, therapists, social workers, residents, and attending physicians regarding patient care is poor, and relationships among them are strained.

The unit generally appears to be in a state of chaos. Patients and their families seek information about their status from physicians, nurses, and other staff and frequently complain that they receive conflicting information from the medical and nursing staffs. At the same time, lengths of stay are unacceptably long due to poor communication among the staff rather than due to unique patient needs.

The organization of the hospital is similar to that of most major teaching facilities, with the major departments representing professional (nursing, social service, dietary) and nonprofessional (housekeeping, security, transportation) functions.

On Unit A, care paths—protocols specifying the sequence and timing of tasks for patients with particular routine conditions—have been introduced to streamline delivery of care. However, they frequently are not followed. Unit A staff stopped holding interdisciplinary rounds several years ago based on the belief that these meetings consume too much valuable staff time. Because many different internal medicine physicians admit patients to the unit, unit staff found it difficult to conduct rounds with the physicians.

Unit B is a general medical unit in a different Eastern teaching hospital. It has a reputation for quality care and responsiveness to both patients and their families. Nurses and other staff express high satisfaction about their work. Communication between nurses, therapists, social workers, residents, and attending physicians is said to be frequent, timely, and accurate, and relationships among them appear to be strong. In general, the unit runs smoothly and responds well to routine situations as well as unusual cases.

Unit B differs from Unit A in several ways. Nursing staff on the unit are organized into teams, with each team responsible for assigned patients from admission to discharge. The house staff in medicine in the hospital also are organized into teams, and except when beds are not available, each team admits patients to one patient care unit. Two house staff teams admit to unit B, and each works primarily with one nursing team. Other health professionals in the hospital, such as social workers, clinical pharmacists, physical therapists, and occupational therapists, care for patients primarily on one unit.

Nurses, physicians, and other health professionals on unit B conduct interdisciplinary rounds daily. Unit B patients are assigned to care paths, and patients' progress on the care paths is reviewed in the interdisciplinary rounds. In addition, the nurse manager and chief resident meet regularly to review unit performance measures, such as patient satisfaction, hospital-acquired infections, and pressure ulcers, and to plan actions to improve care.

CHAPTER PURPOSE

Many administrators and clinicians see the differences between the effectively functioning Unit B and the chaotic Unit A as arising from differences in leadership or staffing. Some attribute the differences to the patients the units care for. Yet others attribute the differences in unit performance to Unit A having been chaotic as long as anyone remembers. But is the chaos on Unit A inevitable? The concepts presented in this chapter illuminate how the effective functioning of Unit B and the chaotic functioning of unit A are affected by differences in the organizational structures of the two hospitals and the mechanisms and process of **coordination** between the two units.

Organization design is the arrangement of responsibilities, authority, and flow of information within an organization, resulting in its **organization structure**. The structure of an organization is analogous to human anatomy, with the caveat that an organization's structure can be changed more readily. The two closely interrelated parts to organization design are (1) how to divide the work and responsibilities and allocate them to units in an organization, and (2) how to coordinate the work of those units to perform the organization's overall work effectively. These two parts of organization design are intimately related, because the division of labor and grouping of responsibilities directly affect the ease of achieving coordination. It is especially important in large organizations, where the arrangement of individuals into separate groupings results in the facilitation of some flows of information and coordination while simultaneously hindering others.

There is no one universally best organization design. What design is best for a given organization depends on characteristics of its environment, work, technologies, and strategy. For example, a large hospital pursuing a strategy of providing the best care in a number of different patient conditions and diseases (e.g., heart disease, cancer, women's health, mental health) might organize into different mini-hospitals, each containing all of the professional and nonprofessional staff required to deliver care to its particular patients. This would facilitate the coordination among staff within each mini-hospital and focus the organization's resource allocation on each mini-hospital. On the other hand, a teaching hospital emphasizing graduate medical education and education of other professions might best organize along the traditional lines of different medical specialties and professions. (Why these are appropriate organization designs for different strategies will be explained later in the chapter.)

WHY IS ORGANIZATION DESIGN IMPORTANT?

Many people, including many senior leaders of major health care organizations, are not fully aware of the effects of organization design. Similar to the physical design of buildings, many health care organizations reflect the incremental addition of new activities in the organization, without rethinking how the organization would be best structured. What results is a design that may no longer fit the organization's strategy or contribute to organization performance. The reference to "silos" in health care organizations has become commonplace, reflected in a dysfunctional design where the different parts function autonomously and do not communicate or coordinate well with each other. There is strong empirical evidence that coordination is related to patient outcomes such as postsurgical complications, hospital readmissions, and patient satisfaction (Gittell, 2016; Gittell et al., 2000; Young, 1997).

At the most micro level in an organization, people are grouped together into work units having a common supervisor. What we call these smallest work units varies from organization to organization. For example, faculty in a medical school may be organized into divisions (e.g. cardiology, medical oncology, infectious diseases), each led by a division chief. These are part of larger units, which in medical schools typically are departments (e.g., medicine, surgery, pathology), led by department chairs. Nurses in hospitals typically are organized into nursing units (here we are using the term "unit" to refer to generic "nursing units" or "patient care units" and not just to "intensive care units"), each led by a nurse manager. In small hospitals, the nurse managers may report directly to the chief nursing officer (often having the title of vice president [VP] for nursing or VP for patient care services). In larger hospitals, there is typically an intermediate level of organization in nursing, with several nurse managers being accountable to each associate director (or associate chief) of nursing, who in turn is accountable to the chief nursing officer. Associate directors typically are responsible for several units based upon the practice specialty (e.g., intensive care, pediatrics, medical, surgical). The variation in position titles used in practice makes it difficult to discuss through example; what is key is understanding that the building blocks of units aggregate hierarchically into larger and larger entities.

Organizations use hierarchies to conduct planning, allocate resources, and hold people accountable for performance and use of those resources. For example, the nursing department in a hospital has an annual budget, most of which is for staff salaries; the chief nursing officer is held accountable for effective management of that budget. The authority and responsibility for staff supervision and budget is typically delegated down the hierarchy to the lowest level managers (e.g., the nurse managers). Different organizational units also have different goals, the achievement of which aggregate up to achieve overall organizational goals. Usually but not always, front-line staff with a common supervisor are located in physical proximity to facilitate supervision. Both the reporting relationship and physical proximity of people affect the frequency of their interactions, which in turn affects the ease or difficulty of coordinating their work. Thus, both common reporting relationships and physical proximity facilitate coordination.

A "table of organization" or "organizational chart," consisting of boxes and lines, provides a shorthand for describing structure. Organizations are complex. No one chart, diagram, or perspective of any organizational model will provide total understanding of all organizational phenomena, nor is taking any single perspective sufficient to manage an organization effectively. Considering structure, however, is an important approach to understanding the complexity of organizations. It helps us understand why some things seem to "fall through the cracks" all too often and not get done properly or at all, even when they are supposed to be the responsibility of capable, motivated people. It also helps us to understand and predict where conflict will occur in an organization, without even considering the people involved, and to manage it better.

In a large organization, it is always necessary to partition the organization into units. One of the most critical design choices is determining where to place the organizational boundaries between units. However, every way of dividing work and responsibilities across units has both advantages and disadvantages. Boundaries not only encourage people within units to work closely together but also create barriers to coordination across units. People within work units tend to develop a common set of goals and perspectives on their work, but the different goals, as well as competition for resources, contribute to conflict across units. When organization design is done well, those trade-offs are made in a way that most facilitates and least hinders the accomplishment of an organization's work. The problems inherent in a good design are those that an organization can live with and interfere as little as possible with its most important work.

TWIN STRUCTURAL ISSUES: DIFFERENTIATION AND INTEGRATION

Every organization design has functional and dysfunctional characteristics. The key question, then, is what is the best design for a given organization? During the first half of the twentieth century, organization researchers sought the one best way. Only in the 1960s did researchers begin to see that the highest-performing organizations in different industries (performing different types of work and having different technologies) were organized and managed differently (Thompson, 1967; Woodward, 1965). Structural contingency theory (Lawrence and

Lorsch, 1967) is based on the premise that there is no one best design; rather, the best way to structure and manage an organization depends on its unique work, environment, and strategy.

Lawrence and Lorsch (1967) extended earlier findings relating organizational performance to the "fit" between an organization's design and its environment. The environment includes not only its physical environment but also the political, financial, technological, scientific, and regulatory conditions that affect it. Environment includes other organizations such as suppliers, competitors, regulatory bodies, professional societies, labor unions, and customers or clients, individually and collectively. Environment also includes the information and resources needed by an organization and the technology needed to process them. Lawrence and Lorsch's key insight was that the environmental demands facing the organization dictated differences across its units in how they were structured and designed.

Differentiation

Different units in an organization perform different tasks, use different technologies, and face different subenvironments. The original research on industrial firms noted that these tasks and subenvironments differ across research, engineering, manufacturing, marketing, and sales departments. Not only do these departments do different work but they also require different interpersonal, time, and goal orientations to do their work most effectively. For example, researchers need relatively long time horizons, whereas manufacturing staff need relatively short time horizons to match the nature of their work and the demands of their subenvironments.

Different departments interact with different subenvironments. Researchers have to keep up with scientific advances in their field and interact with a scientific subenvironment. The marketing staff, in contrast, has to focus on a market subenvironment. They need to keep in touch with what their customers are looking for, what competitors are doing, and what market trends are. Lawrence and Lorsch found that the highest-performing industrial firms encouraged each subunit in the organization to develop orientations and operating practices tailored to their particular tasks and subenvironments. This means that they had different goals and recruited and developed staff with different time and interpersonal orientations. Since generally people in the same workgroup interact most frequently with each other, have similar goals, and are evaluated on similar objectives, they tend to develop a common way of thinking and common view of their work and subenvironment.

Lawrence and Lorsch's finding that internal structures and management styles varied among organization units built on work of earlier researchers (Burns and Stalker, 1961; Miller and Rice, 1967; Woodward, 1965).

Units with tasks that were highly uncertain (such as research), largely staffed by highly educated professionals, should not be closely supervised or expected to produce results in short time periods. The structure most appropriate for supervising researchers is one in which each supervisor has a large span of control—i.e., many subordinates—with few hierarchical levels. In contrast, manufacturing, with its shorter time frames (you do not want a manufacturing process to be out of control for very long, lest you have much waste and inefficiency), requires a closer level of supervision and control, smaller spans of control, and more hierarchical levels. Lawrence and Lorsch referred to these needed differences in unit structure and employee orientations as **differentiation**.

One aspect of differentiation is **specialization**. Each part of an organization performs a specialized function. It does this best if it is organized and managed to meet the unique requirements of its specialized work. Different specialties within medicine relate to different subenvironments, and different specialists have different personal characteristics. For example, internists are often referred to as being more cerebral with somewhat longer time orientations, whereas surgeons are more action-oriented with shorter time spans. Psychiatrists are more people-oriented, while radiologists focus more on technology. As a reflection of the different scientific bases of their work, different specialties also belong to different professional organizations and read different journals. Different professions (physicians, nursing, social workers) also have different orientations, accrediting bodies, and journals.

Integration

In addition to the relationship between differentiation and organizational performance, Lawrence and Lorsch found a strong relationship between integration and performance. **Integration** is the coordination of activities among organizational units, including the management of interunit conflict. Differentiation and integration are antagonistic to each other: the greater the differences among units, the more difficult it is for them to integrate their efforts. This reflects their different orientations, activities, and goals. According to Lawrence and Lorsch, the highest-performing organizations achieved joint levels of differentiation and integration commensurate with environmental demands. How they did so, we will address below.

COORDINATION AT THE MACRO LEVEL

Coordination needs to be addressed at two organizational levels: At the macro level, the focus is on the overall coordination needs and structural approaches to address those needs; at the micro level, the focus is more on the actual processes used to achieve coordination in specific situations. The specific needs for coordination are driven by the specific types of **interdependence** among organizational units.

Interdependence

If different organizational units could work independently of each other, there would be little need for coordination. However, total independence is never the case in complex organizations. One way to examine interdependence is to ask questions such as, "For what reasons, and how often, do various people or organizational units need to work together?" "How critical is it that they coordinate their efforts?" and "To what extent can the work of one unit affect the work of another?" In addressing these questions, first and foremost one should examine the flow of work, particularly that work which directly contributes to the central goals of the organization. In health care organizations, this is the direct delivery of patient care. Second, but also important, is to examine work that supports direct patient care, such as performance of diagnostic tests. Third are back-office functions that support the functioning of the overall organization (e.g., accounting, finance, human resource management).

Three factors should be considered in assessing the needs for coordination:

1. Interconnectedness of the work of the organization units
2. Uncertainty of the tasks
3. Size of the organization

According to Galbraith (1973), increases in each factor increase the information-processing requirements (i.e., the amount and richness of information that needs to be exchanged) within the organization and thus the need for coordination.

Interconnectedness of Work

Interconnectedness is an attribute of work itself. To the degree that work efforts need to fit together, we refer to them as being interconnected. This consideration is quite separate from the number of people or units performing these efforts. To the extent the organization structure separates work efforts that are highly interconnected, such efforts must be coordinated for successful task accomplishment. A few examples ranging from low to high interconnectedness illustrate this point. At the low end of the scale, hospital outpatient clinics typically have different staff and serve different patient populations. The work of any one clinic inherently has little connection with the work of other clinics, reducing their need to coordinate care delivery. These same clinics may have greater interconnectedness in the presence of (1) education of medical students, nursing students, and house staff; and (2) treatment of patients having multiple diseases and requiring visits to multiple clinics. At the other end of the continuum, specialized inpatient units require medical staff, nurses, and therapists to work together to serve a patient population in a particular clinical area. Similarly, the work efforts performed by different members of a surgical team are highly interconnected.

Task Uncertainty

The need for coordination in the presence of **task uncertainty** is central in the writing of the early contingency theorists (Burns and Stalker, 1961; Duncan, 1972; Galbraith, 1973; Lawrence and Lorsch, 1967; Perrow, 1967, 1972). Where there is a high degree of certainty in a task, few things arise that cannot be planned in advance. Different organizational units can perform their work in a predetermined manner, with few exceptions that require redirecting efforts to assure coordination. For example, most of the work done by clinical laboratories in conducting diagnostic tests has little inherent task uncertainty; routine lab work requires little coordination between clinical units and laboratories. Uncertainty is introduced when a patient's condition changes rapidly, necessitating immediate laboratory tests at unanticipated times. Uncertainty related to changes in a patient's condition can also require greater coordination among the different providers caring for that patient as well as between caregivers and support services.

Relatively little uncertainty also exists in the task of postoperative care for simple, uncomplicated surgical procedures. Even when some complications arise (e.g., a patient with urinary retention), the actions needed to address them are well known. In such cases, there is a low need for coordination between surgeons and nursing personnel providing postoperative care. By contrast, the very nature of many medical diagnoses reflects high clinical uncertainty and requires greater coordination between nursing and medical staff on an inpatient medical unit. While interconnectedness and uncertainty are conceptually distinct, they may exert an interactive effect calling for greater coordination.

Size

Increased size also calls for greater coordination. As more organizational units are involved in a particular task, the challenge of coordinating their effort increases in complexity. Work is also more specialized in larger than in smaller organizations, requiring greater integration to achieve concerted action. In the absence of coordination, increased size and specialization can impede organizational performance in the form of reduced quality of care, complications of treatment, delays and extended length of hospital stays, and duplication of effort.

Sharing Resources

Interdependence among organizational units also stems from *sharing of resources* such as space, people, and equipment. Greater efficiency in use of resources can be attained by sharing among units but at a cost of requiring coordination. If units share resources (e.g., a social worker), conflicts in availability inevitably arise. If no one coordinates these activities, both efficiency and effectiveness can suffer.

Slack resources and duplicated resources can also be used to reduce information-processing requirements. One example in a health care setting is having excess capacity in support services: additional staff permit easier and rapid fulfillment of requests but at the cost of additional personnel and equipment. (The concept of slack resources is discussed in greater detail in Chapter 9.)

Types of Interdependence

Thompson (1967) defined three types of organizational interdependence: **pooled interdependence**, **sequential interdependence**, and **reciprocal interdependence**. The three types required increasing coordination costs. The least costly type, pooled interdependence, is characterized by low interconnectedness in the work of different units. The work efforts of different units simply do not need to fit together directly but jointly affect the overall organization. The outpatient clinics treating different patient populations described earlier have pooled interdependence. Although there are not direct connects in the work of the clinics, the reputation of any clinic may affect the hospital's reputation, which in turn affects the reputation of all other clinics. Compared with pooled interdependence, sequential and reciprocal interdependence exhibit greater interconnectedness in the work efforts of the different units. The requirement for direct linkages between the work of two units (as in a sequential assembly line) is more difficult and therefore more costly to coordinate than needing only indirect links. The requirement for direct linkages in two directions (reciprocal) is even more difficult to coordinate. Van de Ven and Delbecq (1974) later added **team interdependence** (also called **simultaneous interdependence**) as a fourth category. Here the reciprocal tasks need to be performed simultaneously, as, for example, in the work among a surgical team. (For more on interdependence, please refer to Chapter 5.)

Structural Approaches to Coordination

In designing an organization's structure, it is necessary to balance the benefits of differentiation (specialization) and those of integration (coordination). Galbraith (1973, 1977) argued that organizations can apply a series of devices to manage increasing levels of interdependence. These include the following:

1. Hierarchy of authority
2. Rules and procedures
3. Planning and goal setting
4. Vertical information systems
5. Lateral relations

Hierarchy of Authority

In the simplest of situations, the **hierarchy of authority** itself acts as an adequate coordinating device to ensure that the efforts of different work units mesh together. Hierarchical coordination allows units to conduct their work relatively independently of each other. Often their need to coordinate stems from sharing common resources. For example, consider the nursing department hierarchy in Figure 3.1. On the few occasions when disagreements among nursing units arise, issues can be referred for resolution to the first common supervisor in the hierarchy. To minimize the number of levels that issues need to be referred up the hierarchy, units with the greatest interdependence that have more occasions to resolve issues should be overseen by the same supervisor in the hierarchy. For example, consider the nursing units labeled A through F in Sample Organization I in Figure 3.2. If A and D were more interdependent than any other units, they should be grouped as shown in Sample Organization II in Figure 3.2, thereby allowing the hierarchy to function more effectively as a coordinating device. An example is placing nursing units serving patients in the same specialty under the responsibility of the same supervisor (often called "associate director" but sometimes called "director"). For classical organization theorists, the hierarchy was the primary coordinating mechanism. However, few health care organizations have coordination needs that can be met solely by the hierarchy. Furthermore, since physicians are typically not employees of community hospitals and long-term care facilities, no common supervisor over nursing and medical personnel exists. Other approaches must be used to achieve coordination.

Rules and Procedures

Frequently, organizations augment the hierarchy of authority with **rules and procedures** specifying how things are to be done and what things should not be done. Examples range from (a) "food is not to be taken from the cafeteria" to (b) procedures for ordering supplies to (c) complex protocols for delivering care. During the last 25 years, there has been a dramatic increase in the use of care protocols and clinical guidelines. These rules specify the services and medications patients should receive and when they should receive them, given a set of clinical indications and circumstances. While clinical guidelines were initially derided by some clinicians as "cookbook medicine," they have become a central feature of the way health care is delivered in the twenty-first century (Hoff, Sutcliffe, and Young, 2016). Another example is checklists, whereby a procedure must follow standards embodied in a list or work may not commence without completing the list. Nurses and physicians often complete these lists together in real time (cf., Gawande, 2010; Haynes et al., 2009). As long as the work is programmable, formal rules and procedures can be developed and applied to facilitate coordination. When predictable exceptions arise, the rules themselves may call for application of additional rules including extending deference to the judgment of the decision maker within certain parameters. When unanticipated exceptions arise, an issue may require referral up the hierarchy.

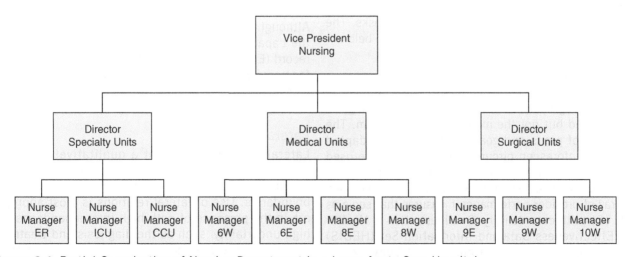

Figure 3.1 Partial Organization of Nursing Department in a Large Acute Care Hospital.

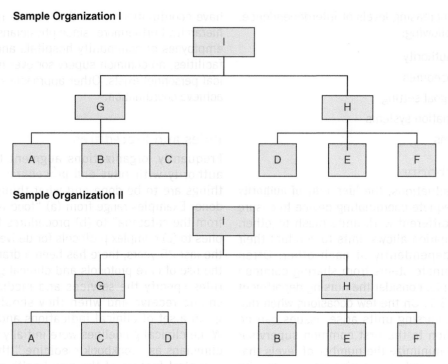

Figure 3.2 Simplified Partial Organization Structures.

The use of hierarchy of authority and rules and procedures is the basis of bureaucratic organizations. Their efficiency lies in the development of optimal policies and procedures, eliminating the need to "reinvent the wheel" each time a situation is encountered. They can be used in two different ways. First, they can provide certainty by delineating and controlling the efforts of those lower in the organization. Second, they can be used to provide guidance in performing work and to promote codification of agreements on how work is to be done, determined by the individuals responsible for interconnected elements. Key limitations of rules and procedures, however, include (a) the difficulty in fully controlling behavior, which is a special problem in professional organizations, and (b) the inability to respond to unprogrammable tasks. The use of rules and procedures is discussed further below.

Planning and Goal Setting

Compared to rules and procedures, the use of **planning and goal setting** reduces the degree of control since goals are specified but not the means to achieve them. The advantage of plans and goals is they can be adapted to new or unforeseen circumstances and can be used in situations that are less programmable. Over the past 25 years, the U.S. health care industry has developed an array of provider performance measures that serve as goals of health care delivery. One illustration is Healthcare Effectiveness Data and Information Set (HEDIS) that encompasses the effectiveness, availability, experience, and utilization of care.

Vertical Information Systems

The integration devices described above can be augmented by vertical information systems, such as planning, budgeting, and information (both manual and computer) systems. Such approaches increase the organization's information-processing capacity by facilitating information flow up and down the hierarchy and by increasing the capabilities of managers to handle that information. In this manner, vertical information systems provide managers with more timely information about what is happening in their units and allow them to better control the units under them. Such systems augment use of the hierarchy and build on the hierarchy itself by vertical interactions across levels in the organization. Although originally viewed as a method for amplifying the capacity of the hierarchy, today electronic health record (EHR) systems are also an important mechanism for transferring information laterally among health care providers (discussed below).

Lateral Relations

Lateral relations represent a qualitatively different approach to coordination whereby members of different units interact directly and laterally across internal boundaries. Use of lateral relations is most appropriate in the presence of both high interdependence and high uncertainty, such as the diagnosis and treatment of patients involving more than one specialist. In these instances, specialists and professionals from multiple units often need to interact frequently. Several different types of lateral relations can be used to coordinate their efforts, such as direct contact, liaison roles, integrators, teams and task forces, and matrix organizations. The most extreme approach is a complete restructuring that groups together the most interdependent activities and people into new organization units. This "program structure" will be described in more detail below.

Building on the work of Galbraith (1973), Charns and Tewksbury (1993) developed a continuum of organizational forms representing increasingly greater emphasis on coordination across traditional specialized departments in health care organizations (Byrne et al., 2004; Greenberg, Rosenheck, and Charns, 2003). An elaboration of their continuum of organizational forms is displayed in Figure 3.3. On the far left of the continuum is the traditional **functional structure**, where the organization design emphasizes each profession and discipline independently. This is graphically indicated in Figure 3.3 by the vertical expanse of the top triangle, "emphasis on differentiation/specialization" being at its greatest extent. On the far right of the continuum in Figure 3.3 is the "program organization," often called a "service line" organization in health care. This design emphasizes each

program independently as well as coordination among disciplines within programs, graphically depicted by the height of bottom triangle, "Program/Service Line Integration." We can use this continuum to compare different organization designs. We first describe these contrasting organizational structures and then describe alternative forms that enhance coordination across disciplines by building on the functional structure.

Functional Structure (1): In this structure, segmentation is based on specialty departments. The structure emphasizes each specialty department functioning relatively independently of the other departments. The functional structure appears on the far left side of the continuum to indicate its extreme emphasis on differentiation by specialty and lack of any emphasis on integration across specialties. In health care, the departments typically correspond to different professional functions (e.g., medical specialties and subspecialties, nursing, social work, etc.) and nonprofessional functions (e.g., environmental services, transportation). These are displayed as the "boxes" in the organization chart in Figure 3.4. This structure only addresses pooled interdependence. The more that senior managers encourage each function to work autonomously, the less that coordination is achieved.

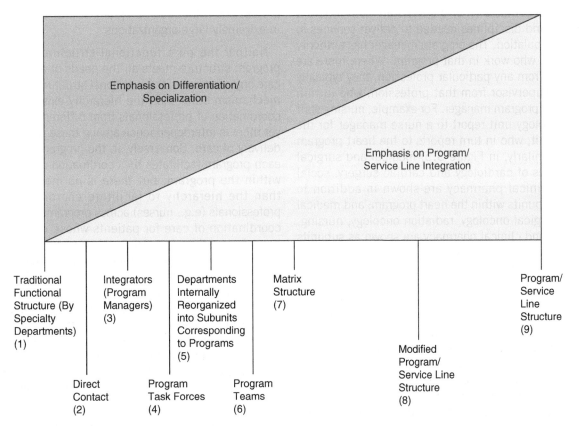

Figure 3.3 Continuum of Organization Structures.

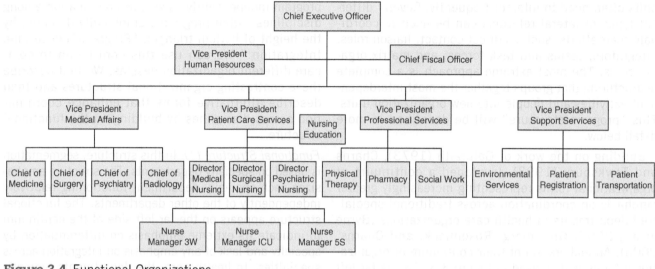

Figure 3.4 Functional Organizations.

Program Structure (9): At the extreme other end of the continuum is the program (or "service line") structure. (Note that some organizations use other terms such as "strategic business unit (SBU)," "institute," or "operating division" for this structure; Porter and Lee, 2018). Here, the emphasis is on individual programs, such as heart, cancer, women's health, and mental health, although there may be as many as 20 such programs in a large hospital. Each program contains all of the key staff from different professions and disciplines needed to deliver services to its patient population. The program manager has authority over the staff who work in that program. Where there are several staff from any particular profession, they typically report to a supervisor from that profession, who in turn reports to the program manager. For example, nursing staff on the cardiology unit report to a nurse manager for the cardiology unit, who in turn reports to the heart program manager. Similarly, in Figure 3.5, medical and surgical subspecialties of cardiology and cardiac surgery, social work, and clinical pharmacy are shown in addition to nursing as subunits within the heart program; and medical oncology, surgical oncology, radiation oncology, nursing, social work, and clinical pharmacy are shown as subunits of the cancer program. These professional subunits are representative; others such as physical therapy and occupational therapy may also be subunits within these programs. Note that Figure 3.5 shows no nursing or other department, as all professions are located within respective programs. By contrast, medical specialties of pathology and radiology are not located within these programs and remain separate to render their ancillary services across all programs. Thus, at the highest level of the pure program organization, there is no differentiation by profession or discipline; such differentiation occurs only *within* each program. In contrast to the functional structure, where staffing decisions are made by each department independently, the program manager can determine staffing mix and levels that are most appropriate for the particular program. In large hospitals, the programs function as "mini-hospitals," having all staff needed to provide care for their patients and sometimes even having their own buildings. The program structure places total emphasis on integration of disciplines and professions within each program. It may only be feasible in extremely large organizations.

Neither the pure functional structure nor the pure program structure meets all the needs of a typical health care organization. In the functional structure (1), no formal mechanism other than the hierarchy exists to facilitate coordination of professionals from different departments, yet there is interdependence among these professionals in delivery of care. Conversely, in the program structure (9), each program facilitates the coordination of professionals within the program, but there is no mechanism other than the hierarchy to facilitate coordination of like professionals (e.g., nurses) across programs or to facilitate coordination of care for patients whose illness requires care of more than one program (e.g., a patient with heart disease and diabetes). While the hierarchy (a vertical coordinating mechanism) can be effective for resource allocation decisions, it is too limited for addressing high levels of interdependence, such as those inherent in the delivery of complex patient care. It is thus common to find health care organizations using various other integrative mechanisms to facilitate coordination across functional departments. These mechanisms, shown as alternatives (2) through (7) in Figure 3.3, are discussed below.

Direct Contact (2): The **direct contact** form is structurally the same as the functional structure but differs in that staff

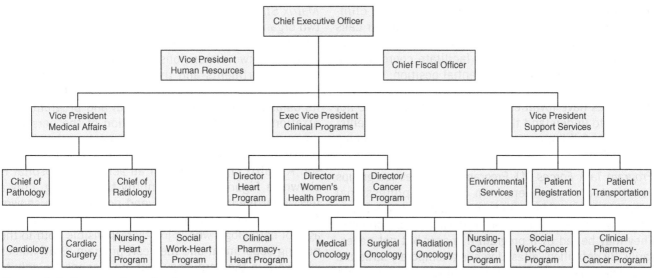

Figure 3.5 Program Organization.

in one functional department may directly contact members of other departments. Direct contact occurs very frequently in health care and other organizations, especially where it is facilitated by having the people who need to interact most frequently located in close physical proximity. This is relatively simple and consumes few organizational resources. The difference between the pure functional structure (1) and direct contact (2) is largely in the way the organization is managed. Among all lateral relations, direct contact is the least powerful integrative mechanism. Factors that limit its effectiveness are the following:

- The people contacted may be occupied with other issues and not motivated to contribute to solving a problem they see as belonging only to the initiator of the contact. This is not unusual and often is exacerbated by an organization's reward system. Thus, what is a high priority for a contacting unit may be a low priority for a unit being contacted.

- In responding to the request of another unit, the work flow of the contacted unit may be interrupted, resulting in reduced efficiencies and thus a cost to the organization. The more a unit is pressed for performance on a particular set of goals unique to itself, the less willing members will be to assist other units. For example, if a maintenance department is held closely to its budget, it will be reluctant to meet the requests of other departments if such requests might jeopardize achievement of the maintenance department's budget objectives. Thus, it is not unusual to find a maintenance department responding more slowly than is desired by nursing or other staff members to a request they see as urgent, even when all parties agree that that is maintenance's responsibility. Often maintenance sees the request as one that

would require either interruption of other activities or use of overtime, both of which would negatively affect its budget.

- Members of one unit may not know whom to contact in a second unit to initiate their requests.

In some organizations, direct contact is discouraged by managers in functional departments for reasons of maintaining control over their personnel. However, historically, the prohibitions on direct contact have diminished. In health care, direct contact among providers from different disciplines and professions is commonplace in the direct delivery of care.

Integrators and Liaison Roles (3): Added to the functional structure are individuals who have responsibility for coordination of program activities across the traditional specialty departments. Sometimes these integrators are called "program managers," even though, by definition, they do not have formal authority over personnel working in a program. Although they are not called "integrators," case managers who coordinate a patient's care across specialties or between a hospital and a skilled nursing facility are another example. Without formal authority for staff in any of the specialty departments, **integrators** must rely upon their interpersonal skills, association with senior managers to whom they report who do have formal authority, and the perception of the value they add to the organization. The characteristics of effective integrators are well described in Lawrence and Lorsch (1967) and Charns and Tewksbury (1993). Integrators are more effective when they have good interpersonal skills and are seen by those they are integrating as being able to understand their points of view. **Liaison roles** are created within departments to facilitate coordination between that department and others. For example, the clinical laboratories may appoint individuals to answer calls from patient care units trying to locate test results. Note that while the liaison role can facilitate coordination, it is typically not a highly influential position. Because it is located within a department, the individuals in those roles have loyalties to their departments, are not as likely to understand the needs of other departments, and do not fulfill a neutral position among parties being coordinated.

Program Task Forces (4): Program **task forces** are groups constituted of members from different professional departments to address a program-related task, such as planning for new services or improving a care process. They may be led by a program manager but not necessarily. By definition, a task force is a temporary structure that disbands once its task is completed. Its strength as an integrating mechanism derives from its bringing together people from different departments so that they can work directly together.

Departments Restructured Internally (5): Departments can reorganize their subunits to correspond to programs. This establishes consistent patterns of interaction and thereby facilitates coordination within each program. An example is organizing nursing into specialized units (e.g., cardiology, oncology, etc.) rather than having general medical-surgical units. This can facilitate the coordination between specialist physicians and corresponding nursing staff on the specialty units. Another example is assigning patients to social workers, physical and occupational therapists, and other professionals based on the patient's condition and the medical specialty treating it (which corresponds to different programs). While staff continue to be accountable to their professional departments, the departments lose some influence over their personnel as they work with other departments in the same program.

Program Teams (6): This structural alternative formalizes the interactions among staff from different professional departments into **teams**. Types of health care teams frequently seen are multidisciplinary patient care teams organized around specialized patient care units, ambulatory care clinics and practices, and program management teams. The latter might consist of one or more physicians, a nurse manager, and an administrator, who are mutually responsible for managing a program. For example, the chief of cardiology, chief of cardiac surgery, the nurse manager for the cardiology unit, and an administrator can have joint responsibility for a heart program. In contrast to task forces, teams endure over time with ongoing responsibility for their mutual work. Typically, program managers have input, but not responsibility, for performance evaluations of staff who work in their program.

Matrix Structure (7): The **matrix organization** consists of two organization structures—the traditional functional structure and the program structure—overlaid on each other. The two dimensions of the matrix are the specialty departments and the programs. It is shown in the middle of the continuum of Figure 3.3 to represent its balance between the functional and program organizations. Typically, a small portion of the personnel are in "matrixed" positions—i.e., they have two bosses of equal authority. Other staff have a single supervisor. A matrix organization for an acute care hospital is shown in Figure 3.6. To simplify the drawing, only a few departments, programs, and positions are shown. An example of a "matrixed" position is the nurse manager of cardiology, who is jointly responsible both to the nursing department and the heart program. Staff nurses who work in the cardiology unit are responsible only to the nurse manager.

Matrix structures have all of the advantages of both the traditional functional structure and program structure, providing management and coordination of both functions and programs simultaneously. The matrix, however, is the most complex organizational form and is costly to manage, having two complete hierarchical structures. Furthermore, having strong advocates for both functional and program perspectives encourages latent conflicts between functions and programs to become manifest. This requires a high level of conflict management skills, which few organizations have. Often the term "matrix" is used incorrectly to refer to a range of structures from task forces to modified program structures on the continuum; using the term in this imprecise way does not convey the necessary detail to determine how an organization is actually structured.

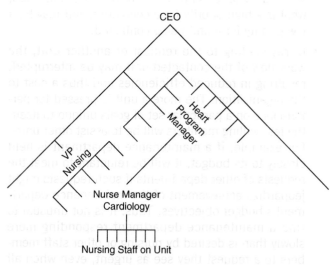

Figure 3.6 Matrix Organization.

Modified Program Structure (8): While the pure program structure (9) is theoretically possible, it is not practical in any but the largest organizations where there are sufficient numbers of staff in each profession and in each program to use resources effectively, to have the needed staff coverage, and to address the maintenance of professional competence and other professional issues (this is the "mini-hospital" described above). This is why organizations that adopt a program structure typically modify it by establishing coordinating mechanisms that cross the programs and address professional needs. A modified program structure for a teaching hospital is shown in Figure 3.7. Note the segregated position of VP for nursing and nursing education with no line authority over nurse managers and nurses in the various programs. The VP for nursing and/or a Nursing Council are responsible for professional issues in nursing, such as setting policy for professional practice, assisting in recruitment, and professional education. Note also the addition of chiefs of medicine and surgery in the modified program structure (Figure 3.7), as compared to the pure program structure (Figure 3.5). They or their subordinates are responsible for professional development of physicians in internal medicine and surgery, respectively, as well as educational activities (e.g., residency programs) within their specialties. Without these or similar positions, there would be no mechanism to coordinate the physicians in the same specialty who organizationally are in different programs (e.g., surgeons in heart, cancer, etc.). The pure program structure (9) and modified program structure (8) can be thought of as mirror images of structural alternatives (1) through (6), with alternatives (2) through (6)

providing coordination across functional departments and alternative (8) providing coordination across programs. In practice, there are fewer systematic variations of coordinating mechanisms across programs (8) than there are coordinating mechanisms across departments (2–6).

Until the 1980s, few health care organizations were structured in matrix or program forms, with most following traditional structures augmented by task forces and teams. In the 1980s, a number of health care organizations adopted program structures represented by families of services. Some organizations maintained their program structures while others returned to traditional structures. Some organizations have adopted program structures to mimic apparent trends or follow the suggestions of consultants. There is little academic evidence to support the benefits of program versus traditional functional structures, although some health care leaders have very strong feelings about the benefits of service line models (Byrne et al., 2004; Charns and Tewksbury, 1993; Greenberg, Rosenheck, and Charns, 2003; Louis et al., 2017; Young, Charns, and Hereen, 1994).

SERVICE LINES

The term "service line" is often used in health care instead of the generic term "program." **Service lines** are interdisciplinary programs that are organized around diseases or conditions, patient populations, or "technologies" (such as transplant). Service lines can be established for several reasons, such as to monitor expenses, facilitate marketing, and/or to manage a service as a business entity,

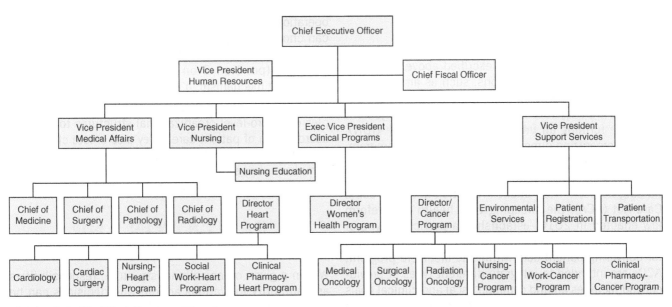

Figure 3.7 Modified Program Structure.

including coordinating delivery of patient care. Each entails different interdependencies among departments and therefore different coordinating needs. Coordination needs are lowest for monitoring costs and marketing and highest for delivery of patient care. The structures on the right side of the continuum in Figure 3.3 are needed only for achieving high levels of coordination across professional departments. Therefore, the matrix and program structures are needed only when the intent is to address coordination of patient care. A detailed discussion of service lines is presented in Charns and Tewksbury (1993).

LINE AND STAFF POSITIONS

Managers who have authority and responsibility for activities and decisions that directly contribute to the provision of goods and services are referred to as "line managers." In the functional structure in health care, these are people in supervisory positions over the various professional and nonprofessional departments; in the program organization, these are the "program managers" and their subordinates (see Figure 3.4). Units that provide support services to the organization, such as human resources, finance, and information systems, are referred to as "staff departments." Individuals in staff departments are not directly involved in care delivery. This is sometimes confusing in health care because we use the term "staff" also to refer to providers of care (e.g., medical staff, nursing staff). In the functional, program, and modified program organizations depicted in Figures 3.4, 3.5, and 3.7, the staff departments are shown with a horizontal line connecting to the side of the box (cf. human resources, finance, nursing education).

INTEGRATED DELIVERY SYSTEMS

The organization structures described above pertain to single health care organizations, such as an individual hospital. The concepts can also be applied to multiple facilities that operate under a common management structure forming an **integrated delivery network** (IDN). The two organizing dimensions, profession and program, are augmented in IDNs that offer different types of services along the continuum of patient care (e.g. hospitals, nursing homes). The Patient Protection and Affordable Care Act (ACA), the sweeping U.S. health care reform law enacted in 2010, established a particular type of IDN, known as the **accountable care organization** (ACO) for delivering patient care within the Medicare program. ACOs are intended to integrate different types of providers and facilities around common fiscal and clinical goals for a defined population of patients. Private-sector health plans have also developed payment models to encourage the formation of ACOs (Fisher et al., 2012).

In addition to having multiple facilities, IDNs may also cover multiple geographic regions, with each region comprising a full spectrum of health care organizations: hospitals, long-term care facilities, rehabilitation facilities, ambulatory care facilities, and home health agencies. A large IDN may have several regions and a regional hierarchical structure in which each facility is accountable to regional management. This allows for resource allocation that considers all of the needs in each region and a perspective that supersedes that of any single facility. This is important to minimize competition among facilities in each region and avoid unnecessary duplication of services. The regional management structure can also provide some coordination among facilities within each region, such as patient transfers among locations.

To augment coordination across facilities and geographic regions, IDNs can use lateral coordinating mechanisms similar to positions 3 through 6 in Figure 3.3. For example, they can establish a senior-level nurse executive to coordinate and set policy for professional practice and disseminate best practices across regions and facilities in the IDN. The nurse executive role can be augmented with task forces or teams, such as a systemwide nursing council, to discuss professional practice issues. Similarly, within a region, program managers can exert oversight for each clinical program, such as those discussed above (heart, cancer, women's health, etc.). This provides greater management focus on each program and helps to coordinate policy and resource allocation decisions from a regional perspective. It can also assist in disseminating best practices for each program across the facilities within each region. This can be done for the IDN as a whole as well as for each region, but the broader focus of the program manager will be a limiting factor in how much attention can be placed on operational, as contrasted with policy, issues. Some IDNs can choose to implement a matrix or program structure at the regional or IDN level; this requires using a program manager (position 3 on the continuum) or stronger integrating mechanism in each facility.

IDNs generally and ACOs specifically represent examples of macro-level organizational structures to promote coordination of patient care. They also create challenges as well as opportunities. Such structures may require complementary structures and mechanisms to coordinate care across facilities and geographic regions.

CENTRALIZATION AND DECENTRALIZATION

Within a given organizational structure, responsibilities and authority for various actions and decisions can be located at different vertical levels in the hierarchy as well as shared horizontally across departments. For example, hospital decisions on equipment purchases can be made by department managers or the C-suite (i.e., chief operating officer, chief executive officer, chief financial officer). They can be made by an individual or a committee. The degree to which decisions are made lower in the organization is referred to as vertical **decentralization**; the degree to which decisions are made at the higher levels of the organization is referred to as **centralization**. Some decisions may be centralized and others decentralized within the same organization. Department managers may make equipment purchases up to a fixed amount, while having to refer larger purchase decisions to higher levels. They may also have authority for hiring decisions but not for financial decisions (or vice versa).

In general, the important question to ask is whether decisions are being made at the organizational level at which the relevant information resides. In high-technology industries such as health care, greater decentralization is expected because of the expertise at lower levels in the organization. As a general rule, decisions should be made at the lowest possible levels, especially when the majority of workers are professionals. In addition, decentralization has positive benefits for motivation of lower-level managers: having authority to make decisions for their departments provides motivation to make those decisions wisely. Decentralization, however, reduces uniformity and standardization in the organization (e.g., in personnel policies and equipment purchases) as each unit can make its decisions independently of others. This can impact organizational performance. Thus, many organizations use a combination of centralization and decentralization, whereby units follow organization-wide policies but retain local authority in specific operating decisions.

In **program organization structures**, the full advantage of managing programs is achieved when decisions are decentralized to the program managers. This way, each program (or mini-hospital) has the overall responsibility for and perspective of its program and can set policy and make operational decisions most appropriate for its area. However, full decentralization of decision making contributes to greater variation in program policies and practices.

In multi-institutional systems (or IDNs), decisions can be centralized in the corporate office or decentralized to the regions or further to the individual operating organizations (hospitals, long-term care facilities, etc.). The organization is said to be vertically centralized when the majority of decisions are centered at the corporate office. An important design factor is deciding upon the extent to which individual operating units can develop their own strategic plans separately from those developed by the corporate office. Typically, major policies are determined at the corporate office to ensure uniformity across the whole system; by contrast, decisions concerning the direct delivery of care and implementation of policies are decentralized to local units.

PARALLEL ORGANIZATION

Parallel organization refers to a part of the organization structure that is parallel to and distinct from the main part of the organization. The concept is used in two different ways. First, a parallel structure of committees and task forces accountable to an oversight committee is often used for large change programs. In this case, the parallel organization is usually temporary but may last for several years. The task forces are drawn from multiple disciplines and often different levels in the organization to combine their perspectives while avoiding parochialism, self-interest, and differences in power and status. The structure seeks to facilitate openness, creativity, and problem solving for the purpose of organizational improvement. Second, parallel structures can arise from the addition of program managers through teams, as depicted by forms (3) through (6) on the continuum in Figure 3.3 (Charns and Tewksbury, 1993). More commonly, however, they are referred to as "integrating mechanisms."

HYBRID STRUCTURES

Another variation in structural designs is the **hybrid organization**. In this case, organizations maintain their traditional functional structures but create completely separate entities for one or two programs. For example, they may develop a freestanding heart center or cancer center (or both), each containing all key personnel required to provide those services. The advantage is the structure's focus on the activities of the freestanding center(s) and facilitation of coordination within each center, while also maintaining the advantages of the functional structure in the main part of the organization. The disadvantage is the barrier this structure introduces between each freestanding center and the rest of the organization.

The Electronic Health Record as a Coordinating Mechanism

The EHR has become a major mechanism to facilitate care coordination through its ability to transfer and store information, facilitate consultations and referrals among providers, report performance measures, and serve as a foundation for electronic care reminders, care pathways, patient registries, and dashboards to monitor care. The EHR can facilitate asynchronous communication but, as compared to other coordinating mechanisms, cannot easily facilitate bidirectional communication. Starting in 2009, the federal government spent billions of dollars in incentive payments to providers to encourage the adoption and use of EHRs. To qualify for these payments, physicians had to demonstrate they were using the EHRs to meet established criteria pertaining to the effective management of patient care ("meaningful use"). While physician adoption of EHRs has increased substantially due to the incentive program, the extent to which the technology has helped to improve patient care is less understood (DesRoches et al., 2013; The Office of the National Coordinator for Health Information Technology, 2017).

Physical Proximity to Facilitate Coordination

As noted above, physical proximity also facilitates coordination. People who work in different departments, units, or service lines often are in physically separate locations, on different floors, wings, or buildings. Some organizations consciously use physical proximity to bridge the gaps among people with the highest interdependence. A prime example of this is placing a mental health professional within the primary care unit. The physical proximity promotes easy access to each other and also facilitates coordination by encouraging the development of working relationships, trust, and effective information exchange. Such access allows for "warm handoffs" in patient referrals from the primary care provider personally introducing the patient to the mental health professional. This increases the likelihood that the patient will obtain mental health care. (Patients oftentimes do not keep appointments for mental health referrals.)

ORGANIZATIONS WITH MULTIPLE GOALS

The literature on organization structure has been developed primarily in industrial organizations whose primary goal is to effectively and efficiently produce products or services. While the organization design problem is more complex in multiproduct compared to single-product firms, the goals of effectiveness and efficiency remain the same. Health care organizations, however, often have the multiple goals of patient care, research, and education. Designing a structure to meet one of these goals often conflicts with designs to meet others. Using teaching hospitals as their primary example, Stoelwinder and Charns (1981) noted that organizing for patient care would result in segmenting the organization into multidisciplinary units, each aligned with a disease or patient population (i.e., a program structure). By contrast, organizing to maintain state-of-the-art competence in each profession and discipline and to recruit and develop new members of each profession and discipline would result in an organization segmented into discipline-based units. Note that the discipline-based organization structure places greatest emphasis on differentiation (as shown on the left in Figure 3.3), while the program organization structure

emphasizes integration (coordination) across professions and disciplines in the delivery of care (as shown on the right in Figure 3.3). Such conflicts among goals and organization designs are often resolved by the differential power among different stakeholders. Optimally, the organization design supports the organization's strategy, while goals that are not well addressed by the chosen structure are met using integrating mechanisms that cut across different interdependent units.

GOVERNANCE AND THE THREE-LEGGED STOOL OF ADMINISTRATION, MEDICAL STAFF, AND THE BOARD

Hospitals also differ from other types of organizations because of the unique position of their medical staffs. Whereas professionals in other types of organizations are typically employed by the organizations, such is not the case in most hospitals. In community hospitals, physicians are organized into a voluntary medical staff, governed by bylaws and rules and regulations, and coordinated through a set of committees. All other hospital personnel are organized hierarchically within clinical and administrative units. The coexistence of separate lines of authority for hospital administration and the medical staff has long been a distinguishing feature of community hospitals. The medical staff is ultimately accountable to the board of trustees, as is the chief executive officer (CEO) and other hospital staff who report to the CEO. Throughout much of the twentieth century, this type of **governance** structure was quite viable for community hospitals, as the reimbursement and competitive environment generally imposed few pressures for greater integration between hospital and medical staff leadership. However, during the last 30 years, significant changes in reimbursement policies and market competition forced hospitals to develop stronger linkages between administration and the medical staff, starting with placing medical staff members on the hospital governing board (Young, 1997). A recent study of three community hospitals having different medical staff arrangements found greater coordination and patient-centered care when the medical staff was more highly engaged in the hospital (Louis et al, 2017).

Traditionally, there have been stronger linkages between medical staff and hospital administration in academic health centers than has been the case with community hospitals. In most academic health centers, the full-time medical staff are faculty of the affiliated medical school and may be salaried employees of the medical school or faculty practice plan, having clinical privileges only at that hospital.

MICRO-LEVEL COORDINATION

The macro-level approaches to coordination discussed above provide the infrastructure for achieving coordination, but it is the micro-level processes through which coordination actually is achieved. In analyzing micro-level needs for coordination, it is helpful first to ask whether the work is programmable work. That is, can specific activities be detailed and assigned to different individuals and groups so that if each piece is performed correctly and according to plan, different people's and units' efforts will mesh together? If so, then the work is programmable. Tasks having inherently high uncertainty, where one cannot fully anticipate the events that might possibly occur, do not lend themselves completely to detailed rules and procedures and are largely not programmable. Neither are tasks for which relationships between causes and effects are not well understood. Examples of unprogrammable work are providers attempting to diagnose a rare disease, developing research hypotheses, and designing programs for educating the public in new health practices.

The second question to ask in assessing micro-level needs for coordination is how familiar the people involved are with a particular action or decision. What is familiar to an experienced worker may be unfamiliar to an inexperienced one. Familiarity with an issue affects understanding of cause-and-effect relationships and how to perform required activities, as well as the chances for successful task completion. For example, familiarity with a patient's problem affects the clinician's understanding of the antecedents and consequences when treating that problem. This, along with a facility with specified clinical technical interventions, enhances the likelihood of successful task completion (e.g., treatment of the patient) (Radwin, 1998). For example, although an appendectomy is a fairly programmable surgical task, coordination among surgical team members who have never performed this procedure would be more complicated than for an experienced team. Familiarity with an issue may also be more than just years of experience performing a particular service or procedure. A recent study examining coordination found that physicians involved in preoperative surgical care lacked familiarity with the perspectives and expectations of patients regarding the process (Malley and Young, 2017). Clearly, providers' familiarity with the clinical issue should extend to an appreciation of patients' needs and desires.

Research on the micro-level coordination of work has shown that coordination affects organizational performance in health care and other settings (e.g., Argote, 1982; Duncan, 1973; Georgopoulis and Mann, 1962; Shortell et al., 1994; Van de Ven and Delbecq, 1974). Knaus et al. (1986) reported a strong association between coordination and mortality in critical care units. Similarly, Young et al. (1998) found a relationship between the pattern of coordination among nurses, surgeons, and anesthesiologists and risk-adjusted rates of postsurgical complications. In addition to clinical outcomes, some studies have found a link between coordination and outcomes such as greater patient satisfaction and shorter lengths of stay (Gittell, 2016; Gittell et al., 2000; Ovretveit, 2011). These performance outcomes are increasingly relevant in a more cost-conscious and patient-centered health care environment.

Research also shows that the most effective way to achieve coordination varies with the characteristics of the work performed, primarily its certainty or uncertainty. In one of the first empirical studies of variation in coordination within work units, Duncan (1972) found that work units change their patterns of interaction in response to differing levels of task uncertainty. Building upon the theoretical work of March and Simon (1958), Van de Ven and Delbecq (1974) found variations in patterns of coordination among units facing different levels of task uncertainty. For example, clinicians in an emergency department generally have more uncertainty in their work than clinicians on a routine surgery unit, thereby requiring greater coordination of their efforts.

Charns et al. (1981) and Charns and Schaefer (1983) extended the findings of Van de Ven and Delbecq (1974) and the theoretical writings of Mintzberg (1979) to suggest that work groups use two primary approaches to coordination: **programming** and **feedback**. Young et al. (1998) found that the joint use of these approaches was related to the patient outcomes of postsurgical complications.

DEBATE TIME: Service Lines

Many health care leaders are proponents of service line organization structures. What are the reasons why hospitals should adopt a service line structure? What are the reasons why hospitals should organize by a functional structure? When do you think task force and team structures, augmenting the functional structure, are most appropriate?

Programming Approaches to Coordination

Programming approaches to coordination include three ways of standardizing the performance of work that are most effective when the work is well understood and programmable. These approaches may also be called "standardized approaches."

Standardization of work encompasses the use of rules, regulations, schedules, plans, procedures, policies, and protocols to specify the activities to be performed. Also included are care plans and multidisciplinary clinical critical paths, which specify for any particular patient condition the interventions required and anticipated results at various times. Although the literatures on coordination and quality improvement have developed separately from each other, "standardized work" is also a central concept in quality improvement.

Standardization of skills is the specification of the training or skills required to perform work. This is often achieved through specification of minimum levels and types of education, certification as evidence of meeting minimum qualifications, or on-the-job training.

Standardization of output specifies either the form of or specifications for intermediate outcomes of work as they are passed from one job or unit to another. It can also set specifications and goals for the service or product being provided.

Feedback Approaches to Coordination

In situations of high uncertainty, programming approaches alone cannot provide the needed coordination. Exchange of information and feedback is needed. Feedback approaches to coordination (also called "personal approaches"), which facilitate the transfer of information in unfamiliar situations, include the following:

Supervision is the basis for coordination through an organization's hierarchy. It is the exchange of information between two people, one of whom is responsible for the work of the other.

Mutual adjustment is the exchange of information about work performance between two people who are not in a hierarchical relationship, such as between two nurses, between a nurse and a physician, or between a case manager and other care providers.

Group coordination is the exchange of information among more than two people, such as through meetings, rounds, and conferences.

Feedback approaches to coordination are more time-consuming and require more effort than programming approaches. However, they are needed to achieve effective decisions and actions in situations characterized by high levels of uncertainty.

Evidence indicates that higher-performing patient care units in teaching hospitals differ from lower-performing units in their greater use of all six types of coordinating mechanisms (Charns et al., 1981; Young et al., 1998). High-performing units utilize plans, rules, procedures, and protocols not as constraints and organizational "red tape" but as guidelines for routine work. Contrary to earlier writings, effective use of programming approaches actually allows staff—especially nurses—greater discretion in their work.

Often, new roles (a macro-coordination approach discussed above) are created in health care organizations to facilitate coordination. Such roles rely upon both programming and feedback approaches to achieve coordination at the micro level. Case management is one example. There has been an explosion of case-management (sometimes called "care management") personnel, employed by hospitals, accountable care organizations, and physician groups. Case managers use both predetermined plans for guiding their work (programming) and interpersonal contacts with other providers and organizations (feedback) to improve care coordination. Case managers play the role of "boundary spanners," helping to facilitate handoffs and helping the patient negotiate the boundaries between different members of the care provider team. Like boundary spanners, case managers also play an information-processing role within organizations (Galbraith, 1977) and between organizations (Aldrich and Herker, 1977) during transitions in care. Organizational scholars have learned that boundary spanners are most successful when they not only process information but also read contextual clues (Tushman and Scanlan, 1981), build trust (Currall and Judge, 1995), and build shared goals, shared knowledge, and mutual respect across boundaries (Gittell, 2002). However, to play these multiple roles effectively requires both technical expertise and time. Research in both the airline and health care industries shows that case managers are more effective in coordinating work when they are responsible for a relatively small number of flights (Gittell, 2003) or patients (Gittell, 2002). Smaller caseloads for case managers can allow other participants to use their time more efficiently, therefore reducing overall resource utilization.

Similarly, one programming approach that is quite prevalent—clinical pathways (Bohmer, 1998)—has the potential to increase the quality of communication and working relationships, rather than replace the need for them, as earlier theory would have predicted. Clinical pathways that included greater numbers of the relevant clinical functions led to higher levels of relational coordination among clinical staff as well as higher-quality and more efficient surgical outcomes (Gittell, 2002). Even in the high-velocity environment of trauma units, programming using protocols plays an important role in the coordination of care (Faraj and Xiao, 2006). Like clinical pathways that are used for surgical patients, these protocols take the form of a standard operating procedure whereby roles, decision points, and event sequences are specified. These programming approaches appear to improve coordination across different members of the patient care team even when actions cannot be fully specified in advance, because they provide a shared cognitive framework of the task. Both studies show, however, that programming approaches do not diminish the need for informal, feedback forms of coordination. Rather, they provide a context within which feedback forms of coordination can more effectively occur.

In addition, when faced with unfamiliar situations, high-performing units increase their use of feedback approaches to a greater extent than low-performing ones. This result is consistent with findings from an earlier study of emergency rooms that nonprogrammed approaches to coordination were more effective under conditions of high uncertainty (Argote, 1982). Other feedback approaches help to improve coordination and patient outcomes. For example, in a study of joint replacement surgery, more inclusive team meetings predicted higher levels of coordination among clinical staff as well as more efficient and higher-quality patient outcomes (Gittell, 2002).

Taken together with the findings about clinical pathways, these findings suggest that even relatively straightforward procedures benefit from using feedback approaches in addition to programming approaches. Consistent with previous findings, feedback approaches to coordination have an even stronger impact on outcomes as the uncertainty in patient conditions increases. Considering that what is familiar work to one person may not be familiar to another, some hospitals recognize that mentoring is needed until staff are familiar with the standard procedures. A positive example of this is the use of experienced nurses to mentor junior nursing staff. A negative example is to cover staffing shortages by moving an inexperienced nurse from one unit to another unit where she or he does not know the standard procedures. Feedback and programming approaches to coordination can both be designed to strengthen working relationships, but there are many practices in health care organizations that work in the opposite direction. Nursing staff turnover and rotation, house staff rotation, and limited involvement by physicians and other professionals in patient care units or outpatient clinics greatly hinder the development of such relationships and can prevent full use of feedback approaches to coordination. Working relationships are also undermined by the professional identities of health care workers (Abbott, 1988) and by the occupational communities that tend to grow up around those professional identities (Van Maanen and Barley, 1984). Coordinating mechanisms, as discussed in the section on macro-level coordination above, can be used to counteract these divisive tendencies and to strengthen key working relationships.

Job design also exerts large, significant effects on patient outcomes and coordination between physicians and other clinicians (Gittell et al., 2008). The physician job of hospitalists (physicians who specialize in hospital-based care) provides them the opportunity to focus on the delivery of acute care and to become familiar with the staff and routines of a particular hospital. This specialization contributes to quality of care and coordination with other hospital staff. The use of hospitalists does, however, fragment the care of patients between the hospital and primary care providers in ambulatory care settings, thus creating a different coordination challenge.

To summarize, coordination affects both quality and efficiency in organizational performance. The types of coordinating approaches that can be used effectively depend somewhat upon the nature of the work performed. Greater advantage can be taken of programming approaches when the unit's work is limited in scope and uncertainty, though even then programming appears to work better in tandem with feedback approaches. Similarly, programming approaches complement, but do not replace, feedback approaches in situations of higher uncertainty. It should be noted that people with greater experience in a particular job will encounter fewer unfamiliar situations than people with less experience. Those with less experience, therefore, need to use feedback approaches to a greater extent than do highly experienced people. This is typically reflected in their greater reliance on discussions with managers, peers, or mentors. Finally, feedback approaches require trust and understanding among people, which in turn requires organizational practices such as consistency in working together, conflict-resolution processes, or selection of staff members skilled at teamwork.

Relational Coordination

Another perspective has emerged in recent years, called **relational coordination**, which captures aspects of both the programming and feedback approaches to coordination. Relational coordination encompasses technical concerns with information flow and task interdependence as well as psychosocial concerns with relational interdependence (or the quality of working relationships). Coordination is not seen as a mechanical process of information exchange but rather as a relational process involving a network of communication and relationship ties among people whose tasks are interdependent (Faraj and Xiao, 2006; Gittell, 2002, 2016; Weick and Roberts, 1993).

Relational coordination takes account not only of the work itself but also the process of people working together and its affective aspects. Relational coordination is comprised of two interacting components: **relationships** and **communication**. Ideal relationships can be seen as consisting of shared goals, shared knowledge, and mutual respect. Communication can be viewed in terms of its frequency, timeliness, accuracy, and focus on problem solving. Relational coordination tends to be weakest among people who carry out different jobs in the same work process, especially when those people are part of different work units and have different professional backgrounds. This includes the work of doctors, nurses, and social workers, reflecting the earlier discussion of differentiation at the macro level. Effective coordination across disciplines in health care is most critical to delivery of effective care, yet is most challenging to achieve. To achieve the quality and efficiency outcomes that health care organizations strive for, managers must invest in relationships where they are hardest to build—where work is highly interconnected among people with distinct, competing professional identities.

Relational coordination, programming, and feedback approaches are complementary ways of looking at coordination at the micro level. Some scholars argue that relational coordination provides in-depth detail to the feedback approach to coordination. Other scholars argue that programming and feedback are mechanisms to achieve relational coordination (in their view, the overarching concept regarding coordination at the micro level). Both conceptual frameworks have found strong relationships with clinical outcomes, task performance, staff satisfaction, and motivation.

The Electronic Health Record as a Micro-Level Coordinating Mechanism

If used effectively, the EHR contributes to coordination by facilitating communication and providing the platform for standardizing work. Examples of how the EHR facilitates programming/standardized approaches to coordination include (a) computerized physician order entry (CPOE), which standardizes prescribing of medications through predefined criteria for selection of medications and dosages, and checks for conflicting medications; (b) the use of electronic reminders for tests and preventive care (e.g., flu vaccinations); and (c) the use of guidelines. It facilitates communication by making patient information available to different providers (as long as they have access to the system and interoperability is present). The use of electronic consults (e-consults) provides for direct exchange of information, typically between primary care and specialty care. Finally, having a patient portal to the system allows for information exchange between patients and providers.

The AHRQ Atlas of Coordination

The Agency for Healthcare Quality and Research (AHRQ) has spent considerable effort in developing an atlas of measures "for assessing care coordination interventions in research studies and demonstration projects" (McDonald et al., 2014). According to the Atlas, "Care coordination is the deliberate organization of patient care activities between two or more participants (including the patient) involved in a patient's care to facilitate the appropriate delivery of health services" (p. 6).

The Atlas also notes that "care coordination means different things to different people; no consensus definition has fully evolved" (p. 6). The Atlas places emphasis on coordination in transitions in care (Snow et al., 2009), as they note, "Ultimately, this Atlas reflects an understanding of care coordination that occurs most often during and in response to care transitions (e.g., transitions across settings, within care teams, among care participants, between encounters or care episodes, as patient needs change). And that involves activities or approaches that bridge gaps arising from those transitions" (p. 6). Using the terminology of this chapter, transitions represent specific situations, typically characterized by high interdependence among providers or among organizations, that therefore require coordination.

The Atlas provides two constructs for understanding the mechanisms by which care is coordinated. One construct comprises "clinician activities" such as communicating, designating accountability, facilitating transitions, and linking to resources. Most of these can be seen through the lens of feedback approaches to coordination. The second construct is "continuity of care," which is further classified as informational continuity, relational continuity (both of these are feedback approaches), and management continuity of the patient by sharing and agreeing on plans for treatment (standardization of output).

Conceptual clarity may be needed here since the Atlas does not necessarily differentiate patient-centered care from care coordination. One solution is to view patient-centered care as both an antecedent and a consequence of care coordination. For example, a patient may enjoy highly patient-centric primary care. Well-coordinated care is required to maintain that high level when a patient is admitted to the hospital (cf., Radwin et al., 2016).

In sum, the Atlas provides a different but complementary perspective on care coordination (e.g., through its emphasis on care transitions) and provides two constructs that are asserted to affect coordination. This chapter is largely based on the organizational literature that has been studied in health care settings and provides a theoretical lens through which to view the Atlas. The Atlas and the subsequent research it stimulates in measure development may help to advance our study and understanding of care coordination.

• • • IN PRACTICE: The Veterans Healthcare System

The Veterans Healthcare System (formally, the Veterans Health Administration, VHA), the largest fully integrated health care system in the United States, began a redesign effort in 1995 (Kizer, 1999; Young, 2000). The overall goal in redesigning was to systematize quality management (QM) to ensure the provision of consistent and predictable high-quality care and access by patients to the entire system. The decision to redesign the organization structure of the VHA came about for a number of reasons, including pressures from the external environment such as the market-based restructuring of health care in general, growth of scientific and biomedical knowledge, general dissatisfaction with health care (especially VHA), consumer expectations for quality, and many managerial and operational problems.

Because of these factors, the VHA embarked on an ambitious process to redesign the health system in order to improve effectiveness and efficiency in day-to-day operations and bring about a quality transformation. During 1994 and 1995, various planning efforts and consensus-building activities were carried out to design and begin to implement a new operating structure. Prior to the redesign, VHA had 172 hospitals and four regions. Approximately 40 to 45 hospitals were accountable to each regional manager. The large span of control in each region allowed the hospitals to function relatively autonomously, with a high degree of decentralization of operations within the system and a low level of supervision and actual accountability. Resources were allocated to hospitals based on the amount of services provided in previous years. The hospitals competed with each other for resources and had a duplication of services in facilities located close to each other.

The structure changed the basic operating unit within the system from individual hospitals and medical centers to 22 regional networks called Veterans Integrated Service Networks (VISNs). Funding of operations was then allocated to VISNs on the basis of their populations, and care patterns began to shift away from acute hospitals. Decisions were centralized from the hospitals to the regions, and simultaneously they were decentralized from headquarters in Washington, D.C., to the regions. These changes were a fundamental shift from the VHA's former disease-oriented, hospital-based, and professional discipline-based paradigms to ones that are patient-centered, prevention-oriented, community-based, and premised on universal primary care. In the new system, multidisciplinary teams had shared responsibility and accountability for patient care.

Results

Results suggest that VHAs transformation contributed to a remarkable level of achievement. Between 1994 and 1998 (approximately), some of the successes were the following:

- Fifty-two percent (27,319 of 52,315) of all VHA acute-care hospital beds were closed.

- VHA's bed-days of care per 1,000 patients decreased 62 percent. The current VHA rate is now about 5 percent lower than the projected Medicare rate for the same time period.

- Universal primary care has been implemented, and by March 1998, 80 percent of patients could identify their primary caregiver.

- Annual inpatient admissions were 32 percent (284,596), while ambulatory care visits per year increased 43 percent (from 25.0 million to 35.8 million per year).

- The management and operation of 50 hospitals has been merged into 24 locally integrated health care systems.

- By 2010, nearly 800 new community-based outpatient clinics were established to improve access to care. The clinics were funded from redirected savings—that is, no "new" funds have been provided for these clinics.

- Surgeries performed on an outpatient basis increased from 35 percent to 75 percent of all surgeries. This change was accompanied by increased surgical productivity and reduced mortality.

- Systemwide staffing was decreased by 11 percent (23,112 of 206,578 full-time employee equivalents), whereas the number of patients treated per year increased by 18 percent. This included 8 percent more psychiatric/substance-abuse treatment patients, 19 percent more homeless patients, and 53 percent more blind rehabilitation patients.

- Telephone-linked care ("call centers") has been implemented at all VA medical centers as well as temporary lodging ("hotel") beds.

- Over 2,700 VHA forms were eliminated (67 percent of the total), and all remaining forms and directives were put into electronic form.

- A pharmacy benefits management program has produced an estimated cumulative savings of $347 million.

• • • IN PRACTICE: The Veterans Healthcare System (Continued)

Jha et al. (2003) reported on an assessment of changes in quality-of-care indicators at VHA from 1994 through 2000 and compared these results for the VHA with the quality of care afforded by the Medicare fee-for-service system using the same quality indicators. Results showed VA patients were receiving appropriate care at 90 percent or greater for 9 of 17 quality indicators. Quality indicators exceeded those for not only the average community hospital but also the average academic health center.

In addition, VHA had implemented the following:

- A national medication administration system (bar coding for medication administration)
- A national electronic medical record
- Computerized drug interaction system
- Computerized physician order entry

These findings suggest that changing an organizational design that matches the characteristics of the external and internal environments and is in keeping with the vision and missions of the organization can increase the outcomes of the organization in terms of quality of services.

SUMMARY AND MANAGERIAL GUIDELINES

1. Organization design is a key factor in affecting behavior, and thus outcomes, of organizations. It operates in several ways. These include focusing people's attention on the work and goals of their units to the relative exclusion of work and goals of other units and facilitating coordination among people in the same unit, while hindering coordination of work across units.

2. All organization designs have both beneficial and dysfunctional characteristics. The functional structure yields benefits of specialization by profession and medical specialties and subspecialties, contributing to high levels of competence and professional development in each profession individually. This structure, however, impedes coordination among different professions. To address the needs for coordination across departments, structural integrating mechanisms can be used.

3. Program structures provide the strongest structures for integrating across professions within each program, but they have the dysfunctional characteristic of a lesser focus on professional specialization and professional development. In addition, the program structure hinders coordination across programs. With a large number of possible ways to structure an organization, it is important to choose a structure that is the best fit for a given organization's purpose and strategy.

4. Within the context of an organization's structure, micro-level process and mechanisms of coordination can facilitate the achievement of coordination.

5. Programming approaches to coordination can be used best when work is predictable and cause-and-effect relationships are well known.

6. Feedback approaches, which rely upon the relationships among people, are most needed when the work is relatively uncertain.

7. Since much clinical work is highly uncertain but much is also predictable and routine, a combination of programming and feedback approaches to coordination yields more effective and efficient delivery of care.

DISCUSSION QUESTIONS

1. In the tale of two units, Unit B functioned much more smoothly that Unit A. Identify the macro-level coordination mechanisms being used in Unit B that were not used in Unit A. What is the nature of task interdependence among staff in the patient care units in the "tale of two units"?

2. Identify the micro-level coordination mechanisms used in Unit B that were not used in Unit A.

3. In the VA case study, reorganizing this integrated delivery system into regional networks (VISNs) and decentralizing authority to the VISN directors seemed to have contributed to a substantial improvement in organization performance. What are the negative aspects of the reorganized structure and decentralization?

4. Describe alternatives for a service line structure internal to each VISN in the VA case.

5. Why is the hierarchical structure limited in its capability to facilitate coordination in health care organizations?

CASE

The vice president for patient care services (VP-PCS) and the vice president for medical affairs (VP-MA) at Northeast Medical Center (NMC) were very concerned about coordination between medicine and nursing in the inpatient medical/surgical units. NMC was a large tertiary-care teaching hospital, affiliated with the Northeast Schools of Medicine (NSOM) and Nursing (NSON). NMC participated in a joint residency program with three other hospitals affiliated with NSOM. Most residents spent six weeks at NMC.

The VPs had observed that coordination sharply decreased after restrictions on resident hours were implemented. The VP-PCS noted, "The residents rotate through our hospital so quickly that the nurses hardly get to know their names, much less establish a working relationship." The VPs also observed that handoffs of patients from one resident team to another were problematic and had become more so, they believed, as a result of the shorter shifts worked by the residents.

The VP-MA suggested expanding NMC's hospitalist program to address the coordination problems. He argued that hospitalists would provide a consistent medical coverage that would compensate for what he called "fragmented" coverage by residents. However, the chief of medicine was opposed to this proposal. He argued that it would negatively affect the educational experience of residents by reducing their responsibilities. He was backed in this argument by the chairman of medicine at NSOM. As was common in academic centers, the chief of medicine reported to the VP-MA at NMC and also to the chairman of medicine at NSOM.

Questions

1. Is it consistent with organizational theory to expect that coordination between nurses and residents would suffer as a result of the change in resident working hours?

2. Would the addition of hospitalists improve coordination?

3. What other changes could improve coordination?

4. What are counterarguments to the position held by the chief of medicine and chairman of medicine that the hospitalists would negatively affect the educational experience of residents?

REFERENCES

Abbott, A. (1988). *The system of professions: An essay on the division of expert labor*. Chicago, IL: University of Chicago Press.

Aldrich, H., & Herker, D. (1977). Boundary spanning roles and organization structure. *Academy of Management Review, 2*(2), 217–230.

Argote, L. (1982). Input uncertainty and organizational coordination in hospital emergency units. *Administrative Science Quarterly, 27*, 420–434.

Bohmer, R. (1998). Critical pathways at Massachusetts General Hospital. *Journal of Vascular Surgery, 28*, 373–377.

Burns, T., & Stalker, G. M. (1961). *The management of innovation*. London: Tavistock.

Byrne, M., Charns, M. P., Parker, V. A., et al. (2004). The effects of organization on medical utilization: An analysis of service line organization. *Medical Care, 42*(1), 28–37.

Charns, M. P., & Schaefer, M. J. (1983). *Health care organizations: A model for management*. Englewood Cliffs, NJ: Prentice-Hall.

Charns, M. P., & Tewksbury, L. S. (1993). *Collaborative management in health care: Implementing the integrative organization*. San Francisco, CA: Jossey-Bass.

Charns, M. P., Stoelwinder, J. U., Miller, R. A., et al. (1981). *Coordination and patient unit effectiveness*. Academy of Management Annual Meetings, San Diego, CA.

Currall, S. C., & Judge, T. A. (1995). Measuring trust between organizational boundary role persons. *Organizational Behavior and Human Decision Processes, 64*(2), 151–170.

DesRoches, C. M., Audet, A. Painter, M., et al. (2013). Meeting meaningful use criteria and managing patient populations. *Annals of Internal Medicine, 158*, 791–799.

Duncan, R. B. (1972). Characteristics of organizational environments and perceived environmental uncertainty. *Administrative Science Quarterly, 17*, 313–327.

Duncan, R. B. (1973). Multiple decision-making structures in adapting to environmental uncertainty: The impact on organizational effectiveness. *Human Relations, 26*(3), 273–291.

Faraj, S., & Xiao, Y. (2006). Coordination in fast response organizations. *Management Science, 52*(8), 1155–1169.

Fisher, E. S., Shortell, S. M., Kreindler, S. A., et al. (2012). A framework for evaluating the formation, implementation and performance of accountable care organizations. *Health Affairs, 31*(11), 2368–2378.

Galbraith, J. R. (1973). *Designing complex organizations*. Reading, MA: Addison-Wesley.

Galbraith, J. R. (1977). *Organization design*. Reading, MA: Addison-Wesley.

Gawande, A. (2010). *The checklist manifesto (HB)*. India: Penguin Books.

Georgopoulis, B. S., & Mann, F. C. (1962). *The community general hospital*. New York: Macmillan.

Gittell, J. H. (2002). Coordinating mechanisms in care provider groups: Relational coordination as a mediator and input uncertainty as a moderator of performance effects. *Management Science, 48*(11), 1408–1426.

Gittell, J. H. (2003). *The Southwest Airlines way: Using the power of relationships to achieve high performance*. New York: McGraw-Hill.

Gittell, J. H. (2016). *Transforming relationships for high performance: The power of relational coordination*. Stanford, CA: Stanford University Press.

Gittell, J. H., Fairfield, K., Bierbaum, B., et al. (2000). Impact of relational coordination on quality of care, post-operative pain and functioning, and length of stay: A nine hospital study of surgical patients. *Medical Care, 38*(8), 807–819.

Gittell, J. H., Weinberg, D., Bennett, A., et al. (2008). Is the doctor in? A relational approach to job design and the coordination of work. *Human Resource Management, 47*(4), 729–755.

Greenberg, G., Rosenheck, R. A., & Charns, M. P. (2003). From professional dominance to service line management in the Veterans Health Administration: Impact on mental health care. *Medical Care, 41*(9), 1013–1023.

Haynes, A. B., Weiser, T. G., Berry, W. R., et al. (2009). A surgical safety checklist to reduce morbidity and mortality in a global population. *New England Journal of Medicine, 360*(5), 491–499.

Hoff, T. J., Sutcliffe, K. M., & Young, G. J. (Eds.). (2016). *The healthcare professional workforce: Understanding human capital in a changing industry*, Chapter 1. New York: Oxford University Press

Jha, A. K., Perlin, J. B., Kizer, K. W., et al. (2003). Effect of the transformation of the Veterans Affairs Health Care System on the quality of care. *New England Journal of Medicine, 348*(22), 2218–2227.

Kizer, K. W. (1999). The "new VA": A national laboratory for health care quality management. *American Journal of Medical Quality, 14*(1), 3–20.

Knaus, W. A., Draper, E. A., Wagner, D. P., et al. (1986). An evaluation of outcome from intensive care in major medical centers. *Annals of Internal Medicine, 104*, 416–418.

Lawrence, P. R., & Lorsch, J. W. (1967). *Organization and environment: Managing differentiation and integration*. Boston, MA: Division of Research, Harvard Business School.

Louis, C. J., Clark, J. R., Gray, B., et al. (2017, June 15). Service line structure and decision-maker attention in three health systems: Implications for patient-centered care. *Health Care Management Review*.

Malley, A. M., & Young, G. J. (2017). A qualitative study of patient and provider experiences during preoperative care transitions. *Journal of Clinical Nursing, 26*(13–14), 2016–2024.

March, J. F., & Simon, H. A. (1958). *Organizations*. New York: John Wiley & Sons.

McDonald, K. M., Schultz, E., Albin, L., et al. (2014). *Care coordination measures Atlas update*. Rockville, MD: Agency for Healthcare Research and Quality. Retrieved from http://www.ahrq.gov/professionals/prevention-chronic-care/improve/coordination/atlas2014/index.html. Content last reviewed June 2014.

Miller, E. J., & Rice, A. K. (1967). *Systems of organization*. London: Tavistock.

Mintzberg, H. (1979). *The structuring of organizations*. Englewood Cliffs, NJ: Prentice-Hall.

Ovretveit, J. (2011). *Does clinical coordination improve quality and save money?* London: The Health Foundation.

Perrow, C. B. (1967). A framework for the comparative analysis of organizations. *American Sociological Review, 32*(2), 194–208.

Perrow, C. B. (1972). *Complex organizations: A critical essay*. Glenview, IL: Scott, Foresman.

Porter, M. E. & Lee, T. H. (2018). What 21st century health care should learn from 20th century business. *New England Journal of Medicine Catalyst*. September 5, 2018.

Radwin, L. (1998). Empirically generated attributes of experience in nursing. *Journal of Advanced Nursing, 27*, 590–595.

Radwin, L. E., Castonguay, D., Keenan, C. B., et al. (2016). An expanded theoretical framework of care coordination across transitions in care settings. *Journal of nursing care quality, 31*(3), 269–274.

Shortell, S. M., Zimmerman, J., Rousseau, D., et al. (1994). The performance of intensive care units: Does good management make a difference? *Medical Care, 32*(5), 508–525.

Snow, V, Beck, D, Budnitz, T., et al. (2009). Transitions of care consensus policy statement: American College of Physicians, Society of General Internal Medicine, Society of Hospital Medicine, American Geriatrics Society, American College of Emergency Physicians. *Journal of Hospital Medicine, 4*(6), 364–370.

Stoelwinder, J. U., & Charns, M. P. (1981). A task field model of organization design and analysis. *Human Relations, 34*(9), 743–762.

The Office of the National Coordinator for Health Information Technology, Health IT Dashboard. (2017). Retrieved July 21, 2017, from https://dashboard.healthit.gov/quickstats/pages/physician-ehr-adoption-trends.php.

Thompson, J. D. (1967). *Organizations in action*. New York: McGraw-Hill.

Tushman, M. L., & Scanlan, T. J. (1981). Characteristics and external orientations of boundary spanning individuals. *Academy of Management Journal, 24*(1), 83–98.

Van de Ven, A. H., & Delbecq, A. L. (1974). A task contingent model of work unit structure. *Administrative Science Quarterly, 19*(2), 183–197.

Van Maanen, J., & Barley, S. R. (1984). Occupational communities: Culture and control in organizations. *Research in Organizational Behavior, 6*, 287–365.

Weick, K. E., & Roberts, K. (1993). Collective mind in organizations: Heedful interrelating on flight decks. *Administrative Science Quarterly, 38*, 357–381.

Woodward, J. (1965). *Industrial organization: Theory and practice*. London: Oxford University Press.

Young. G. (1997). Insider representation on the governing boards of nonprofit hospitals: Trends and implications for charitable care. *Inquiry, 33*, 352–362.

Young, G. (2000). Managing organizational transformations: Lessons from the Veterans Health Administration. *California Management Review, 43*(1), 66–82.

Young, G., Charns, M., & Hereen, T. (1994). Product line management and employee assessments of their work environments: A study of hospitals. *Academy of Management Journal, 47*(5), 723–734.

Young, G., Charns, M., Desai, K., et al. (1998). Patterns of coordination and clinical outcomes: A study of surgical services. *Health Services Research, 33*(5), 1211–1236.

Chapter 4

Motivating People

Thomas D'Aunno, Mattia Gilmartin, and Sumit Kumar

CHAPTER OUTLINE

- Motivation and Management
- The What and How of Motivation
- Process Perspectives
- Motivating Health Care Professionals
- Motivational Problems

LEARNING OBJECTIVES

After completing this chapter, the reader should be able to:

1. Define motivation and distinguish it from other factors that influence individuals' performance
2. Recognize popular but misleading myths about motivation
3. Discuss how motivation depends heavily on the situations in which individuals work
4. Explain managers' roles in motivating individuals
5. Identify key characteristics of individuals and their work that motivate them
6. Identify important processes involved in motivating individuals
7. Discuss how to deal with motivational problems

KEY TERMS

Empowerment

Expectancy

Fairness

Feedback

Goal Setting

Intrinsic Motivation

Job Redesign

Motivation

Pay-for-Performance

CHAPTER PURPOSE

This chapter aims to develop readers' ability to effectively motivate individuals, including subordinates and coworkers, in health care organizations. The chapter consists of four major sections. First, we define motivation, distinguish it from other factors that can affect individuals' performance, and describe common myths about motivation. The second section identifies several important factors that managers can influence to improve or maintain individuals' motivation. The third section discusses motivational issues that are particular to specific professional groups, particularly physicians and nurses. Last, we examine common motivational problems and discuss how to deal with them.

The principles and practices of motivation that we describe in this chapter are excellent tools for ensuring that health care organizations' most expensive resources, staff members, are also the most valuable assets. Empirical evidence indicates that human resource practices, such as those that improve motivation, can positively influence an organization's performance, including its financial performance (Noe et al., 2006; Pfeffer, 1998). Consequently, a highly motivated workforce can serve as a difficult-to-replicate competitive advantage.

MOTIVATION AND MANAGEMENT

Defining and Distinguishing Motivation

We define **motivation** as a state of feeling or thinking in which one is energized or aroused to perform a task or engage in a particular behavior (Kanfer, Chen, and Pritchard, 2008). This definition focuses on motivation as an emotional or cognitive state that is independent of action. This focus clearly distinguishes motivation from the performance of a task and its consequences. Notice, too, that motivation can be a state of either feeling or thinking, or a combination of the two.

Myths about Motivation—And Some Antidotes

There are several common myths about motivating individuals. Our view is that these myths are more harmful than helpful and, as a result, we confront them early in this chapter. Four particular myths are addressed below.

Myth 1: One can assess motivation by productivity. To illustrate this myth, consider this conversation.
Supervisor: Tom just isn't motivated anymore!
Foreman: How can you tell?
Supervisor: His productivity has fallen off by more than 50 percent.

Motivation should not be confused with performance. Individuals can be highly motivated but still have limited productivity and poor performance. Performance depends on far more than motivation, including, but not limited to, availability of resources needed to perform a job well (Humphrey, Nahrgang, and Morgeson, 2007).

Myth 2: Some individuals are just motivated and others are not. This myth is based on the view that motivation is a personality trait or characteristic that remains relatively stable from time to time and place to place.

Although some evidence suggests that individual traits are linked to motivation (Chang et al., 2012), the vast majority of empirical evidence indicates that situational factors (e.g., relationships with coworkers, supervisor behavior, access to needed materials) are more important in shaping individuals' motivation and behavior (Kanfer, Frese, and Johnson, 2017).

Myth 3: Motivation can be mass produced. A third myth about motivation is that it can be influenced by actions that appeal to large numbers of individuals at once, such as speeches by charismatic leaders, or by placing motivational posters throughout a workplace.

Most often these approaches do not work (Laurinaitis, 1997). To motivate individuals effectively, managers typically need to treat them as individuals. Contrary to the myth of mass production, individuals vary widely from each other in many ways. As a result, it is a central theme of this chapter that managers must motivate coworkers and subordinates on an individual basis, tailoring actions to individuals' circumstances and needs, particularly their job position or occupation, career stage, and personal or family concerns.

Occupation. Managers should understand how their ability to motivate individuals may vary according to their occupation or job category. For example, union contracts often prohibit certain types of changes in job design and responsibilities; managers need to know what occupational groups are covered by such contracts and how they affect certain approaches to motivation.

Career stage. A second important way in which individuals vary is their career stage. To illustrate, consider a recent graduate of a health care management program. She may be highly motivated by assignments that provide opportunities for learning new technical skills. In contrast, her colleague who has more experience may wish to take on responsibilities to develop leadership skills. Managers need to be sensitive to such career stage needs, motives, and values (Kanfer and Ackerman, 2004).

Personal factors. Perhaps more than we generally recognize, a variety of factors from their personal lives influence individuals at work. For example, personal factors sometimes parallel career stages. A recent graduate may have few family ties that would limit his interest in work that involved travel, whereas a manager with young children may be less motivated by opportunity for travel on the job. Other important personal influences that can affect motivation include family illness, divorce, substance abuse, health problems, child care, and financial stress. These are clearly delicate areas for managers to tread; yet, managers need to be aware that such personal factors can affect work motivation.

Myth 4: Money makes the world go 'round. Many scholars agree that financial rewards motivate individuals (Stajkovic and Luthans, 2001); however, managers make a mistake if they do not broaden instruments of motivation to include nonmonetary motivators as well.

Particularly in the health care sector, money is not typically the most important motivator (World Health Organization, 2008). In the next sections, we address nonfinancial factors that motivate individuals.

• • • IN PRACTICE: A Cry for Help

Working and keeping motivated on a busy 24-bed general intensive care unit, a charge nurse tells her story:

ICU nursing is stressful. It is stressful to be there, to work so closely with patients, to do so much to keep them going, and then have someone else get all the credit. The nurses do the work, they act as the eyes and ears monitoring and responding to the patients' condition, but oftentimes it is the physician who saves them and gets all the credit.

The ICU is also becoming a more dangerous place to work. In addition to tuberculosis, HIV, and hepatitis, there are more blood-borne and communicable diseases that we are exposed to. Patients who come here are often under the influence of drugs or alcohol. They often react to the medications we administer to them. Because the atmosphere is unfamiliar, they frequently get violent.

Another stressful aspect of the job is heightened consumer expectations about the patient experience. Everyone is an expert. The families continually remind me to wash my hands. The managers have been demanding more consumer-friendly behavior from the ICU nurses. They recently instituted a 24-hour visiting hours. They told us, "You will tolerate someone being here 24 hours a day as long as there is no bonafide reason that they shouldn't be there." For the most part this is fine with us. We are part of a very family- and community-oriented health system, and families can really help. Spending time in the ICU allows families to reassure kids that all is well, make certain their elderly parents or grandparents don't fall out of bed and are comfortable. In some cases, if a family member is not available, we have to hire sitters for $12 an hour to keep an eye on the patient. Generally, the sitters are unskilled individuals who can't participate in the patient care process. Usually they knit, eat chips, read, watch TV, or sleep.

Although family members can assist us, more often than not, they can also impede our ability to do our work. We have one "frequent flyer" who is in here all the time. His wife will not leave. She insists on doing his care. The husband has severe diabetes, and she insists on doing the glucose monitoring and dressing changes. We can't get rid of her. She makes the nurses very uncomfortable. Sometimes you have to take care of the entire family, not just the member in the bed. Many families are already dysfunctional to begin with; they don't usually function any better in the ICU setting.

The managers recently restructured our system by focusing less on financial rewards and more on recognizing our contributions to meeting clinical quality targets, like fall or infection rates. The ICU nurses do receive a higher pay differential, because the work is more demanding and specialized. However, managers want to get away from differential pay because, as they say, "Everything is getting to be a specialty." But believe me, money still talks!

A year ago, the managers cut back ICU staffing in an effort to save money. Shortly after that time, we went into a 10-month period of very high census and very high acuity. The highest anyone could ever remember and we were understaffed! Work became horrible. I didn't want to go. Every time it would be hellish. The 24 ICU beds were always full of seriously ill individuals.

As the demands and stresses became greater, the necessary ICU "collaboration and team behaviors" were just put aside. The nurses weren't motivated to work as a team anymore; they began focusing only on "their" patients. However, we all have to keep watch on the telemetry banks and the arrhythmia alarms. Phones ring that have

• • • IN PRACTICE: A Cry for Help (Continued)

to be answered. The pneumatic tubes [which transport lab results, blood samples, and medications] need to be attended to. These activities are not assigned, but need to be done as a team.

Often, nurses that were scheduled to work twelve hours would have to stay for mandatory overtime. For a while, we had to work every weekend and holiday. To help ease the staffing void, the hospital began to rely on external agency nurses that are paid a higher wage. When the agency nurses come here, they are not 100%. They might be totally unfamiliar with our practice protocols, and we don't necessarily know their skill level. Naturally, these nurses take a lot of time to orient to the unit and our routines. Furthermore, because agency nurses are not given computer passwords, we have to do their charting, which creates more work for us. The agency nurses are hired guns who are paid about $18 more per hour than we are. They also work whenever they want to.

Although we are a nonprofit, we have a gain-sharing plan. Managers think money is not an issue with us. They played with the equations. We worked very hard—all out—for 10 months in a very difficult and understaffed environment. We did receive our gain-share checks, but it was practically nothing. Because of the high patient census and acuity, coupled with staff cutbacks, the external agency staff was used heavily. They are paid a premium. Apparently, that is where most of our gain-share went. We didn't feel that the gain-share checks rewarded us at all. In the end, it had nothing to do with all the extra effort. That was our reward for being full-time, committed, extremely hard working, and concerned for quality.

I can go down to the agency tomorrow and make $18 an hour more than I do now.

To learn more about the nursing workforce and labor shortages, see the American Association of Colleges of Nursing website: http://www.aacn.nche.edu/media-relations/fact-sheets/nursing-shortage.

Manager's Role

The "individual-in-situation" perspective indicates that managers should take a comprehensive approach when evaluating factors that motivate individuals (Kanfer, Frese, and Johnson, 2017). Managers can assess motivation levels in informal interviews, using open-ended questions to learn about individuals' needs, perceptions, and values. These discussions need not be lengthy. What matters more is that they are timely, that individuals feel comfortable in openly expressing their concerns, and that managers use the opportunity to problem solve and set agreed-on goals. Managers can play a critical role in motivating others not only by assessing current motivation but also by altering conditions that may reduce motivation.

THE WHAT AND HOW OF MOTIVATION

What factors energize individuals to work? How are individuals energized? How can managers enable individuals to build and maintain high levels of energy for their work? Based on results from studies conducted in the past 70 years (Kanfer, Frese, and Johnson, 2017), several principles and practices have emerged to guide managers as they seek to effectively motivate individuals at work.

The Role of Individual Characteristics

Research shows that several individual characteristics are associated with work motivation (Kanfer, Frese, and Johnson, 2017). These characteristics fall into two categories. First, there are so-called "universal motives," which are understood to be widely shared across individuals. These are a need for fairness and the need to engage in work that is meaningful, interesting, and enjoyable (termed "intrinsic motivation"). Second, there are traits that vary in strength across individuals. These include the need to learn, develop competence, and achieve. We focus first on universal motives.

The Importance of Fairness

Adams proposed a theory of work motivation that focuses on individuals' desire for equity, or **fairness**, in their relationships (Adams, 1963, 1965). Relationships are fair when individuals perceive that their outcomes (e.g., pay) are proportionate to their perceived contributions or inputs (e.g., task effort). Further, Adams argued that individuals evaluate fairness by comparing themselves to similar coworkers. Hence, individuals contrast their perceived inputs and outcomes with their perceptions of others' inputs and outcomes. Individuals experience tension when they perceive this comparison to be unequal. Adams also proposed that individuals are motivated to reduce tensions that result from perceived inequity: the greater the perceived inequity and resulting tension, the greater the motivation to reduce it.

Depending on the magnitude of the perceived inequity, individuals may use one of several approaches to restore balance in their relationships with others and organizations. These approaches include altering their perceptions of their own or others' inputs or outcomes, changing their inputs or outcomes, getting others to change their inputs or outcomes, and leaving the inequitable work situation altogether (Campbell and Pritchard, 1976).

Research also shows that individuals are motivated by perceived fairness in procedures and processes that managers use to determine outcomes (Brockner, 2015). For example, an individual who does not receive a promotion he or she believes he or she earned is likely to be concerned about fairness in the process that his or her manager used to make the decision. In sum, much research suggests that perceptions of fairness contribute substantially to work motivation (Brockner, 2015).

The equity and fairness perspective provides useful insights and guidelines for health care managers. First, individuals compare themselves to others, and this comparison influences motivation. Second, managers may change perceptions of inequity by explaining differences between jobs or other conditions that make it necessary to reward or treat individuals differently (Kim and Mauborgne, 2003). In other instances, managers may find ways to compensate for perceived differences; however, it is not always possible to restore perceptions of equity, and they may persist as a source of motivational problems (Brockner, 2006). Last, because individuals value fairness in the processes and procedures that managers use to make decisions, taking time to be transparent about processes of evaluation and decision making may enhance employees' motivation (Brockner, 2015).

Intrinsic Motivation

Intrinsic motivation exists when we complete tasks because they are meaningful, interesting, and enjoyable—as compared to situations in which motivation derives from extrinsic rewards such as money or status (Kanfer, Frese, and Johnson, 2017). In general, intrinsic motivation has been linked to better performance on complex tasks and those involving quality of work, while extrinsic motivation has been found to be better for performance on routine tasks and those involving quantity of production (Cerasoli, Nicklin, and Ford, 2014; McGraw and McCullers, 1979). This may explain why efforts to improve the performance of health care providers with pay-for-performance models (i.e., extrinsic motivation tools) have been disappointing (Damberg et al., 2014). Greater use of intrinsic incentives may prove more effective for many of the tasks that physicians, nurses, and other clinicians perform.

Trait-Based Motives

Among individual traits that researchers have examined to understand their role in work motivation, results from several studies show that a few are particularly important. These include the need to learn, develop competence, and achieve.

Murray (1938) and his student McClelland (1961, 1965) pioneered research on achievement motivation, which refers to an individual's need to accomplish something difficult by attaining high standards of excellence. It reflects the desire to achieve a goal more effectively than in the past. Research shows that, in general, individuals with higher levels of achievement motivation set more challenging goals and attain higher levels of performance (Phillips and Gully, 1997).

Higgins (1997) proposed a model of motivation that elaborated on achievement motivation. He posed an intriguing question: What causes individuals to strive for achievement? He argued that individuals vary in their motives as they pursue work-related goals. Some focus on maximizing gains to ensure success and achievement; he termed this a promotion focus. In contrast, other individuals focus on minimizing losses to prevent failure, which is termed a loss prevention focus. Research shows support for this distinction (Lanaj, Chang, and Johnson, 2012). Specifically, individuals who have higher levels of motivation to learn and achieve, and who show a greater promotion focus, have higher performance levels than individuals who are motivated to prevent failure or protect against losses (e.g., to their reputations) at work (Kanfer, Frese, and Johnson, 2017; Wallace and Chen, 2006).

PROCESS PERSPECTIVES

Though understanding individual characteristics is useful for managers to promote motivation, this knowledge does not shed much light on the "how" of motivation. For example, individuals' needs for achievement do not explain how they select particular goals or how they make choices to allocate their time and effort to achieve them. These questions involve behaviors that are addressed by perspectives on the processes involved in motivation. It is to these perspectives that we now turn.

Specifically, we examine two different approaches to motivation that share a focus on goals, that is, ends that individuals strive to attain. One approach, based in expectancy theory (Mitchell, 1982), focuses on how individuals select particular goals to attain. The other approach, based in goal-setting theory (Latham and Locke, 2006), focuses on how individuals make decisions to change their aim to achieve a particular goal and the level of intensity with which they pursue goals (Kanfer, Frese, and Johnson, 2017).

• • • IN PRACTICE: Motivating a Primary Care Physician in a Community Health Center

Susan Smith, MD, a primary care physician, is employed by an urban community health center. Because such a large proportion of her patients are diabetic, she has been intimately involved in the development of a new diabetic disease-management program for the center. The center wants the disease to be managed in such a way that it is kept under control so that patients can maintain a higher quality of life and longer-term costs do not rise as a result of the need for more extensive medical interventions.

Dr. Smith is very confident that between her own ability and the detailed guidelines for managing the disease developed by the center, she will be able to do a good job of keeping her diabetic patients' disease under control. The disease-management guidelines require her to get patients to test their blood sugar levels four times per day using testing strips and to frequently order laboratory tests, glaucoma screenings, and podiatric referrals throughout the course of a year.

The center uses financial incentives to motivate primary care physician behavior, primarily through the use of a bonus pool of dollars from which the physicians can share at the end of the year. The more productive a physician is over the course of the year (as measured by the number of patients she or he sees), the bigger the bonus check at year's end. Although the disease-management guidelines recently went into effect, the center's financial incentive system for its primary care physicians has not changed in any way. Dr. Smith realizes that since a large percentage of her patients are diabetic, if she is to vigorously adhere to the guidelines, she may not receive any bonus at year's end because following the guidelines will require her to take more time with each patient, thus reducing the number of patients she sees overall.

Expectancy Theory

An early, prominent, and useful view of motivation, termed "expectancy theory" (Georgopoulos, Mahoney, and Jones, 1957; Vroom, 1964), assumes that individuals make rational calculations about how to expend work effort. In these calculations, individuals know what rewards they want from work and understand that their performance will determine the extent to which they attain the rewards they value. Expectancy theory has four central components: job outcomes or goals, valences, instrumentality, and expectancy (Mitchell, 1982) (see Figure 4.1). Valences are how individuals

feel about outcomes or goals, instrumentality is the extent to which individuals believe that attaining a job outcome depends on performance, and **expectancy** is the perceived link between work effort and performance.

Using expectancy theory, we can illustrate the degree to which the primary care physician described in "In Practice: Motivating a Primary Care Physician in a Community Health Center" might be motivated to adhere to the community health center's disease-management guidelines. This physician is confident that by following the guidelines she will be able to do a reasonably good job of controlling the disease among her patients;

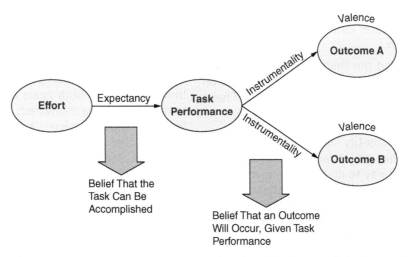

Figure 4.1 Common Motivation Problems and Potential Solutions.

however, the physician knows that due to the additional time required to effectively managing her patients, there also is a high probability that she will not share in any financial bonuses paid out at year's end. Because this is a job outcome she does not favor, it receives a negative valence. Instrumentality, or the probability that performance will lead to outcomes, is fairly high, but the outcome has a forceful negative valence. Because the outcome (no end-of-year bonus) is not related to performance, the physician's motivation to carry out high-quality diabetes disease management has been substantially reduced.

Motivation is the end product of valence, instrumentality, and expectancy. Individuals are motivated when a combination of factors occurs: They value an outcome (i.e., valence is high and positive), they believe that good performance will be rewarded with desired outcomes (i.e., instrumentality is high), and they believe that their efforts will produce good performance (i.e., expectancy is high). In contrast, motivation is likely to be low if the components of expectancy theory have low values. If individuals do not care about their job outcomes, then they have less reason to work for them. Or, if organizations do not link outcomes to performance (e.g., pay raises are linked to seniority rather than performance), then individuals have less reason to care about their performance. Similarly, if effort and performance seem unrelated, then there is less reason to try hard.

The theory of planned behavior (Ajzen, 1991) has usefully extended expectancy theory by recognizing the influential role that the social context of work plays in individuals' motivation. Specifically, this view emphasizes that social pressure often influences individuals' decisions about their course of action, including how they might weigh valence, instrumentality, and expectancy. This view has a good deal of empirical support (Armitage and Conner, 2001) and suggests that managers who create supportive social environments, including organizational and unit-level cultures, may increase levels of worker motivation.

Expectancy theory and the theory of planned behavior provide useful guidelines for managerial action (Pritchard, De Leo, and Von Bergen, 1976). These include the following:

1. Managers should identify incentives, rewards, and job outcomes that are attractive to individuals. Perhaps the best way to do this is to involve subordinates and coworkers actively in shaping these key features of their work, for example, by asking individuals directly about their preferences using surveys and one-to-one meetings.

2. The rules for attaining incentives or rewards must be clear to all involved. For example, expected levels of performance should be spelled out in as much detail as possible. Such rules should be stated in job descriptions and employee orientations. These rules should also be reviewed periodically, both informally and formally. We add here a note from equity theory: The rules should be perceived as fair.

3. Individuals must perceive that their efforts will lead to the desired level of performance.

4. Social pressure from peers often shapes individuals' perceptions about incentives and rewards, and their link to outcomes. Managers should aim to create environments in which there are shared positive views of these issues.

Striving for Goals: Goal Setting and Feedback

Locke (1968) and his colleagues (Latham and Locke, 2006; Locke and Latham, 2004) developed an especially useful motivation theory that focuses on the role of goals and **goal setting**. Goals are powerful because they direct individuals' attention, focus effort on tasks related to goal attainment, and encourage individuals to persist in such tasks. In short, a goal provides guidelines for how much effort to put into work.

Empirical support for key parts of goal-setting theory is impressive and shows that several conditions should be met for goals to have a positive influence on performance (Latham and Locke, 2006). First, individuals should be aware of goals and know what must be done to attain them. Second, individuals should accept goals as something that they are willing to work for. This is why it is often important to involve individuals in setting goals for their work.

Third, research shows that goal setting is more effective, and usually only effective, when goals are specific and **feedback** is given to individuals so that they can monitor their performance in relation to goals. Indeed, goal setting without feedback seems to have little long-term effect on performance (Becker, 1978). On the other hand, feedback without goal setting is also ineffective. Individuals need both goals and feedback on progress toward goals to be motivated. Furthermore, self-created feedback appears to exert a greater effect on motivation than feedback from external sources (Ivancevich and McMahon, 1982).

Fourth, for goal setting to be effective, individuals must have the ability to reach the goals (Locke, 1982). Importantly, individuals also need to have self-efficacy, that is, they need to *believe* that they have the ability to perform particular tasks and to achieve goals for their motivation levels to remain high (Bandura, 1977; Phillips, Hollenbeck, and Ilgen, 1996).

Last, the complexity of a task and the difficulty of goals matter. The beneficial effects of setting goals are reduced when individuals face goals and tasks that are too demanding or complex (Wood, Mento, and Locke, 1987). One likely explanation for these results is that when individuals engage in a particularly difficult, complex, or novel task, their lack of knowledge or skills diminishes their motivation (Kanfer, Frese, and Johnson, 2017).

The implications for managers are the following:

1. Work collaboratively with individuals to set goals that are adequately difficult and specific; revise and update goals as necessary.
2. Provide timely and specific feedback to individuals on their progress toward goals.
3. Build commitment to goals by helping individuals believe they can attain goals and by selecting goals that are congruent with their values.
4. Rewards should be given contingent on goal attainment.

MOTIVATING HEALTH CARE PROFESSIONALS

Health care organizations typically have a varied and large number of professionals working within them, including, for example, clinical professionals (physicians, nurses, physical therapists, social workers), financial managers, and specialists in data management and quality improvement. Professionals are distinct from other occupational groups in the extent to which (1) they control who may become a member of the group by means of rigorous selection and licensure—this typically results in a high degree of cohesion among members and a strong sense of identity with, and loyalty to, the profession; (2) their work is based on codified, often scientifically based, knowledge and standards; (3) they adhere to a service-focused code of ethics; and (4) they are autonomous and control their own activities (O'Connor and Lanning, 1992). Autonomy is perhaps the most important of these defining characteristics.

Because health care professionals generally are educated and socialized to think and act with a great deal of individual discretion and autonomy in their day-to-day work, managers often find it difficult to motivate them to change their behavior. Indeed, professionals may resent managerial or organizational forays into their activities. Yet, because professionals, especially physicians and nurses, carry out so much of the day-to-day work in health care organizations, managers will be more effective if they learn how to motivate clinicians to provide high-quality, cost-effective services,

for example, by abandoning detrimental behaviors such as excessive use of resources (e.g., unnecessary diagnostic testing).

Physician Motivation

Research and practice suggest several important guidelines for motivating physicians. Merely distributing guidelines, protocols, or other tools to improve clinical practice often results in little or no change in behavior (Smith, 2000). In contrast, more useful approaches include the use of reminders and feedback, especially feedback that is data-driven and provides benchmarks (Agency for Healthcare Research and Quality [AHRQ], 2010; Centers for Medicare & Medicaid Services, 2017). Because of their professional socialization, intrinsic motivation, and strong achievement needs, most physicians want to deliver not only high-quality but also exceptional care to their patients. For them to know the extent to which they are achieving these objectives, they need to be able to assess how well they are doing with respect to peers, their own past performance, and to benchmark goals. One way of accomplishing this is to develop high-quality information systems that provide feedback on a frequent basis. Such a system can allow medical professionals to not only know how well they are doing but also enhance their confidence that they are doing things right (McKethan and Jha, 2014).

Though feedback can be a powerful tool to assist managers in motivating physician behavior, there are several factors that should be considered to maximize the effectiveness of feedback. First, for feedback to be of value, physicians must recognize that their behavior needs to change. Second, feedback needs to be frequent, timely, and given at precise time intervals to sustain new behaviors. Third, feedback must be useable, consistent, correct, and of sufficient diversity. It should contain important and valid data, for example, on finances and quality of care. Otherwise, behavior problems can intensify as rewards flow to improvements based on flawed feedback data (Charns and Smith-Tewksbury, 1993). Last, managers should not portray the feedback as "good" or "bad."

Another approach that may prove quite effective is the use of principles from behavioral economics, including the use of nudges (Thaler and Sunstein, 2008). To nudge is to coax or gently encourage someone to do something. Results from a recent study show how powerful relatively simply interventions using nudges can be. The study involved an experiment in which physicians prescribing antibiotics using an electronic health record (EHR) system were randomized to different treatments. Results show that merely suggesting an alternative medication to physicians when the electronic system flagged a prescription as questionable did not reduce inappropriate prescriptions. But, asking physicians to provide a short, written justification reduced inappropriate prescriptions by 75 percent (from 23.2 percent to 5.2 percent) (Meeker et al., 2016).

Last, it is important to involve physician leaders in efforts to change physician practices; indeed, physicians are likely to respond more favorably to projects in which they can participate heavily or control entirely (D'Aunno et al., 2016). It is more effective to motivate physicians to change their behavior when they are partners who share in a project's mission, investment, and returns.

Nurses

Unfortunately, high levels of job dissatisfaction and voluntary turnover among nurses are a chronic problem that threatens quality of care in health care organizations across the United States (see "In Practice: A Cry for Help") (American Association of Colleges of Nursing, 2007; Institute of Medicine, 2003). Although rates of turnover have improved in recent years, in 2015 the national rate of voluntary nurse turnover in hospitals was still quite high at 17 percent (NSI Nursing Solutions Inc., 2016). Furthermore, more than 20 percent of hospital nurses are dissatisfied with their jobs and more than 30 percent report symptoms of burnout (McHugh et al., 2011).

Nurses, like others, voluntarily leave their jobs for many reasons. For some, life circumstances precipitate a job change (e.g., children, illness, relocation, retirement). Many nurses, however, leave their jobs because they can no longer take the work pressure, long hours, ineffective managers and unhelpful colleagues, limited opportunities for advancement, or the lack of recognition for their accomplishments. As a leading nurse management researcher, Linda Aiken, put it in a commentary on the state of the nursing workforce crisis, "It's the poor work environment, stupid!" (2002, p. 220). Indeed, results from research in both general management and health care settings show that job satisfaction and turnover are consistently and positively related to several characteristics of work environments, many of which we have discussed above (Kovner et al., 2006). In particular, inadequate nurse staffing and consequent high workloads are major problems motivating nurse turnover (McHugh et al., 2011).

In response to poor working environments for nurses, the American Nurses Association developed the Magnet hospital model in the 1980s. This program, which has expanded significantly since its inception, aims to improve the work environment for nurses and thus increase their motivation, satisfaction, and performance, while reducing turnover. The name "Magnet" conveys that good work environments will attract and retain nurses.

MOTIVATIONAL PROBLEMS
Nature and Causes

The key sources of motivational problems include unclear expectations about desired performance; impediments to performance, such as inadequate resources and support from coworkers or managers; and a mismatch between individuals' skills and job requirements. Determining the specific causes of a particular individual's motivation problem is often difficult. The most effective approach is for managers to develop a strong professional relationship that enables effective two-way communication. Listening to and encouraging individuals to speak frankly are particularly effective approaches (Nembhard and Edmondson, 2006). Research indicates that upward communication systems can have several benefits, including reduced absenteeism and turnover, increased productivity, and higher profits (Pfeffer, 1998).

Potential Solutions

Most motivational problems require multiple strategies to address effectively. Successful motivation programs might include several integrated and mutually reinforcing approaches (Locke and Latham, 1990, 2004). At a minimum, these approaches should include some combination of goal setting, with sufficiently specific and challenging goals; valued rewards contingent upon performance; clear and shared expectancy of success; feedback, individual involvement, or participation; and job redesign (Hackman and Oldham, 1976; Humphrey, Nahrgang, and Morgeson, 2007). The long-run goal should be to develop and retain a "culture of performance." (See "In Practice: Memorial Hermann Sugar Land Hospital.")

Job redesign is a particularly useful approach to promote motivation. It is based on the premise that altering certain aspects of jobs to satisfy individuals' psychological needs will motivate them to exert more effort. According to Hackman and Oldham (1980), satisfaction of higher-order needs occurs when an individual experiences the following psychological states. First, the job allows an individual to feel personally responsible for a significant segment of his or her work outcomes. Autonomy or personal control is the key job dimension contributing to feelings of personal responsibility for job outcomes. Second, the job involves doing something that is perceived as meaningful by the individual. The three core dimensions that can make jobs meaningful are task identity (i.e., completion of a whole task), skill variety (i.e., utilization of different skills), and task significance (i.e., substantial impact). Third, the job provides an individual with knowledge of results. Feedback from the job itself or from another individual is the core job dimension, which provides knowledge of results.

Steffen, Nystrom, and O'Connor (1996), for example, examined job redesign for nurses and nurses' aides employed in long-term care settings. The results showed that family members' satisfaction with the quality of services received was positively influenced by nurses' level of organizational commitment, which, in turn, was positively correlated with autonomy, task identity, and skill variety. This study indicates that redesigning nursing jobs in long-term care settings can serve to motivate these individuals to be more committed to the organization as well as to provide higher levels of service quality.

Job redesign is most appropriate when it is feasible given the structure of jobs, legal constraints, and individuals' characteristics and values. Job redesign in health care is certainly feasible but may be subject to more legal and professional constraints than most other industries (Blayney, 1992).

Research in both nonhealth care and health care organizations generally supports the validity of the job characteristics model in enhancing motivation, especially for individuals who strongly value personal feelings of accomplishment and growth (Grant and Parker, 2009; Humphrey, Nahrgang, and Morgeson, 2007). However, the success of any job redesign effort is likely to depend on other reinforcing factors such as the reward system and top management support.

Indeed, many strategies to improve motivation depend on the **empowerment** of individuals. Empowerment involves "directed autonomy" whereby individuals or teams are given an overall direction, yet considerable leeway concerning how they go about following that direction. Empowerment also involves sharing information with individuals, enabling them to understand and contribute to organizational performance and giving them the autonomy to make decisions that influence organizational outcomes.

Empowerment is a matter of degree rather than an absolute (Ford and Fottler, 1995). Managers could choose to provide higher degrees of empowerment for some individuals and teams doing certain tasks than for others. Managers can empower individuals by giving them control over any or all of the following: identifying problems, developing alternative solutions, evaluating alternative options, choosing an option, or implementing a solution.

Table 4.1 outlines the three motivational problems discussed in the beginning of this section together with potential solutions.

Table 4.1 Common Motivation Problems and Potential Solutions

Motivational Problems	Potential Solutions
1. Inadequate performance definition (i.e., lack of goals, inadequate job descriptions, inadequate performance standards, inadequate performance assessment)	• Well-defined job descriptions • Well-defined performance standards • Goal setting
2. Impediments to performance (i.e., bureaucratic or environmental obstacles, inadequate resources or support from coworkers and managers, poor individual-to-job matching, inadequate information)	• Feedback on performance • Improved employee selection and matching to jobs • Job redesign
3. Inadequate performance–reward linkages (i.e., inappropriate or inadequate rewards, poor timing of rewards, low probability of receiving rewards, inequity in distribution of rewards)	• Enhanced opportunities for achievement (i.e., individual involvement-participation, job redesign, career planning, professional development opportunities) • Enhanced autonomy or personal control, self-management, modified work schedule, recognition, praise or awards, opportunity to display skills or talents, opportunity to mentor or train others, promotions in rank or position, information concerning organization or department, preferred work activities or projects, preferred work space • Enhanced social support (i.e., work teams, task groups, social activities, professional and community group participation, personal communication or leadership style)

DEBATE TIME: What Do You Think?

Pay-for-performance programs (also termed "value-based purchasing") of various kinds have increased substantially in number and importance in the last decade. The reason for the rising prominence of pay-for-performance programs is that payers, consumers, and other stakeholders believe that health care organizations are not providing services at a satisfactory level of quality or cost, and that strengthening the link between performance and financial rewards will produce better results.

Nonetheless, critics of these programs argue that they will not meet their aims for several reasons. First, pay-for-performance may focus providers narrowly on performance measures, potentially crowding out important work that is not rewarded by pay-for-performance schemes. Second, measures used in these programs may not be adequately aligned with desired outcomes. Third, pay-for-performance programs may erode physician autonomy—this is especially a problem when patients' needs do not match particular protocols and require alternative processes of care to improve outcomes. Fourth, pay-for-performance programs may penalize (e.g., by withholding payments) individuals and organizations for work processes or outcomes that are not under their control. Fifth, pay-for-performance programs put too much emphasis on extrinsic rather than intrinsic rewards for work, potentially displacing intrinsic motives for work. Last, the rewards associated with pay-for-performance programs may be too small, or criteria for receiving rewards may conflict with each other, resulting in a weak signal and little impact on motivation.

How do various motivation theories help us understand whether pay-for-performance programs will work? What do the theories predict might go wrong?

SUMMARY AND MANAGERIAL GUIDELINES

1. Health care managers can motivate individuals by determining what needs and rewards they view as most important. This can be accomplished through formal and informal means of communication.

2. Rewards should be both monetary and nonmonetary. They should be relevant to the priority needs of particular individuals or groups. If at all possible, solicit individuals' views on rewards and involve them in developing and implementing reward and incentive systems.

3. Goals should be set at the time of hiring and at periodic performance evaluations. Set or encourage individuals to set goals that are challenging and specific; revise and update goals as necessary.

4. Expectations about goal attainment and consequences also should be set at the time of hiring and reviewed periodically. Build commitment to goals by helping individuals believe that they can attain them and by selecting goals that are consistent with their values.

5. Make sure that the rules for attaining rewards are clear to everyone.

6. Check individuals' perceptions of the fairness of their work and rewards. Address perceived inequities as best as possible, given resource constraints. Note that perceptions of inequity are especially likely when managers try to take individuals' different needs into account.

7. Provide timely and specific feedback to individuals on their progress toward goals.

8. Reward individuals contingent on performance.

9. Redesigning jobs is a useful approach for increasing the match between individuals' needs and motives and their work. Redesigning offers much potential for increased motivation to the extent that it involves building-in responsibility, decision making,

DISCUSSION QUESTIONS

1. How can managers distinguish a motivational problem from other factors that affect an individual's performance?

2. In situations such as the ICU faced in "A Cry for Help" (In Practice), what role can managers and clinical leaders play to improve staff morale and motivation?

3. What approaches other than a productivity bonus could the management team at the community health center have used to change Dr. Smith's practice patterns (see "In Practice: Motivating a Primary Care Physician in a Community Health Center")?

4. If you wanted to implement a motivational program in your organization, what elements would you include in your implementation plan? What metrics would you use to measure the success of the initiative?

CASE

Memorial Hermann Sugar Land Hospital: 2016 Malcolm Baldrige National Quality Award Winner

Memorial Hermann Sugar Land Hospital (MHSL) is a 149-bed, not-for-profit hospital located in Fort Bend County, one of the fastest growing and most ethnically diverse counties in the nation, in the greater Houston, Texas area. Founded as a for-profit hospital in 1982, the Fort Bend Hospital, as it was then known, quickly developed a reputation for delivering high-quality care in a family-friendly environment. The Houston-based Memorial Hermann Health System (MHHS) acquired the Fort Bend Hospital in 1999.

After the acquisition, the senior leadership team set its sights on becoming one of the nation's leading community hospitals. Guided by the mantra "Why Not Us," the leaders set out to create an organization known for outstanding clinical care, zero harm, and delivering an amazing patient experience. In 2016, the MHSL Hospital won the prestigious Malcolm Baldrige National Healthcare Quality award in recognition of its exemplary level of patient care.

The MHSL Hospital provides inpatient and outpatient services in the specialties of general medical and cardiovascular, surgical, intensive care, orthopedics, sports medicine and rehabilitation, diagnostic, and woman's and children's services. It is 1 of the 14 hospitals in the larger Memorial Hermann Health System. Each of the 14 hospitals in the system operates as a strategically located business unit that provides services tailored to support the needs of its local community.

Unlike other health systems in which individual hospitals might compete with each other by offering the same services, MHHS has developed a highly integrated system to deliver community-based comprehensive care. As patients' needs change, they are referred to the appropriate business unit within the larger health system. Health care services are aligned across the MMHS's strategic business units so that each unit is able to focus, improve, and innovate on a select set of services.

Vision and Values and Operating Framework

MHSL seeks to become the preeminent community hospital in the nation by providing exemplary family-centered care that is highly reliable, safe, and effective. To achieve this vision, the MHHS core values emphasize *accountability*, *compassion*, *collaboration*, *empowerment*, *innovation*, *results orientation*, and *one Memorial Hermann system*. The MHHS leaders also created the ADVANCE model as the overarching framework to design, implement, and evaluate programs and services across the system and to guide work on a daily basis.

The ADVANCE model components are the following:

A—Align with Physicians

D—Delivery Quality Care

A—Achieve Operational Targets

N—Nurture Growth and Innovation

C—Consumer-Centric

E—Enhance Population Health

Workforce Development and Engagement

The MHSLH workforce is the foundation for its success: much emphasis is placed on workforce development and engagement at all levels of the health system. In particular, the MHHS uses a workforce lifecycle model to recruit, retain, and develop professional staff and employees. The focus is on finding individuals who share systemwide values to support the family-oriented culture and the goals of safe and high-quality clinical care. The workforce engagement phases include the following:

Phase 1 Discover and Recruit. The model begins with attracting new employees to the Sugar Land Hospital. This phase emphasizes attracting individuals who can contribute to, and enrich, the organizational mission, vision, and culture, and who reflect the ethic and cultural diversity of the community. The ideal employee brings diverse thought and possesses strong technical skills needed to achieve the organization's performance goals. New employees are recruited though a variety of methods including events and job fairs, referrals, direct marketing, out-of-state recruitment, and social media. Executive-level and highly specialized roles are handled by professional recruiting firms.

Similarly, physicians are recruited to MHHS hospitals in collaboration with the Memorial Hermann Medical Group, the University of Texas, and the MHSLH executive team including the director of business development.

Phase 2 Welcome and Connect. All potential employees are screened for cultural fit with the MHHS values as well as the skills and competencies required to perform in positions. Once individuals have passed the initial screening phase, they participate in a three-step hiring process that includes an in-depth assessment by trained recruiters to determine alignment with the organization's values. Skills and expertise are further assessed and background checks are completed at this time. In the second step, candidates complete either the Hartman Value Profile, to gauge their capacity to make value judgments about themselves and the world, or the Prophecy Assessment, designed to evaluate nurses' clinical, situational, and behavioral competencies.

The final phase of recruitment includes behavioral interviews conducted by a panel of trained employees who assess the candidate for fit with organizational values and specific roles within departments. Recruitment concludes with additional background checks, physicals, and other mandatory preemployment requirements. New employees attend a systemwide "Culture Day," followed by a multiday new employee orientation and a department-specific orientation that concentrates on helping new employees acclimate to the surroundings, understand expectations, and how to function in departments.

Physician recruitment and retention are handled in a similar manner, beginning with rigorous interviews and credentialing to identify and attract physicians who share the MHHS values and possess clinical and leadership skills to contribute to the goals of patient care quality and safety. Physician onboarding includes welcome sessions with the senior leadership team and a review of hospital policies, procedures, clinical priority areas, and equipment. The concepts of the ADVANCE model and the core organizational competency of patient safety are the focus of the physician orientation programs. New physicians are invited to participate in 30-60-90-day follow-up meetings with managers that provide opportunities to offer support and further clarify clinical and operational goals and expectations.

Phase 3 Enrich and Energize. This phase focuses on enriching and energizing the workforce through performance feedback. The core value of accountability is foundational to the workforce engagement strategy at MHSLH. Leaders energize and motivate the workforce by setting high expectations and performance targets, working collaboratively toward a common purpose, empowering individuals to innovate and try new ideas, providing access to an open and visible leadership team, and conducting formal and informal feedback sessions.

The MHSL organizational culture encourages individuals and teams to exceed performance goals and expectations through distinguished achievement levels. In turn, exemplary performance and achievements are rewarded with financial incentives, performance evaluations, and formal recognition. To support high performance, managers and leaders at all levels provide individuals with ongoing feedback to identify opportunities for improvement. Managers provide feedback in daily interactions to reinforce expectations and to guide individual performance improvement. Individuals who fall below the expected performance levels are required to follow an improvement plan.

Phase 4 Recognize and Refuel. This phase focuses on recognizing and rewarding accomplishments. Recognition programs are used to celebrate individual and collective successes. Peer recognition programs such as Employee Partner of the Year, Physician Partner of the Year, Volunteer Partner of the Year, Employee Appreciation Days, and Doctor's Days are examples of programs that recognize a job well done and further support the MHSLH culture of excellence. High-performing individuals at all levels are eligible for a merit raise that is managed through each department's incentive budget. To reinforce the *One Memorial Hermann* model, each employee receives quarterly incentives as system-level goals on each of the ADVANCE strategies are met.

Phase 5 Growth. Individual growth and development are an important part of the MHSLH employee engagement model and a key driver of sustainable high performance. Specific workforce development needs are segmented and tailored to take education, job responsibilities, and organizational change needs into account. Examples of workforce growth and development programs and opportunities include tuition reimbursement/loan repayment, flexible scheduling, and opportunities to participate in change and performance improvement efforts as well as governance councils and committees. Flexible scheduling is offered so that individuals are able to balance the responsibilities of their work and family life, which reinforces the MHHS Family Caring for Family culture.

Fort Bend is a rapidly growing metropolitan area that requires an agile approach to workforce management. Change management strategies are used to design and execute job duties so that each employee is supported and empowered to provide the highest levels of service and clinical care. The workforce management approach includes (1) a workforce plan; (2) professional development and educational programs to develop knowledge, skills, and competencies; (3) employee involvement in process improvement and design efforts; and (4) reward and recognition programs. The overall workforce management plan is managed by the system-level human resource management group. When reductions in workforce are needed within one business unit, the affected individuals are given the opportunity to move to another unit in the system. Cross-training, continuing education, and mentoring programs are also used to ensure that the workforce possesses the knowledge and capabilities that support the organization's performance goals.

Performance Management

The ongoing performance management and feedback model ensures that individuals have a clear understanding of how they contribute to performance goals and the ways in which they can improve their contributions to the patient experience. A formal employee engagement survey and annual review provide data and insights about changes in behaviors required to ensure high performance in the areas of clinical care, patient safety, and exemplary service. Additionally, the annual workforce engagement survey is used to identify the top factors associated with high performance and engagement across different employee groups. In turn, the leadership team uses the data to make corrections and improvements to the overall workforce engagement strategy.

Employees contribute to the performance evaluation process by completing a self-assessment at the end of each year that is used to guide the development of mutually agreed-on personal and team performance goals and objectives during the formal performance review. The effectiveness of the informal and formal feedback methods is assessed against measurable changes in patient care quality and operational efficiency measures.

Each year managers across the MHSLH review the skills and competencies of the employees in their units. The annual review is used to identify individuals who are ready to assume leadership positions or new career opportunities as well as gaps in the current workforce composition necessary to support organizational goals. The data gathered though the annual review inform succession planning, leadership development, and continuing education programs for the coming year.

Questions

1. What are the key factors in Memorial Hermann Sugar Land Hospital's successful approach to motivation?

2. Do you see weaknesses in the Memorial Hermann Sugar Land Hospital's approach?

3. Can the Memorial Hermann Sugar Land Hospital's approach be replicated in other health care organizations? What are some important barriers and facilitators to using the Memorial Hermann Sugar Land Hospital's approach?

SOURCE: Memorial Hermann Sugar Land. (2016). 2016 Baldrige National Quality Award Application. Available at https://www.nist.gov/baldrige. For more information about the Malcolm Baldrige National Quality Award and to view the previous health care award winners, see https://www.nist.gov/baldrige.

REFERENCES

Adams, J. S. (1963). Toward an understanding of inequity. *Journal of Abnormal and Social Psychology, 67*(5), 422–436.

Adams, J. S. (1965). Inequity in social exchange. In L. Berkowitz (Ed.), *Advances in Experimental Social Psychology, II* (pp. 267–299). New York: Academic Press.

Agency for Healthcare Research and Quality (AHRQ). (2010). *2010 National Quality and Disparities Reports.* Retrieved July 24, 2017, from https://archive.ahrq.gov/research/findings/nhqrdr/nhqrdr10/qrdr10.html.

Aiken, L. H. (2002). Commentary. *Medical Care Research and Review, 59*(2), 215–222.

Ajzen, I. (1991). The theory of planned behavior. *Organizational Behavior and Human Decision Processes, 50,* 179–211.

American Association of Colleges of Nursing. (2007). Nursing shortage resource fact sheet. Retrieved July 24, 2017, from http://www.aacn.nche.edu/Media/shortageresource.htm#about.

Armitage, C. J., & Conner, M. (2001). Efficacy of the theory of planned behavior: A meta-analytic review. *British Journal of Social Psychology, 40*(4), 471–499.

Bandura, A. (1977). Self-efficacy: Toward a unifying theory of behavioral change. *Psychological Review, 84*(2), 191–215.

Becker, L. J. (1978). Joint effect of feedback and goal setting on performance: A field study of residential energy conservation. *Journal of Applied Psychology, 63*(4), 428–433.

Blayney, K. D. (Ed.). (1992). *Healing hands: Customizing your health team for institutional survival.* Battle Creek, MI: W. K. Kellogg Foundation.

Brockner, J. (2006). Why it's so hard to be fair. *Harvard Business Review, 84*(3), 122–129.

Brockner, J. (2015) *The process matters: Engaging and equipping individuals for success.* Princeton, NJ: Princeton University Press.

Campbell, J. P., & Pritchard, R. D. (1976). Motivation theory in industrial and organizational psychology. In M. D. Dunnette (Ed.), *Handbook of industrial and organizational psychology* (pp. 63–130). Skokie, IL: Rand McNally.

Centers for Medicare & Medicaid Services. (2017). *The physician feedback program & quality and resource use reports (QRURs)* [PDF document]. Retrieved July 24, 2017, from https://www.cms.gov/Medicare/Medicare-Fee-for-Service -Payment/PhysicianFeedbackProgram/downloads/QRUR _Presentation.pdf.

Cerasoli, C. P., Nicklin, J. M., & Ford, M. T. (2014). Intrinsic motivation and extrinsic incentives jointly predict performance: A 40-year meta-analysis. *Psychological Bulletin, 140*(4), 980–1008.

Chang, C.-H., Ferris, D. L., Johnson, R. E., et al. (2012). Core self-evaluations: A review and evaluation of the literature. *Journal of Management, 38*(1), 81–128.

Charns, M. P., & Smith-Tewksbury, L. J. (1993). *Collaborative management in health care: Implementing the integrative organization.* San Francisco, CA: Jossey-Bass.

Damberg, C. L., Sorbero, M. E., Lovejoy, S. L., et al. (2014). *Measuring success in health care value-based purchasing programs: Findings from an environmental scan, literature review, and expert panel discussions.* Santa Monica, CA: Rand Corporation. Retrieved July 24, 2017, from http://www.rand. org/pubs/research_reports/RR306.html.

D'Aunno, T., Broffman, L., Sparer, M., et al. (2016). Factors that distinguish high-performing accountable care organizations in the Medicare Shared Savings Program. *Health Service Research, 53*(1), 120–137. doi:10.1111/1475-6773.12642.

Ford, R. C, & Fottler, M. D. (1995). Empowerment: A matter of degree. *Academy of Management Executive, 9*(3), 21–29.

Georgopoulos, B. S., Mahoney, B. S., & Jones, N. W. (1957). A path-goal approach to productivity. *Journal of Applied Psychology, 41*(6), 345–353.

Grant, A. M., & Parker, S. K. (2009). Redesigning work design theories: The rise of relational and proactive perspectives. *Academy of Management Annals, 3*(1), 317–375.

Hackman, J. R., & Oldham, G. R. (1976). Motivation through the design of work: Test of a theory. *Organizational Behavior and Human Performance, 16*(2), 250–279.

Hackman, J. R., & Oldham, G. R. (1980). *Work redesign.* Reading, MA: Addison-Wesley.

Higgins, E. T. (1997). Beyond pleasure and pain. *American Psychologist, 52*(12), 1280–1300.

Humphrey, S. E., Nahrgang, J. D., & Morgeson, F. P. (2007). Integrating motivational, social, and contextual work design features: A meta-analytic summary and theoretical extension of the work design literature. *Journal of Applied Psychology, 92*(5), 1332–1356.

Institute of Medicine. (2003). *Patient safety: Achieving a new standard for care.* Washington, DC: The National Academies Press.

Ivancevich, J. M., & McMahon, J. T. (1982). The effects of goal-setting, external feedback, and self- generated feedback on outcome variables: A field experiment. *Academy of Management Journal, 25*(2), 359–372.

Kanfer, R., Chen, G., & Pritchard, R. D. (2008). The three Cs of work motivation: Content, context, and change. In R. Kanfer, G. Chen, & R. D. Pritchard (Eds.), *Work motivation: Past, present, and future* (pp. 1–16). New York: Routledge.

Kanfer, R., Frese, M., & Johnson, R. E. (2017). Motivation related to work: A century of progress. *Journal of Applied Psychology, 102*(3), 338–355.

Kanfer, R., & Ackerman, P. L. (2004). Aging, adult development and work motivation. *Academy of Management Review, 29*(3), 423–439.

Kim, W. C., & Mauborgne, R. (2003). Fair process: Managing in the knowledge economy. *Harvard Business Review, 81*(1), 127–136, reprint number RO301K.

Kovner, C., Brewer, C., Wu, Y.-W., et al. (2006). Factors associated with work satisfaction of registered nurses. *Journal of Nursing Scholarship, 38*(1), 71–79.

Lanaj, K., Chang, C.-H., & Johnson, R. E. (2012). Regulatory focus and work-related outcomes: A review and meta-analysis. *Psychological Bulletin, 138*(5), 998–1034.

Latham, G. P., & Locke, E. A. (2006). Enhancing the benefits and overcoming the pitfalls of goal setting. *Organizational Dynamics, 34*(5), 332–340.

Laurinaitis, J. (1997). Actions speak louder than posters. *Psychology Today, 30*(3), 16.

Locke, E. A. (1968). Effects of knowledge of results, feedback in relation to standards, and goals on reaction-time performance. *American Journal of Applied Psychology, 81*(4), 566–574.

Locke, E. A. (1982). Relation of goal level to performance with a short work period and multiple goal levels. *Journal of Applied Psychology, 67*(4), 512–514.

Locke, E. A., & Latham, G. P. (1990). Work motivation and satisfaction: Light at the end of the tunnel. *Psychological Science, 1*(4), 240–246.

Locke, E. A., & Latham, G. P. (2004). What should we do about motivation theory? Six recommendations for the twenty-first century. *Academy of Management Review, 29*(3), 388–403.

McClelland, D. C. (1961). *The achieving society.* Princeton, NJ: Van Nostrand.

McClelland, D. C. (1965). Achievement and entrepreneurship: A longitudinal study. *Journal of Personality and Social Psychology, 1*(4), 389–392.

McGraw, K. O., & McCullers, J. C. (1979). Evidence of a detrimental effect of extrinsic incentives on breaking a mental set. *Journal of Experimental Social Psychology, 15*(3), 285–294.

McHugh, M. D., Kutney-Lee, A., Cimiotti, J. P., Sloane, D. M., & Aiken, L. H. (2011). Nurses' widespread job dissatisfaction, burnout, and frustration with health benefits signal problems for patient care. *Health Affairs (Millwood), 30*(2), 202–210.

McKethan, A., & Jha, A. K. (2014). Designing smarter pay-for-performance programs. *Journal of the American Medical Association, 312*(24), 2617–2618.

Meeker, D., Linder, J. A., Fox, C. R., et al. (2016). Effect of behavioral interventions on inappropriate antibiotic prescribing among primary care practices: A randomized clinical trial. *Journal of the American Medical Association, 315*(6), 562–570.

Memorial Hermann Sugar Land. (2016). 2016 Baldrige National Quality Award Application. Retrieved July 24, 2017, from https://www.nist.gov/baldrige.

Mitchell, T. R. (1982). Motivation: New directions for theory, research, and practice. *Academy of Management Review, 7*(1), 80–88.

Murray, H. A. (1938). *Explorations in personality.* New York: Oxford University Press.

Nembhard, I. M, & Edmondson, A. C. (2006). Making it safe: The effects of leader inclusiveness and professional status on psychological safety and improvement efforts in health care teams. *Journal of Organizational Behavior, 27*(7), 941–966.

Noe, R. A., Hollenbeck, J. R., Gerhart, B., & Wright, P. M. (2006). *Human resource management: Gaining a competitive advantage.* New York: McGraw-Hill.

NSI Nursing Solutions, Inc. (2016, March). *2016 National Healthcare Retention & RN Staffing Report.* Retrieved from https://avanthealthcare.com/pdf /NationalHealthcareRNRetentionReport2016.pdf.

O'Connor, S. J., & Lanning, J. A. (1992). The end of autonomy? Reflections on the post-professional physician. *Health Care Management Review, 17*(1), 63–72.

Pfeffer, J. (1998). Six dangerous myths about pay. *Harvard Business Review, 76*(3), 109–119.

Phillips, J. M., Hollenbeck, J. R., & Ilgen, D. R. (1996). Prevalence and prediction of positive discrepancy creation: Examining a discrepancy between two self-regulation theories. *Journal of Applied Psychology, 81*(5), 498–511.

Phillips, J. M., & Gully, S. M. (1997). Role of goal orientation, ability, need for achievement, and locus of control in the self-efficacy and goal-setting process. *Journal of Applied Psychology, 82*(5), 792–802.

Pritchard, R. D., De Leo, P. J., & Von Bergen, C. W. (1976). A field experimental test of expectancy-valence incentive motivation techniques. *Organizational Behavior and Human Performance, 15*(2), 355–406.

Smith, W. R. (2000). Evidence for the effectiveness of techniques to change physician behavior. *CHEST, 118*(2, suppl.), 8S–17S.

Stajkovic, A. D., & Luthans, F. (2001). Differential effects of incentive motivators on work performance. *Academy of Management Journal, 4*(3), 580–590.

Steffen, T. M., Nystrom, P. C, & O'Connor, S. J. (1996). Satisfaction with nursing homes: The design of employees jobs can ultimately influence family members' perceptions. *Journal of Health Care Marketing, 16*(3), 34–38.

Thaler, R. H., & Sunstein, C. R. (2008). *Improving decisions about health, wealth, and happiness.* New Haven, CT: Yale University Press.

Vroom, V. (1964). *Work and motivation.* New York: Wiley.

Wallace, C., & Chen, G. (2006). A multilevel integration of personality, climate, self-regulation, and performance. *Personnel Psychology, 59*(3), 529–557.

Wood, R. E., Mento, A. J., & Locke, E. A. (1987). Task complexity as a moderator of goal effects: A meta-analysis. *Journal of Applied Psychology, 72*(3), 416–425.

World Health Organization. (2008). *Guidelines: Incentives for health professionals.* Geneva, Switzerland: World Health Organization.

Chapter 5

Teams and Team Effectiveness in Health Services Organizations

Bruce J. Fried and Amy C. Edmondson

CHAPTER OUTLINE

- Introduction
- Teams in Health Care
- A Typology of Teams in Health Care
- Understanding Team Performance
- A Model of Team Effectiveness
- Conclusions

LEARNING OBJECTIVES

After completing this chapter, the reader should be able to:

1. Discuss the role and value of teams in health care organizations
2. Distinguish among different types of teams in health care organizations and how these differences affect team processes and performance
3. Identify the factors associated with high-performing teams
4. Describe the potential impact of team characteristics, nature of the work, environmental context, and team processes on team performance
5. Explain alternative methods of decision making in teams, including both functional and dysfunctional decision-making processes
6. Describe the importance of psychological safety to effective team decision making and performance
7. Describe how organizations can develop a culture and processes such that temporary teams, virtual teams, and teams whose composition rapidly changes can succeed
8. Discuss how factors external to the team may affect team processes and performance
9. Discuss the multiple impacts of team cohesiveness on team performance
10. Describe key aspects of group process including leadership, the communication structure, decision making, and stages of team development

KEY TERMS

Accountabilities in Teams

Ambassador Activities

Behavior Norms

Boundary Permeability

Boundary-Spanning Roles

Communication Networks

Communication Technology

Decisional Authority

Delphi Technique

Diversity and Inclusion

Environmental Context

Formal Leadership

Free Rider Syndrome

Groupthink

Informal Leadership

Intergroup Relationships

Management Teams

Membership Fluidity

Nominal Group Technique

Organizational Culture

Parallel Teams

Performance Norms

Pooled Interdependence

Project Teams

Psychological Safety

Reciprocal Interdependence

Scaffolding

Scout Activities

Sequential Interdependence

Skill- and Knowledge-Based Pay
   Social Capital

Social Loafing

Stages of Team Development

Status Differences

Support Teams

Task Coordinator Activities

Task Interdependence

Team-Based Rewards

Team Cohesiveness

Team Composition

Team Goals

Team Interdependence

Team Leadership

Team Learning

Team Norms

Team Performance

Team Processes

Team Size

Teaming

Temporal Nature of Teams

Tenure Diversity

Work Teams

• • • IN PRACTICE: Improving Preventive Services in a Pediatrics Practice: A Less-Than-Successful Team

Glendale Pediatrics is a nine-clinician pediatric group practice. The practice serves a largely middle-class suburban population and prides itself on the provision of preventive services. One of the physicians recently attended a continuing medical education program on preventive services. Upon her return, she decided to assess the practice's performance in this area. She and the other physicians were surprised when she distributed the results. Among the findings were the following:

- Sixty percent of children were behind schedule in at least one immunization.
- Vision screening was conducted and recorded for only 15 percent of children.
- Fifty percent of children were screened for anemia.
- Twenty-five percent of children had their blood pressure recorded in the patient record.
- Thirteen percent of children were screened for lead.

While the pediatricians were bewildered by these findings, the medical record and nursing staff found them consistent with their impressions. The findings were presented and discussed at the monthly staff meeting. Two physicians who together saw about 40 percent of all patients were adamant that their patients were current in their preventive services, and there was no need for a practice-wide effort to improve their preventive service rates. Unfortunately, the data were not linked to individual physicians and thus there was no way to verify their claim. Nonetheless, it was agreed that staff, including the two reluctant physicians, work as a team to address the problem.

The first meeting was scheduled over the noon hour. One of the physicians arrived at 12:20 while two others left early at 12:45. One of the nurses was out sick. No decisions were made, and the entire meeting was spent attempting to find a date and time for follow-up meetings.

At the next meeting, one physician stated that during an acute visit, physicians do not have time to go through the medical record to determine if a patient was behind on any preventive services. The other physicians agreed

• • • IN PRACTICE: Improving Preventive Services in a Pediatrics Practice: A Less-Than-Successful Team (Continued)

and decided that an electronic form should be developed listing all preventive services, and this should be linked to the electronic medical record. The nurses worked together after the meeting to design the form, known as the Preventive Services Chart (PSC).

When the physicians saw the form, they indicated that it was poorly designed. Not all relevant services and immunization schedules were included. The form was eliminated, and the physicians asked the nurses to redesign the form. The nurses consulted with the physician who attended the continuing education seminar to obtain information on the recommended preventive protocols. Based on this information, the form was redesigned with the immunization schedule and other information added. Confident that this was the right form, the new electronic form was rolled out. When presented to the physicians, it was discovered that there was little agreement among the physicians, and an argument broke out at the next meeting about the immunization schedules and protocols for screening.

After this meeting, one of the nurses in consultation with two physicians developed yet another form with separate columns for each physician's preventive services preferred protocol. The medical records staff, hearing about this new procedure informally over lunch, was skeptical about its feasibility. Moreover, when one of the nurses asked a physician when nurses would record this information, she was told that "nurses have it too easy in this practice . . . you have a great deal of down time and you certainly can find time to prepare charts for the next day's patients."

During the next three weeks, the following events transpired:

1. Nurses complained to the physicians that medical records staff were not making records available to them in time to do the preventive services review.

2. Medical records staff complained to the physicians that nurses were unrealistically requesting the next day's charts at 9:00 a.m. so that they could spend the day preparing for the next day's patients. They also reported that nurses were rude in their requests.

3. Physicians complained among themselves that preventive services information was absent for almost half of the patients, and they suspected that the information was inaccurate for a significant number of cases for which information was provided.

4. Nurses were spending an additional one to two hours in the office preparing for the next day's patients. They requested, and were denied, overtime pay.

5. Confusion was rampant when files were prepared for one physician, but another physician ended up seeing the patient. An even more difficult problem was caused by drop-in patients, for whom record reviews were not prepared. Nurses spent up to 30 minutes looking over these drop-in charts and recording the information on the PSC.

6. Two weeks after the system was implemented, one nurse quit abruptly at 3:00 and walked out.

7. One physician gave each parent a hard copy of the PSC and asked parents to record preventive services themselves since the physicians were "too busy to keep track of this."

After a month, the team met again. The physicians decided that the "solution" caused more problems than it solved. They decided to disband the team and work on the preventive services problem individually.

CHAPTER PURPOSE

Teams represent the bedrock of health care organizations, whether we are delivering clinical care or preventive care services, teaching health professionals, or conducting clinical or health services research. The effectiveness of teams can have a direct impact on the effectiveness of the entire organization. A highly skilled professional may be unable to apply her training and skills without an effective team to support her work. Similar to the need to manage information, financial resources, and people, teams also need to be managed. They rarely function to their full potential without appropriate organization and leadership. The purpose of this chapter is to help managers to draw on the full potential of teams and to overcome the most common obstacles to optimal **team performance**. The chapter presents evidence about team effectiveness and team management strategies that may be applied by managers to strengthen their competency in managing and improving teams.

INTRODUCTION

The "In Practice: Improving Preventive Services in a Pediatrics Practice: A Less-Than-Successful Team" case illustrates the variety of ways that teams can run into difficulty. Nonetheless, teams are a mainstay of life in health care and can be useful vehicles for improving quality—if they are organized and managed in an effective manner.

Teams are a mainstay in how we work in society, whether we are involved in business, health care, sports, education, or virtually any other endeavor. Teams are central to twenty-first-century culture, and have been enabled and expanded significantly by globalization, digitalization, and every more sophisticated and efficient modes of communication. Technological and spatial barriers to communication have all but dissolved to the point that it is difficult for many people to recall a time when these barriers existed.

In health care, teams are an indispensable means of work and are present in every venue in which health services are planned, delivered, or evaluated. Within a health care organization, for example, planning for building or renovating a facility may involve a mix of engineers, clinicians, financial analysts, architects, and a variety of technical experts. Carrying out any surgical procedure requires a team of individuals with specialized expertise. Teams are also employed to develop and evaluate quality improvement initiatives, recruit and select new employees, run an emergency department (ED), provide training to employees, and develop and exercise disaster management plans. Some teams, such as a team running a clinical trial, may extend over relatively long periods of time with relatively stable membership, whereas other teams, such as a team of professionals in an ED, may form and reform several times over the course of a day. Team members may work in close proximity to each other, and others may include members from multiple time zones.

Teams represent a method of working, and like any other tool or technology, they can be enormously productive and efficient. They have the potential to improve patient outcomes, reduce costs, solve complex problems, and increase patient satisfaction. Effectively organized and managed teams can raise the level of morale, job satisfaction, and employee engagement. Teams can be a source of learning for the organization, where information is generated about ways to improve processes and outcomes. Conversely, teams can have pathological effects on an organization and its members. Poorly functioning teams can be destructive to morale and relationships and sources of abuse and harassment. Dysfunctional teams may lead to members covering up serious problems and errors, which may lead to catastrophic impacts

on patients. In the clinical realm, effective patient care and management are dependent upon teams. This is the case whether we are dealing with a patient undergoing a surgical procedure in an operating room, or a frail elderly patient with multiple chronic medical conditions living at home. In clinical situations, teams are required to not only provide effective medical solutions but also recognize and address situations that may lead to medical errors. In fact, the entire quality improvement movement—whether in automobile manufacturing or in an operating room—is dependent upon teams. Team training and effective team management are central to quality improvement initiatives (Institute for Health Improvement [IHI], 2016). In reality, there are few, if any, individual heroes or heroines in organizations saving the day. In fact, even the most gifted and talented people need a supportive team to sustain their performance. In most situations in health care, the organization will not reap the full benefits of a talented person unless he or she is supported by, or part of, a strong, competent, highly functional team.

The goal of this chapter is to provide the reader with an understanding of what makes teams effective. To do this, we provide background on the many types of teams that exist in health care, how teams differ in their functions and processes, the common pathologies facing teams, and strategies for improving team performance. While common discourse about teams is often based on a static view of an established group of people who intensively interact in pursuit of a common goal, in many situations, this model no longer holds. For example, the sports team is frequently used as a model for describing teams. With globalization, advances in technology and communication, and new organizational forms have come new approaches to team organization, such as virtual teams. Virtual teams include an array of unorthodox team arrangements, including teams where team members rarely or never actually have face-to-face contact, teams where members are geographically dispersed, and teams that are dispersed over time (Foster et al., 2015). For example, the authors of this chapter rarely interact in person; our collaboration is mediated by information technology. Additionally, many teams are temporary and may form and disband in a matter of days or hours. Consider the example of a multiorganizational emergency response team formed to respond to a community emergency. In many instances, team members may have never met before yet are required to develop trust and cooperate in response to an incident (Moldjord and Iversen, 2015). The emergence of new type of teams challenges organizations to develop new ways to organize and manage such teams. Later in this chapter, we discuss how organizations can develop structures to enable teams to form and function effectively for short periods even where team members may have never met.

For many decades, teams have been the focus of extensive research, and much has been learned about team effectiveness. Some of this research has been conducted in health care organizations, but the vast majority has been carried out in other settings, ranging from sports teams to product development teams to airline pilot crews. A remarkable aspect of this research is that lessons learned from one type of team are often applicable to other types of teams. This provides the opportunity to use the results of research carried out in diverse settings to inform this discussion of teams in health care. Thus, this chapter will present some of the most important research findings related to high-performing teams. The discussion will begin with a description of the types of teams found in health care organizations.

TEAMS IN HEALTH CARE

Teams are groups, but not all groups are teams. While there is a wide variety of type of teams, overall teams have a defined purpose, membership, or composition that may be static or quite fluid over time, structure, specific processes to guide the team's work, and leadership. Groups (that are not teams) may possess some characteristics of teams but lack one or more key elements. Key characteristics of teams are having a common purpose, defined members (although membership may change frequently), structure of positions or roles, processes of working together, and at least one person in the leadership role. Teams may have formal and informal leaders, leadership functions that rotate among team members, and at times, leaders who are external to the team (Morgeson, DeRue, and Karam, 2010). In fact, team leadership can emerge simultaneously from multiple sources. A surgical team clearly meets the characteristics of a team; it has a purpose, defined members, structure, processes, and leadership. A group of nurses who go out

to dinner together would likely not be considered a team, although meeting some of the characteristics of a team.

In this chapter, we focus on teams whose purpose is directly related to the goals of the organization. We apply the definition of teams developed by Cohen and Bailey (1997) as "a collection of individuals who are interdependent in their tasks, who share responsibility for outcomes, who see themselves and who are seen by others as an intact social entity embedded in one or more larger social systems . . . and who manage their relationships across organizational boundaries." While there is much variation in teams, we view teams as intact social systems with boundaries, interdependence among members, and differentiated member roles or structure. Organizationally based teams are task-oriented with a specific purpose. They generally have one or more tasks to perform and produce measurable outcomes. Last, they operate within an organizational or, in some instances, a multiorganizational context and interact with a larger organization or organizational subunits (Hackman, 1990a).

We include in our discussion teams that are time-limited, such as project or product development teams, as well as those that are more permanent in nature. It is important to note that in addition to the permanence dimension, teams vary across many other dimensions as well. The most important of these are discussed below. We sometimes use the term "group" instead of "team." This is usually because research in a particular area has been dominated by researchers who have examined groups in a generic sense (i.e., with no distinctions between teams and groups), and therefore refer to groups rather than teams. We employ the original language of their research, although much of this earlier work may be applied to teams as we define them.

• • • IN PRACTICE: Can We Create a Team Culture?

As chair of a subspecialty department in a medical school, Dr. Rideout understands that patients are treated not just by individual physicians but by teams of people in the department. For example, when a patient enters the clinic, she confronts a team of individuals—a desk clerk, nurse, technician, physician, a patient business associate, and so forth. He has found, however, that these teams have dysfunctional characteristics and result in low levels of patient satisfaction and poor morale. He has consulted with his staff and is struggling to create a department that is supportive of teamwork. Consider the following comments:

From a Physician: They're typical state employees. When I need a technician to prep a patient in the clinic, they're nowhere to be found. What do these people do all day? It's my job to treat patients, and since we're now paid partially on the basis of patient satisfaction scores, when a patient is left waiting, this brings down our scores and we all suffer. These state employees don't realize that we're in a teaching hospital, and I have responsibilities for research and teaching, not to mention being part of all of these hospital committees. These technicians have no sense of accountability. And don't even ask me about the patient business associates and the schedulers. We should fire them all and start from scratch.

From a Technician: Many of these physicians treat the clinic as if it is their private practice. They think that all they have to do is snap their fingers and a technician will magically appear. Never mind that each technician works for three or four physicians and, when a physician needs me to prep a patient, I am usually in the process

• • • IN PRACTICE: Can We Create a Team Culture? *(Continued)*

of prepping another patient for someone else. The physicians are worried about patient waiting time. Most of them show up around 8:45 in the morning for their 8:00 appointment, so we're already behind schedule by 8:01. Then they disappear midday without telling us where they are or when they'll be back. And they're blaming us for our dismally low patient satisfaction scores.

From a Patient Business Associate: This is a difficult job. I do everything from answering phones, registering new patients, dealing with payment and insurance issues with patients, communicating with patients in person and by phone, and solving or trying to solve problems. When a patient is angry, it's my job to calm her and diffuse her anger. When a physician gets angry with me or someone else, I grin and bear it. The worst situation is when physicians argue with staff in front of patients. We provide excellent quality care, but patients do have other options. We need to think of the patient in customer terms. My days are filled with multitasking and being accountable to physicians and the clinic directors—and also advocating for patients. I must be focused, attentive to details and friendly. This is a stressful and unpleasant place to work. I've been here five years, and last week I started sending my resume out.

From the Clinic Director: I am caught right smack in the middle. Everyone complains to me. The technicians complain about the physicians and schedulers, the patient business associates complain about the physicians, and they probably all complain about me. My co-director and I have worked hard to get some team spirit around here. We have social events on holidays and birthdays, but only the Chair and one or two physicians ever attend. As I see it, everyone here has turned into a caricature. Physicians and staff don't speak to each other as individuals, but as stereotypes. "Technicians are lazy, schedulers are incompetent, patient business associates are do-gooders who try to get patients seen even if they can't pay, and physicians are arrogant." The only thing positive here is the Chair. Everyone likes Dr. Rideout, but he doesn't like confrontation and has let things go too far. He should have been stronger and gotten these people into line long ago. We're a teaching hospital, and these people behave as if they're 6-year old brats. I love the mission of this hospital, but I could get a job in a private medical practice for better pay and far less stress.

As the chair of the department in a Midwestern medical school, Dr. Rideout realizes that this situation has deteriorated. The department is among the lowest in the health system in patient satisfaction scores, and staff morale is at its lowest point in the 10 years that he has been chair. "Our employees are loyal, but we scare away many good potential employees. On several occasions, new staff members have left after two weeks here."

Dr. Rideout is a firm believer in teamwork, but he has become exceedingly frustrated because of deterioration in whatever teamwork there may once have been. This was a tough place when he came 10 years ago and has not improved. He is weary and skeptical of the complaining and thinks they are all to blame—or no one is to blame. He is a good listener and has hoped that his listening will diffuse the anger felt by physicians and staff. This has not worked. He is planning to retire in two years and wants to leave the department in better shape than it was when he arrived.

Dr. Rideout is sincere and well-meaning but does not know where to turn. He feels he is dealing with some very difficult personalities, and perhaps this is just the way of the world. Dr. Rideout has consulted with other department heads, his wife, a psychiatrist, and with his clinic directors. He has even spoken with his minister. These people were kind and supportive but could provide no real help. However, at the Christmas party two weeks ago, he happened to be talking with a student working on her MHA. Being in the holiday mood, he shared some of his problems with her. She had some interesting comments and observations. Most memorable were two specific comments: The first was the following: *Many health care organizations are filled with good people working in bad processes.* The other comment, which really caught his attention, was the following: *Every system is perfectly designed to achieve the results that it produces.*

A TYPOLOGY OF TEAMS IN HEALTH CARE

A discussion of team characteristics can be confusing because of the multiple ways teams have been described over time. Using a typology (i.e., grouping by dimensions) generally facilitates this type of discussion; therefore, in this chapter, we use the subsequent typology along with a description of each element:

1. Function or purpose
2. Decisional authority
3. Temporal nature
4. Time and space

5. Diversity and Inclusion
6. Accountabilities
7. Membership fluidity and boundary permeability

Function or Purpose: Why a Team?

The first element in our typology is function or purpose. Teams are employed for multiple purposes in health care and have become a primary mechanism for getting work done. An important question worthy of attention is whether it is desirable to have a team, rather than an individual, accomplish a particular task. In many settings, it is routine for a manager, faced with a difficult decision, to assign a team to analyze the options and make a recommendation. That is, if a complex task is to be accomplished, a team may be most the appropriate vehicle for accomplishing the work. It is not an exaggeration to say that teams are the building blocks of organizations.

Teamwork offers many potential advantages. Assuming that teams are functioning effectively, they have the potential to create synergy among its members. The term "synergy" is typically used to summarize the idea that the productivity of a team may exceed the sum of individual member contributions. In the area of decision making, synergy also refers to the generation of ideas to improve decision making. The interplay of ideas among team members can generate innovation, particularly when members build on and critically evaluate the work and ideas of others on the team. In this way, if one member of a team overlooks a factor critical for decision making, under the right conditions, other members can supplement such gaps with the information necessary to make an effective decision. In addition, teams can be a source of empowerment and satisfaction for employees, which, in turn, may lead to lower turnover and absenteeism, and greater commitment to the goals of the organization. Perhaps of greatest importance is that teams bring together diverse expertise and perspectives from multiple disciplines. As a result, this knowledge is brought to bear on complex problems, decisions, or tasks.

Despite their advantages, teams can also have drawbacks. For example, teams may diffuse talent in an organization. Is the organization asking its most talented people to spend time on a team when their efforts could be better used for other tasks? Teams also require a team-oriented culture and level of infrastructure and processes to function effectively. An organization that is not team-focused may not be prepared to make accommodations and structures required for effective team performance. For example, most organizations are structured under traditional unity of command principles. That is, each person is accountable to one person, typically the chief of a particular functional area, such as nursing or information technology. However, when an organization moves to cross-functional teams, employees may have multiple **accountabilities**, perhaps to project

team managers as well as their functional manager. As a result, the organization must be prepared to train managers to supervise teams, while also training employees to work in a team-focused environment. Following from this, individuals within the organization must have **team leadership** competencies related to effective team management, such as conflict management, communication, and meeting management. Put simply, although teams have the potential to increase productivity and improve quality, they also have the potential to increase costs and stress if they are initiated in an organization unprepared to develop the necessary mechanisms to support teams.

In determining if a team is appropriate for a particular task or decision, it is important to understand the multiple purposes of teams. Below, we describe work teams, support teams, parallel teams, project teams, and management teams in the following paragraphs.

Work teams are groups of people responsible for producing goods or providing services. These teams are directed toward the primary mission and objectives of the organization such as treating ED patients, providing immunizations and other preventive services to children, managing patients on an intensive care unit (ICU), and developing a new pharmaceutical product. These teams may be directed by supervisors or manage themselves. In the health care environment, work teams include treatment teams, research teams, home care teams, and community-based crisis intervention teams. Work teams are usually ongoing and relatively permanent in nature, although membership and leadership may vary. Work teams can consist of members of the same discipline, or they can be multidisciplinary. They may also involve people at multiple levels in the organization and people with significantly different levels of education. The term "microsystem" is used to describe small groups of people who work together on a regular basis to provide care to patient subpopulations (Nelson et al., 2002). These are freestanding clinical units with both clinical and business aims designed to maximize performance outcomes (Batalden et al., 2003). We can say that work teams do the fundamental work of the organization, whether this means providing services, producing products, or generating new knowledge.

Support teams enable others to do their work and serve many functions such as quality improvement, strategic planning, and personnel search committees. Note that individuals who serve on work teams may also have a role on support teams. In this situation, they may be referred to as **parallel teams**—teams typically composed of people from different work units who carry out functions not regularly performed in the organization. They usually have limited authority and generally make recommendations to individuals higher in the organizational hierarchy. In the health care system, parallel teams may be involved in such activities as continuous quality improvement (CQI), task forces, community health needs assessments, and staff search committees. By their nature, they are often multidisciplinary. As suggested by the diversity of teams falling into this category, these teams may be temporary or permanent features of the organization.

Project teams are usually time-limited, producing one-time outputs such as a new product or service. In health care, such teams may exist for purposes of planning a new hospital, developing a new Alzheimer's unit in a nursing home, developing a new information system, writing a new employee handbook, or preparing a hospital disaster preparedness plan.

Last, management teams coordinate and provide direction to the subunits under their jurisdiction. Management teams may exist at multiple levels, such as board, senior management, or departmental levels. Management teams may also include members from multiple levels of the hierarchy. Members of management teams have defined line responsibilities, although management teams may at times include individuals who are in nonline staff positions. Such individuals may play roles that are different from those of managers. For instance, they may serve the team in an advisory capacity with limited decisional authority.

Note that team purposes described in this section may overlap; therefore, teams often include elements of different team types. For example, a support team can be established to complete a particular project, and a treatment team might function in a quality improvement capacity.

Decisional Authority

Perhaps one of the most misunderstood aspects of teams is the element we call decisional authority. Decisional authority refers to a continuum of roles that teams may play in decision making. At one end of the continuum, teams may have the authority to make decisions. The hospital board of trustees generally fits into this category. A self-managed work team comes close to having full decisional authority, although even these teams ultimately report to a higher authority, which may veto or otherwise alter a decision.

At the other extreme are teams with no decisional authority. These types of teams are frequently established to make recommendations or to generate options for decision making. For example, an organization seeking to install a new information system may assign a team composed of administrative support personnel and IT professionals to provide input on its information technology needs. Alternatively, such a team may be asked to assess the benefits and drawbacks of information systems from different vendors. They may or may not be asked to make a recommendation. In any event, final decision-making authority rests with senior management or a specific person or team higher in the hierarchy.

Misunderstandings about a team's decisional authority usually result from a team having vague or misinformation about its decisional role. Often, the decision-making authority of the team is not made clear, and teams may assume they have more authority than they actually have. The lesson for managers is apparent: the role of a team should be clear, particularly the role that it plays in decision making. However, even when decisional authority is made clear, team members may become disillusioned if they perceive that their recommendations or input have been ignored by the decision maker. In a team-focused organization, it is critical that managers respect team members' work and time. Where a decision is made that contradicts a team's recommendation, communication with team members is critical to avoid the frustration that may result from such situations. When unmanaged, disillusionment may inhibit future efforts to engage teams in similar work.

Temporal Nature

Teams vary in their temporal nature or permanence. As noted earlier, teams can be relatively permanent and ongoing or time-limited and focused on a particular project or task. The use of time-limited teams has become more common in large part because of the rapidity of change and the need to respond quickly to changing circumstances. In the area of new product development, for example, changes in technology, shorter product life cycles, and globalization require quick and efficient development of new products (Edmondson and Nembhard, 2009). The health care industry faces similar changes brought on by technological and other environmental changes. A new strain of influenza, for example, may affect multiple segments of a hospital. On a global scale, the West Africa Ebola outbreak required the rapid training and deployment of multidisciplinary rapid response teams consisting of, among others, anthropologists, community engagement experts, social mobilizers, doctors and nurses, sanitation workers, and safe and dignified burial teams (WHO, 2016).

Whether a team is temporary or not has no bearing on its importance to the organization. What is important, however, is that team processes accommodate the speed that is sometimes required of temporary teams. Group process and leadership issues, discussed later in this chapter, may need to be resolved more efficiently than in teams that are more traditional.

Time and Space

The vast quantity of research and literature on teams is predicated on teams that exist and function in a particular time and place. Advice offered on managing team meetings is based on the idea that meetings have set starting and ending times; some of this literature prescribes physical details of team management, such as optimal seating arrangements, mechanisms for ensuring full participation, and methods of dealing with people who arrive late and leave early.

With advances in communication and the ease with which **communication technology** can be used, rules of time and space often do not hold. Teams can communicate and work efficiently over any distance. Teams need not meet at a specified time, but virtual meetings can extend over several days if necessary, feasible, and appropriate to the team task. Team members can take hours or days to respond to a question from another team member, and one's response can be made at any time during the day or night.

Technology affords the opportunity for even physically constrained teams to have extended communication outside of the formal team setting. The term "virtual teams" implies that much or all communication among team members takes place outside of traditional face-to-face meetings through such mechanisms as e-mail, fax, and multiple forms of video teleconferencing. Teams operating through telemedicine-type approaches are used for education, consultation, diagnosis, and treatment, and they have the advantage of making available to virtual team members complex information in real time over virtually infinite distances. Team members can obtain specialized advice from experts at any distance. Thus, a radiologist in Mumbai can be a virtual member of a treatment team in rural Oklahoma. There is great potential using virtual teams in health care, including providing care to chronically ill patients (Wiecha and Pollard, 2007) and in ICUs (Hoonakker, McGuirem, and Carayon, 2011).

A study conducted at Rush University Medical Center found that a virtual health care team reduced emergency room visits by high-risk diabetes patients. Carried out under the auspices of the "Virtual Integrated Practice" (VIP) model, teams consisting of pharmacists, social workers, and dieticians communicated via multiple technologies to help coordinate care for these patients (Rush University Medical Center, 2008). Communication technology provides many new opportunities for enhanced teamwork, including the active inclusion of patients on virtual teams.

While there is potential for growth in virtual teams, it is important to note that virtual teams require additional rules and guidance. Virtual teams enhance the ability for teams to fluidly shift team membership according to particular needs. This may involve the inclusion of people from outside the organization, including patients. These dynamics present additional challenges for managers. New or modified processes for team management must be designed, tested, and refined. These dynamics may also have implications for traditional reporting relationships, accountability, and reward systems in the organization. Modified measurement and control systems need to be put in place to ensure that performance is effectively monitored. Finally, since technology plays a central role in virtual teams, it is necessary for team members to be comfortable with the multiple communication technologies used by a virtual team. This is not a trivial point, particularly since virtual team members may come from different organizations (or no organization at all) and backgrounds.

Diversity and Inclusion

Diversity provides both opportunities and challenges for teamwork. The advantages include the opportunity to obtain multiple perspectives and expertise that may be required for effective decision making. A major challenge resulting from diversity is managing multiple viewpoints and worldviews and the conflicts that may result from interactions among diverse team members.

It is important to note that having a team with diverse membership does not guarantee that the team will benefit from the knowledge and insights of its members. Diverse membership is an appropriate starting point for obtaining multiple ideas, but an inclusive and safe environment is required for team members to feel comfortable expressing their views. For example, one dimension of diversity is having team members from different hierarchical levels in the organization. This is common in quality improvement teams, where the insights of people at lower levels are particularly important because they are often closest to where the impact of quality gaps appears. It should not be assumed that team members at lower levels of the organization would feel sufficiently secure to disagree or question the views of others in the team. In other words, it is important for team leaders to create and reinforce an inclusive culture where members are encouraged to participate without fear of having their views discounted or ignored by others.

Diversity itself is multidimensional, and depending upon the team and its needs, diversity may be defined differently. In society at large, we tend to think of diversity in terms of ethnic and racial diversity, and in health care, diversity in professional backgrounds is often used when discussing teams. Among the challenges faced by multidisciplinary teams are differences in social status between professions, different worldviews, and differences in language and professional terminology and jargon. However, diversity extends into other relevant domains, including the following:

- Diversity based on age and generation. This has particular relevance in organizations as they work to accommodate the work styles of baby boomers, Gen Xers, millennials, retired persons, and others.
- Gender diversity. This type of diversity requires an understanding of how gender may affect one's

worldview and perceptions of problems and solutions. In health care, gender is often correlated with social status in the organization—specifically, the fact that nurses are predominantly female and physicians are now split about equally between male and female.

- Diversity in hierarchical level. This is particularly relevant in health care teams, where **team composition** may specifically require people from different levels in the organization as well as different departments.

- Consumer and professional diversity. Teams sometimes include consumers as team members. Consumers may feel intimidated on health care teams because they lack familiarity with behavioral norms and the language used on professionally dominated teams. Consumers may also come from different socioeconomic backgrounds than professionals on a team, adding yet another diversity domain.

- Demographic and cultural diversity. Our health care organizations should optimally mirror the heterogeneous nature of society. As society in general struggles toward greater inclusiveness, organizations and teams confront the tensions, misunderstandings, and prejudices that sometimes result from a multicultural environment. Because many teams require close collaboration among their members, cultural differences may become magnified in a team setting.

Diversity can yield great benefits to organizations, but as Edmondson and Roloff (2009) discuss, obtaining these benefits requires that teams establish an environment of trust and psychological safety. That is, team members must feel comfortable expressing their views without fear of being unnoticed or worse being ostracized or demeaned.

Accountabilities

Just as teams have different levels of decisional authority, they also vary in the types of accountability required of them. Teams may be internally accountable, externally accountable, or both. A manager may assign a team the responsibility to complete a task; therefore, the team is externally accountable to that manager. On a project team, team members are accountable to the project team leader, but the project leader, representing the team, may be externally accountable to a manager outside of the team. Similarly, team members on a project team may also be accountable to their functional managers, a situation known as a program or matrix structure.

In well-functioning teams, team members perceive that they are accountable to *each other* for their individual contributions. Team communication, coordination, team outcomes, and discipline become the responsibility of team members, largely eliminating the need for external team management. In fact, in certain circumstances,

an effective team leader should strive for a team that is self-managing or has self-managing characteristics.

Membership Fluidity and Boundary Permeability

This final dimension deals with the nature of membership and team boundaries. It was noted earlier that teams might be temporary or permanent. Membership may also be relatively stable over time or fluid. In a medical school residents' advisory committee, team membership will change quite frequently as residents leave and new ones arrive. There are liabilities to **membership fluidity**, including lack of cohesiveness among team members. Teams with fluid membership may have to continuously reorient team members, and new team members may require considerable time before they are able to make significant contributions to the work of the team. On the other hand, fluid membership may bring a continuous influx of new ideas that may benefit team performance and keep the team from becoming so inwardly focused that it loses touch with changes in the external environment. On the downside, long-standing team members may resent "young Turks" who may be perceived as seeking to change the way things are done.

Related to membership fluidity is team **boundary permeability**. Some teams have a specific core membership that is sustained over time. The board of trustees of a hospital has a relatively stable set of team members, perhaps with a few members beginning and ending their terms each year. A team that is planning a new hospital wing will likely have a core membership that is relatively stable but may require additional team members as the need for new areas of expertise arises. Some members of this team may enter and exit the team several times according to the team's needs. Consider as well the team of professionals in a hospital ED. Team membership changes quite frequently during the course of a 24-hour day, just as the flight crew of a commercial passenger jet changes its composition with every flight. How do these teams function with such rapid turnover? The difference is that the work in an ED or passenger jet is highly standardized, and the professionals who work in these settings are highly trained in the roles they play in those settings. Even in a setting as unpredictable as an ED, employees are trained to respond in a planned way to the unexpected. Therefore, while teams may have permeable boundaries and membership, they may still exhibit high levels of performance.

In sum, teams vary along multiple dimensions. As discussed throughout this chapter, where teams locate themselves on these dimensions has important implications for team performance and team management. Teams strive for high levels of performance, and the following section addresses team performance.

UNDERSTANDING TEAM PERFORMANCE

We described earlier how teams represent the building blocks of organizational life and that the performance of a single employee is often determined by how well the team performs. Some may argue that too much importance is placed on how individual performance is affected by team performance. This may be true in certain types of work settings where an individual can outperform team performance. This would have its highest likelihood in a situation where there is a relative lack of interdependence between employees. For example, one could make the case (although it would contain many holes!) that an excellent elementary schoolteacher is unaffected by the overall quality of teaching in the school. We do have occasions in which excellent teachers teach in "bad" schools. It is difficult to come up with a similar situation in health care because the work of health care employees is so dependent upon the quality of others' work.

Moving beyond individual and team levels—to the organizational level—what is the impact of team performance on the overall performance of the organization? Here, the answer is much less ambiguous than the previous discussion about the impact of teams on individual performance. Everyone in a health care organization is a member of a team, and in most cases, employees are members of multiple teams, some of which may overlap in membership. Thus, teams are the entity that makes any kind of productivity possible. It is highly likely that a health care organization with poorly functioning teams will have lower productivity as well as lower levels of other effectiveness measures than an organization whose teams are well constituted and well managed. Given a choice, a surgical patient needing three days of postoperative care would certainly prefer a nursing unit where nurses communicate with each other accurately and where physicians and nurses respect each other's views. In a word, an informed patient would prefer a nursing unit that has the attributes of a strong team.

Some years ago, health care entered the era of accountability. Health care organizations have always had "reputations" for high or low quality, but the idea of actually measuring performance according to agreed-upon measures is relatively new. Private organizations and the U.S. government publicize quality ratings and rankings for hospitals (see https://www.medicare.gov/hospital-compare/search.html), nursing homes (see http://www.medicare.gov/NHCompare), and other health care organizations. While measurement and reporting are still incomplete and in need of further development and refinement, measurement of organizational performance in health care will be a constant feature of the health care environment, with teams playing a major role.

Consider some of the most important measures used by the Department of Health and Human Services to assess hospital quality (Medicare.gov, 2017):

- Rate of readmission for patients with pneumonia
- Rate of complications for patients receiving hip or knee replacements
- Health care workers given influenza vaccination
- Patients who reported that their nurses "always" communicated well

Each of these measures is based on professionally developed guidelines. Implementation of these procedures requires that the appropriate people in the hospital have an understanding of the guidelines and the evidence that informs them. However, knowing the guidelines and the supporting evidence is very different from taking the correct action based on those guidelines. For these and other measures, it is easy to demonstrate the role played by teams.

With hospitals eager to earn good ratings on such quality measures, it is somewhat surprising that they do not pay more attention to those "building blocks" of quality—teams. Much attention is given to assessing the quality of clinicians through review of credentials and past work experience. This provides necessary information about hospital staff members' technical competence, but it is inadequate to ensure that appropriate evidence-based procedures are implemented. Should hospitals have the same type of "credentialing" of teams? Given the importance of teams in implementing evidence-based practices and organizational performance, it seems advisable—at a minimum—for health care organizations to engage in periodic team audits that would address such questions as the following:

- What is the level of communication among team members in our organization? What are the strengths and weaknesses of communication on our teams?
- How satisfied are team members with how members communicate and how teams are managed? To what extent do team members feel as if they have input into decision making?
- What mechanisms do teams have in place to promote **team learning** and improvement in team processes and outcomes?
- To what extent do team members feel that it is safe to express themselves to other team members?
- What are the dominant leadership styles in our teams, and are these styles appropriate to the work of the team?
- Are we training team members and team leaders, and is there evidence that this training has resulted in improved team functioning and outcomes?

• What is the level of communication and coordination among teams? What are the specific areas that require improvement in interteam relationships? Do our teams have specific measures to assess their effectiveness in producing desired outcomes? Are team members aware of these measures, and are they reviewed periodically by team leaders?

Whether we are examining sports teams, surgical teams, or public health surveillance teams, it is clear that not all teams are equal. Some exhibit higher levels of performance than others do. Why do teams vary in their performance? Some variation may be due to differences in the skills of individual members, an explanation that may be salient in teams with little interdependence among their members; however, in many situations, individual team members may be highly talented, yet the team makes poor decisions that lead to suboptimal outcomes. Later in this chapter, for example, we discuss the concept of **groupthink**, in which disastrously poor advice may be generated and acted upon by a team of highly talented and skilled individuals.

In the following section, we present a model of team effectiveness. Using this model, we incorporate existing evidence of the major factors that make certain teams more effective than others.

A MODEL OF TEAM EFFECTIVENESS

What makes some teams more effective than others? We know that teams are not naturally effective by simply bringing people together who are highly skilled at their assigned tasks. Basic team member competence is important and necessary but insufficient to predict effective team performance. There is obviously not a single action that team leaders can take to ensure that their team will perform at peak levels. Nevertheless, there are actions and decisions that leaders can take to improve the probability that a team will perform at a high level and improve its performance over time. We adopt in this section a model of team effectiveness that includes a range of these actions, decisions, and processes. Some of these are interdependent, where implementation of one strategy is dependent upon another necessary strategy.

Notwithstanding the usefulness of this model, we also need to accept—as all managers must—that certain factors are outside of the control of the organization or manager. For example, we know that **team cohesiveness** is generally a positive team attribute, but a manager cannot always control events that may reduce team cohesion, such as turnover among team members. It is vital, however, that managers and team leaders understand and anticipate how uncontrollable factors may affect team performance. If such uncontrollable factors can

be planned for, negative impacts may be minimized. At the same time, uncontrollable factors can have a positive impact on team processes and outcomes. For instance, recessionary times, not controllable by managers, can nonetheless lead to lower employee turnover and potentially increase team cohesion. A manager can take advantage of such "silver linings" by using the opportunity to strengthen teams and improve working conditions.

Figure 5.1 provides an overview of the multiple factors associated with team effectiveness. In the interests of simplicity, the multiple interrelationships among these factors are not included in the model, although they are addressed in the text. Moving from left to right, the model sets out three sets of factors, referred to as Team Characteristics, Nature of the Work, and the Environmental Context within which the team is situated. For each item listed, note that most are at least partially controllable by the manager, the noted exceptions being Organizational Culture and External Environment.

Farther to the right of Figure 5.1 is a set of Team Process factors, many of which may be modified or controlled by the manager. Finally, Team Effectiveness factors are indicated. These include both performance outputs, such as patient outcomes, as well as team process measures, such as team member satisfaction and the capacity for team effectiveness to be sustained over time. As noted above, not illustrated in the model are potential interrelationships among these outcomes, such as the potential impact of team member satisfaction on patient outcomes.

Team Characteristics
Team Size, Composition, and Diversity

Team size has been a subject of research for many years. In general, **team size** has an inverted U-shaped relationship to effectiveness so that too few or too many members may reduce the level of performance (Cohen and Bailey, 1997). As teams grow in size, communication and coordination problems tend to increase, and a climate of cohesiveness may decrease (Colquitt, Noe, and Jackson, 2002; Liberman et al., 2001). However, a team must be sufficiently large to accomplish its work. A useful rule of thumb is that teams should be staffed to the smallest number to accomplish the work (Hackman, 1987).

The U-shaped relationship between size and effectiveness is not precise. In treatment teams, performance has been found to be negatively affected by size (Alexander et al., 1996; Vinokur-Kaplan, 1995b); in quality improvement teams, the effect was curvilinear (Shortell et al., 2004). Most likely, this is due to smaller teams being less cumbersome and having fewer social distractions. Smaller teams also experience a lower incidence of **social loafing**, a phenomenon in which a team member benefits from the work of the team without making a commensurate contribution to the work of the team

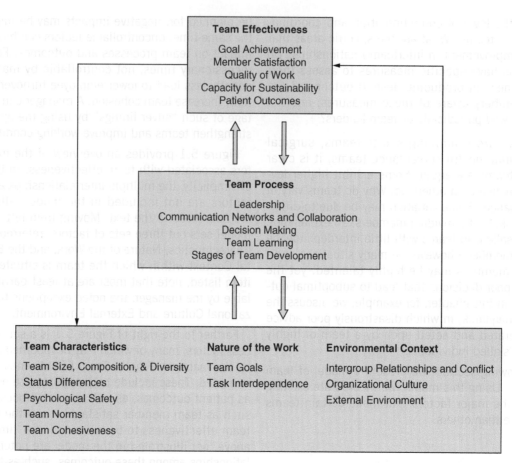

Figure 5.1 A Model of Team Effectiveness.

(Liden et al., 2004). A member's lack of work is more visible on a small team, while individuals in larger teams may be able to maintain anonymity and gain from the work of the group without making a suitable contribution.

However, team size is often out of the control of the manager, particularly when democratic representational norms pervade an organization. In these situations, constituencies may demand to be represented, and the leader may need to design strategies to make the group more manageable (e.g., forming subcommittees). Otherwise, teams may be *overstaffed.* Overstaffed teams may perform work in a perfunctory, lackadaisical manner. Overstaffed teams may also lead to competition and jealousy among team members, with individuals guarding their particular domain. Alternatively, members of large teams may distance themselves from the team's efforts and lack commitment to the team. On the other hand, breaking a team into subgroups or subcommittees has its own set of problems. When large teams are divided into smaller ones, subgroups may become cliquish and, while cohesive within themselves, may become isolated from the rest of the team.

As noted above, the impact of team size on performance is dependent upon a number of factors. Although

the empirical evidence on the relationship between team size and performance is less than definitive, it is useful for managers to keep in mind the potential problems and benefits that may emerge because of team size.

Team composition and diversity are important determinants of team performance as well. For certain types of teams, it is relatively easy to control team membership. The CEO of a hospital can select from a wide variety of employees to serve on a strategic planning task force, while the director of nursing may be highly constrained in the nurses chosen for a self-managed nursing team in a pediatric oncology unit. In the latter situation, the director of nursing is limited by the pool of nurses in the unit or trained in such a specialty area. However, an awareness of likely problems related to membership helps, at least, to identify potential problems and to develop strategies to manage them. In our examination of team composition, we consider the following diagnostic questions (Hackman, 1990b):

• Is the team appropriately staffed? Is the diversity of members appropriate?

• Do members have the expertise required to perform team tasks well?

- Are the members so similar that there is little for them to learn from one another? Alternatively, are they so heterogeneous that they risk having difficulty communicating and coordinating with one another?

- Is the team composed of members who have worked together before, and if not, how will team members learn about each other and their work styles?

Team composition may vary along a number of dimensions, such as age, occupation, gender, tenure, abilities, personality, and experience. Diversity, or the distribution of personal attributes among team members, is likely to affect the way individuals perceive each other and how well they work together (Jackson, Joshi, and Erhardt, 2003). These, in turn, may affect team performance. Most research on group composition concludes that diversity in a team is particularly desirable when the work is complex and has a limited time span (Campion, Medsker, and Higgs, 1993). Thus, diversity in team members' abilities and experiences is particularly important (Athanasaw, 2003). However, one study found that a balance between different levels of managerial experience was needed in entrepreneurial teams in the medical and surgical instruments industry (Kor, 2003). That is, the more effective teams were composed of members who had a balance between industry and team experience; too much of either created conflict and decreased the ability of the team to seize new growth opportunities.

Diversity has become a very important concern in health care organizations. Diversity can help to promote quality and competitive advantage by including staff who can best understand diverse cultures. As noted earlier, strategies aimed at inclusion help organizations reap the potential benefits of diversity. Diversity can also generate a broader perspective on a problem, which may lead to superior problem analysis and suitable solutions. From a legal perspective, diversity is a concern in relation to equal employment opportunity law. Thus, it has become so important that the Joint Commission has instituted requirements for staff diversity and cultural competence (Joint Commission, 2005). Although diversity brings many advantages, it also comes with problems, such as the potential for increased conflict and a loss of cohesiveness. Researchers, finding a negative relationship between diversity and performance in new product development teams, suggest that group heterogeneity might reduce social integration and cohesion (Ancona and Caldwell, 1992b). As a result, conflict begins in the initial stages of group formation and affects performance throughout the team's existence. In multidisciplinary health care teams, this is especially prevalent due to the differences between disciplines in basic philosophy and values, treatment modality, and terminology.

Tenure Diversity, or the length of time members have been on the team, is also an important consideration in teams. For instance, new members coming into an already functioning team must be socialized to **team norms** (standards shared by team members that regulate team members' behavior) and procedures, which can take valuable time away from the work of the team. Although continuity of staffing is important, boundaries of some teams are, by necessity, more permeable than others. For example, hospital teams may include different physicians and nurses corresponding to the needs of the patients at certain points in their treatment and recovery. Having a clear mission and set of task priorities would decrease many problems associated with tenure diversity, while the use of core and peripheral members and full-time and alternate members will increase team continuity and stabilize the process (Ancona and Caldwell, 1998; Topping, Norton, and Scafidi, 2003). The diversity "liability" can also be alleviated if members have previous experience working in teams or have been given training in team-building techniques (Athanasaw, 2003; Topping, Norton, and Scafidi, 2003). Katzenbach and Smith (1993) note that successful teams do not just happen; they become effective when members have certain skills that permit them to function positively in a group situation. Training and previous group experience—especially if members have worked together before—can provide these skills and reduce the potential for conflict.

Status Differences

Status is a measure of worth conferred on an individual by a group. **Status differences** are seen throughout organizations and occur in all teams. It may have the effect of motivating people and providing them with a means of identification; it may be a force for stability in the organization (Scott, 1967). Status differences can also be a negative force and a source of conflict and tension. These differences exist in all teams and can have a profound effect on team functioning and individual behavior on teams. Status differences cannot be eliminated but, if well managed, can mitigate negative impacts. In this section, we discuss some of the ways that status differences affect teams and suggest strategies for managing status differences.

Status differences in health care are common and well entrenched (Lemieux-Charles and McGuire, 2006; Nembhard and Edmondson, 2006; Topping, Norton, and Scafidi, 2003). Multidisciplinary teams benefit from operating as a company of equals, yet the reality may make this very difficult. For example, in a study of end-stage renal disease teams in which most team participants accepted the equal participation ideology, it was clear that the physicians, who had higher professional status than other groups, had greater involvement than others in decision making (Deber and Leatt, 1986). The mismatch between expectations and reality made many team members, particularly staff nurses, feel a sense of role deprivation. That is, they were inhibited in their ability to fulfill completely their role as health professionals. This in turn led to a decrease in morale and job satisfaction. Status issues may be exacerbated in teams characterized by gender diversity, particularly when men comprise the higher status group. High-status members tend to initiate communication more often, are provided more opportunities to participate, and have more influence over the decision-making process. Thus, a lower-status team member may feel intimidated or ignored by higher-status team members. The group, as a result, may not benefit from this person's expertise.

Status differences can profoundly affect team effectiveness. They may impede someone with less authority or status from challenging someone with more authority. Similarly, status differences may inhibit someone of higher status from hearing input from those with lower status. The term "authority *gradient*" has been used to describe differences in status and authority. Authority gradients have been identified in the airline industry as one of the causes of aviation accidents. That is, coordination and communication within the cockpit may be inhibited by differences in authority and status. In health care, authority gradients have been discussed among physicians, between residents and attending physicians, and between physicians and nurses, pharmacists, and social workers. Cosby (2009) notes as well the authority gradients between physicians in different specialties.

Status differences may affect patient outcomes. From the well-regarded IOM report, *Keeping Patients Safe: Transforming the Work Environment of Nurses*, "counterproductive hierarchical communication patterns that derive from status differences" are partly responsible for many medical errors (Institute of Medicine, 2004). Further, a review of medical malpractice cases from across the country found that physicians (higher-status team members) often ignored important information communicated by nurses, who had lower status on the team. Nurses in turn withheld relevant information for diagnosis and treatment from physicians (Schmitt, 1990). In a status-consciousness environment such as health care, opportunities for learning and improvement can be missed because of unwillingness to engage in communication necessary for improvement.

Some teams have developed positive norms of equality, which can certainly help to minimize the negative impact of status differences. However, norms of equality may run counter to the formal or informal status of individual group members in the larger organization. For example, within a hospital, a physician may possess and exercise his or her power. Within a CQI team, that same physician may be expected to serve as an equal in analyzing problems and recommending solutions. Is it possible for such an individual to adjust his or her attitudes and behaviors according to the norms of the particular social milieu? As discussed later in the section on Environmental Context,

this is an example of the larger environment (the hospital) potentially affecting the behavior of individuals on a particular team. This discrepancy between the status one has outside of the team and with the status one has within the team may pose team management challenges.

CQI teams often use training early in the team development process to cope with problems brought about by status differences. In well-managed multidisciplinary teams, lower-status individuals should feel elevated by being part of such high-profile, effective teams. If status inequality exists, it is advisable for leaders to build a trusting environment in which members can disagree with the leader and others on the team without repercussions. In other words, the team leader should strive to achieve a climate of psychological safety for his or her members. In a study of 23 neonatal intensive care units (NICUs), NICU medical directors who were more attentive to other professions' ideas and concerns mitigated perceptions of status differences, increased unit psychological safety, and had success implementing quality improvement projects in the units (Nembhard and Edmondson, 2006).

Psychological Safety

Psychological safety describes individuals' perceptions about the consequences of interpersonal risks in their work environment—largely taken-for-granted beliefs about how others will respond when one puts oneself on the line, such as by asking a question, seeking feedback, reporting a mistake, or proposing a new idea in the team context. In psychologically safe teams, people believe that if they make a mistake, other team members will not penalize or think less of them for it. This belief fosters the confidence to experiment, discuss mistakes and problems, and ask others for help. Psychological safety is created by mutual respect and trust among team members, and leader behavior is a powerful influence on the level of psychological safety in teams (Edmondson, 1999, 2003).

Management research on psychological safety started with studies of organizational change, when Schein and Bennis (1965) discussed the need to create psychological safety for individuals if they are to feel secure and capable of changing. Psychological safety helps people overcome the defensiveness, or "learning anxiety," that occurs when people are presented with data that disconfirm their expectations or hopes, which can thwart productive learning behavior (Schein, 1985). However, the need for a team climate conducive to learning does not imply a cozy environment in which people are close friends nor does it suggest an absence of pressure or problems. Team psychological safety is distinct from group cohesiveness; team cohesiveness can reduce willingness to disagree and challenge others' views, creating groupthink (Janis, 1972). This represents a *lack* of interpersonal risk-taking. Psychological safety describes instead a climate in which the focus is on productive discussion that enables early prevention of problems and the accomplishment of shared goals, because people feel less of a need to focus on self-protection.

Although few people are without concern about others' impressions, our immediate social context can mitigate—or exacerbate—the reluctance to relax our guard. Research in hospitals and other organizations has found differences across teams in people's willingness to engage in behavior for which the outcomes are uncertain and potentially harmful to their image. When psychological safety is high, teams are much more likely to engage in learning, which in turn promotes team performance (Edmondson, 1999). Just as compelling goals are necessary to motivate learning, psychological safety enhances the power of such goals by facilitating less self-conscious interpersonal interactions. Without a goal, there is no clear direction to drive toward and no motivation to exert the effort; without psychological safety, the risks of engaging wholeheartedly in learning behaviors and other key team processes in front of other people are simply too great. In a study of NICUs noted earlier, ICU psychological safety was associated with implementation success of quality improvement projects; when unit members were able to raise questions and concerns, they were better able to understand the rationale behind proposed changes and more able and willing to implement them quickly (Tucker, Nembhard, and Edmondson, 2007).

Team Norms

Team norms are defined as standards that are shared by team members and that regulate member behavior. **Behavior norms** are rules that standardize how people act at work on a day-to-day basis, while **performance norms** are rules that standardize employee output. Behavioral norms in teams are far-reaching and may vary substantially from one team to another in the same organization. Norms may govern how much each individual participates in the team's work, how humor is used, the use of formal group procedures (e.g., Robert's Rules of Order), and responses to absence and lateness. In their study of operating room nurses, Denison and Sutton (1990) describe their surprise at the behavioral norms present in the operating room:

> At first we were surprised by the norms of emotional expression in the operating rooms. The first time we entered the room where a coronary bypass operation was being done, for example, we were surprised by the loud rock music blaring from the speakers, the smiles on the faces of the surgical team, and the constant joking. Denison observed one surgeon who joked and told a series of funny stories as he performed the complicated task of cutting the veins out of a patient's leg—veins

that would be used to bypass clogged coronary arteries. Similarly, one reason that Sutton almost passed out during a tonsillectomy was that he became very upset when the surgeon laughed, joked, and talked about "what was on the tube last night" while blood from an unconscious child splattered about.

Norms are powerful influences in organizations and teams, and the existence of norms is necessary for effective group functioning. In Hackman's (1976) classic *Work Redesign*, he suggests that norms have the following characteristics:

1. Norms summarize and simplify team influence processes. They denote the processes by which teams regulate member behavior.

2. Norms apply only to behavior, not to private thoughts and feelings. Private acceptance of norms is not necessary; only public compliance is required.

3. Norms are generally developed only for behaviors that are viewed as important by most team members.

4. Norms usually develop gradually, but members can quicken the process. Norms usually are developed by team members when the occasion arises, such as when a situation occurs that requires new ground rules for members in order to protect team integrity.

5. Not all norms apply to all team members. Some norms apply only to newer members, while others may be applied to individuals based on seniority, gender, race, economic status, or profession.

Teams generally have norms related to equity in member participation and rewards. One common problem related to this norm is that of the **free rider syndrome**. This term refers to a situation where a team member obtains the benefits of group membership but does not accept a proportional share of the costs of membership (Albanese and Van Fleet, 1985). The free rider is seen as someone who promotes self-interest (the personal acquisition of benefits) over the public interest (the need to contribute to the activity that produces those benefits). It is often observed that the larger the group, the greater the free rider effect (Roberts and Hunt, 1991). What can managers do to minimize free riding? Through effective use of power, design of organizations (including the size of the organizational units), and control of the incentive system, managers can influence team member behavior (Albanese and Van Fleet, 1985). At a routine level, this influence may be achieved by offering financial incentives or special forms of recognition to particular group members. In the longer term, it is important for managers to deal with the free rider problem by attempting to broaden the individual's concept of self-interest by creating, communicating, and maintaining a group culture that views effort expended on team processes as contributing to a shared goal that is meaningful to each team member.

Team norms may not always be positive from the perspective of team performance. For example, a team may have a norm that relegates women to second-class status; this is unlikely to be an explicitly stated norm, but it may be a norm nevertheless. Similarly, teams may establish a norm that silence among team members represents agreement and consensus on a decision. Silence may in fact indicate agreement; alternatively, it can be an indication that team members are pressured to agree with a team's decision and to withhold opposition. Because of the significance of norms in team functioning, it is important to clarify team norms and to identify unwritten norms that may negatively affect team performance and team member satisfaction. This is particularly important for multidisciplinary teams in health care settings (Deeter-Schmelz and Ramsey, 2003), where norms about status and assertiveness can minimize the chance of the team being dominated by one discipline (Vinokur-Kaplan, 1995a).

Team Cohesiveness

Team cohesiveness is among the most widely studied aspects of teams and team effectiveness (Salas et al., 2015). Team cohesiveness refers in general to the degree to which members of a group are *attracted* to other members and, thereby, are motivated to stay in the group. One can think of cohesion as having two components: affective and instrumental. The affective dimension refers to a composite of interpersonal attraction, liking, trust, or positive attitudes toward team members. Related to this is team pride or "the extent to which group members exhibit liking for the status or the ideologies that the group supports or represents, or the shared importance of being a member of the group" (Beal et al., 2003, p. 995). Based on the idea that groups come together to maximize rewards and minimize penalties, instrumental cohesion refers to the social bonds between group members that are bound by the group's working relationship. In this way, group members are drawn together by a shared commitment to the group's tasks. A more limiting definition views cohesiveness as the extent to which members are committed to the group (Goodman, Ravlin, and Schminke, 1987). This approach acknowledges that members can be committed to a common task but not necessarily be attracted to each other. This is a pragmatic view of cohesiveness that is particularly important for focusing on the management of teams in which members, such as nurses, physicians, psychologists, and social workers, are already highly committed to professional standards.

Cohesion is an important component in understanding team processes and effectiveness. Highly cohesive teams may exhibit higher levels of performance, greater member satisfaction, and lower levels of turnover (Gully, Devine, and Whitney, 1995; Hoegl and Gemuenden, 2001; Yang and Tang, 2004). The relationship between cohesion and effectiveness is particularly strong when the work of the team is complex and requires high levels of coordination, communication, and mutual accountability. An investigation of treatment teams in psychiatric hospitals, where members are highly interdependent on each other, found that cohesive teams had higher performance levels than less cohesive ones (Vinokur-Kaplan, 1995a). Similar findings resulted from a study examining the effectiveness of geriatric rehabilitation teams (Wells et al., 2003). Related to our earlier discussion of virtual teams, cohesion has also been found to be a binding factor that can reinforce connections where members are physically and culturally disconnected (Lim, 2018).

Related to team norms, cohesiveness can promote better enforcement of team norms and general control over team members; however, taken to an extreme, this can lead to undue or dysfunctional conformity. For instance, there are circumstances under which high levels of cohesiveness can lead to *lower* levels of productivity. That is, if a team's norms favor low productivity, then having a highly cohesive group will likely lead to high levels of conformity to this norm and, hence, lower productivity. Similarly, a highly cohesive team may work against a manager's efforts to involve new team members or to encourage interaction with other teams. Cohesiveness, therefore, should be evaluated in context. In most circumstances, it is a positive attribute, while in other situations, it can lead to conformity and counterproductive norms and practices.

What are the sources of cohesiveness? A central tenet of social psychological theory is that individuals are attracted to others who are similar to them; therefore, homogeneous groups should be more cohesive than heterogeneous ones. All-female groups, for instance, tend to be more cohesive than all-male and mixed sex groups (Bettenhausen, 1991). The lack of conflict, team training, a positive predisposition for teamwork, and the presence of trust among members also lead to increased cohesiveness (Deeter-Schmelz and Ramsey, 2003). To complicate matters, some research suggests that conflict may be beneficial to group performance, particularly when a group is dealing with complex problem-solving tasks (Cosier, 1981; Janis, 1972; Schwenk, 1983). In this sense, multidisciplinary teams and culturally diverse teams, while potentially exhibiting higher levels of conflict and less cohesiveness, may also be more creative and innovative in their approach to problem solving (Mitchell et al., 2010).

The cohesiveness of a team is also influenced by the goal orientation or reward structure of the team. Let us consider two conditions. First is the situation of goal interdependence in which members are evaluated and rewarded as a team (i.e., equal reward structure). Here, progress to each member's professional/personal goals is identical to progress to **team goals**. The second condition is one in which group members are judged and rewarded as individuals (i.e., unequal reward structure). In essence, one member may reach his or her goal at the expense of another team member. In general, the findings support the first or cooperative condition (Parker, McAdams, and Zielinski, 2000; Yang and Tang, 2004). Team members in the second situation are more likely to be highly competitive, leading to lower cohesiveness due to the following:

- Less intermember influence and acceptance of other's ideas
- Greater difficulty in communication and understanding
- Less coordination effort, less division of labor, and less productivity

Following from this, cohesive groups tend to have levels of interaction that are greater and more positive, strengthened by conditions of high interdependence. That is, groups that have equivalent reward structures not only perform more efficiently but also develop cooperative strategies such as teamwork and pooling of information that facilitate achievement of jointly shared goals.

Nature of the Work

Organizational research has for many years adopted the principle of contingency; specifically, that there is no one best way to organize—rather, organizational structures and processes must be aligned with a number of factors, including environmental factors, the technology used by the organization, and the nature of the work done by the organization. Among the underlying themes in research on teams is that team tasks can be classified according to their critical demands; that is, critical features of a task dictate particular team behaviors essential to successful performance. These specific behaviors include not only individual effort but also cooperative and interdependent endeavors. This means that effective performance is a function of matching team processes to task demands. In this section, we identify key aspects of the tasks confronting teams and the manner in which teams adapt to different task characteristics. In addition, we consider two aspects of the work of a team: goals and the level and type of task interdependence.

Team Goals

Team goals and their accompanying tasks can be categorized according to goal clarity, complexity, and diversity. Each of these dimensions has implications for the manner in which a team is organized and managed. For example, some teams work toward goals and engage in activities that are repeated over time. In these situations,

communication and coordination mechanisms among team members can be routinized. Although they face variations and some uncertainty, obstetrical teams face a defined set of goals, namely the safe delivery of newborns and the health and well-being of mother and child. The goals and accompanying tasks for such teams and for individual team members are well structured and understood by team members. Where goals and tasks are relatively predictable, and where team members understand exactly what is to be done, the work of a team can become routine. In fact, with the right organizational supports, team members who have never met can quickly and effectively coordinate their work based on well-defined roles and organizational supports.

Valentine and Edmondson (2015) use the term **scaffolding** (a term first used in the education sector) to describe a light meso-level organizational structure that enables desired behaviors. These structures do not require consistent individual members but rather bind a set of roles, for example, physicians and nurses, giving them collective responsibility for a defined set of tasks. The authors described how scaffolding operated in a busy academic medical center ED that had been generating poor performance metrics in comparison with benchmark medical centers. The original design of the ED was a common approach in many EDs:

> When patients arrived at the ED waiting room, they would be triaged, and their chart would be placed on a counter. Any available nurse could take the chart to begin the patient-care work and then return the chart to the counter. Any available resident could then take the chart and begin her work, returning the chart to the counter when done, signaling that the patient case was ready for an attending. Finally, any attending could take the chart to join the case. This design was intended to match the first available nurse, resident, and attending to each new patient. (Valentine & Edmondson, 2015)

The difficulty with this design is that for any given patient, nurses, residents, and attendings needed to coordinate their work and have follow-up conversations about patients. The essentially random allocation of patients to nurses, residents, and attendings was frequently confused about which triad of professional was responsible for a patient. Moreover, nurses often struggled to find or approach an attending physician, reluctant to impose—especially on someone not well known to them.

The new design organized the ED into pods, where each pod had an assigned group of professionals. Arriving patients were assigned to a pod, so it became clear who was responsible for which patients. The design was referred to by Valentine and Edmondson as team scaffolds because the pods were not actually teams but instead lightweight structures that enabled coordination among team members based on their defined professional responsibilities. Pods enabled professionals to replace others as shifts changed, but any professional entering a pod knew his or her responsibilities, and could easily assimilate into the flow of work. As noted earlier, professionals were bounded together not because they were friends or had prior relationships but because they had a collective task and clear professional tasks and responsibilities.

Goal and task clarity were significant variables in determining the performance of hospital treatment teams, allowing them to meet the hospital's standards of quality, quantity, and timeliness (Shaw, 1990; Vinokur-Kaplan, 1995a). Task complexity is related to team interaction; the more complex the task, the greater the need for interaction. Thus, it is important that managers plan for enhanced communication among the team members under conditions of complexity. Others have found that an increase in task diversity, as defined by the number of different conditions treated within ICUs, challenges caregivers since their expertise and knowledge can be applied across a wider range of conditions and leads to better outcomes (Shortell et al., 1994).

Task Interdependence

The hospital ED case described above provides an example of intensive task interdependence. **Task interdependence** refers to the interconnections between tasks or, more specifically, the degree to which team members must rely on one another to perform work effectively. A useful way of classifying task interdependence is through a hierarchy of task interdependence based on the extent and manner in which information or resources are exchanged (Thompson, 1967; Van de Ven, Delbecq, and Koenig, 1976):

- **Pooled interdependence** is a situation in which each member makes a contribution to the group output without the need for interaction among members. Since each group member completes the whole task, team performance is the sum of the individual efforts. Standardized rules and procedures are needed to enhance coordination of team outputs.

- **Sequential interdependence** is a situation in which one group member must act before another one can. Group members have different roles and perform different tasks in some prescribed order, with the work flowing in only one direction. There is always an element of potential contingency since readjustment is necessary if any member fails to meet expectations. Coordination using schedules and plans is needed to keep the team on track.

- **Reciprocal interdependence** is a situation in which the outputs of each member become inputs for the others such that each member poses a contingency for the other. Group members often are specialists with different areas of expertise and have structured roles; therefore, they perform different parts of the task in a flexible, "back-and-forth" order. Leaders must provide for open communication between members and scheduled meetings as necessary.

- **Team interdependence** is a situation in which team members must actively coordinate to diagnose and solve problems or otherwise carry out work or work-related activities. The workflow is simultaneous and multidirectional. Coordination requires mutual interactions with group autonomy to decide the sequencing of inputs and outputs among members. Leaders should plan frequent meetings while also encouraging unscheduled ones.

Higher levels of interdependence frequently imply greater uncertainty faced by team members. Therefore, as the degree of interdependence among team members increases, so does the need for information exchange and processing, coordination, communication, and cooperation. Implicit in this is the need for matching the information exchange and processing needs requirements with appropriate interaction and coordination patterns that facilitate information exchange. If team members perceive low interdependence when high interdependence actually exists, then too little effort will go toward coordination. On the contrary, when interdependence is perceived as higher than it really is, too much effort may be expended in coordination behavior at the expense of performance. For this reason, interdependence and the level and type of coordination must be appropriately matched. Some researchers go so far as to suggest that successful teams are the ones that match interdependence in terms of task, goal, and feedback. That is, a successful team is one in which reciprocal work is matched with group goals and group feedback. Group goals and feedback mean that rewards would be based on the group goal and feedback given on the group's performance as a whole. Conversely, pooled interdependence should be matched with a situation of individual goals and feedback.

Regardless of the task characteristic, the important point for managers is the need to match team tasks with process and structure. One study demonstrating this matching described the reengineering effort in a large urban hospital system that used teams for overcoming care delivery problems, particularly fragmentation and discontinuities in delivery (Schweikhart and Smith-Daniels, 1996). Focused teams, or relatively autonomous operating units, were formed by merging multidisciplinary clinicians into patient care units so that pharmacists, respiratory therapists, nurses, and other caregivers were integrated through shared governance and cross-training. The teams were given high levels of autonomy and accountability, while sharing responsibility for both care production work—execution of the patient's care plan—and care management work—planning and coordinating the care. In this case, high levels of task complexity and interdependence were matched with a team structure that allowed increased levels of communication and interaction.

In virtual teams, team members may be separated not only by geography and time but also by culture and language. In this situation, managers are faced with the dual challenges of coordinating work among individuals from different disciplines and from different cultures (Barczak and McDonough, 2003). In health care, this type of team is most common in product development (e.g., pharmaceuticals and medical equipment) and in clinical research.

Environmental Context

Teams do not exist and function in a vacuum but operate within a broader environmental context. Pressures and events from outside of the immediate team affect the team and its members. In this section, we examine several critical external factors that may affect team performance: intergroup relationships and conflict, organizational culture, and the larger external environment.

Intergroup Relationships and Conflict

An important part of a team's external environment is the presence of other teams. In many situations, effective team performance is dependent upon a team's ability to form intergroup relationships with other teams in a positive and productive manner. In complex organizations, one of the most challenging tasks of many teams is to interact with other teams whose work is related to theirs (Edmondson, 2002). For example, consider the myriad intergroup interactions among teams that must occur in the merging of two hospitals (see Dooley and Zimmerman, 2003; Sidorov, 2003; Yang and Tang, 2004). Teams assembled to deal with staffing issues, technology, finances, architectural concerns, and countless other factors must work with other teams in both their own group and the merging organization. One could only imagine the confusion if each team chose to work without the advice and input of other teams.

What happens when teams must coordinate their efforts? What are the factors responsible for effective and ineffective intergroup relationships in this context? Intergroup relationships are often lateral, or peer, relationships rather than hierarchical ones. As health care organizations have moved away from rigid hierarchical structures to manage work, and as they have become more specialized, the need for new coordination mechanisms has increased such as cross-team training, virtual team updates, and joint meetings for planning and coordination.

In the process of working out intergroup challenges and coordination issues, intergroup conflict is perhaps inevitable. Given the uncertainty and heterogeneity of inputs in health care, it is virtually impossible to design all work processes in advance in such ways as to ensure that the work of all groups mesh perfectly with the work of other groups. When conflicts or disagreements occur among groups, it is important that team members possess a repertoire of conflict resolution strategies. In some cases, the interfaces among teams require only fine-tuning; in the worst situations, work processes may need to be overhauled to achieve functional intergroup relationships.

Some intergroup conflict results from interpersonal differences or animosities. However, most intergroup conflict emerges because of factors related to the interdependence of multiple teams. This is especially true for health care organizations that are known for high levels of interaction and, therefore, present more opportunities for conflict. Conflict between groups cannot usually be addressed at an individual level; one member of a group can rarely resolve an intergroup conflict in a unilateral manner. If intergroup conflict is viewed as resulting from problems in the *interface* between groups, then the analysis of the causes and sources of conflict should examine the nature of relationships.

First, intergroup conflict is more likely to occur when there is ambiguity about the team's respective task responsibilities and roles. This situation largely explains conflicts that occur between professional groups with overlapping practice domains, such as between psychologists and psychiatrists (Brown and Keyes, 2000; Weist et al., 2001). Task and role ambiguity may also be common in organizations undergoing rapid growth or change, where different groups may have divergent understandings of the nature and implications of change. Consider the conflict that may occur when an organization is in the midst of a merger (Dooley and Zimmerman, 2003). This type of conflict points to the need to articulate team roles clearly and distinguish precisely the responsibilities of similar groups. Conflict may also arise from intergroup differences in work orientation. Every team develops its own set of norms regarding the manner in which work is accomplished.

Related to differences in work orientation is the problem of goal incompatibility among teams. Teams whose goals are in conflict, or perceived to be in conflict, must sometimes work together. A common conflict in health care is between teams whose orientation is primarily cost containment and teams whose orientation is focused more on quality concerns. At other times, differences in group culture may cause conflict between teams. Each group develops its own unique norms, communication network, and values, which collectively is referred to as a team culture. Conflict may emerge when there are culture conflicts between teams. Last, intergroup conflict may occur when there is competition for resources. Teams may have much in common and be oriented toward the same goals, yet experience conflict because they are competing for the same limited financial, human, or physical resources.

Perhaps of greatest importance for the organization as a whole, as conflict emerges between groups, cooperative relationships may be replaced by a win-or-lose mentality. In this case, victory becomes more important than solving the problem that may have caused the conflict in the first place. Because of this, it is important to develop strategies to manage and reduce intergroup conflict.

Organizational Culture

Among the most important environmental factors affecting team performance is the **organizational culture** of the larger organization. For teams to function to their maximum potential, it is extremely important that a suitable culture exists—one that values and emphasizes teamwork and participation (Zárraga and Bonache, 2005). Among the most common complaints about teams in organizations is that they do not receive adequate support from the larger organization. While many organizations claim a commitment to a team-based organization, they often lack effective culture and strategies for accomplishing this transition.

How does senior management of an organization adopt a team-based culture? First, it is important for senior management to internalize the concept of a team culture and to understand fully how a team culture is consistent with and supportive of its overall strategy. Furthermore, this needs to be communicated throughout the organization. Senior management also needs (1) to believe that employees want to be responsible for their work, (2) to be able to demonstrate the team philosophy, (3) to articulate a coherent vision of the team environment, and (4) to have the creativity and authority to overcome obstacles as they surface (Moorhead and Griffin, 1998; Orsburn et al., 1990).

As with other aspects of organizational life, teams require strong support from senior management to be effective (Liberman et al., 2001). By support, we refer to resources such as money, human resources, training, and time, as well as philosophical support for the work of the team. Once senior management has made a commitment to teams, it may be necessary to develop a detailed implementation plan. This plan might include a clarification of the organization mission to focus on such things as continuous improvement, employee involvement, and customer satisfaction; selecting sites for teams; preparing a design team to assist with team staffing and operation; planning the transfer of authority from management to teams; and drafting a preliminary plan for implementation. To be successful, teams need an internal champion who can provide motivation, encouragement, and work to acquire the resources and support required (Cohen and Bailey, 1997; Shortell et al., 2004).

Training constitutes a key part of implementing and supporting teams, and to be effective, the organizational culture must support its use (Liberman, et al, 2001). No one would ever consider the possibility of a soccer team being successful without substantial training or practice. Based on the experience of countless nonsports teams, the need for training—in fact, continuous training—is very apparent. There is a vast literature on selecting and training individuals to work in teams and the knowledge, skills, and abilities necessary for effective teamwork. Such training may include cognitive content, including the rationale or raison d'être of having a team-based organization. Affective content should also be addressed, including the roles and responsibilities of team members and team norms as well as logistical issues dealing with meeting management and the reward system (Moorhead and Griffin, 1998). Other examples include team interaction training that can lead to shared mental models (Marks, Zaccaro, and Mathieu, 2000); problem-solving and decision-making training, which can enhance interdisciplinary team interactions (Doran et al., 2002); and newcomer training, which can speed the socialization process (Chen and Klimoski, 2003). Overall, for team training to be comprehensive, it optimally should include requisite technical, administrative, and interpersonal skills.

The reward system of the organization should optimally reflect the organizational culture. Thus, a challenge facing all managers is the structure of reward system. To what extent should the organization allocate team, as opposed to (or in addition to) individual, rewards? The organization also needs to address one of the unanswered questions in organizational research: do team-based rewards improve team and/or individual performance? Despite the equivocal nature of the literature in this area (Kirkman et al., 2016), there seems to be a natural tendency for team-oriented organizations to consider **team-based rewards**.

Team-based rewards may come in several forms, including deadline-driven rewards where a team reaches a particular goal by a specified time, incentive bonuses that are most common among sales groups for achieving a financial goal, and profit-sharing and gain-sharing plans, the latter referring to rewards for achieving cost-saving targets.

Team-based rewards may motivate people to work collectively and consider team and organizational goals as well as goals related solely to one's job. Among the greatest downsides is the risk that not all members of a team will contribute equally to the team's success, referred to earlier as the free rider syndrome, leading to a situation of inequity and resentment. Reward systems where teams compete against each other are generally not recommended because they can have the dysfunctional impact of withholding information and creating destructive tension in the organization.

We can also indirectly reward teams through a variety of other mechanisms. **Skill- and knowledge-based pay** may be used to reward team members for mastering new skills that contribute to meeting team performance goals. It should be stressed that while there are many options for rewarding team performance, the number of organizations that actually use team-based incentives is relatively small, and some organizations have abandoned team-based pay systems. One reason for this is the complexity of such schemes and lack of agreement about the link between incentives and performance. While there is an intuitive appeal to performance-based compensation, there exists substantial dissent regarding its premise. Many managers and scholars believe that such schemes are highly destructive to individual, team, and organizational performance. In addition, there are a number of critical questions that need to be resolved to ensure that a team payment system does not yield unintended negative consequences, including (Pascarella, 1997) the following:

- Does the team as a whole receive rewards, or are team members rewarded solely on the basis of their individual performance?

- If rewards are not uniformly distributed among team members, how does management assess the relative contributions of different team members?

- Should team members be compensated for results, behaviors, or both?

- How should people be rewarded when they have membership on multiple teams?

These are critical questions, the answers to which depend upon the manner in which teams are used in the organization as well as the culture of the organization (Beersma et al., 2003). However, several hybrid compensation structures have been successful in simultaneously motivating low-performing team members to improve while encouraging high-performing members to help in this process (Katz, 2001). An example of a hybrid plan involves a team threshold; once the team as a whole reaches this level, pay increases are based on individual performance. This is especially relevant when there are enough highly skilled workers on the team to teach their less-skilled or less-knowledgeable colleagues.

External Environment

Like organizations as a whole, teams are affected by the external environment in which they operate. This makes it important to understand how external factors influence team processes and effectiveness (Ancona, 1990; Arrow, McGrath, and Berdahl, 2000). Most research has involved organizational factors that affect teams (e.g., support from senior levels of the organization), so there is little known about the effect of other external factors (Lacey and Gruenfeld, 1999). For many teams, the greater external environment may exert influence equal

to or greater than the internal organizational environment (Hackman, 2003; Salas, Burke, and Cannon-Bowers, 2000). This is particularly true for multidisciplinary, interagency groups that interact with and depend on not only member organizations but also the community environment and local service network for critical resources and support. These teams often are used in low-resource rural areas to extend services, making it critical to understand how these conditions affect teams and how to develop strategies to override the effects.

In several studies (Fried et al., 1998; Topping and Calloway, 2000), the findings indicated that resource scarcity was an important issue in the development of mental health delivery systems in rural environments. In areas with high levels of resource scarcity, only a few core providers took a central or gatekeeper role, thereby implying that organizations in that system act more autonomously than a system with more resources. This, in turn, will affect the collaborative behavior or **social capital** existing in the provider network, in specific, and community, as a whole. Social capital can be best defined as the web of cooperative relationships between providers in a service system that involve interpersonal trust, norms of reciprocity, and mutual aid (Veenstra, 2000). In situations of scarce resources where social capital may be low since organizations tend to interact less, there will be little impetus to use teams to solve interorganizational problems. For instance, teams including acute care hospital nurses and community providers are used to provide care to older people discharged from the hospital (Robinson and Street, 2004). In these situations, collaboration among team members would be much more difficult.

Another contextual factor influencing collaboration between team members is the history of the provider network or community. Interagency teams, whose members have a long history of service coordination, tend to report a remarkably easy process of forming and becoming a cohesive, effective team (Topping, Norton, and Scafidi, 2003). There may also be rural and urban differences. Many rural areas report that "everyone knows each other and have worked together before." Thus, a sense of "teamness" is there from the beginning. In addition, urban communities tend to include a larger number of service organizations so that interagency teams usually are composed of many professionals, while rural areas have to depend on nontraditional groups, such as the YMCA, churches, and Boys and Girls Clubs, for members. This, of course, increases diversity, which may also increase team conflict (Jackson, 1992; Kor, 2003).

Team Processes

Up until this point, we have discussed such team characteristics as composition and norms, the type of work done, the environment within which teams operate, and interrelationships among these factors. In this section, we focus on *how* teams do their work—how they are led, the manner in which communication is handled, how they make decisions, and other processes and procedures. Team processes thus refer to the methods of interacting and performing work by team members alone and in interaction with each other. Processes addressed in this section are leadership, communications, decision making, learning, and how the work of the team is affected by its stage of development.

Leadership

Leadership in teams refers to the ability of individuals to influence other members toward the achievement of the team's goals. This definition permits us to include formal and informal leadership. By **formal leadership**, we refer to legitimate, or officially designated leadership authority given to a team member. In some cases, an external individual in a position of authority can assign leadership, or in other instances, leaders may be designated through voting or other forms of consensus. By **informal leadership**, we refer to individuals who assume leadership roles based on some personal characteristics, such as expertise, experience, or personal charisma.

Related to but distinct from leadership is power. Some team members may acquire and exert power in a team through their relationships with individuals outside of the team. For example, in an academic medical center, a team member whose spouse is a vice president may be in a position to wield considerable power. A team member may also obtain power because he or she is perceived to be nonsubstitutable, or difficult to replace, in the organization. Some people may also achieve power because they have the ability to cope with uncertainties faced by the organization. An IT staff member may achieve an inordinate amount of power because her skills and knowledge are scarce *and* because of her ability to cope with a major uncertainty—the risk that the information system will fail, causing potentially widespread disruption to the work of the organization.

Some teams have multiple leaders. For instance, there may be a formal leader as well as several informal ones. Informal leaders can be supportive of the formal leader or can undercut the authority of the formal leader. Examples of formal leaders are head nurses, department managers, and project committee chairs. As noted before, formal leaders have legitimate authority in the team. That is, the organization has granted these individuals power along with some ability to use formal rewards and sanctions to support that authority. However, the formal leader may not be the most *influential* person on the team. The extent to which team members accept the formal leader's wishes is, in large part, determined by the attitudes of the informal leader(s).

Leadership in teams has been studied extensively and has included both formal and informal leadership. That is, the important distinction is often not between formal and informal leadership but between effective and ineffective leadership. In one study, leadership in ICUs was positively related to efficiency of operation, satisfaction, and lower turnover of nurses (Shortell et al., 1994). Successful leaders adopted a supportive formal or informal leadership style, emphasizing standards of excellence, encouraging interaction, communicating clear goals and expectations, responding to changing needs, and providing support resources when possible. In another study, surgeon leadership was critical to the successful implementation of a new technology (Edmondson, 2003). Successful leaders communicated a compelling rationale for the change, motivating others to exert the necessary effort, and minimized the status difference between themselves and other members of the operating room team, to facilitate others' ability to speak up with questions, observations, and concerns.

Team leaders vary in the leadership style they adopt, and different circumstances call for different approaches. In deciding upon a leadership style, therefore, group leaders need to consider in realistic terms their formal and informal authority within the group. Use of a coercive or forceful style may backfire when the individual does not have the power to back up decisions. Such a leader may find that the informal leader is able to veto, modify, or sabotage demands. Webster et al. (1998), using case management teams, found that "powerless leaders" were faced with the formation of cliques and competition from more influential members. It is best, therefore, for the formal leader not only to consider the views of informal leaders but also to collaborate with them if possible. It is therefore wise for a formal team leader to know the identity of the informal leader(s) and positively engage him in the work of the team.

Communication Networks and Collaboration

A team cannot function effectively unless members can exchange information in an accurate and timely manner. Team leaders are usually best positioned to help manage communications within a team and between the team and external teams and other entities (Hackman, 1982). Consider the case of a nurse in a NICU, who has just met with a patient's physician and must pass on vital information to the nurse on the next shift as well as to the parents who will visit during the next shift. How is information conveyed? Without workable communication processes, important information may be lost or inaccurately communicated. In fact, the evaluation and design of communication processes are important components of many quality improvement projects (Tucker, Nembhard, and Edmondson, 2007).

Communication speed and accuracy in a team are influenced by the nature of the team's communication network and by the complexity of its task. When a task is simple and **communication networks** are centralized (e.g., a wheel-and-spoke structure), speed and accuracy are enhanced in a team. However, when tasks are relatively complex, centralized communication networks lower both speed and accuracy because people serving as network hubs (i.e., information disseminators) may suffer from information overload. In this situation, communication networks are best decentralized (e.g., a star-shaped structure), relieving a manager of the need to filter (and possibly unintentionally distort) information before it is passed on. In the example of the NICU, it would be inefficient and risk error to have a nurse on the earlier shift communicate needed information to a head nurse first, who would then pass it on to the next shift's nurse. Timeliness and accuracy are both served by direct communication between the two nurses on the front lines of care. The team should thus use communication processes that encourage direct interaction between nurses on sequential shifts.

The team communication network can be best described in terms of process behavior and interaction strategies (Coopman, 2001; Stewart and Barrick, 2000). This involves the type of interaction that occurs between members (Stewart and Barrick, 2000). Most measurement of this behavior is based on the classic work of Bales (1950), who separated group process into either maintenance behaviors or task behaviors. The maintenance category includes interpersonal activities that lead to open communication, supportiveness, and reduction of interpersonal conflict. Task behaviors are those that relate directly to the team's work on its task. Using such a classification system, it should be possible to determine how team interactions develop and to assess the effectiveness of the process (Hackman, 1987). In a study of multidisciplinary, interagency teams coordinating services to youth with serious emotional disturbances, it was found that new teams engaged in more maintenance behavior than older, more experienced teams (Topping, Breland, and Fowler, 2004). Moreover, the focus on maintenance interactions occurred throughout team meetings indicating that teams in the forming stage interact differently. As a result, the new teams had less task-oriented interaction; therefore, they reviewed fewer cases and engaged in less task-oriented behavior.

Although most of the focus in teams is on internal communications, teams also rely on external relationships (Gladstein, 1984). Boundary-spanning activities help teams coordinate with other teams in the organization and ensure that team activities serve the needs of the organization as a whole. New product or new technology teams, for example, use a diverse array of members, including researchers from the marketing department, physicians from the medical staff, and senior managers. All members take on **boundary-spanning roles**, because all members are responsible for representing and communicating with their external function while also working interdependently with other members of the team. Ancona and Caldwell (1992a) use the following classification to describe the range of boundary-spanning activities observed in their research:

- **Ambassador activities**: Members carrying out these activities communicate frequently with those above them in the hierarchy. This set of activities is used to protect the team from outside pressures, to persuade others to support the team, and to lobby for resources.

- **Task coordinator activities**: Members carrying out these activities communicate frequently with other groups and persons at lateral levels in the organization. These activities include discussing problems with others, obtaining feedback, and coordinating and negotiating with outsiders.

- **Scout activities**: Members carrying out these activities are involved in general scanning for ideas and information about the external environment. These differ from the other two in that these activities relate to general scanning instead of specific coordination issues.

Generally, effective teams engage in high levels of ambassadorial and task coordinator activities and low levels of prolonged scouting activities. They found that other, "isolationist" teams neglected external activity altogether and thus tended to do quite poorly, probably due to being out of touch with the environment in which they work. In addition, some groups such as R&D teams use boundary spanning as an effective means of communication but have found that stakeholder (customer) ratings were highest when the project leader—not the team—was the source of information (Hirst and Mann, 2004).

Throughout this chapter, we have made frequent reference to temporary teams and teams whose membership is fluid and may change over short periods of time, for example, the length of a hospital shift. In a rapidly changing environment, teams may need to form quickly and may disband, alter their goals, or change composition over a short period of time. This type of situation is increasingly common, and is certainly true in health care. Edmondson states that organizations need to be able to create and disband teams when the team's specific purpose has been achieved. Edmondson suggests that today's organizations need to be prepared to form teams "on the fly," and that organizations need to have the competency to "team" (Edmondson, 2012). Using the term **teaming**, she explains that teams need to be able to coordinate and collaborate "without the benefit of stable team structures, because many operations, such as hospitals, power plants, and military installations, require a level of staffing flexibility that make stable team composition rare" (Edmondson, 2012). Having the competency to form teams on short notice is supported by our earlier discussion of scaffolding or establishing enabling structures and processes to develop teams when the traditional requisite for team effectiveness is absent.

Decision Making

Most teams are involved in making decisions at some point. This does not mean that all team members are involved in making all decisions, or even that the team itself makes decisions. To illustrate, a hospital president may ask for a recommendation on a decision from his or her senior management team but retain the right to make the final decision. Similarly, a physician may obtain input from a variety of professionals but make the final determination on treatment. Managers and team leaders can decrease the chance of misunderstandings by clarifying the role of the team and the role of each member in a particular decision. Team members can generally accept limitations on their influence as long as the boundaries of their influence are clear.

In contrast, decision making in a multidisciplinary research team—set up to produce high-quality research by leveraging a diversity of inputs—calls for a highly participative approach, with considerable dialogue and discussion prior to coming to a decision. Decisions in this setting may be based on consensus and compromise (Edmondson, Watkins, and Roberto, 2003).

Decision making in teams can be particularly challenging when time is limited. Under these circumstances, it may not be possible to obtain extensive participation for a particular decision. For example, decision making in an emergency triage team may be made without full consultation because time is critical and decisions must be made quickly and often by a single individual. Clearly, we would not want to use an elaborate team decision-making process (such as one that might be used by the multidisciplinary research team described above) in an ED! Conversely, given the ambiguities faced in research and the need for multiple perspectives (and few urgent time constraints), we would not want one individual making unilateral decisions in that context.

Critical is clarifying to team members the distinction between problem solving and decision making. Some groups, such as some process improvement teams, are established to solve problems or seek methods for improving a particular organizational process. However, they may not be given authority to actually implement their solutions, particularly when substantial resources are required.

The processes by which information is exchanged and decisions are made are distinct and of central importance. Teams naturally attempt to make correct decisions, applying all available information to the issue at hand. However, there is also an important distinction between gathering information related to a decision and applying that information for decision making. Information may be available in a team, but effective use of that information for decision making does not always occur. Unique information (known by only one member) may not surface in group discussions (Stasser, 1999). Experimental studies have demonstrated that groups tend to dwell on common information (that held by all members) such that privately held information fails to surface; further, when it does surface, its impact is often muted (Larson et al., 1996). Additionally, teams can become polarized on an issue in ways that do not reflect the full range of information and opinion in the group. As team members compare their positions on an issue with those of others on the team, pressures emerge to accept one position or the other as the *team* position. Furthermore, when one position is more forcefully argued than another, it gains support, despite initial discussion that revealed no clearly favored argument (Cartwright and Zander, 1968), or revealed contradictory information. Sunstein and Hastie (2015) argue that groups that do not correct their errors actually amplify those errors; groups may experience cascade effects, where group members follow the views of those who spoke and acted first. This can lead to increased polarization within a group. "Groups focus on shared information—what everybody knows already—at the expense of unshared information and thus fail to obtain the benefit of critical and perhaps troubling information that one or a few people have" (Sunstein and Hastie, 2015, p. 25).

A manifestation of the poor use of information is the groupthink phenomenon, which can lead to premature convergence on a poor decision (Janis, 1972). The concept emerged from Janis's studies of high-level policy decisions by government leaders, including decisions about the Vietnam War, the Bay of Pigs, and the Korean War. Groupthink can occur at all levels of decision making, from the level of a family to high-profile policy decisions. Essentially, groupthink occurs when the desire for harmony and consensus overrides members' rational efforts to appraise the situation. In other words, groupthink occurs when maintaining the pleasant atmosphere of the team implicitly becomes more important to members than reaching a good decision. Some or all of the following symptoms may indicate the presence of groupthink (Janis, 1972):

1. *The illusion of invulnerability.* Team members may reassure themselves about obvious dangers and become overly optimistic and willing to take extraordinary risks.

2. *Collective rationalization.* Teams may overlook blind spots in their plans. When confronted with conflicting information, the team may spend considerable time and energy refuting the information and rationalizing a decision.

3. *Belief in the inherent morality of the team.* Highly cohesive teams may develop a sense of self-righteousness about their role, making them insensitive to the consequences of decisions.

4. *Stereotyping others.* Victims of groupthink hold biased, highly negative views of competing teams. They assume that they are unable to negotiate with other teams, and rule out compromise. This refusal to compromise is also related to their belief in the inherent morality and "rightness" of the team, as described above.

5. *Pressures to conform.* Group members face severe *pressures* to conform to team norms and to team decisions. Dissent is considered abnormal and may lead to formal or informal censure or punishment.

6. *The use of mindguards.* Mindguards are members who withhold or discount dissonant information that interferes with the team's current view of a problem and its solution.

7. *Self-censorship.* Teams subject to groupthink pressure members to remain silent about possible misgivings and to minimize self-doubts about a decision. This and other symptoms are particularly prevalent when a team has a member with a great deal of power and influence.

8. *Illusion of unanimity.* A sense of unanimity emerges when members assume that silence and lack of protest signify agreement and consensus. Lack of disagreement does not necessarily mean there is not serious disagreement.

The consequences of groupthink are that teams may limit themselves, often prematurely, to one possible solution and fail to conduct a comprehensive analysis of a problem. When groupthink is well entrenched, members may fail to *review* their decisions in light of new information or changing events. Teams may also fail to consult adequately with experts within or outside the organization and fail to develop contingency plans in the event that the decision turns out to be wrong.

Team leaders can help avoid groupthink. First, leaders can encourage members to critically evaluate proposals and solutions. Where a leader is particularly powerful and influential (yet still wants to get unbiased views from team members), the leader may refrain from stating his or her position until later in the decision-making process. Another strategy is to assign the same problem to two separate work teams. Most importantly, groupthink can be avoided by proactively engaging in a process of *critical appraisal* of ideas and solutions and by understanding the warning signs of groupthink. Managers might also consider alternative systematic methods of decision making that emphasize member participation. **Nominal group technique** and **Delphi technique** elicit group members' opinions prior to judgments about those opinions. These

and other approaches help generate ideas and facilitate objective debate (Gustafson, 1975).

Team Learning

In a changing and uncertain world, a team's ability to learn is essential to its ongoing effectiveness (Edmondson, 1999). In the organizational literature, some discuss learning as an outcome, others as a process (see Edmondson, 1999). This chapter joins the latter tradition in treating team learning as a process, and we describe the behaviors and activities through which teams learn. Team learning is defined as an iterative process of reflection and action through which teams may discover and correct problems and errors in their work processes.

Learning processes consist of activities carried out by team members through which a team obtains and processes data that allow it to adapt and improve. Examples include seeking feedback on how well the team's outputs meet its customers' needs, talking about errors, and experimenting. It is through these activities that teams detect changes in the environment, better understand customer requirements, develop members' collective understanding of the situation, or discover unexpected consequences of previous team actions.

A study of cardiac surgery operating room teams learning to use a new technology for minimally invasive surgery found that the teams that were successful did a great deal more reflecting aloud on what they were learning, on how the process was going, and what changes might be made going forward than other teams (Edmondson, 2003). The learning for these teams involved acquiring knowledge and skills related to technical aspects of the new technology. It also involved practicing new interpersonal behaviors, such as speaking up in the operating room in new ways.

The behaviors through which teams learn may involve personal risk. For instance, other team members may think less of an individual for raising a concern, admitting an error, or asking a question for which the answer seems obvious to some. For this reason, learning in teams is greatly enabled by a climate of psychological safety, in which people believe that others will not think less of them for well-intentioned mistakes. This is an element of team climate and is described further later in this chapter.

In health care, team learning is particularly important for two reasons. First, medical knowledge is constantly developing; individual providers must keep up with new care protocols, medications, and technologies. Physicians maintain their currency with new developments in biology and medical technology by scanning the medical literature, attending conferences, and consulting with trusted colleagues. In fact, developments in science and medicine have always required continuing education for physicians and nurses. At the same time, however, the organizational context of health care delivery has changed in ways that increase the interdependence of the care delivery process so that groups must learn how to better coordinate their activities to reflect changes in care protocols and to adjust to the unexpected. One recent study of teams, mentioned above for its findings related to psychological safety, also found that quality improvement teams had greater success implementing new practices when they had found support in the medical literature for the efficacy of the proposed changes (Tucker, Nembhard, and Edmondson, 2007).

Another vital element of team learning in health care is the detection and correction of errors. One way this learning occurs is through Morbidity and Mortality (M&M) rounds; however, physicians may be uncomfortable openly discussing errors with their colleagues such that much learning about error remains private and individual. The current medicolegal environment, which tends to hold the individual accountable for medical outcomes, together with the ethic of professional conscientiousness, serves to reinforce a model of learning focused on private learning by individual practitioners (Bohmer and Edmondson, 2001). Yet, team learning, where new insights are rapidly shared among providers, is a critical part of the new environment of health care, and increasingly, health care organizations are learning how to learn from their own failures. For example, Children's Hospital and Clinics of Minneapolis instituted "blame-free reporting" and safety action teams to encourage the reporting of mistakes and near misses to learn how to prevent them. Intermountain Health Care in Utah uses an integrated system that blends information technology and behavioral norms to allow the hospitals to learn from error and continuously improve the quality of care (Bohmer and Edmondson, 2002; Edmondson, 2004). Recently, Cincinnati Children's Hospital has embarked upon a similar and highly successful change effort, in which errors and sentinel events are thoroughly analyzed and publicly discussed for the lessons they contain (Tucker and Edmondson, 2009). In these cases, managers have worked hard to help people overcome the stigma of error to facilitate continuous, collective learning.

Stages of Team Development

The effectiveness of a team is affected to varying degrees by its maturity or **stage of team development**. Teams go through predictable stages of development, although the speed with which they mature varies. The familiar model presented below should not be used as a guaranteed way to understand team development, but the model provides a framework for a team leader who may be facing frustration because a team has not been achieving its potential. . It may be due to the team's immaturity or because it has not gone through the five stages of team

development described below (Tuckman, 1965; Whetten and Cameron, 1998). Not all teams follow this precise pattern, but maturity and the age of a team need to be taken into consideration as a team leader plans and works. The following sequence of team development is summarized below:

1. *Forming.* During the first stage, members become acquainted with each other and with the team purpose and goals. Members attempt to discover what behaviors are acceptable and unacceptable, while establishing trust and familiarity. This early stage is characterized by polite and tentative interactions. Establishing a clear direction is critical.

2. *Storming.* At this stage, the team may face disagreement, power struggles, and the need to manage conflict. Members may attempt to influence the development of group norms, roles, and procedures; therefore, the stage has high potential for conflict. Focusing on process improvements, team achievement, and collaborative relationships can help overcome emergent conflicts.

3. *Norming.* During this stage, the team grows more cohesive and aligned in purpose and actions. Agreement is achieved on rules and processes of decision making, roles and expectations, and team commitment emerges. Emphasizing the team's direction or goals is essential for forward progress.

4. *Performing.* Once team members agree on the purpose and norms of the group, they can move forward to the task of defining separate roles and establishing work plans. The team is faced with the need for continuous improvement, innovation, and speed. Leaders must be ready to sponsor new ideas, orchestrate their implementation, and foster extraordinary performance from members.

5. *Adjourning.* For temporary teams, the adjournment stage may be characterized by a sense of task accomplishment, regret, and increased emotionality.

As noted, teams may deviate from this model; not all teams pass through all stages as described. Some teams may begin at a norming or performing stage (e.g., members who have worked together before), while some may never move beyond the storming stage. Moreover, teams may not move in a linear fashion through the stages but exhibit long, stable periods in which little occurs, interspersed with relatively brief periods of dramatic progress—a "punctuated equilibrium" model (Gersick, 1989). Last, some teams may revert to earlier stages of development, sometimes resulting from new tasks or responsibilities given to the team, a change in formal or informal leadership, the addition of a new member, or the loss of a valuable member. Managers should consider the stage of team development in establishing team expectations. For example, research has shown that managers of virtual teams need to be cognizant of the challenges associated with each stage of the life cycle and implement appropriate intervention strategies accordingly (Furst et al., 2004). An example of such a strategy is the active involvement of a senior sponsor in clarifying team mission and goals during the early stages of team development.

Team Processes as Intermediary between Structure and Outcomes

Team processes are thus the intermediary between team structures and the outcome of team effectiveness. Through ineffective processes, teams composed of highly talented individuals can be dysfunctional. Conversely, effective processes help a team to achieve its potential. Team processes are important because unlike relatively unchangeable inputs, such as the team's composition and task, team processes can be altered and improved upon by team members and leaders. Teams can learn how to better communicate, leaders can improve their ability to manage meetings and coach other team members, members can experiment with different types of

decision making, and teams can learn and improve. The extent to which these and other processes are appropriately used can have a profound impact on team outcomes. Last, what constitutes effective team processes is contingent on the context. As noted above, saving lives in an ED requires extraordinary and rapid communication, and a unilateral decision-making style, while a medical research team can benefit from a participative consensus-seeking approach. In sum, no single set of team processes meets every team's needs; team processes are dependent upon structural aspects of the team, including team size, the nature of team tasks, and the larger context within which the team operates.

CONCLUSIONS

One of the most important managerial tasks in health services organizations is the development and management of teams. It is now common wisdom that organizations as a whole, as well as individuals, are dependent upon well-functioning teams. As noted, however, teams do not naturally perform at a high level. Nor do teams naturally develop and improve. In fact, their level of

DEBATE TIME: The Individual versus the Team?

Managers often preach the importance of teams, yet our workforce management systems continue to be oriented largely on the individual. If teams are that important, shouldn't we reengineer our workforce management practices around teams rather than individuals? Consider the following aspects of management:

- Individual employees are given a job description, and this job description is often supported by a comprehensive job analysis. Teams, on the other hand, often have vague goals and unclear work processes.
- Individual employees are optimally provided with an orientation to their job and ongoing training to improve their performance. How often are teams provided with a similar orientation to their work and training to improve team performance?
- Complex systems have been established to select job applicants for work in an organization. With some exceptions, technical qualifications are deemed to be of paramount importance in the selection process. Systematic evaluation techniques are used to assess technical qualifications. If organizations are truly interested in improving team performance, should we not employ similar methods to determine the "teamworthiness" of job applicants?
- Organizations orient their motivational and reward systems around individual employee performance. Given the importance of teams and team performance, should we spend energy developing effective ways of motivating and improving team performance? If so, how should such reward systems be structured, and what are the risks around team-based reward systems?
- Performance management systems are designed to provide feedback, coaching, and goal setting for individuals. How often are teams provided with feedback on their performance, along with strategies for improving team performance?

The question is not whether we should ignore the individual and individual reward systems. The larger question is how do we design the workforce management process in our health care organizations to truly do justice to the prominent role of teams, now and in the future? Can our culture change from one that views the individual as the sole unit of value to one where the work team is recognized as having similar value? Is it possible for our bureaucratic organizational systems—such as personnel systems—to recognize and accommodate the value of teams? Are the obstacles insurmountable: is it worth the effort?

performance may even erode and become dysfunctional over time without deliberate and continuous supportive efforts. Effective managers understand that improving a team's performance is a complex endeavor and that improvement strategies need to emphasize team structures and processes. Managers must also understand the

challenges and contributions of individual members of the team (see Debate Time). Finally, while we can make general theoretical statements about teams, each team develops in a distinct way, at its own pace, making its own mark in the organization. Thus, there is both science and art to managing and working with teams.

SUMMARY AND MANAGERIAL GUIDELINES

Effective team management requires understanding of fundamental team principles and theories as well as an ability to translate those concepts into management action and behavior. The following managerial guidelines provide specific applications of theory with the goal of improving team effectiveness:

1. Team members are both individuals and team members. To ensure a sustained level of motivation, reward systems should be constructed so that individual and team contributions are recognized. Rewards need not be financial in nature, and care should be taken to avoid compensation systems that create inequity among team members.

2. Ongoing teams usually have a set of group norms, some of which are functional, while others dysfunctional. Team leaders need to be aware of both positive and negative norms and develop strategies to reinforce positive norms and eliminate norms that limit team effectiveness.

3. Conflict is common in teams, and managers must be able to accurately diagnose the causes of conflict. To resolve team conflict, managers should also be comfortable with a range of conflict resolution strategies.

4. Team leadership is complex, partly because teams often have both a formal leader as well as one or more informal leaders. Managers should be aware of these often unspoken dynamics because they can have a profound impact on team processes and effectiveness. In addition, there are instances in which a formal team leader may have limited formal authority.

5. Managers should clarify to team members the role of a team. In particular, team members must understand clearly the team's role in decision making. Some teams provide input to decision makers, while other teams have the authority to make decisions. Team leaders should clearly understand the decisional authority of the team and communicate this accurately to team members.

6. Managers should understand the applicability of a variety of approaches to building team consensus and decision making. They should avoid prematurely moving to arbitrary approaches to decision making, such as imposing a decision or voting. Full airing of perspectives and the identification and discussion of team members' interests (rather than positions) may help to identify areas of agreement among team members.

7. Managers should be aware of status differences among team members and how these differences may affect the fullness of discussion and the airing of differences.

8. Managers should employ specific techniques for managing meetings, including the following:

    a. Team leaders should prepare an agenda, with time limits for each item, and the placement of the most critical agenda items early on the agenda. Some managers include an indication of the purpose of each item, whether it is for information, discussion, decision making, or other purpose.

    b. If specific team members are expected to address an issue at a meeting, the manager should brief those individuals prior to the meeting to be sure there is agreement on the agenda item and the role of the team member during the meeting.

    c. Team leaders should review the progress made to date and establish the purpose of the meeting. When appropriate, ask subcommittee representatives to review the progress of their work to date.

    d. Team members should be provided with needed materials prior to meetings.

    e. Team leaders should manage team discussions to ensure full participation. For example, it is advisable to ask more junior team members for their input prior to asking for the views of more senior team members.

    f. It is important to keep a record of team deliberations, in particular decisions that were made and the discussion that supported each decision.

g. Team leaders should utilize delegation for complex decisions and information-gathering tasks. Managers should maintain an awareness of the flow of discussion and close off discussion when it becomes apparent that further progress requires more information and/or more extensive analysis.

h. Close the meeting by summarizing what has been accomplished and reviewing assignments for the next meeting. Team meetings should start on time and, except for extenuating circumstances, end at or prior to the expected ending time. Should the meeting's business be concluded prior to the announced end time, the meeting should end. Team members will likely be delighted to be finishing early.

DISCUSSION QUESTIONS

1. To foster teamwork and a culture of quality improvement, a new director of an ambulatory care center in a hospital has begun holding twice-monthly management team meetings, consisting of several physicians, nurses, physician assistants, financial managers, and others. Attendance at these meetings has been erratic, and enforcing attendance is difficult because many of these people report to their discipline chiefs rather than to the director of the center. What advice would you give to this person to promote more consistent participation?

2. A community task force has been formed to improve the coordination of care for the frail elderly. Given the large number of people and agencies involved in providing services to this population, how would you balance the need for representation with the need to keep the task force size to a manageable level?

3. You are a member of a hospital project team assigned to develop a new pediatric oncology service line. Your team is expected to develop a business plan for presentation to the senior management team and the hospital board. A specific timetable has been established for producing a set of deliverables. The team leader is a well-known oncologist with a very strong clinical background and reputation. However, his team leadership skills leave something to be desired. Among other problems, meetings are cancelled at the last minute, delegation of tasks is ambiguous, and the focus and direction of the project changes scope at virtually every meeting. As a team member, what alternatives do you have to improve team management? Which alternative would you select as having the best chance of success?

4. Along with other hospital business managers, you have been a member of a management team. Recently, you have been promoted, and your former business manager team members now report to you. As the new leader of the management team, what challenges will you face in managing the team? How would you approach these challenges?

5. As described in this chapter, teams go through stages of development. As a team leader, what is the practical value to understanding these stages? How could this knowledge improve your effectiveness as a team leader?

CASE

Using Teams to Achieve Millennium Development Goals

Childhood mortality continues to be a major health problem in developing countries. A child born in a developing country is over 13 times more likely to die within the first five years of life than a child born in an industrialized country. Sub-Saharan African countries account for about half the deaths of children under five in the developing world. Between 1990 and 2006, about 27 countries—the large majority in sub-Saharan Africa—made no progress in reducing childhood deaths.

The country of Ghana had set a goal of decreasing childhood mortality from 110 per 1,000 live births to 20 per 1,000 live births by 2015. The most common causes of death among children under age five in Ghana are malaria and neonatal diseases, primarily asphyxia, sepsis, and prematurity. Tragically, most of these deaths are preventable. Among other initiatives, Project Fives-Alive! was established to reduce childhood mortality in Ghana. The approach taken by this nationwide project was guided by the IHI Breakthrough Series Improvement Collaborative Network. Through this multiyear project, teams of frontline health providers and their managers met periodically in learning sessions where they acquired quality improvement knowledge and skills. Teams tested system improvement changes and learned from each other. This is one of the first applications of IHI improvement initiatives in Africa. When the project was fully scaled up, hundreds of teams in Ghana participated in this improvement effort.

Among the most important factors associated with under-five mortality is underutilization of health services. For example, many women do not receive antenatal care, preventive measures (such as neonatal tetanus protection and folate/iron supplements) are inconsistently provided, and many women lack knowledge about oral rehydration therapy and other life-saving procedures.

Why the focus on teams? The answer is that frontline providers are often in the best position to understand the obstacles that women face in accessing services—and to suggest and test potential solutions. As with quality improvement initiatives elsewhere, teams need training, knowledge, and skills, as well as a framework for applying quality improvement methods. Throughout the country, teams were trained in quality improvement methods: setting measurable goals, implementing tests of change, identifying best practices, and—perhaps of greatest significance from a country development perspective—sharing their experiences with other teams and disseminating this knowledge to the larger global health community.

Results are encouraging. Teams enthusiastically shared their knowledge through collaborative meetings, and evidence emerged of improvements in the processes of care and, hopefully, in health outcomes. Even more encouraging is evidence that teams learned how to function as teams and to apply a systems improvement perspective to other health system problems. Development of well-functioning and highly trained teams could be a key part of achieving important global health goals.

Questions

1. One feature of the teams in this case is frequent turnover among team members. How might turnover among team members affect team performance? What approaches can team leaders take to minimize potential negative impacts of turnover and gain advantages, if any?

2. Consumers or patients are sometimes involved in quality improvement teams, but in this role, they may feel that their voices are unimportant, or that their participation is symbolic rather than substantive. Do you think that consumers should be involved in the improvement teams in this case? Why or why not? If consumers are involved, how can team leaders and members most effectively utilize their knowledge and insights?

3. Even when team improvement efforts achieve change, the sustainability of change remains a pervasive challenge. In fact, sustainability of the teams themselves may be problematic. What are the particular obstacles to sustaining the improvements achieved by teams in this case? Similarly, what factors might lead to the dissolution of the improvement teams over time? As a team leader, what strategies might be used to sustain change and to uphold the vitality of the team over time?

REFERENCES

Albanese, R., & Van Fleet, D. D. (1985). Rational behavior in groups: The free riding tendency. *Academy of Management Review, 10,* 244–255.

Alexander, J. A., Jinnett, K., D'Aunno, T. A., & Ullman, E. (1996). The effects of treatment team diversity and size on assessments of team functioning. *Hospital & Health Services Administration, 41,* 37–53.

Ancona, D. G. (1990). Outward bound: Strategies for team survival in an organization. *Academy of Management Journal, 2,* 334–365.

Ancona, D. G., & Caldwell, D. F. (1992a). Bridging the boundary: External activity and performance in organizational teams. *Administrative Science Quarterly, 37,* 634–665.

Ancona, D. G., & Caldwell, D. F. (1992b). Demography and design: Predictors of a new product team performance. *Organization Science, 3,* 321–341.

Ancona, D. G., & Caldwell, D. F. (1998). Rethinking team composition from the outside in. In D. H. Gruenfeld (Ed.), *Research on managing groups and teams* (pp. 21–37). Stamford, CT: MAI Press.

Arrow, H., McGrath, J. E., & Berdahl, J. L. (2000). *Small groups as complex systems.* Thousand Oaks, CA: Sage Publications.

Athanasaw, Y. (2003). Team characteristics and team member knowledge, skills, and ability relationships to the effectiveness of cross-functional teams in the public sector. *International Journal of Public Administration, 26,* 1165–1204.

Bales, R. F. (1950). *Interactive process analysis: A method for the study of small groups.* Chicago, IL: University of Chicago Press.

Barczak, G., & McDonough, E. F. (2003, November–December). Leading global product development teams. *Research Technology Management, 46*(6), 14.

Batalden, P. B., Nelson, E. C., Edwards, W. H., et al. (2003). Microsystems in health care: Part 9. Developing small clinical units to attain peak performance. *Joint Commission Journal on Quality Improvement, 29*(11), 575–585.

Beal, D. J., Cohen, R. R., Burke, M. J., et al. (2003). Cohesion and performance in groups: A meta-analytic clarification of construct relations. *Journal of Applied Psychology, 88,* 989–1004.

Beersma, B., Hollenbeck, J. R., Humphrey, S. E., et al. (2003). Cooperation, competition, and team performance: Toward a contingency approach. *Academy of Management Journal, 46,* 572–591.

Bettenhausen, K. L. (1991). Five years of group research: What we have learned and what needs to be addressed. *Journal of Management, 17*, 345–381.

Bohmer, R., & Edmondson, A. (2001, March–April). Organizational learning in health care, *Health Forum Journal, 44*(2), 32–35.

Bohmer R., & Edmondson, A. (2002) Intermountain health care. Harvard Business School Case #9-602-145. Boston, MA: HBS Press.

Brown, B., & Keyes, M. (2000). Blurred roles and permeable boundaries: The experience of multidisciplinary working in community mental health. *Health and Social Care in the Community, 8*(6), 425–435.

Campion, M. A., Medsker, G. J., & Higgs, A. C. (1993). Relations between work group characteristics and effectiveness: Implications for designing effective work groups. *Personnel Psychology, 46*, 823–850.

Cartwright, D., & Zander, A. (1968). *Group dynamics: Research and theory* (3rd ed.). New York: Harper & Row.

Chen, G., & Klimoski, R. J. (2003). The impact of expectations on newcomer performance in teams as mediated by work characteristics, social exchanges, and empowerment. *Academy of Management Journal, 46*, 591–607.

Cohen, S. G., & Bailey, D. E. (1997). What makes teams work: Group effectiveness research from the shop floor to the executive suite. *Journal of Management, 23*(3), 239–290.

Colquitt, J. A., Noe, R. A., & Jackson, C. L. (2002). Justice in teams: Antecedents and consequences of procedural justice climate. *Personnel Psychology, 55*, 83–100.

Coopman, S. J. (2001). Democracy, performance, and outcomes in interdisciplinary health care teams. *The Journal of Business Communication, 38*(3), 261–281.

Cosby K. S. (2009). Authority gradients and communication. In P. Croskerry, K. S. Cosby, S. M. Schenkel, & R. L. Wears (Eds.), *Patient safety in emergency medicine* (chap. 28). Philadelphia, PA: Wolters Kluwer/Lippincott Williams & Wilkins.

Cosier, R. A. (1981). Dialectical inquiry in strategic planning: A case of premature acceptance? *Academy of Management Review, 6*, 643–648.

Deber, R. B., & Leatt, P (1986). The multidisciplinary renal team: Who makes the decisions? *Health Matrix, 4*(3), 3–9.

Deeter-Schmelz, D. R., & Ramsey, D. R. (2003). An investigation of team information processing in service teams: Exploring the link between teams and customers. *Journal of the Academy of Marketing Science, 31*(4), 409–425.

Denison, D. R., & Sutton, R. I. (1990). Operating room nurses. In J. R. Hackman (Ed.), *Groups that work (and those that don't): Creating conditions for effective teamwork (pp. 293–308).* San Francisco, CA: Jossey-Bass.

Dooley, K. J., & Zimmerman, B. J. (2003). Merger as marriage: Communication issues in postmerger integration. *Health Care Management Review, 28*, 55–68.

Doran, D., Baker, R., Murray, M., et al. (2002). Achieving clinical improvement: An interdisciplinary intervention. *Health Care Management Review, 27*, 42–57.

Edmondson, A. (1999). Psychological safety and learning behavior in work teams. *Administrative Science Quarterly, 44*, 350–383.

Edmondson, A. C. (2002). The local and variegated nature of learning in organizations. *Organization Science, 13*(2), 128–146.

Edmondson, A. C. (2003). Speaking up in the operating room: How team leaders promote learning in interdisciplinary action teams. *Journal of Management Studies, 40*(6), 1419–1452.

Edmondson, A. C. (2004). Learning from failure in health care: Frequent opportunities, pervasive barriers. *Quality and Safety in Health Care, 13*, 3–9.

Edmondson, A. C. (2012). *Teaming: How organizations learn, innovate, and compete in the knowledge economy.* San Francisco, CA: Wiley.

Edmondson, A. C., & Nembhard, I. M. (2009). Product development and learning in project teams: The challenges are the benefits. *Journal of Product Innovation Management, 26*, 123–138.

Edmondson, A. C., Roberto, M., & Watkins, M. (2003). A dynamic model of top management team effectiveness: Managing unstructured task streams. *Leadership Quarterly, 219*, 1–29.

Edmondson, A., & Roloff, K. (2009, Fall). Leveraging diversity through psychological safety. *Rotman Magazine, 47–51.*

Foster, M. K., Abbey, A., Callow, M. A., Zu, X., & Wilson, A.D. (2015, June). Rethinking virtuality and its impact on teams. *Small Group Research, 46*(3), 267–299.

Fried, B. J., Johnsen, M. C., Starrett, B. E., Calloway, M. O., & Morrissey, J. P. (1998). An empirical assessment of rural community support networks for individuals with severe mental disorders. *Community Mental Health Journal, 34*(1), 39–56.

Furst, S. A., Reeves, M. Rosen, B., & Blackburn, R. S. (2004). Managing the life cycle of virtual teams. *Academy of Management Executive, 18*, 6–20.

Gersick, C. J. G. (1989). Marking time: Predictable transitions in task groups. *Academy of Management, 32*, 274–309.

Gladstein, D. (1984). Groups in context: A model of task group effectiveness. *Administrative Science Quarterly, 29*, 499–517.

Goodman, P. S., Ravlin, E., & Schminke, M. (1987). Understanding groups in organizations. *Research in Organizational Behavior, 9*, 121–173.

Gully, S. M., Devine, D. J., & Whitney D. J. (1995). A meta-analysis of cohesion and performance. *Small Group Research, 26*, 497–520.

Gustafson, D. H. (1975). *Group techniques for program planners.* Glenview, IL: Scott Foresman and Company.

Hackman, J. R. (1976). Work design. In J. R. Hackman & J. L. Suttle (Eds.), *Improving life at work.* Santa Monica, CA: Goodyear.

Hackman, J. R. (1982). *A set of methods for research on work teams* (Technical Report No. 1). School of Organization and Management. New Haven, CT: Yale University.

Hackman, J. R. (1987). The design of work teams. In J. Lorsch (Ed.), *Handbook of organizational behavior (pp. 315–342).* New York: Prentice-Hall.

Hackman, J. R. (1990a). *Groups that work (and those that don't).* San Francisco, CA: Jossey-Bass.

Hackman, J. R. (1990b). Introduction. Work teams in organizations: An orienting framework. In J. R. Hackman (Ed.), *Groups that work (and those that don't): Creating conditions for effectiveness teamwork (pp. 1–14).* San Francisco, CA: Jossey-Bass.

Hackman, J. R. (2003). Learning more by crossing levels: Evidence from airplanes, hospitals, and orchestras. *Journal of Organizational Behavior, 24*(8), 905–1013.

Hirst, G., & Mann, L. (2004). A model of R&D leadership and team communication: The relationship with project performance. *R & D Management, 34*, 147–161.

Hoegl, M., & Gemuenden, H. G. (2001). Teamwork quality and the success of innovative projects: A theoretical concept and empirical evidence. *Organization Science, 12*, 435–449.

Hoonakker, P., McGuirem K., & Carayon, P. (2011). Sociotechnical issues of tele-ICU technology. In D. M. Haftor, & A. Mirijadotter (Eds.), *Information and communication technologies, society and human beings: Theory and framework* (Chapter 18). Hershey, PA: Information Science Reference.

Institute for Health Improvement (IHI). (2016). Science of improvement: Forming the team. Accessed June 5, 2017, from http://www.ihi.org/resources/Pages/HowtoImprove/ScienceofImprovementFormingtheTeam.aspx.

Institute of Medicine (US) Committee on the Work Environment for Nurses and Patient Safety. (2004). *Keeping patients safe: Transforming the work environment of nurses.* In A. Page (Ed.) Washington, DC: National Academies Press.

Jackson, S. E. (1992). Team composition in organizational settings: Issues in managing an increasingly diverse work force. In S. Worchel, W. Wood, & J. A. Simpson (Eds.), *Group process and productivity.* Newbury Park, CA: Sage.

Jackson, S. E., Joshi, A., & Erhardt, N. L. (2003). Recent research on team and organizational diversity: SWOT analysis and implications. *Journal of Management, 29*(6), 801–830.

Janis, L. L. (1972). *Victims of groupthink.* Boston, MA: Houghton-Mifflin.

Joint Commission on Accreditation of Healthcare Organizations. (2005). *2005 comprehensive accreditation manual for hospitals: The official handbook (CAMH).* Oakbrook Terrace, IL: JCAHO.

Katz, N. (2001). Getting the most out of your team. *Harvard Business Review, 79*, 22.

Katzenbach, J. R., & Smith, D. K. (1993). The discipline of teams. *Harvard Business Review, 71*, 111–120.

Kirkman, B., Li, N., Zheng, X, Harris, B., & Liu, X. (2016, March 14). Teamwork works best when top performers are rewarded. *Harvard Business Review.*

Kor, Y. (2003). Experience-based top management team competence and sustained growth. *Organization Science, 14*(6), 707–720.

Lacey, R., & Gruenfeld, D. (1999). Unwrapping the work group: How extra-organizational context affects group behavior. *Research on Managing Groups and Teams, 2*, 157–177.

Larson, J., Christensen, C., Abbott, A., et al. (1996). Diagnosing groups: Charting the flow of information in medical decision making teams. *Journal of Personality and Social Psychology, 71*, 315–330.

Lemieux-Charles, L., & McGuire, W. L. (2006). What do we know about health care team effectiveness? A review of the literature." *Medical Care Research and Review, 63*(3), 263–300.

Liberman, R. P., Hilty, D. M., Drake, R. E., et al. (2001). Requirements for multidisciplinary teamwork in psychiatric rehabilitation. *Psychiatric Services, 52*(10), 1331–1342.

Liden, R. C., Wayne, S. J., Jaworski, R. A., et al. (2004). Social loafing: A field investigation. *Journal of Management, 30*, 285–305.

Lim JoAnne Yong-Kwan (2018). "IT-enabled awareness and self-directed leadership behaviors in virtual teams." *Information and Organization.* 28(2), 71–88.

Marks, M. A., Zaccaro, S. J., & Mathieu, J. E. (2000). Performance implications of leader briefings and team-interaction training for team adaptation to novel environments. *Journal of Applied Psychology, 85*, 971–987.

Medicare.gov. (2017). *Hospital compare.* Accessed June 5, 2017, from https://www.medicare.gov/hospitalcompare/search.html.

Moldjord, C., & Iversen, A. (2015). Developing vulnerability trust in temporary high performance teams. *Team Performance Management, 21*(5/6), 231–246. doi: 10.1108/TPM-08-2014-0050.

Moorhead, G., & Griffin, R. W. (1998). *Organizational behavior: Managing people and organizations.* Boston, MA: Houghton Mifflin.

Morgeson, F. P., DeRue, D. S, & Karam, E. P. (2010). Leadership in teams: A functional approach to understanding leadership structures and processes. *Journal of Management, 36*(1), 5–39.

Nelson E. C., Batalden P. B., Huber T. P., et al. (2002). Microsystems in health care: Part 1. Learning from high-performing front-line clinical units. *Joint Commission Journal on Quality Improvement, 28*(9), 472–493.

Nembhard, I. M., & Edmondson, A. C. (2006). Making it safe: The effects of leader inclusiveness and professional status on psychological safety and improvement efforts in health care teams. *Journal of Organizational Behavior, 27*(7), 941–966.

Orsburn, J. D., Moran, L., Musselwhite, E., et al. (1990). *Self-directed work teams: The new American challenge.* Homewood, IL: Business One Irwin.

Parker, G., McAdams, J., & Zielinski, D. (2000). *Rewarding teams: Lessons from the trenches.* San Francisco, CA: Jossey-Bass.

Pascarella, P. (1997, February). Compensating teams. *Across the Board* (pp. 16–22).

Roberts, K. H., & Hunt, D. M. (1991). *Organizational behavior.* Boston, MA: PWS-Kent Publishing Co.

Robinson, A., & Street, A. (2004). Care of older people: Improving networks between acute care nurses and an aged care assessment team. *Journal of Clinical Nursing, 13*(4), 486–497.

Rush University Medical Center. (2008, May 26). Reduced emergency room visits for elderly patients attributed to virtual health care team approach. *Diabetes Week* (p. 222).

Salas, E., Burke, C. S., & Cannon-Bowers, J. A. (2000). Teamwork: Emerging principles. *International Journal of Management Reviews, 2*(4), 339–356.

Salas, E., Shuffler, M. L., Thayer, A. L., et al. (2015). "Understanding and improving teamwork in organizations: A scientifically based practical guide." *Human Resource Management*, 54(4), 599–622.

Schein, E. H. (1985). *Organizational culture and leadership.* San Francisco, CA: Jossey-Bass.

Schein, E. H., & Bennis, W. (1965). *Personal and organizational change through group methods.* New York, Wiley.

Schmitt, M. H. (1990). Medical malpractice and interdisciplinary team dynamics. *Proceedings of the 12th*

Annual Interdisciplinary Health Care Team Conference (pp. 53–66). Indianapolis: Indiana University

Schweikhart, S. B., & Smith-Daniels, V. (1996). Reengineering the work of caregivers: Role redefinition, team structures, and organizational redesign. *Health Care Management Review, 41,* 19–36.

Schwenk, C. R. (1983). Laboratory research on ill-structured decision aids: The case of dialectical inquiry. *Decision Sciences, 14,* 140–144.

Scott, W. G. (1967). *Organization theory.* Homewood, IL: Irwin.

Shaw, R. B. (1990). Mental health treatment teams. In J. R. Hackman (Ed.), *Groups that work (and those that don't)* (pp. 320–348). San Francisco, CA: Jossey-Bass.

Shortell, S. M., Marsteller, J. A., Lin, M., et al. (2004, November). The role of perceived team effectiveness in improving chronic illness care. *Medical Care, 42*(11), 1040–1048.

Shortell, S. M., Zimmerman, J. E., Rousseau, D. M., et al. (1994). The performance of intensive care units: Does good management make a difference? *Medical Care, 32,* 508–525.

Sidorov, J. (2003). Case study of a failed merger of hospital systems. *Managed Care, 12*(11), 56–60.

Stasser, G. (1999). The uncertain role of unshared information in collective choice. In L. Thompson, J. Levine, & D. Messick (Eds.), *Shared cognition in organizations* (pp. 49–69). Mahwah, NJ: Lawrence Erlbaum Associates.

Stewart, G. L., & Barrick, M. R. (2000). Team structure and performance: Assessing the mediating role of intrateam process and the moderating role of task type. *Academy of Management Journal, 43*(20), 135–148.

Sunstein, C. R., & Hastie, R. (2015). *Wiser: Getting beyond groupthink to make groups smarter.* Boston, MA: Harvard Business Review Press.

Thompson, J. D. (1967). *Organizations in action.* New York: McGraw-Hill.

Topping, S., Breland, J., & Fowler, A. (2004). Inter-agency teams: The nature of collaboration, interaction, and effectiveness in serving children and youth with SED. Working Paper.

Topping, S., & Calloway, M. (2000). Does resource scarcity create interorganizational coordination and formal service linkages? A case study of a rural mental health system. *Advances in Health Care Management, 1,* 393–419.

Topping, S., Norton, T., & Scafidi, B. (2003). Coordination of services: The use of multidisciplinary, interagency teams. In S. Dopson, & A. L. Mark (Eds.), *Leading health care organizations* (pp. 100–112). New York: Palgrave Macmillan.

Tucker, A. L., Nembhard, I. M., & Edmondson, A. C. (2007). Implementing new practices: An empirical study of organizational learning in hospital intensive care units. *Management Science, 53*(6), 894–907.

Tucker, A., & Edmondson, A. (2009). Cincinnati Children's Hospital Medical Center. Boston, MA: HBS Publishing Case # 9-609-109.

Tuckman, B. W. (1965). Developmental sequences in small groups. *Psychological Bulletin, 63,* 384–399.

Valentine, M.A., & Edmondson, A.C. (2015) Team scaffolds: How mesolevel structures enable role-based coordination in temporary groups. *Organization Science, 26*(2), 405–422. Retrieved from http://dx.doi.org/10.1287/orsc.2014.0947.

Van de Ven, A. H., Delbecq, A. L., & Koenig, R. (1976). Determinants of coordination modes within organizations. *American Sociological Review, 41,* 322–338.

Veenstra, G. (2000). Social capital, SES and health: An individual-level analysis. *Social Science & Medicine, 50,* 619–629.

Vinokur-Kaplan, D. (1995a). Enhancing the effectiveness of interdisciplinary mental health treatment teams. *Administration and Policy in Mental Health, 22*(5), 521–530.

Vinokur-Kaplan, D. (1995b). Treatment teams that work (and those that don't): An application of Hackman's group effectiveness model to interdisciplinary teams in psychiatric hospitals. *Journal of Applied Behavioral Science, 31,* 303–327.

Webster, C. M., Grusky, O., Young, A., et al. (1998). Leadership structures in case management teams: An application of social network analysis. *Research in Community and Mental Health, 9,* 11–28.

Weist, M. D., Lowie, J. A., Flaherty, L. T., et al. (2001). Collaboration among the education, mental health, and public health systems to promote youth mental health. *Psychiatric Services, 52*(10), 1348–1351.

Wells, J. L., Seabrook, J. A., Stolee, P., et al. (2003). State of the art in geriatric rehabilitation. Part I: Review of frailty and comprehensive geriatric assessment. *Archives of Physical Medical and Rehabilitation, 84*(6), 890–897.

Whetten, D. A., & Cameron, K. S. (1998). *Developing management skills* (4th ed.). Reading, MA: Addison-Wesley.

Wiecha J., & Pollard T. (2004, September). The interdisciplinary eHealth team: Chronic care for the future. *Journal of Medical Internet Research Electronic Resource, 6*(3), e22.

World Health Organization. (2016). Ebola outbreak 2014–present: How the outbreak and WHOs response unfolded. Accessed June 5, 2017, http://www.who.int/csr/disease/ebola/response/phases/en/.

Yang, H., & Tang, J. (2004). Team structure and team performance in IS development: A social network perspective. *Information & Management, 41,* 335–350.

Zárraga, C., & Bonache, J. (2005). The impact of team atmosphere on knowledge outcomes in self-managed teams. *Organization Studies, 26*(5), 661–681.

Chapter 6

Communication

Mario Moussa and Derek Newberry

CHAPTER OUTLINE

- Who Says What to Whom?
- Barriers to Communication
- Patient Care Teams
- Stakeholders
- Tools for Managing Organizational Communication
- Social Networks and Social Media
- Communication Networks
- Organizational Politics
- Communication as a Leadership Art

LEARNING OBJECTIVES

After completing this chapter, the reader should be able to:

1. Discuss the classical sender–receiver communication model and later elaborations of it
2. Identify stakeholders and choose the means for effectively communicating with them
3. Describe the most recent research on social networks and apply it in their work settings
4. Explain the importance of organizational politics
5. Discuss the importance of effective communication in leading health care organizations

KEY TERMS

Barriers to Communication

Communication Networks

Curse of Knowledge

Distortion

Ethos, Pathos, Logos

Feedback

Leadership

Message

Organizational Learning

Organizational Politics

Psychological Safety

Receiver

Sender

Social Media

Social Networks

Speaker–Listener Model

Stakeholder

Stakeholder Analysis

• • • IN PRACTICE: The Debate over Health Care Reform

At a meeting of the American Medical Association (AMA), in June 2009, President Barack Obama addressed a group of the most influential doctors in the country about health care reform (Text: Obama's Speech on Health Care Reform. June 15, 2009). Many people in the audience were skeptical about his plans. Seeking to win them over, the president emphasized a few key points:

- The health care system needs better record-keeping. The government should therefore continue investing in electronic medical records. Better records, he claimed, will lead to "lower administrative costs" and "reduce medical errors."

- Americans need to take more responsibility for their own health. They need to quit smoking, go for a run, and encourage their kids to turn off their video games and spend more time playing outside.

- Everybody needs to eat better and swear off the fatty foods that cause obesity. To show he was following his own advice, the president told the doctors he had planted a vegetable garden on the White House lawn.

- Employers should adopt incentive programs like Safeway's. Safeway has a program called "Healthy Measures" that offers rewards, in the form of reduced premiums, for lowering cholesterol levels and blood pressure.

The payoff of these reasonable proposals, claimed the president, is that consumers can reduce the dollars they spend on medical care, make fewer unnecessary visits to their doctors and the hospital, and be healthier. President Obama made it clear that even the doctors in the audience would benefit, too. Research-based treatment guidelines will make their practices more effective, and the cost burden of the entire health care system will become more sustainable.

Sounds like a win–win. Who could object?

But people did—lots of them. Most notably, Sarah Palin, the Republican vice presidential candidate in the 2008 national election, almost singlehandedly derailed President Obama's arguments for reform by raising the specter of "death panels." Two months after the President's AMA speech, Palin famously declared, "The America I know and love is not one in which my parents or my baby with Down syndrome will have to stand in front of Obama's 'death panel' so his bureaucrats can decide, based on a subjective judgment of their 'level of productivity in society,' whether they are worthy of health care. Such a system is downright evil" (Palin doubles down on death panels, 2009). Somehow, the president's suggestions about invigorating jogs and home-grown vegetables were getting lost in the debate over reform.

Even though leading bipartisan policy analysts made it clear that the notion of death panels was fiction rather than fact, the image of somber dark-suited government officials making life-and-death decisions that affect powerless citizens was too gripping to be forgotten. By the end of August, most news outlets were treating the "death panel" question as one of the central issues in the reform debate.

CHAPTER PURPOSE

Disregard, for the moment, the political jockeying that went on in the arguments over death panels in the Affordable Care Act. The public debate on health care in 2009 served to highlight an essential characteristic of health care information: for technical as well as political reasons, it is astoundingly complex. This complexity is a problem for any professional in communicating about issues related to clinical delivery, financing, outcomes, safety, professional expertise, and patient choice. Whether you are a politician advocating a policy, an administrator managing a hospital, or a physician treating a patient, it is likely that at least some part of your message—the information or feeling you seek to communicate—will be misunderstood.

The purpose of this chapter is to review the communication concepts and frameworks you can employ as an executive or health care provider to avoid this unfortunate outcome. By applying the key concepts described in this chapter, you will increase the chances that you actually get your point across. You will learn:

1. How to think about the act of communication.

2. The theory and practice of managing stakeholders—the people and groups who have an interest in your ideas.

3. The science of relationships and its practical value in health care settings.

4. The importance of organizational politics and how to lead in complex political environments.

WHO SAYS WHAT TO WHOM?

One of the dominant figures in communication theory is the ancient Greek philosopher Aristotle (2006). His model of communication, which he called "rhetoric," has influenced the way theorists have thought about the topic for over 2,000 years. Aristotle described communication as a mostly linear process involving a speaker and a listener—the speaker–listener model. Figure 6.1 shows a simplified version of this process. Effective speakers "package" their **message** using one or more of the three persuasive means of conveying a message: **ethos** (character), **pathos** (emotion), and **logos** (logic).

Aristotle's means of persuasion are still relevant today. Consider, for example, the enduring importance of character—or "credibility"—in modern terms. People tend to believe facts stated by someone whom they see as trustworthy or knowledgeable and discount information coming from those whom they mistrust. Indeed, character often trumps logic, as you can see in most political debates. Whether or not you worried about death panels probably had a lot to do with your political leanings: Supporters of prominent Obama critic Sarah Palin were more likely than others to be suspicious, simply because it was she who had raised a concern about government bureaucrats making life-and-death decisions. Similarly, since people have especially strong reactions to emotion, it is an especially powerful way of making a point—often more powerful than logic alone. Just consider the recent examples of Ronald Reagan or Bill Clinton, who are considered masters of using stories and emotional appeals to win support for complicated policies. But emotion is not always enough. Logic matters most when someone is really paying attention to your ideas. Psychologists have identified a principle called "the power of because," which refers to the fact that arguments backed by logic or reasons tend to be more persuasive than those for which the speaker offers no supporting evidence (Langer, 1989).

The well-known management theorist Nitin Nohria captured the importance of rhetoric and persuasion for modern leaders in a widely cited quote: "Communication is the real work of **leadership**" (Blagg and Young, 2001; Eccles, Nohria, and Berkely, 1994; Nohria and Harrington, 1993). The most effective leaders, Nohria says, know how and when to use each of Aristotle's means of persuasion. Most important, they listen and observe carefully before they communicate, paying attention to social clues that reveal the underlying interests and values of a particular audience: middle managers, front-line staff, external groups, and others. Effective leaders recognize that communication is more than "just words." As the philosopher and linguist C. W. Morris said, language is the "subtlest and most powerful tool" for controlling behavior (Morris, 1949). Modern corporate leaders such as General Electric's former CEO Jack Welch and Apple's CEO Tim Cook have a deep appreciation for this point, crafting and rehearsing their public statements with the utmost care.

Recent communication theorists have built on Aristotle's **speaker–listener model**, adding an element that Aristotle only implied: **distortion**. The sociologist

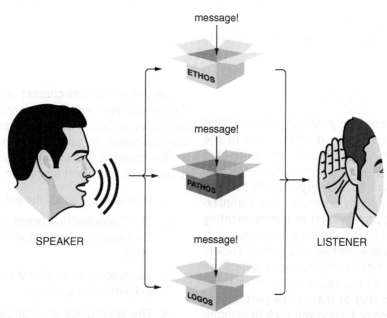

Figure 6.1 Aristotle's Means of Persuasion.

Harold Laswell, in summarizing his perspective on communication, famously asked, "Who says what in which channel to whom?" (Laswell, 1948). Laswell recognized that many factors affected how listeners understood a message: the **sender** of the message, the content of the message, the medium (face-to-face, written, or electronic communication), and the listeners themselves. All of these factors influence "impact," which might be completely different from the literal or intended content of a message (Croft, 2004). Later scholars went further and incorporated this possibility of misunderstanding into their theories, leading to the more complex **feedback** model illustrated in Figure 6.2 (Longest and Young, 2006).

The feedback model takes account of psychological, cognitive, and contextual factors in communication. From a practical perspective, it shows that you need to pay attention not only to your intended meaning but also to the entire context in which communication takes place and which ultimately determines how your meaning is construed.

The philosopher of language Ludwig Wittgenstein underscored the centrality of context and the likelihood of misunderstanding in a brief, provocative quote that has stimulated decades of discussion: "If a lion could speak, we could not understand him" (Wittgenstein, 1973). Basically, Wittgenstein's insight is that to communicate effectively, you have to understand the other's situation: their history, social context, values, and psychology. There is no way a human can understand a being so utterly different as a lion. By extension, if another person's values and experience differ dramatically from yours, you will have a hard time communicating with him or her. The practical implication, for managers and leaders, is that they need to understand the context in which others hear their words and construct and adjust their communication strategies accordingly.

For organizations large and small, it takes work to construct a communication strategy. The key to an effective strategy is to identify specific audiences within and around your organization, analyze their contexts in terms of values and interests, and choose a means of engaging in two-way interaction with them. Figure 6.3 shows how to organize such a strategy (Argenti, Howell, and Beck, 2005).

This framework makes it clear that a "one-size-fits-all" communication strategy is doomed to fail. In any organization, there are multiple audiences, each of which has its own set of values, interests, and assumptions that require highly customized methods. A standard set of questions helps organize a communication strategy: What is the goal? What is the message? Who is the audience? What is the right "channel"? What are the feedback mechanisms? (Norton and Coffey, 2007).

The consensus among contemporary scholars is that today's leaders need to engage in robust, targeted two-way communication. The era of autocratic, top-down communication is over. Markets and consumer preferences change so fast that organizations must be constantly learning and adapting to internal and external environments. Leading management theorists use the term **organizational learning** to describe the range of communication methods designed to engage people in a collective process of problem solving, planning, and implementation (Senge, 2006).

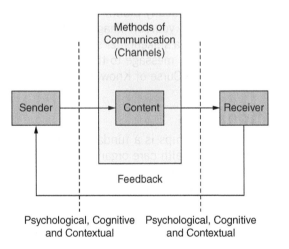

Figure 6.2 Sender, Receiver, and Feedback Model.

Purpose	Audience	Method
Manage public relations	Employees, media, analysts	Press releases, interviews
Build internal support for initiatives	Employees	Town hall meetings, memos, newsletters
Marketing	Physicians, consumers, payors	Sales calls, advertising, promotions
Government relations	Regulators	Lobbying, one-on-one meetings

Figure 6.3 Organizing a Communication Strategy.

Each audience is a **stakeholder**—a person or group of people who are affected by your ideas and will have a reaction to them. The full context in which they live and work encompasses their psychological and cognitive biases, their social networks, and the **organizational politics** that represent their interests. Skillful executives know that they must actively manage stakeholders, tailoring messages to their context and cultivating their support for policies and programs. Otherwise, even the best plans will encounter resistance that slows down or derails execution.

BARRIERS TO COMMUNICATION

Even when you, the sender, know exactly what you want to say, the distortion within the **receiver** often blocks your message. As George Bernard Shaw quipped, "The single biggest problem in communication is the illusion that it has taken place."

A game created at Stanford University shows why it is that communication so often goes awry. A researcher assigned people two roles: "tappers" and "listeners." Each tapper was asked to tap out a well-known song to a listener. Before this exercise, the tappers were asked to estimate the odds that the listener would recognize the song. The average reply was 50 percent. In actuality, only 1 in 40 listeners recognized the song. The explanation is that the tappers have trouble imagining what the listeners are hearing. The songs seem obvious to the tappers, but to the listeners, they are anything but. The tappers suffer from the **Curse of Knowledge**—the problem of imagining another person's state of mind when you have a piece of knowledge that he or she lacks (Heath and Heath, 2007).

The Curse of Knowledge is evident every day at work, in presentations that hospital CEOs give to staff, in meetings that professionals conduct with colleagues from other disciplines, and in conversations that physicians have with patients. When a CEO announces that his or her hospital generated $200 million in annual profit, many of his or her listeners, no matter how educated or sophisticated they might be, imagine that the sum is tidily stored in a bank account somewhere. Some will complain that if the hospital "made" so much money, they should get some of it. Only those who have experience working with income statements or have an MBA degree really understand that profit is actually an accounting concept and not a pile of dollars waiting to be spent. Physicians, nurses, and technical specialists are trained in clinical settings, so their frame of reference makes it difficult to understand the practical import of the CEO's message about operational performance. A similar problem occurs in clinical encounters, where misunderstandings are surprisingly common. There is evidence that patients misunderstand up to 80 percent of the information conveyed by their physicians (Britten et al., 2000). Uncertainty, anxiety, and lack of clinical training all get in the way. This is especially consequential when patients leave the clinical environment and may quickly forget or misinterpret care instructions. For this reason, taking the time to develop an awareness of the patient's frame of reference directly impacts quality of care. Improvements in discharge planning have proven to be effective in reducing readmission rates because they ensure clinicians are mindful about communicating to patients and their family members in a way they are able to understand (Shepperd et al., 2013).

Extensive research has revealed that one typically encounters a small number of **barriers to communication** when sending a message (Shell and Moussa, 2007). As an organizational leader, to increase the likelihood that important stakeholders will pay attention to you and your idea, you need to assess each situation, decide which barriers are relevant, and employ strategies to turn them into assets. There are five barriers: negative or ambiguous relationships, poor credibility, conflicting belief systems, conflicting interests, and communication mismatches. By systematically planning to turn the barriers into assets, you help yourself imagine what it is like to view a situation from a stakeholder's perspective and how to communicate your message to them. This is the best way to overcome the Curse of Knowledge.

Relationships

Developing relationships is a fundamental skill in managing and leading health care organizations and in delivering clinical treatments. Relationships give people a level of trust and confidence in each other, facilitating communication and making it easier to cooperate. People respond well to others who take an interest in them, especially when there is no obvious benefit that flows from it.

Even in today's wired world, where you can communicate using e-mail, Slack, Facebook, and many other **social media**, face time matters in building relationships. In a 1987 experiment, R. F. Bornstein and two other psychologists showed that, in the most literal terms, a face makes all the difference (Bornstein, Leone, and Donna, 1987). They flashed photographs of several people on a screen so quickly that subjects were not even aware of having seen them. Then the subjects had conversations with the people whose photographs had been displayed. Consistently, subjects found those people "likeable" and, even more striking, persuasive. In staged disagreements, subjects sided with them more often than with others they had never seen before.

Similarly, in clinical settings, many patients who value relationships need to feel the connection that comes with a face-to-face encounter. As one patient put it, "I think that if I meet a new doctor and we don't have that face-to-face contact, I would not feel comfortable telling him all my ills" (Armstrong-Coben, 2009). The following true story about an elderly patient vividly illustrates this preference. One morning, he was touching up the paint on his sailboat. Nearby, another boat owner, who happened to be an emergency medical technician, noticed the man was struggling to breathe and that his lips had turned purple. A trip to the local community hospital led to a barrage of high-tech tests and procedures, a diagnosis of emphysema, later complications with cerebral hematomas, and hospitalizations and rehospitalizations that brought him into contact with a neurologist, a neurosurgeon, a cardiologist, and a pulmonologist. Throughout this medical ordeal, the team of specialists stayed in touch with each other and the primary care physician via various electronic media. But one person remained out of the loop—the patient. One day, six months into the experience, the primary care physician phoned his wife to check on his patient. The patient recalls thinking, "Why was he calling *her*?" The physician was communicating, but he was emotionally disconnected. He was not paying enough attention to the relationship. Feeling intense frustration, the patient was likely to ignore some or all of the physician's prescriptions, even if he understood them in the first place.

Because of the importance of relationships, you should take the time to get to know what is important to the people you work with. Successful stakeholder management depends upon your ability to establish, maintain, and deepen your connections with people.

Credibility

As Aristotle first noted, credibility ensures that people take you and your ideas seriously. Most modern experts agree that credibility is based on others' perceptions of three characteristics: competence, expertise, and trustworthiness. Thus, your credibility resides in a subjective experience that others have of your character rather than your objective qualities. Moreover, credibility is highly fragile. You can lose your credibility in a single moment of poor judgment, miscalculation, or misconduct.

You establish competence by reliably making good on your commitments. When you promise that a department chair will receive another assistant professor position, you should be sure that you can actually follow through on the pledge. In health care organizations, agreements big and small hinge on reliability. Once you gain a reputation for it, your words carry tremendous weight.

When it comes to expertise, you must choose your sources carefully. You may consider your experience as an administrator to be an important source of authoritative knowledge, but the surgeon you want to influence may consider administration to be simply applied "common sense." In this case, you must find some other way of establishing your credibility. In beginning a conversation, you may need to acknowledge that the *surgeon's* expertise is extremely valuable to the success of the hospital. This shows that at least you know enough to value his or her efforts. As Dale Carnegie pointed in his classic *How to Win Friends and Influence People*, the need to feel important is one of the most powerful desires that everyone has.

Management expert Stephen Covey says that trust is "the one thing that changes everything" (Covey and Merrill, 2008). With it, almost any stakeholder can be won over. Without it, you have a hard time getting anything done. Trust-building will become even more important as the physician workforce continues to diversify. The push for diversity in health care organizations makes sense not only for moral reasons but because of its effect on performance as well. Research on decision making tells us that groups with more diverse and independent perspectives tend to achieve better outcomes (Levine et al., 2014). But higher performance does not come automatically. To leverage the benefits of diversity, you need to be able to develop a shared perspective and a sense of mutual commitment with colleagues—in other words, you need trust (Polzer, Milton, and Swarm, 2002).

Similarity is one of the foundations of trust in a relationship; if someone sees you as being "one of us," he or she is more likely to give you the benefit of the doubt (Levin, Whitener, and Cross, 2006). To build trust, try to find common ground with others, whether it be through similar aspects of your background, shared experiences, or shared goals. Listening carefully to others is a good way to identify these similarities and is also a good rapport-building tool in itself. Neuroscientists have confirmed what we intuitively know to be true: We enjoy talking about ourselves and sharing our opinions (Tamir and Mitchell, 2012). By just developing your listening skills, you make yourself more charismatic to others and also better equipped to communicate effectively in a diverse work environment.

Beliefs

Whenever you can, you should couch your messages in terms that resonate with the core beliefs and values of your stakeholders. These deeply held principles exert a strong influence on their opinions and actions. Psychologists have a variety of explanations for why appeals to core beliefs work: belief bias (the tendency of people to accept any and all conclusions that fit within their systems of belief), the consistency principle (the need for people to behave in ways that are consistent with previously declared values and norms), and the pull of "power" or "God" terms (the tendency of people to respond to appeals invoking ultimate values such as safety, connection, community, or truth). These explanations all point to the same conclusion: if an idea promises to reinforce one of your stakeholder's core beliefs or the values related to them, the idea gains traction (Gardner, 2006).

Surprisingly, this phenomenon affects researchers as well as dogmatic ideologues. For example, in the historic effort to map the human genome, virtually everyone in the scientific community believed that a painstaking, gene-by-gene mapping process, destined to take decades, was the only way to assure a complete, accurate map. When geneticist James Weber and computational biologist Eugene Myers made a landmark presentation at a 1996 conference in Bermuda outlining a "shotgun sequencing" method for speeding up the process, leading scientists refused to take it seriously. "Flawed and unworkable," said the experts. But one man—a little known researcher and former surfer named Craig Venter—was not so sure. He called Myers, and together they made history, turning the human genome mapping effort into a high-profile race that they won a short four years later in 2000.

The inventor of the theory of evolution, Charles Darwin, once remarked that it was so difficult for him to overcome his own beliefs when he was gathering data that he made a conscious effort to seek out contrary examples. The temptation to skip over evidence that contradicted his beliefs was so strong that Darwin made a habit of immediately writing all such evidence down. Otherwise, he reported, he was sure to forget it.

If even committed scientists have trouble overcoming the biases caused by their own beliefs, imagine the problems such beliefs cause in ordinary organizational life. Under such circumstances, it will not matter how much formal authority you may have as an executive or department administrator. Ideas that violate basic beliefs will simply be rejected. Because belief bias is so powerful, you should frame your ideas using key phrases that honor your stakeholders' core values. In the health care setting, such phrases include "quality care," "patient satisfaction," "scientific rigor," and "outcomes." Hot-button phrases likely to stimulate resistance are "bottom-line performance," "market-based competition," and "efficiency."

When you advocate an idea that seems contrary to some core belief, you should break your proposal into small bites that reduce the amount of dramatic change required from your stakeholders. Psychologists have discovered that people sometimes have what they call "anchor positions" on various beliefs and opinions, and their willingness to be flexible on these positions can depend on how much they are asked to change. The less you ask of your stakeholders, the more willing they are to move in your direction.

Another example from the research world illustrates this point. In the early 1980s, it was hard for anyone in the IBM research department to get a hearing for ideas that took personal computers seriously. Senior leaders believed that there were no competitive markets left to conquer. IBM was so dominant that the only measure of real success left to them was promotion within the company. Low-level internal task forces had forecast that the industry was about to change, but the people at the top, blinded by their beliefs, refused to take these warnings seriously. Nevertheless, an IBM senior manager named Bill Lowe succeeded in obtaining development funds for an experimental PC project that set the stage for IBM's entry into that market. He did it by keeping the project so small that nobody could be bothered to oppose it. When it became clear that Lowe's little program would take no resources away from the focus on the company's corporate customers, the IBM Management Committee let it pass as one of the dozen or so things it approved in a given week. The PC initiative, in short, flew in under the radar screen of IBM's core beliefs.

Interests

At the very center of stakeholder management, like the bull's eye in the middle of a target, are their self-interests, problems, and needs. If you can show your stakeholders that your idea furthers their interests, you will usually have a much easier time gaining their support.

Academic studies in psychology confirm two important findings about the role of self-interest in communication. First, people pay much closer attention to messages they see as having important personal consequences for them than ones that do not. Even a glance at nonfiction bestseller lists in publishing, which is perennially littered with titles such as *You on a Diet*, *Why We Want You to Be Rich*, and *Younger You*, confirms this basic truth. Second, self-interest biases the way people think about proposals. Naturally enough, people tend to favor ideas that benefit them and oppose those that will force them to shoulder significant costs. But research has also shown that audiences see arguments as *more persuasive* when they stand to gain from an idea and less persuasive when they stand to lose. In short, people's interests serve as windows through which they see your ideas. When you can find and address their interests, they open their window to let your ideas in; if they see your idea as running against their needs, the windows close.

To think about your stakeholders' interests in a systematic way, you should ask three important questions:

1. Why might it be in the other party's interests to support my idea?
2. What do other parties want that I can give them to gain their support?
3. Why might they say no?

Your answers to these questions will help you frame your idea so that it appeals to others' underlying interests and gets their attention.

For example, a medical center faced a serious crisis when a change in government regulations forced the hospital CEO to take away a major insurance benefit enjoyed by a low-paid but important group of workers: hospital residents (doctors in training). As the CEO prepared his formal announcement to make this change, rumors spread that the residents were organizing a job action to demand compensation to make up for the loss. The hospital, meanwhile, was in no position to give this group a raise without also raising the pay of many other workers, something it could not afford to do.

Finding himself between a rock and hard place, the CEO asked the residents' leaders to join a committee to explore their overall situation at the hospital. His charge to the administrator leading this committee was simple: find out as much as possible about what the residents' real interests were. His hope was that something would turn up that he could take action on. After a week of meetings, his administrator reported back that the residents would be willing to accept their reduced insurance benefit if the hospital would agree to one very important demand: they wanted to wear the same, somewhat longer white coats that full-fledged physicians wore so that patients would treat them with the same respect. The CEO ordered the new coats without delay.

Communication Styles

Jim Collins wrote in his best seller *Good to Great* that one of the best practices of the best organizations is a willingness to gather data, analyze it, and "confront the brutal facts" (Collins, 2001). It sounds easy, but this advice is much easier to give than to follow. You must constantly remind yourself that your audience's point of view is much more important than your own. And you need to return to the questions about your own credibility: How do stakeholders see you, and do you have credibility?

When it comes to communicating the substance of your message, the most important thing you can do is define it simply. Charles Kettering, the great engineer and inventor, stated, "A problem well stated is a problem half solved." And according to noted communications expert David Zarefsky, "Definition is the key to persuasion." By providing a crisp answer to the question, "What is the problem?" you establish the context in which your ideas will be evaluated. Cognitive psychologists call this the act of *framing,* and it powerfully affects people's perceptions, the standards they will call to mind, the evidence they will consider relevant, the emotions they will feel, and the decisions they will ultimately make. As the American journalist and commentator Walter Lippman once said, "For the most part, we do not first see, and then define.

We define first and then see." How you state the problem defines what your audience will see in their mind's eye.

At the World Economic Forum in Davos, Switzerland, in 2005, social activist Bono used framing to influence the AIDS debate. Bono sat on a stage with British prime minister Tony Blair, former U.S. president Bill Clinton, presidents Olusegun Obasanjo of Nigeria and Thabo Mbeki of South Africa, and Microsoft CEO Bill Gates. Bono listened as the others detailed all of the difficulties Africa faced in overcoming AIDS, poverty, and political corruption. Then the moderator asked Bono what he would like to see changed. Instead of continuing with the panel discussion, Bono decided to reframe the issue. What he wanted changed, he said, was "the tone of the debate." He continued,

> Here we are, reasonable men talking about a reasonable situation. I walk down the street and people say: "I love what you're doing. Love your cause, Bon." [But] I don't think 6,000 Africans a day dying from AIDS is a cause; it's an emergency. And 3,000 children dying every day of malaria isn't a cause; it's an emergency.

Bono's message got through. The audience of corporate executives, government ministers, and cultural luminaries burst into loud applause. Poverty and AIDS in Africa were not business-as-usual issues for public officials. They were global "emergencies." Emergencies require action, not analysis. They affect everyone, not just specialists.

To return to the earlier example of health care reform in the United States, the biggest mistake that the Obama administration may have made in managing communications on this issue was overcomplication. As one critic put it after passage of the Affordable Care Act (ACA), "The White House has taken an issue more intimate and immediate than perhaps any other in a voter's life and transformed it into an abstract, technical argument about long-term actuarial projections. It's a peculiar kind of reverse political alchemy: transforming gold into lead" (Pinkerton, 2010). Palin knew what she was doing when she adopted a different communication strategy. When asked about her "death panels" remark, she said, "[It's] a lot like when President Reagan used to refer to the Soviet Union as the 'evil empire.' He got his point across. He got people thinking and researching what he was talking about. It was quite effective. Same thing with the death panels." A follow-up comment reveals that she made a conscious choice in emphasizing the phrase, "The term I used to describe the panel making these decisions should not be taken literally" (Davis, 2009).

After simplicity, the second-most important quality of your message is vividness. Consider, for example, the strategy used in communicating the importance of hand washing at Cedars-Sinai Medical Center in Los Angeles (Dubner and Leavitt, 2006). Bacterial infections are a serious problem in hospitals, with thousands of people dying each year from germs carried from one patient to another on the hands of doctors and nurses. But getting hospital staff—especially physicians—to wash their hands after each examination is surprisingly difficult, even though everyone knows it is the right thing to do. Hospital hygiene poses, in short, a classic problem of organizational communication: getting people to adopt a new "best practice" when old habits are deeply ingrained.

At Cedars-Sinai, there were several causes for lax hand washing: physicians said they were too busy, the sinks were not always conveniently located, and, even more perversely, the doctors actually believed they *were* washing their hands. Each physician was convinced that "someone else" was the source of the bacteria problem. This presented administrators with a delicate issue of organizational politics: how could they sell doctors on the idea of washing their hands without insulting or alienating them? Administrators tried data-based, inspirational appeals using e-mails, faxes, and posters, but hospital staff assigned to spy on the doctors reported no change in behavioral habits. The hospital then switched to the self-interest persuasion channel and offered doctors $10 gift certificates

at the local coffee shop when they were seen washing up by hand-washing "spies." This program had a moderately positive effect, but compliance still fell far short of what the hospital needed to protect its patients.

Finally, the hospital decided to try a vivid, visual way to deliver the hand-washing message. At a formal luncheon for the senior medical staff, the administrator in charge of the handwashing initiative surprised everyone by bringing out a set of lab trays and asking the doctors to press their hands into these trays to record the bacterial cultures residing on their hands at that moment. The hospital used these hand prints to create full-color, graphic images of the bacterial colonies residing there. They made sure these pictures were as disgusting as possible.

Their final step was to transform these images into screen savers and load them on every computer in the hospital. Thus, no matter where physicians were, these images stalked them. Compliance with the handwashing rule immediately shot up to nearly 100 percent and stayed there. The pictures of the actual bacteria on the doctors' own hands, as Dubner and Levitt put it, "was worth 1,000 statistical tables."

• • • IN PRACTICE: Using Communication to Manage Chronic Illness

Chronic illness is a growing problem in U.S. health care, with 26 percent of adults experiencing multiple chronic conditions (MCCs) in recent studies (Ward, 2013). Qualitative research on MCC indicates that patient–provider interactions create pivotal moments that make the difference between effective and ineffective treatment (Thorne, 2006). Patients often leave conversations with their physicians feeling that they are lower-priority than others with acute needs. On the other hand, physicians may fail to understand the broader context of their MCC patients' symptoms. These miscommunications lead to dissatisfied and frustrated patients who are less likely to adhere to treatment.

A communication technique developed by clinical psychologists called motivational interviewing has been shown to improve outcomes by increasing mutual understanding and giving MCC patients a sense of ownership over treatment plans. The process shown in Figure 6.4 helps clinicians to identify and remove the barriers to communication described in this chapter.

Ask permission to discuss with the patient

Begin with an open-ended question

Reflect back the patient's opinion

Explore the importance of this topic from the patient's point of view

Ask them what would make that increase or decrease

Ask how confident the patient is that if they wanted to make a change, they could

Ask them what would make that rise or fall

Expose the ambivalence

Reflect to them

When they are ready, work out a plan together

Figure 6.4 The Steps of Motivational Interviewing.

SOURCE: Falcone et al. (2014).

This story is an extreme example of a more general truth about human perception: People respond to ideas that are easy to visualize because they can be recalled from memory more readily. Psychologists call this the "availability" phenomenon. The more "available" an idea is, the more people believe it to be true. The beauty of the Cedars-Sinai screen savers was that the bacteria displayed actually had been found on the physicians' hands.

PATIENT CARE TEAMS

Effective communication is all the more important in patient care teams where it has an even greater impact on health outcomes. When communication happens frequently and openly between patients and providers as well as within clinical teams, there tends to be greater adherence to treatment plans and lower likelihood of error, leading to reduced hospitalizations and lower costs. This is especially the case for transitional programs, where handoffs of patient care can increase the risk of miscommunication (Peikes et al., 2009).

Teams with good interpersonal communication tend to be characterized by a shared belief that individual members are accepted and valued by each other—a phenomenon called **psychological safety** (Edmondson and Lei, 2014). Clinical teams with a high degree of psychological safety are more open to learning from mistakes, giving honest feedback, and trying out new practices, all of which have been shown to reduce mortality rates (Nembhard and Tucker, 2011). When nurses feel comfortable pointing out oversights made by attending physicians, and established clinicians view new ideas as a learning opportunity rather than a threat to their status, their teams perform better.

To create an environment of psychological safety and improve the openness of communication on your team, an important first step is to do what is called "priming": Explicitly tell your team that their input is valuable and necessary for your collective success. We assume others believe this, but it is not always a shared perception, especially in teams with clear hierarchies. For example, one study indicates that when clinical teams prioritize safety and explicitly encourage members to speak up about mistakes, they have lower rates of medical errors (Leroy et al., 2012). Priming critical thinking in this way makes the implicit explicit and makes it much more likely that team members will feel comfortable communicating openly (Sunstein and Hastie, 2014).

Another effective strategy for encouraging open communication in care teams is for leaders to acknowledge their own fallibility to the group (Edmondson, 2002). One of our colleagues who heads up an aerial emergency response team at Penn Medicine told us in an interview that he uses this strategy regularly to maintain a high level of interpersonal trust. He does this at critical moments, such as during feedback discussions following a high-risk rescue, in which emotions are volatile and team members may become defensive about admitting mistakes. As he begins these conversations, he makes a point of being the first person to list anything he could have done better during the mission and asks his colleagues to offer him further feedback. By showing a little vulnerability, this highly accomplished physician demonstrates to his more junior subordinates that being similarly open is not only acceptable but also desirable.

Having one-on-one conversations before discussing sensitive team issues as a group can also encourage better, more transparent communication. Group discussions increase the risk of embarrassment and fear of ostracism for offering unpopular opinions or acknowledging mistakes. Having individual conversations with team members first can help air issues that would have otherwise stayed hidden. In one case study of a rock band that was experiencing internal strife, the lead singer found that her band members shared honest criticisms of her leadership style in one-on-one conversations that they were unwilling to voice to the whole group (Roussin, 2008). What is true for rock stars is true for high-performing patient care teams: Good communication only happens if you can create the right environment for it.

STAKEHOLDERS

The "stakeholder" is one of the most important concepts in health care. Effective leaders know their stakeholders, paying close attention to the barriers that distort communication.

The concept of a stakeholder goes back to management research done in the 1960s about the environment in which corporate executives do strategic planning. Building on the idea of a "stockholder," stakeholder theorists recognized that owners—the stockholders—were just one group among many that influenced a corporation's decisions and actions. There were others who had legitimate or at least de facto "claims" on the corporation: customers, employees, citizens, legislators, and activists, to name a few. Each of these groups has an interest in a corporation's investments, projects, environmental policies, and other commitments because they all have consequences that extend far beyond the narrow circle of profit-and-loss statements (Freeman and McVea, 2001).

Health care organizations are located in especially complex stakeholder environments. Take, for example, a large academic hospital. It can easily have more than two dozen stakeholders, as illustrated by Figure 6.5. Each stakeholder group has interests that predispose it to support or contest the hospital's initiatives.

To understand stakeholder management in action, consider the quality initiatives that hospitals across the country have recently undertaken. A centerpiece of many endeavors is unit-based clinical teams, composed of a physician, a nurse manager, and a quality specialist.

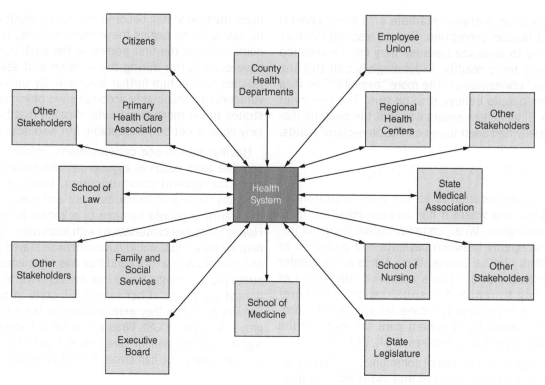

Figure 6.5 Stakeholder Map for a Large Academic Hospital.

These teams have produced stunning results, decreasing average length of stay, improving the effectiveness of care in a broad range of clinical areas, and reducing patient wait times for scheduled appointments. In the abstract, no one would claim that these are undesirable outcomes. Yet there may be reasons that certain groups might be lukewarm supporters, if not outright opponents, of quality efforts in specific situations. Physicians might feel, for example, that working in a team-based environment rather than the more traditional hierarchical structure in which they were trained compromises their professional status. Or unit staff might resist the introduction of new quality guidelines because they entail learning whole new ways of doing their jobs, with little or no benefit to be gained in compensation or job satisfaction. Other groups may have other reasons for opposing the initiative that, on the face of it, seem unassailable. As a hospital administrator championing the quality initiative, you would need to assess just who has a stake in it, whether they support or oppose it, and whether they have enough power to make a difference.

This is the essence of **stakeholder analysis**, which is the first step in stakeholder management. A useful tool to guide the analysis is a Power/Interest matrix, such as the one in Figure 6.6 (Block, 1991). By systematically mapping the stakeholders, you can begin to articulate communication strategies for each group.

This matrix reveals that you need to pay a lot of attention to those three people who are powerful and have a strong interest in the initiative. Assume that two of them

(Dr. Jones and Dr. Smith) are top-producing physicians—if they become unhappy, you should respond quickly with some well-crafted message points. If there is one particular physician among them who wields influence with physicians across the hospital (Dr. Black), you should make a special effort to sit down with him or her and understand how you can address his or her concerns. You can adopt more of a maintenance strategy for those powerful stakeholders who have little interest in the quality initiative. The finance officers in departments that are not directly involved in the initiative fall into this category. Because of their position, they are generally powerful players, but they have no immediate reason to get involved. For the time being, you want to keep it that way, so you should make sure nothing happens to disrupt their peace of mind. As for those stakeholders who have an interest but wield little power, such as junior residents, you can communicate with them on a "need to know" basis. Finally, you can safely expend the minimum effort on communicating with stakeholders who have neither interest nor power in this situation. As valuable as they might be to the hospital's operations, maintenance workers, who fall into this category, should not be at the top of your mind in leading this particular initiative. But you would need to pay a lot of attention to them in a different setting—for example, in a process-improvement project aimed at optimizing the facilities management function.

This kind of analysis, if you are not used to doing it, might seem overly calculating. But your ultimate goal is a practical one—managerial effectiveness. By understanding

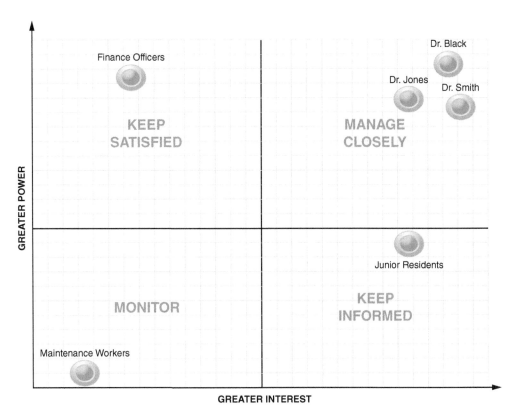

Figure 6.6 Power-Interest Matrix.

exactly with whom you need to communicate and how, you can maximize the impact of your ideas. There are two important reasons why broad involvement of many different stakeholders is crucial to your success as a communicator. First, stakeholders can offer their knowledge, expertise, attitudes, and suggestions about your ideas. By organizing this collective intelligence, you sharpen your own thinking. Second, stakeholders will be more committed and knowledgeable through being involved. And the more committed stakeholders are, the more willing they will be to support your ideas.

important as an organizational initiative moves into the implementation phase.

The methods can be divided between those most appropriate for small- and large-group communication—with the methods listed farther down in the table generally being more appropriate for larger, less personal settings. The methods or mix of methods that work best vary according to the situation. But your managerial focus should always be on tailoring communication as much as possible to fit the profile of a particular person, group, or organizational culture.

TOOLS FOR MANAGING ORGANIZATIONAL COMMUNICATION

After identifying stakeholders, assessing their interests, and developing strategies for overcoming potential communication barriers, the next step is to select methods for consulting with them. Table 6.1 describes various tools for engaging stakeholders in an organizational communication process. You should choose methods on the basis of your goals. "Nominal Group Technique," for instance, helps draw out ideas from a small group of stakeholders, while questionnaires are more successful at representing the opinions held by a larger population. The issue of broad representation generally becomes more

SOCIAL NETWORKS AND SOCIAL MEDIA

The most recent research on communication has highlighted the importance of **social networks**—the connections among a group of people and the broader environment in which they live and work. In settings of all kinds, people get things done and spread information through these informal channels (Burt, 2007; Christakis and Fowler, 2009; Powell, 1998). The extent of your network constitutes your "social capital" and is one of your most important assets as a communicator. An invaluable addition to stakeholder analysis, a social network map is like an X-ray that reveals the inner workings of your organization and its environment.

Table 6.1 Tools for Engaging Stakeholders

Consulting Modes	Time Required	Objectives	Description	Representative	Strengths	Weaknesses
Open-ended interviews	30 minutes–1 hour	To obtain responses to relatively complex issues and alternatives	Interviewer poses questions to respondent	No	Complicated questions may be entertained; may suggest other questions to be explored in more structured formats	Dependent on the interviewing skills of the interviewer, time-consuming, expensive
Structured interviews	15 minutes–1 hour	To obtain responses to relatively complex issues and alternatives	Interviewer poses questions to respondent	Yes, with appropriate sampling	Complicated questions may be entertained. Valuable for generating questions for more standardized formats	Dependent on the interviewing skills of the interviewer, time-consuming, expensive
Nominal Group Technique	1/2 hour–2 hours	To increase and balance participation among meeting participants	Individual generation of ideas in writing, followed by group discussion and ranking of ideas	No	Easy to learn, easy to use, produces broad participation	No interaction among ideas and issues
Interview design	1–2 hours	To stimulate interaction among large groups (16–200) and reveal similarities and differences among their ideas	Several rounds of one-on-one interviewing by group members, followed by summaries of interviews	No	Active involvement of group members, rapid generation of ideas	Not appropriate for exploring a particular idea or proposal in depth
Focus group	2–3 hours	To generate hypotheses about the way members and customers think	Open discussions among 6–12 people, facilitated by a trained moderator	No	Flexibility, open to unexpected responses, good for exploring unfamiliar terrain	Dependent on facilitator's ability, peer pressure can silence some participants, interpretation can be difficult
One-minute essays	1–3 minutes	To provide a brief opportunity for reflection on a discussion	Brief writing exercise or key takeaways from a discussion	No	Quick, easy to do, offers a chance to digest information	Not appropriate for sorting out complex proposals

Table 6.1 Tools for Engaging Stakeholders (continued)

Consulting Modes	Time Required	Objectives	Description	Representative	Strengths	Weaknesses
Short questionnaire	15–30 minutes	To solicit information about specific topics	Prepared questions with limited range of responses	Yes, with appropriate sampling	Respondents have opportunity to reflect on responses, no chance of interviewer influencing	Low response rate, no opportunity for interviewer to clarify questions, small amount of information gathered, takes time to develop effective questions
Long questionnaire	1/2 hour–1 hour	To solicit information about specific topics	Prepared questions with limited range of responses	Yes, with appropriate sampling	More information gathered with brief questionnaires	Same disadvantages as brief questionnaires, except length further reduces response rate
Mini Delphi	15–30 minutes (for each round)	To produce a consensus ratio-scaled evaluation of alternatives	Respondents prioritize alternatives, then repeat exercise after seeing the average rankings from previous rounds	No	Gives geographically dispersed respondents the chance to interact with each other; anonymity prevents bias	Assumes the desirability of the average response
Workshop designs	1/2 day–1 1/2 days	To provide a structured setting where participants collectively explore issues in depth	Events where small and large groups engage in facilitated discussions and exercises	No	Participants have time to focus on a set of topics, collaborative efforts can produce richer ideas and proposals	Time-consuming, requires careful design work, difficult to meet participants' heightened expectations
Exploring strategic options	1/2–1 day	To develop a strategic agenda	Derives key alternatives from open-ended interviews, then sets data on current state, desired future state, and relative importance	No	Helps build common strategic agenda, identifies quickly areas of disagreement	Time-consuming, depends on skill in extracting key choices from interviews

In a recent study of treatment guidelines for hypertension, a group of researchers compared two primary care practices. Figure 6.7 shows the pattern of relationships for each one. The one on the left has much greater "density"—a measure of the number of connections per person. Other measures reveal that the physicians in this practice spend more time working together collaboratively and engaging in two-way communication. As the researchers predicted, this practice was much more successful at implementing treatment guidelines among its physicians.

Two concepts explain the differences between the practices in adhering to the treatment guidelines: connection and contagion. "Connection" refers to the pattern of relationships that a group of people have. Some networks have mainly a hub-and-spoke configuration, where one person resides at the center of several relationships. There may be several hubs and a few connections between the hubs. Another configuration is mainly hierarchical, where a few people sit "atop" others and send information "down" through a network. And then there are networks like the first primary care practice, characterized by lots of interconnections between people. These patterns influence whether and how information spreads through a network.

"Contagion" explains how the information spreads. Biologically, people have evolved to mimic others' behavior. In mimicking behavior, they also pick up corresponding emotions. As the authors of *Connected* note, there is a lot of truth in the saying, "When you smile, the world smiles with you." In one of the strangest epidemics ever recorded, in 1962, an outbreak of uncontrollable laughter spread in Tanzania from one person to another until it "infected" over 1,000 people. Four schools were forced to close, and villages were paralyzed. Just like this "illness of laughing," new treatment guidelines spread among professionals who work closely with each other. You are much more likely to "catch" them than someone who spends most of their time working in isolation.

The practical value of a social network map is that it shows how you should manage the flow of information in your organization and its environment. If you know that it has a hub-and-spoke structure, then you should target the "hubs." You can bring them together for a

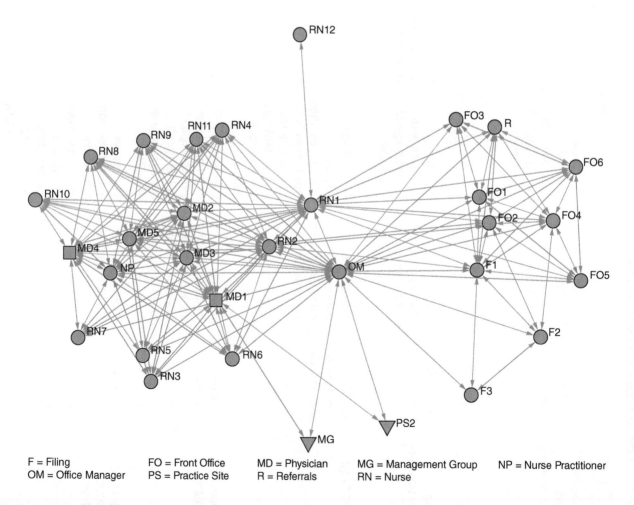

F = Filing   FO = Front Office   MD = Physician   MG = Management Group   NP = Nurse Practitioner
OM = Office Manager   PS = Practice Site   R = Referrals   RN = Nurse

Figure 6.7 Density of Connections per Physician.

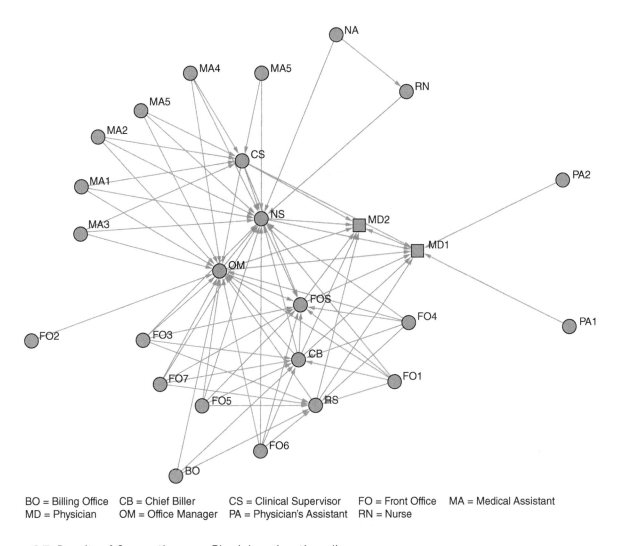

Figure 6.7 Density of Connections per Physician. *(continued)*

meeting, using one or more of the consultation methods described earlier. Once the "hubs" have bought into your proposal, you can rely on them to spread it through the surrounding "spokes." Or, if you work in a more hierarchical environment, you should focus on reaching out to those at the "top." They will facilitate the flow of information "down" through the rest of the organization.

A Michigan study of health care outreach organizations is a good example of using a social network map in this way (Michigan Department of Community Health, 2009). Researchers assessed the effectiveness of several Diabetes Outreach Networks (DONs), organizations dedicated to promoting diabetes prevention, detection, and treatment. Their findings reveal that, as illustrated in Figure 6.8, the most successful DONs had a central, "hub" position in their social networks.

From a policy perspective, one of the most important implications is that the DONs play an invaluable role in spreading clinical information and should continue to be funded. The data also suggest a particular set of management practices will maximize the DONs' impact as "hubs": establishing regional advisory councils, offering professional development courses, and disseminating information resources online.

The point about online information sharing raises an important issue related to social networks: social networking. Modern communication technology offers a dizzying array of options for using social media for building social networks: e-mail, tweets, chat messages, online forums, and other electronic tools that continue to appear with amazing speed. As a manager and health care provider, which channels should you choose? Research into communication has shown that people have different preferences for how they like to give and receive information, online and offline. One size does not fit all. What counts as "connection," therefore, differs from person to person, depending on their psychological and technological preferences.

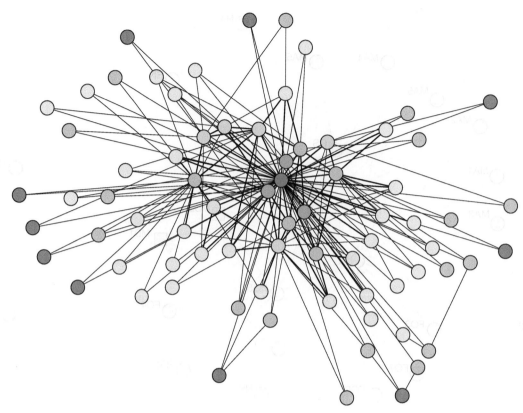

Figure 6.8 A Social Network Map.

You need to be sensitive to these differences in building relationships and disseminating information. Every situation is different, so you need to exercise judgment in choosing the appropriate communication strategy. But in every case, it pays to ask a key question: What is the right balance of psychological and informational needs? When the need for psychological contact is high, you should lean toward "high-touch" encounters. If informational needs are strongest, you should rely more on social media tools.

Consider, for example, patient communication. Since patients do better when they are knowledgeable and actively involved in their care, health care providers must give them the information they need to make the best decisions. Today, this often requires striking the right balance between virtual and face-to-face communication for each patient. The researchers Ben Gerber and Arnold Eiser found that, as decision makers, patients fall into two broad categories: the "knowledge acquirer" and the "informed decision maker" (Gerber and Eiser, 2001). The knowledge acquirer is the more passive one—more comfortable with the physician as the ultimate authority. But this patient may still want to learn about his or her condition. In this case, you can "prescribe" a website that provides background on healthy diets or home care. These patients are more likely to comply with behavioral advice if a health provider has "primed" them before they review online material that supplements other information sources. The informed decision maker wants to participate more fully in making

decisions. You can make face-to-face meetings with these patients more productive by directing them to sites where they can use credible information to educate themselves.

Patients who are comfortable working online can handle routine informational issues using social media tools. At Patientsite.org, at Boston's Beth Israel Deaconess Medical Center, patients read and send e-mail, make appointments, see personal test results, and refill prescriptions. They also access information about wellness services, medication management programs, and decision-making tools. In this setting, social media are useful in "broadcasting" information to a whole population of patients.

In managing organizational communication, you should design a system that includes both face-to-face and virtual channels. Stakeholder preferences should guide your choices about which ones to use and with whom. The benefit for you as a manager will be a social network—an "invisible" but powerful organization existing "inside" the formal hierarchy—that amplifies the impact of your programs and initiatives.

COMMUNICATION NETWORKS

Another way to view your communication strategy is through the concept of **communication networks** (Longest and Young, 2006). You can create these networks to achieve various objectives. Figure 6.9 illustrates five basic patterns that scholars have identified. Each pattern is appropriate to different managerial situations.

The following examples illustrate the practical uses to which you can put the concept of a communication network:

- *Chain*: Simple hierarchical communication is most like a chain. Messages flow downwards and upwards from one level to another. Basic factual information, like work schedules or requests for vacation days, can be communicated in this way.

- *Y*: In a Y pattern, people report up to a superior, who in turn has a dual reporting relationship to two separate superiors. As a chief operating officer, for instance, you might recommend that a senior nurse in a large clinical department report directly to the department chair and to the chief nursing officer, each of whom has a "stake" in his or her performance at the departmental level. This ensures that both departmental and enterprise-wide "interests" are represented in the reporting relationship.

- *Wheel*: A wheel is suitable when you have to communicate with several people who have no need to communicate directly with each other. When you keep important stakeholders from different parts of an organization "in the loop"—department chairs, administrators, and staff—you are following this pattern.

- *Circle*: Peers, such as division chiefs, often communicate in a "circle" between regular meetings and events. Anyone can communicate with anyone else, but no one is formally managing or controlling the communication. As a senior administrator, you might encourage this kind of self-managing information flow as a conscious strategy.

- *All-Channel*: Real-time team meetings are venues where "all-channel" communication takes place. Information flows freely as team members speak directly to each other.

Like social networks, communication networks are conceptual tools for managing the flow of information across large and complex organizations. They help organize your thinking about communication strategies.

ORGANIZATIONAL POLITICS

Even if you are a master of stakeholder management, know how to manage the flow of information through social and communication networks, and are comfortable with social media tools, you cannot avoid organizational politics. There is plenty of evidence showing that politics is a reality in most workplaces. Studies have found that some political activity takes place in nearly all organizations. And in nearly half, it takes place to a "very great" or "fair" extent. If you consider yourself "above" politics, you condemn yourself to being dominated by those who are willing to get into the trenches and fight. As the ancient philosopher Plato said, "Those who are too smart to engage in politics are condemned to being governed by those who are dumber." As a leader, therefore, you must be prepared to get involved in this often rough-and-tumble activity.

A good example of the skillful combination of communication finesse and political savvy is Richard Shannon, a physician who led an effort at Allegheny General Hospital to reduce the incidence of lethal infections in the ICU (Institute for Healthcare Improvement, 2005). He started small, realizing that there would be too much resistance among many stakeholder groups to making large-scale procedural changes all at once. With seed money

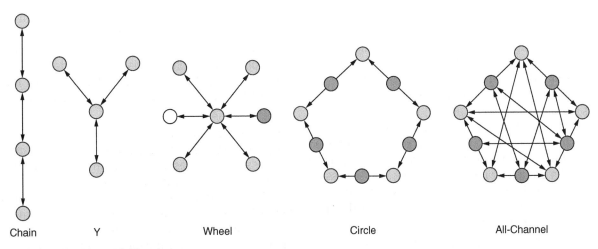

Figure 6.9 Social Network Typology.

for a small pilot project, Shannon implemented a zero-defect problem-solving process inspired by Toyota's lean production techniques. The results were stunning: Catheter-related bloodstream infections (CRBLIs) and ventilator-associated pneumonias (VAPs) were reduced by 87 percent and 83 percent, respectively. Then Shannon focused on getting traction with two key stakeholder groups: the nurses and residents. "We estimate that our efforts probably saved 47 lives," he said. "Once the staff saw we could have that kind of impact, they were immediately on board."

Next, Shannon turned his attention to getting support from senior management. He adjusted his communication strategy accordingly. He noted that this group of stakeholders had a distinctive perspective: "Their job is to look at costs, but they don't get to see the consequences of poor quality care case by case. They see aggregated data, which blunts the financial impact." Shannon thus highlighted the financial impact of a case involving a single patient who suffered from multiple complications caused by a catheter infection. "The hospital had to absorb more than $41,000 on that one case," Shannon noted. In addition, he discovered, "30 to 70 percent of the total went for treating the infection or the complications it caused." In total, the hospital could save millions by controlling infections—specifically, $2.2 million. This figure got the attention of senior management as well as the hospital's largest insurer, who ponied up a $2.1 million bonus to keep the work going.

Paul Levy was similarly skilled in responding to the bare-knuckles politicking at Beth Israel Deaconess Medical Center. Soon after he took over as CEO, he laid out his communication ground rules (Grey, 2006). Anybody could criticize his plans, as long as they did so openly and offered constructive alternatives. Following a meeting with department chiefs, Levy received a rude challenge to this principle. One of the chiefs had sat silently through a discussion of operational problems. Afterwards, he sent a harshly critical e-mail to Levy lambasting his plans and copied all of the other chiefs and the chairman of the hospital's board. Rather than address the chief's criticisms in private, as earlier administrators might have done, Levy openly confronted the chief in a bluntly worded e-mail. Levy made it clear he was not going to be bullied. The other chiefs, who were tired of endless sniping and wanted action, became even stronger allies of Levy. But Levy knew when to respond with softer gestures, too. When one group of nurses rebelled over work rules, leading to scores of resignations, Levy established a group of task forces to look into the issue. Once the nurses had an opportunity to work collaboratively on solving their own problems, turnover dropped from 15 percent to 4 percent.

The stories of Richard Shannon and Paul Levy show that effective communication requires that you think carefully about the political interests of key stakeholder groups. For Shannon, the key group was the senior administrators, who had the power to expand the small-scale initiative into an enterprise-wide initiative. Shannon tailored his communication to speak directly to their financial perspective. Levy made an attention-getting point about his leadership in standing up publicly to a disrespectful department chief. But Levy also knew when to back off and let an important stakeholder group—the nurses—find its own solution to a dispute over work rules. Organizational communication is like basketball—skill, timing, judgment, and even luck are all part of the game.

Overcoming Inertia

Strong political skills can get an initiative or idea moving forward but may still be insufficient to make change stick due to the powerful force of inertia in organizations. Our reliance on habits and established routines to get things done gives us a bias toward the status quo and makes it very difficult to change, even if we have compelling reasons to do so. Behavioral scientists like Richard Thaler and Cass Sunstein (2009) have developed a whole area of study called "choice architecture" dedicated to addressing this challenge. Their research on the psychology and neuroscience of decision making provides us with insights on how to influence stakeholders who do not care to change their routines or do not understand what they are expected to do differently.

Choice architecture is all about "nudging" people toward changing behaviors rather than trying to force them, which is more likely to incite stubborn resistance. Nudging means changing your stakeholders' environment in subtle ways so that it becomes easier for them to implement your strategy or initiative. For example, Penn Medicine has its own Nudge Unit, and one of its successful projects involved increasing the administration of flu shots to patients. The team altered the hospital's electronic medical records system to display a pop-up window during regular clinical visits that would ask the physicians if they wanted to order a flu shot for their patients. This simple, minimally intrusive request led to a 37 percent increase in vaccination rates (Patel et al., 2017).

Nudges are also useful in overcoming inertia because they tend to have a multiplier effect: Examples of successful changes in one team or division tend to circulate and encourage others to buy in. You can accelerate this process by telling stories about these "small wins" to others. Stories are an important communication device because they make abstract changes tangible and they leverage the power of social consensus to gain support.

When colleagues are set in their ways, it can be hard to get them to adopt new habits, but a combination of creating nudges, getting small wins, and circulating stories about them can help you break the inertia driving most organizational behavior.

COMMUNICATION AS A LEADERSHIP ART

Most health care organizations are complex, high-pressure work settings that include multiple disciplines and professional belief systems. To communicate successfully in this environment, you must learn to adapt to the "local culture" and speak many different "languages."

The need to adapt to stakeholders raises an important leadership issue: authenticity. Will you lose credibility and self-respect if you become a shape-shifter, changing yourself for each new audience? As actress Judy Garland once said, "Always be a first-rate version of yourself instead of a second-rate version of somebody else."

The English philosopher and politician Francis Bacon, who rose to become one of the most powerful men in England in the late 1500s under Queen Elizabeth I, tried to manage virtually every impression he made with people at the royal court. He filled his journals with observations and advice to himself on how he should appear to others in pivotal encounters and drew lessons from each success and failure to take to his next meeting. For example, he once wrote that he needed to "suppress at once my speaking with panting and labor of breath and voice" in conversing with one of the queen's closest advisors. Bacon's goal was to create a separate and distinct "public self" as an instrument of persuasion.

Behavioral experts Rob Goffe and Gareth Jones have wrestled with the apparent paradox that impression management presents (Goffe and Jones, 2005). Your personal credibility, which has its roots in perceived consistency and trustworthiness, provides the foundation for influence. Yet effective communicators are, as these authors say, "like chameleons, capable of adapting to the demands of the situations they face."

Is it really possible to be a "credible chameleon"? Yes, in the following sense: You play many roles in your life—spouse, parent, professional, employee, boss, sports fan, customer, community leader, student, and teacher. In each of these roles, you naturally display different aspects of yourself. Your child's third-grade teacher sees a different side of you than does your boss, and your brother or sister probably sees a different person than does your child. Nevertheless, it is always just "you."

Thus, the authenticity paradox diminishes somewhat when you see that you cannot help being a somewhat "different person" depending on who you are communicating with. And your awareness of these various roles gives you a range of "authentic selves" to draw from in each encounter. The art of communicating as a leader involves knowing which "self" to be: sympathetic listener, master of ceremonies, social networker, or harsh taskmaster.

DEBATE TIME: Is Strategic Communication Really Just Manipulation?

There are many examples in this chapter of leaders who adapted their messages and communication styles to fit a particular situation. Take the case of Dr. Richard Shannon. While he used the language of finance when he was communicating the benefits of lean production techniques to senior administrators at Allegheny General Hospital, he emphasized clinical outcomes when he sought the buy-in of medical staff. In another show of adaptability, Paul Levy at Beth Israel Deaconess Medical Center used strong-arm tactics in dealing with a disruptive surgeon, but he used a much gentler approach with nurses who were upset over work rules. When does "adaptability" become "inauthenticity"?

The very concept of a "stakeholder analysis" might raise a similar question. In using a "Power-Interest Matrix" to categorize stakeholders, you are assigning different levels of importance to people and groups. In executing a communication strategy based on such an analysis, you will pay more attention to some groups than to others. Is this fair?

Finally, management experts Rob Goffe and Gareth Jones propose that leaders should work to become "credible chameleons," adapting themselves to each situation so that they increase the likelihood of being understood. This advice may make some people uneasy. Shakespeare said, "To thine own self be true." Shouldn't you follow this principle rather than trying to be all things to all people?

From the perspective of an organizational leader, weigh the pros and cons of "being yourself" versus being a politically savvy "credible chameleon." In what kinds of situations might it be advisable to show flexibility, and when, if ever, should you simply speak your mind without carefully crafting a communication strategy?

SUMMARY AND MANAGERIAL GUIDELINES

1. In any managerial situation, pay attention not only to the substance of your intended message but also to the ways your message can be distorted.

2. Map the stakeholders of an organization, creating communication strategies appropriate to each stakeholder group.

3. In designing a communication strategy for an entire organization, use different channels for each purpose and audience: town hall meetings, one-on-one briefings, written memos, e-mails, etc.

4. Use multiple communication styles in disseminating organizational policies and strategy: data-oriented, emotional, and visionary.

5. Maximize "organizational learning" by engaging in robust, two-way communication with staff and external stakeholders.

6. Always work to enhance your credibility as a leader, building your reputation for trustworthiness, competence, and expertise.

7. Analyze and actively manage social networks to influence the flow of information within and around your organization.

8. Be willing, when necessary, to engage in "organizational politics" even if you have implemented a highly structured communication strategy.

9. Work hard to be a "credible chameleon" by getting in touch with your multiple "authentic selves" that enable you to make contact with many different kinds of people.

DISCUSSION QUESTIONS

1. Describe Aristotle's model of communication.

2. How did recent communication theorists build on Aristotle's model?

3. What are the five barriers to communication, and how do you remove them?

4. Identify three different methods for consulting with stakeholders in a complex communication process. Explain the objective as well as the strengths and weaknesses of each method.

5. How is the National Cancer Institute's "Patient Centered Communication Model" different from the simple sender–receiver model?

6. How does the concept of "contagion" help explain how information spreads in social networks?

7. Why do leaders need to take account of organizational politics?

CASE: THE CASE OF JESICA SANTILLAN

It is extraordinarily difficult to manage communications in health care settings. Few cases offer a better illustration of that difficulty than Jesica Santillan's. She was a 17-year-old girl who died in 2003 after undergoing a heart and lung transplant at one of the nation's top medical centers in which she received organs with the wrong blood type.

Her tragic story shows how social, technical, and organizational complexities combine to create daunting communication barriers for health providers and administrators. Consider the complicating factors in this situation and the related leadership questions they raise:

- The Family. Jesica's parents smuggled her into the country from Mexico, hoping to find a cure for a heart and lung disorder that doctors in her home country could not treat. The family settled in North Carolina, settling down in a trailer. They soon came to the attention of a local builder, who started a charity that eventually raised enough money for her to receive a transplant at Duke Medical Center. The procedure went terribly wrong, leading to severe and irreversible brain damage. When the doctors informed Jesica's mother that they planned to stop treatment, she announced at a press conference, through a translator, "They are taking her off of the medicine little by little in order to kill her. They want to rid themselves of this problem."

Questions

1. **Leadership question:** What social and cultural barriers may have made it difficult for the doctors to communicate with Jesica's family? What might have the doctors done to increase the chances that Jesica's family understood the true nature of the problems in this terrible circumstance?

   • **The Procedure**. A heart and lung transplant is obviously a challenging procedure. Though Dr. James Jaggers, the chief of pediatric surgery at Duke University, was a highly skilled and well-regarded physician, he was just one among many professionals involved in a multistep process that began with the location of suitable organs somewhere in North America and continued through transferring the patient to the intensive care unit (ICU). The many handoffs required in this process meant there was a risk of important information being lost or garbled at key transition points, as in the "whisper down the lane" game. This is in fact what happened. Jesica Santillan's blood type was O, while the organs' was A. Carolina Donor Services located the organs and, they claimed, informed Dr. Jaggers of the organs' blood type. Dr. Jaggers does not remember the conversation about it. Another physician was sent to pick up the organs in Boston. He was informed three times of the blood type, but since he did not know Jesica's blood type, he was not aware there was a mismatch.

2. **Leadership question:** How would you organize the complex set of steps required in this transplant process to ensure that misunderstandings do not occur in handoffs between professionals?

   • **The Stakeholders**. Following the string of errors leading to the mistaken transplant, the Duke Medical Center had to manage a whole set of stakeholders: the Santillan family, the family's lawyers, the community, the press, and the health provider community. Each stakeholder group had its own interests, influenced by its cultural, social, and professional backgrounds.

3. **Leadership question:** If you were the Duke Medical Center CEO, what general communication strategy would you put in place to manage the stakeholders in this case? In particular, how would your messages to each group differ from the others?

Adapted from a *New York Times* story. Original text retrieved from https://www.nytimes.com/2003/02/23/us/girl-in-transplant-mix-up-dies-after-two-weeks.html.

REFERENCES

Argenti, P., Howell, R. A., & Beck, H. A. (2005). The strategic communication imperative. *MIT Sloan Management Review, 46*(3), 83–89.

Aristotle. (2006). *On rhetoric: A theory of civic discourse.* New York: Oxford University Press.

Armstrong-Coben, A. (2009, March 5). The computer will see you now. *New York Times.* Retrieved October 2, 2018, from https://www.nytimes.com/2009/03/06/opinion/06coben.html.

Blagg, D., & Young, S. (2001). What makes a good leader? *Harvard Business School Working Knowledge.*

Block, P. (1991). *The empowered manager.* San Francisco, CA: Jossey-Bass.

Bornstein, R., Leone, D., & Donna, J. (1987). The generalizability of subliminal mere exposure effects. *Journal of Personality and Social Psychology, 53*(6), 1070–1079.

Britten, N., Stevenson, F., Barry, C., et al. (2000). Misunderstandings in prescribing decisions in general practice: Qualitative study. Retrieved August 12, 2010, from http://www.ncbi.nlm.nih.gov/pmc/articles/PMC27293/?tool=pubmed.

Burt, R. (2007). *Brokerage and closure: An introduction to social capital.* Oxford: Oxford University Press.

Christakis, N., & Fowler, J. (2009). *Connected: the surprising power of our social networks and how they shape our lives.* New York: Little Brown.

Collins, J. (2001). *Good to great: Why some companies make the leap ... and others don't.* New York: HarperBusiness.

Covey, S. & Merrill, R. (2008). *The speed of trust: The one thing that changes everything.* New York: Free Press.

Croft, R. (2004). Communication theory. Retrieved August 12, 2010, from https://cs.eou.edu/rcroft/MM350/CommunicationModels.pdf.

Davis, S. (2009). Palin's "death panels" charge named "Lie of the Year." Retrieved August 12, 2010, from http://blogs.wsj.com/washwire/2009/12/22/palins-death-panels-charge-named-lie-of-the-year/tab/article/.

Dubner, S., & Levitt, S. (2006, September 24). Selling soap. *New York Times.* Retrieved August 12, 2010, from http://www.nytimes.com/2006/09/24/magazine/24wwln_freak.html.

Eccles, R. G., Nohria, N., & Berkely, J. D. (1994). *Beyond the hype: Rediscovering the essence of management.* Boston, MA: Harvard Business School Press.

Edmondson, A. C. (2002). Managing the risk of learning: Psychological safety in work teams. CiteSeerX. Retrieved May 17, 2015, from http://citeseerx.ist.psu.edu/viewdoc/download?doi=10.1.1.118.1943&rep=rep1&type=pdf.

Edmondson, A. C., & Lei, Z. (2014). Psychological safety: The history, renaissance, and future of an interpersonal construct. *Annual Review of Organizational Psychology and Organizational Behavior, 1*(1), 23–43. https://doi.org/10.1146/annurev-orgpsych-031413-091305.

Falcone, T, Dickstein, L, Sieke, E. H., et al. (2014). *Coping with chronic medical illness. Cleveland Clinic Center for Continuing Education.* Cleveland Clinic.

Freeman, R. E., & McVea, J. (2001). A stakeholder approach to strategic management. Working Paper 01-02, Darden Graduate School of Business Administration.

Gardner, H. (2006). *Changing minds: The art and science of changing our own and other people's minds (leadership for the common good).* Boston, MA: Harvard Business School Press.

Gerber, B. S., & Eiser, R. A. (2001). The patient-physician relationship in the internet age: Future prospects and the research agenda. *Journal of Medical Internet Research, 3*(2), e15.

Goffe, R., & Jones, G. (2005). Managing authenticity. *Harvard Business Review, 83*(12), 86–94.

Grey, P. B. (2006). Rx for merger trauma. CFO.com. Retrieved August 12, 2010, from http://www.cfo.com/printable/article.cfm/5598469?f=optionss.

Heath, C., & Heath, D. (2007). *Made to stick.* New York: Random House.

Institute for Healthcare Improvement. (2005). Doing better, spending less. Retrieved August 12, 2010, from http://www.ihi.org/resources/Pages/ImprovementStories/DoingBetterSpendingLess.aspx.

Langer, E. (1989). *Mindfulness.* Reading, MA: Da Capo.

Laswell, H. (1948). The structure and function of communication in society. In L. Bryson (Ed.), *The communication of ideas.* New York: Harper.

Leroy, H., Dierynck, B., Anseel, F., Simons, T., Halbesleben, J. R. B., McCaughey, D., & Sels, L. (2012). Behavioral integrity for safety, priority of safety, psychological safety, and patient safety: A team-level study. *The Journal of Applied Psychology, 97*(6), 1273–1281. https://doi.org/10.1037/a0030076.

Levin, D. Z., Whitener, E. M., & Cross, R. (2006). Perceived trustworthiness of knowledge sources: The moderating impact of relationship length. *The Journal of Applied Psychology, 91*(5), 1163–1171. https://doi.org/10.1037/0021-9010.91.5.1163.

Levine, S. S., Apfelbaum, E. P., Bernard, M., et al. (2014). Ethnic diversity deflates price bubbles. *Proceedings of the National Academy of Sciences, 111*(52), 18524–18529. https://doi.org/10.1073/pnas.1407301111.

Longest, B. B., Jr., & Young, G. (2006). Coordination and communication. In L. Burns, E. Bradley, & B. Weiner (Eds.), *Health care management: Organization design and behavior* (5th ed.). Clifton Park, NY: Delmar Cengage Learning.

Michigan Department of Community Health. (2009). *An interorganizational social network analysis of the Michigan Diabetes Outreach Networks.* Written by L. Corteville & M. Sun. Retrieved August 12, 2010, from http://dpacmi.org/documents/SNA_Report_Final.pdf.

Morris, C. W. (1949). *Signs, language and behavior.* New York: Prentice Hall.

Nembhard, I. M., & Tucker, A. L. (2011). Deliberate learning to improve performance in dynamic service settings: Evidence from hospital intensive care units. *Organization Science, 22*(4), 907–922. https://doi.org/10.1287/orsc.1100.0570.

Nohria, N., & Harrington, B. (1993). *Six principles of successful persuasion.* Boston, MA: Harvard Business School Note: 9-494-037.

Norton, D. P., & Coffey, J. (2007). Building an organized process for strategy communication. *Harvard Business Review, 9*(3), 1–5.

Palin doubles down on "death panels." (2009). Yahoo! News. Retrieved August 12, 2010, from http://www.politico.com/story/2009/08/palin-doubles-down-on-death-panels-026078.

Patel, M. S., Volpp, K. G., Small, D. S., et al. (2017). Using active choice within the electronic health record to increase influenza vaccination rates. *Journal of General Internal Medicine, 32*(7), 790–795. https://doi.org/10.1007/s11606-017-4046-6.

Peikes, D., Chen, A., Schore, J., et al. (2009). Effects of care coordination on hospitalization, quality of care, and health care expenditures among Medicare beneficiaries: 15 randomized trials. *Journal of American Medical Association, 301*(6), 603–618. https://doi.org/10.1001/jama.2009.126.

Pinkerton, J. (2010). Why Obamacare is doomed: The Hollywood version. Retrieved August 12, 2010, from http://www.foxnews.com/opinion/2010/01/26/james-p-pinkerton-extraordinary-measures-obamacare-review/.

Polzer, J. T., Milton, L. P., & Swarm, W. B. (2002). Capitalizing on diversity: Interpersonal congruence in small work groups. *Administrative Science Quarterly, 47*(2), 296–324. https://doi.org/10.2307/3094807.

Powell, W. W. (1998). Learning from collaboration: Knowledge and networks in the biotechnology and pharmaceutical industries. *California Management Review, 40*(3), 228–240.

Roussin, C. J. (2008). Increasing trust, psychological safety, and team performance through dyadic leadership discovery. *Small Group Research, 39*(2), 224–248. https://doi.org/10.1177/1046496408315988.

Senge, P. (2006). *The fifth discipline: The art and practice of the learning organization.* New York: Broadway Business.

Shell, G. R., & Moussa, M. (2007). *The art of woo: Using strategic persuasion to sell your ideas.* New York: Penguin. (8). Portions of this chapter were adapted from the book, with the publisher's permission.

Shepperd, S., Lannin, N. A., Clemson, L. M., et al. (2013). Discharge planning from hospital to home. *The Cochrane Database of Systematic Reviews,* (1), CD000313. https://doi.org/10.1002/14651858.CD000313.pub4.

Sunstein, C. R., & Hastie, R. (2014). Making dumb groups smarter. *Harvard Business Review, 92*(12), 90–98.

Tamir, D. I., & Mitchell, J. P. (2012). Disclosing information about the self is intrinsically rewarding. *Proceedings of the*

National Academy of Sciences, 109(21), 8038–8043. https://doi.org/10.1073/pnas.1202129109.

Text: Obama's speech on health care reform. (2009). *New York Times.* Retrieved August 12, 2010, from http://www.nytimes.com/2009/06/15/health/policy/15obama.text.html?pagewanted=1&_r=1&sq=obama%20on%20health%20care&st=cse&scp=21.

Thaler, R. H., & Sunstein, C. R. (2009). *Nudge: Improving decisions about health, wealth, and happiness.* New York: Penguin.

Thorne, S. (2006). Patient-provider communication in chronic illness: A health promotion window of opportunity. *Family & Community Health, 29*(1 Suppl.), 4S–11S.

Ward, B. W. (2013). Prevalence of multiple chronic conditions among US adults: Estimates from the National Health Interview Survey, 2010. *Preventing Chronic Disease, 10.* https://doi.org/10.5888/pcd10.120203.

Wittgenstein, L. (1973). *Philosophical investigations.* New York: Prentice Hall.

Chapter 7

Power, Politics, and Conflict Management

Timothy Hoff and Kevin W. Rockmann

CHAPTER OUTLINE

- The Uses of Power in Organizations
- What Is Power and Where Does It Come From?
- Key Power Relationships in Health Care Organizations
- The Political Nature of Power
- The Abuse of Power in Health Care Organizations
- Power as a Key Source of Conflict
- Types of Conflict
- Negotiation as a Conflict Management Tool
- Common Mistakes in Managing Conflict via Negotiation
- Negotiation Strategies and Tactics
- Conclusion

LEARNING OBJECTIVES

After completing this chapter, the reader should be able to:

1. Identify what power is and how it is used within health care organizations
2. Describe and compare the major sources of power within health care organizations
3. Identify the differences between individual and subunit sources of power within organizations
4. Identify the differences between managerial and professional sources of power within health care organizations
5. Summarize the interrelationship between power and politics within organizational settings
6. Describe the demographic and contextual factors that affect how power is distributed within health care organizations
7. Classify the various conditions that give rise to power abuses in health care organizations
8. Identify the different roles played by trust, fairness, and transparency in preventing power abuse in health care organizations
9. Describe the different types of conflict and how they might be present in various health care organizations
10. Describe how emotions affect individuals attempting to manage conflict
11. Describe the various mistakes relating to how individuals think about negotiation and how they think about relationships
12. Identify the difference between interests and positions and describe why understanding that difference is critical in negotiation
13. Compare the benefits of compromise, competition, and collaboration as three distinct strategies for negotiation
14. Describe the tactics to find a better solution, the tactics to acquire information, and the tactics to influence others

KEY TERMS

Anchoring Bias

BATNA

Coalitions

Coercion

Collaborating

Competing

Compromising

Confirming Evidence Bias

Contingent

Culturally Derived Power

Emotional Contagion

Fixed-Pie Bias

Fractioning

Functional Fixedness

Individual Sources of Power

Knowledge-Based Sources of Power

Logrolling

Network Centrality

Nonspecific Compensation

Organizational Politics

Power

Power Abuse

Power Stratification

Reciprocity

Relationship Conflict

Self-Fulfilling Prophecy

Structural Sources of Power

Structurally Derived Power

Study of Conflict Management

Task Conflict

Threat Rigidity Effect

Value in Negotiation

Winner's Curse

• • • IN PRACTICE: Pay-for-Performance and Power: Influencing and Negotiating the Murky Measurement Waters of Value-Based Purchasing

The concept of "value-based purchasing" (VBP) has gained traction as a potential means to better link health care outcomes to payment. Numerous national demonstration projects are underway, and the concept's flagship philosophy, "pay-for-performance" (P4P), has been integrated into the majority of physician practices and many hospitals across the United States. VBP rests on a fundamental principle—that practitioners and institutions that produce the best outcomes, from both an efficiency perspective and a quality-of-care perspective, should be rewarded financially, while those who underperform should be subject to earning less. This approach is innovative because traditionally everyone in health care got paid the same, regardless of their performance excellence, for the services they provide.

However, the VBP approach unleashes the potential for many power dynamics within the health care setting and for conflict among different stakeholders. For example, the issues of how to measure cost-effectiveness and quality become front and center to making VBP work. Because there can be substantial disagreement as to the "right" ways to measure these outcomes, the use of power can become an integral component of making decisions in this regard. When one stakeholder such as the Centers for Medicare and Medicaid Services (CMS) uses its power to try to influence the kinds of measures used, conflict may erupt. This conflict can undermine the success of pay-for-performance programs by promoting an adversarial relationship among the parties involved. Insurance companies, employers, and government—all of whom pay for health care services—may seek to exhibit greater influence over the measurement debate because of the dependence by providers such as physicians and hospitals on that payment for their economic survival. This may cause consternation and resistance among providers such as physicians and hospitals, especially if they have differing opinions on the measurement issue.

On the other hand, physicians may use their own advantages of control over clinical knowledge and the public's trust in them to counteract the influence of payers in deciding which measurements will form the basis for paying on the basis of quality and value. Hospitals, because they possess the infrastructure that everyone in the system relies upon to deliver complex care, can exert their own influence to shape measures in a way favorable to their interests and constituencies. Moreover, patients may have little ability to influence the measurement debate, simply because they do not have a source of power upon which to draw in getting the other stakeholders to comply with their preferences. In fact, these overall power dynamics have been seen in the current value-based purchasing movement, where many major decisions around how to measure become drawn-out exercises in power use and influence tactics (Centers for Medicare and Medicaid Services, 2017).

• • • IN PRACTICE: Pay-for-Performance and Power: Influencing and Negotiating the Murky Measurement Waters of Value-Based Purchasing (Continued)

The conflict that arises around identifying the best way to measure outcomes in a pay-for-performance incentive program is often managed through a political process in which different stakeholders attempt to use their power in shaping how the debate is conducted. For example, health care payers may push for the establishment of public reporting of clinical outcomes through devices like "report cards," in part as a means to get consumers on their side and to put physicians and hospitals on the defensive. They may want measurements reported that they feel more in control over, i.e., care processes that can be more easily standardized across different providers. The use of tactics like report cards and care standardization may be promoted overtly as a rational means to achieve performance transparency. However, these tactics may also be used covertly to exert and enhance the payers' control over how "value" and "quality" should be defined and measured in the eyes of the general public. Alternatively, health care providers may put forth a message of "we know best because we deliver the care" to patients and advocacy groups to try to convince them that they should be allowed to exert greater influence over which measures are used.

This is where conflict management and, more specifically, the process of negotiation can play a role in moving the use of power and politics to a productive end. By treating the discussion around measurement within a VBP approach as one in which multiple stakeholders can simultaneously "win," there is a higher probability that the outcome will have something favorable in it for everyone (including patients) and, as a result, will be more easily accepted by all the relevant parties in the negotiation. In this way, negotiations around how to measure "cost-effectiveness" or "quality" that consider multiple viewpoints, provide voice to a diverse group of stakeholders for input, and seek to achieve a level of acceptance and satisfaction among all constituencies are likely to create a more favorable climate for implementing pay-for-performance programs and to enhance the chances for their long-term success. The use of power and politics goes hand in hand with the use of negotiation, simply because power and politics create the potential for conflict among stakeholders, and this conflict is best managed through a more rational approach that seeks to find the most optimum outcome that can be accepted by all.

CHAPTER PURPOSE

As the first In Practice example illustrates, perhaps nothing is as potent a force in organizational life as **power**. Power is the ability to exert influence or control over others. It dictates a significant degree of what goes on in organizations, from decision making to performance outcomes. In health care, where there is greater uncertainty around how to best deliver and pay for care, power looms large as a key variable enabling various stakeholders to control decision making. Power involves two key dynamics—influence and dependence—and when these dynamics are present in large quantities, power may be wielded by individuals, groups, and organizations in ways that allow them to achieve their preferred vision and goals. Those at the sharp end of its use may find themselves unable to pursue their own agenda.

The purpose of this chapter is to provide students with a clearer understanding of what power is, how and where to look for it, where it comes from, and how it plays out in health care organizations. In addition, emphasis is placed on how power relates to the political aspects of organizational action in settings such as hospitals, insurance plans, and physician practices, and the conditions and circumstances that give rise to power abuse

are featured as important factors for managers to keep in mind at all times. The ethics of wielding power effectively should not be understated. A key focus in the second half of the chapter is on the role of conflict management in managing the role of both power and politics. A practical guide is offered for how to use the process of negotiation to achieve mutually satisfactory outcomes among organizational stakeholders.

Power and politics can be implemented in dysfunctional, self-interested ways by a variety of organizational stakeholders. This chapter touches upon this issue. But it also stresses the important and necessary functions played by power and politics in getting organizations and workers to perform effectively. In the case of health care, power and politics are necessary dynamics for getting things done. The use of power and politics heightens the level of conflict that may occur in organizations, and such conflict is best managed, this chapter argues, through a more strategic perspective that focuses on an ethical, rational, and results-oriented process of conflict management and negotiation. In other words, power and politics are the forces that move change and enhance effectiveness in health care, but these forces are managed best through proven tactics associated with skilled conflict management and negotiation.

THE USES OF POWER IN ORGANIZATIONS

Power can be used for different purposes within organizational settings. Perhaps the most ubiquitous use of power in organizations involves determining the key choices made at an organizational level to guide overall company strategy (Finkelstein, 1992). The types of choices in this regard most amenable to the use of power include those that involve higher levels of uncertainty and innovativeness (Mintzberg, Raisinghani, and Theoret, 1976). The use of power by chief executive officers, boards of directors, and other top leadership to guide the direction in which the organization moves, how it chooses to compete, which products or services to offer, and the type of business model employed for pursuing profit has existed as long as the concept of the corporation. Leaders can and do use power effectively to make strategic decisions in efficient ways.

Power may also be used to influence the actions of others, be they workers, professionals, other organizations, or the customers that use the organization's products. In this way, power is thought of as a highly coercive mechanism alongside other influence-wielding tactics such as trust, co-optation, and conformity (Hart and Saunders, 1997). Power in this regard is simply another in a toolbox of tactics individuals in organizations employ to get other people to behave in desired ways. It requires a certain degree of effort and resource use like any other influence approach. While it is worth noting that the use of power in this regard may be no more effective than other "softer" tactics such as gaining people's trust to believe that what is being asked of them is the correct thing to do (McEvily, Perrone, and Zaheer, 2003), nonetheless, it is often viewed as a quick, reliable form of control that can be employed across a diverse array of organizational situations (Pfeffer, 1981).

Power can control, allocate, and redistribute resources of all types within organizations (Pfeffer and Salancik, 1978). These resources include human capital such as clinical staff, financial resources such as budget allocations to hospital departments, and knowledge resources like innovations or awareness of external markets that enable a production process to be done better or a competitive advantage to be gained. For example, power can be used to decide which part of a health care system should have a fully integrated electronic medical record to use first in its everyday work. By being the first to use

• • • IN PRACTICE: The Quality Improvement Department, Accreditation, and Power

Organizations in the health care industry gain a great deal of their legitimacy from accreditation. Many different types of accrediting processes exist, from the Joint Commission for hospitals and other health providers, to the National Committee for Quality Assurance (NCQA) for insurance plans, and to more specialized accreditation for niche providers like laboratories and radiology facilities.

Nothing shifts the power structure more in a health care organization, at least temporarily, than the process of gearing up for one of these many accreditations. Much of the time, the power shift moves favorably in the direction of quality improvement (QI) staff and units within the organization. These staff and units are often the nerve centers of data collection, analysis, and reporting for the kinds of things accrediting organizations request and verify when they visit. Thus, accreditation offers them an opportunity to gain greater control over scarce resources, influence strategic decision making, shape organizational culture, and change the manner in which the organization's workforce does its jobs.

For example, there may be a particular area or work output of the organization where quality measures lag and a problem regarding quality is thought to exist. While a QI department may be involved over time in addressing the issue, if the issue impacts accreditation, greater resources may be made available to QI staff, and greater freedom provided to them by top management, to try to correct the issue in a timely manner. The resources given to QI may be taken away from some other part of the organization, lessening the influence of other stakeholders in the process.

The QI function may be emboldened by the organization to reshape how work is performed in the particular area, how workers do and think about their jobs, what performance data should be collected, and how that data must be evaluated. In this way, QI staff come to be relied upon by top management and the organization as a whole to help ensure that not only are quality problems identified and fixed but also the all-important external accreditation is not jeopardized in any substantive way. This may also represent an opportunity for the QI function to solidify its influence within the organization, acquire greater resources for itself, and gain greater control over others competing for the same resources. Thus, even a short-term shift in power and influence within an organization can have long-term consequences.

such a system, favorable benefits may accrue to that part of the system earlier and in greater quantity than later adopters. Resource control and allocation is perhaps the most widely used application of power within organizations. As the sociologist Charles Perrow asserts, this use of power deals with "the size of the pie" within organizations and how it is sliced—i.e., who wins and who loses in getting more of something that they want, while at the same time preventing others from doing the same thing (Perrow, 1989).

Power may also be wielded for purposes of shaping or transforming organizational or work cultures in ways top management desires or to move the organization toward being more competitive and effective in the marketplace. For example, leaders of both General Electric and IBM used their positions and authority, along with that of their top managers, to help transform these companies during the 1980s and 1990s into global, innovative firms (Gerstner, 2002; Slater, 1999). They did this in large part through a focus on shifting the meaning systems among employees within each of the organizations toward beliefs and values that could support a new way of doing business, one that would enable the companies to meet the challenges of a changing marketplace.

Other companies, particularly in the new gig economy, have strong leaders who use power to push their companies in directions they believe are necessary for success, even at the expense of both public and worker approval (Isaac, 2017; Kantor and Streitfeld, 2015). Using power to change organizational culture carries risks, because culture is difficult to change (Martin, 1992). In addition, the overuse of power by a single leader may stifle a diversity of ideas that may be needed to help the company grow, change its culture, enhance its workforce, or align better with the competitive marketplace. Companies such as Uber and Amazon, while successful because of strong leaders using their power, nonetheless put themselves at risk if that power crowds out other important voices in the organization.

WHAT IS POWER AND WHERE DOES IT COME FROM?

Power has been defined in a variety of ways. However, common to all definitions is the notion of one stakeholder's ability to exert influence over others in ways that, among other things, influence them to do things they normally would not do (Pfeffer, 1981). In short, power is defined by the level of control one group has over another's behavior (Hickson et al., 1971). Central to this definition of power is the idea of influence—i.e., that an individual, group, subunit, or organization has both the ability and opportunity to control how another acts either directly or indirectly (Dahl, 1957). In this way, power by definition involves **coercion**. Coercion is the use

of subtle influence dynamics to achieve desired goals. This means that all power brings with it the potential for heightened tension and conflict within the organizational setting. This is one of the reasons why the use of power is often filtered through a political process within organizations (described later in the chapter). It is also a key reason why negotiation and conflict management, a primary focus of this chapter, are at the center of a more pragmatic view of how to think about, use, and regulate power within organizations.

If influence is at the core of defining power, then this implies that all power is also relational in the sense that its existence, magnitude, and use rely upon an ongoing social exchange between two parties (Dahl, 1957). For example, power can be attributable to a given individual based on another individual's perception of that person's relative influence. However, that perception is likely strengthened or weakened over time as the two individuals interact. The perception of power gets validated through the social experience within organizations. In this way, power requires two or more parties interacting with each other on an ongoing basis to be fully realized. While it may be understood that one group or unit has power over another, for example in a hospital or insurance company, by this definition power would exist in its fullest form only when the powerful group or unit behaves with others in a way specifically designed to control or alter their behavior. In this way, a group of self-employed surgeons working collectively in the same practice may be presumed to have the ability to influence Hospital A's behavior toward them, such as better reimbursement rates or preferred operating room times, because there is an equivalent Hospital B in the same geographic area where these surgeons can take their business. But as a relational dynamic, power would be evident most during moments when the surgical group, through direct communication or posturing during contract negotiations with Hospital A, actually convinces Hospital A to give them higher reimbursement or better operating room times, and Hospital A complies in this regard (see the "In Practice" case study "Pay-for-Performance and Power").

Power comes from several different sources. Three major sources of power within an organization are structural-, cultural-, and individual characteristics. **Structural sources of power** are sources that derive from the formal or bureaucratic aspects of an organization (Wilson, 1989). Examples of these aspects include the organizational chart, written policies and procedures, job titles and descriptions, and budgets. Structural sources of power can be used by individuals, groups, or entire organizations. The potential for power is built into every organization through the existence of a formal structure that orders social relations and provides a guide for behaving to organizational actors. In examining how structure gives rise to power, one need only examine how one or more of these bureaucratic components instill in specific people and groups the ability to exert influence over others.

For example, a simple job title and job description provides insight into the power and influence associated with that position. A job title that includes the word "manager" or "supervisor" means that the person filling the position will have formal authority over one or more persons in the organization. Alternatively, this authority may be implied in the job title (e.g., medical director, chief executive officer, vice president in charge of compliance) and articulated in more detail in the description itself (e.g., "hires, supervises, and evaluates all physicians working in the medical group"). From the title and job description, an individual gains the legitimacy to direct others' actions, evaluate their performance, and serve as the conduit for information between higher levels of the organization and the workers under their direct supervision.

Structurally derived power gains its stability and legitimacy by creating resource dependencies that place some individuals or groups in positions to influence others (Pfeffer and Salancik, 1978). This is seen clearly in the situation in which one department or unit in an organization is relied upon to help produce the work of other departments. In health care, such situations abound. For example, all hospital work from emergency medicine to surgery relies heavily upon departments like radiology and laboratory services for its effective completion of work. The need to test and monitor patient blood levels, screen for infection and disease, and examine bones and organs in detail for proper assessment gives both the radiology and laboratory departments the ability to influence how other work in the hospital is performed and how other actors request and get services from these departments. Without the timely, high-quality assistance of these latter units, both surgical and emergency services can take longer to do, be of lower quality, and cost more. This creates a dependency situation in which radiology and laboratory services, because they are vital to all other work in the hospital, gain additional ability to determine their own work patterns and resource needs. In this instance, the "resource" depended upon is the knowledge and technology associated with radiology and lab work. In other situations, the resources may be financial.

Power also is derived culturally within organizations. Culture is defined as the shared meaning systems that arise out of ongoing interaction between two or more entities (Schein, 1992). Whereas structure represents the formal aspects of organization, culture is associated with the informal aspects, i.e., norms, values, beliefs, and assumptions. **Culturally derived power** is power that derives from these informal aspects and is less visible but no less potent than structurally derived power. In some situations, power deriving from existing norms or beliefs may become more influential than structural power, in part because it seeks to influence organizational behavior in ways that are less visible to public view.

Cultural sources of power cannot easily be identified through formal artifacts such as organizational charts or budgets. Instead, they are discerned from an implicit understanding and appreciation for "how things work" in the organization. An example of culturally derived power might be seen in a group of surgeons, where one surgeon in particular who is widely understood to be "the best cutter" or "have the best hands" is deferred to by other surgical colleagues across a variety of work situations, in large part due to the collective belief that such a surgeon must know and be good at a variety of things if he or she is perceived as the best in this core skill all surgeons value. In this instance, this surgeon gains power and influence due to a shared meaning system within the group that may or may not mirror reality. Similarly, physicians who believe a particular nurse working with them has great sway with other nurses may defer more to that nurse across different work situations, giving the nurse more power to influence not only those physicians but also her fellow nursing colleagues.

Finally, there are several different **individual sources of power** (French and Raven, 1959). These include power rooted in an individual's legitimate authority, ability to reward another, knowledge or expertise, charisma, coercive ability, and informational centrality. According to French and Raven (1959), both expert and reference bases of power involve personal qualities of the individual. In health care particularly, these two sources of power are commonly leveraged by professionals. **Knowledge-based sources of power** are particularly ubiquitous. Knowledge-based power derives from an individual's control over the expertise needed to make key decisions and organize production. This power source is common in health care because much of the work contains higher degrees of uncertainty in terms of both processes and outcomes. Some health care work can be standardized and routinized, but much of it cannot, providing ample opportunity for those with a knowledge advantage to assert control.

Knowledge-based power in the health care industry currently plays out in two major ways. Traditionally, the medical profession has been the primary source of knowledge power-based. Physicians have been able to define how clinical work should be performed, how patients should be treated, and what success and failure mean in different types of delivery situations (Freidson, 1970). Physicians still remain the most powerful group of health care workers in large part because they retain heavy control over the most important forms of clinical and scientific knowledge available, and others defer to them in setting the terms under which that knowledge is applied on an everyday basis.

More recently, however, knowledge-based power through structural rather than individual sources has proliferated. This diffusion is an example of the commodification of knowledge-based power and the transferring of power from professionals like doctors to the organization by standardizing and making it transparent throughout the organization. In one sense, this modern-day quality movement represents an attempt to garner knowledge-based power for the organization and its administrators, either by taking it away from or sharing it with physicians. For example, a clinical care guideline that is developed to treat a diabetic or hypertensive patient, where specifics of the diagnostic process, preferred means of treatment, and identification of risk factors are all included in it, can transfer knowledge previously within the exclusive domain of the physician to the organization, reducing the physician's power in the process.

Finally, it is important to note that none of these three power sources acts alone to generate power in an organization. Sources of power can and do interact with each other, as in the case above where knowledge-based power may be wielded by individuals even as some of that power is embedded formally in the organizational structure through guidelines, policies, and "best practices." The concept of **network centrality** is another illustration of interaction occurring between knowledge-based and structural sources of power. Network centrality refers to a situation within an organization in which one work group or unit lays at the intersection of many other work groups or units, as a result becoming a repository of knowledge and understanding about how the entire organization works (Ibarra and Andrews, 1993). This makes them indispensable sources of information for other parts of the organization and provides them with a greater ability to influence the actions of others.

• • • IN PRACTICE: The Pursuit of Power among Managers and Physicians

Managers and physicians working in the same health care organization might draw upon different sources for establishing and maintaining their power. Managers work in positions typically associated with the formal organization—i.e., the bureaucratic chain of command that exists to help coordinate work in standard and routine ways. If one examines an organizational chart for a department or the entire organization, it may be clear that persons occupying management or supervisory positions possess specific degrees of influence over different organizational functions, budgets, or staff. Physicians, especially those not occupying formal administrative positions, derive their power mainly from knowledge-based and cultural sources. These sources are not specific to any single organization, as might be the case for management power, which relies upon formal policies or organizational charts. Rather, physician power derives similarly across all organizations from the wider societal belief that doctors "should be in charge," possess the most valuable knowledge for effective health care delivery, and are more likely to represent the views of the customer, i.e., patients and their families.

Within the hospital setting, for example, a "dual hierarchy" still exists that recognizes the power of both managers and physicians to direct staff, control work, and make decisions for the organization. One part of the hierarchy recognizes the role played by management personnel in these areas, while the other bestows that same recognition on physicians. Thus, we have "medical directors" who retain control over clinical staff and delivery and department or unit managers whose formal domain is overseeing budgets, nonclinical staff, and often quality improvement reporting. It is this dual hierarchy and its everyday implementation that gives rise to ongoing tension between the two groups within settings such as a hospital. With each having power and influence, and each seen as legitimate by key stakeholders within the organization, the imperative becomes one of advancing the positive contributions of each group to organizational functioning while minimizing the conflict and confusion potentially arising from both groups asserting their power in the same situations.

And assert power they do. Managers may use formal devices to both assert and pursue power, such as the creation of new organizational policies; reorganization; the collection, analysis, and reporting of data around clinical work; and establishment of new domains of authority such as quality assurance or accreditation. They may not be viewed as "knowing what physicians know," but they can seek to offset some of this knowledge advantage by gaining access to the knowledge, standardizing it, and making it transparent throughout the organization. Physicians may counter in their pursuit and assertion of power by making more overt their knowledge advantage in specific work situations, moving to make portions of their work more complex, or look more complex, so it is less subject to management cooptation, and getting others like patients and nurses to believe that they are the most legitimate group to direct care and make decisions. In each case, different sources are drawn upon to promote the group's power and influence. This reality makes health care settings particularly fluid in terms of how such a dual hierarchy works, how power is distributed between the two groups, and which group accomplishes its preferred goals for the organization and itself at a given period in time.

The quality improvement (QI) department of a hospital, insurance plan, or medical group is the clearest example of this in health care. By collecting and analyzing information on each work process in the organization—e.g., what works in one area of the hospital or practice and could be transferred for use to another part—of the QI department gains legitimacy and power. Departments and personnel that require knowledge or understanding held by other parts of the organization will come to depend on such a "network-central" entity like the QI department to help improve their own production processes.

KEY POWER RELATIONSHIPS IN HEALTH CARE ORGANIZATIONS

Health care is a service industry. This means that the key production inputs are the individuals who provide the services—physicians, nurses, and a variety of clinical and nonclinical support staff. Since all power is relational, understanding power within a service industry like health care requires examination of the major stakeholders and their interactions with each other. There are three key power relationships in health care organizations: physician–patient, physician–nurse, and physician–administrator.

The most important relationship in health care involves that of physician and patient. All health care service delivery is built around this relationship, because patients are the ultimate consumers of all health care services. Traditionally, physicians have held great authority over patients, and the main reason for this has been the significant asymmetries in knowledge, information, and access. Physicians possess the clinical knowledge and skills patients seek when accessing care and historically, such knowledge and skills were not available for access in any manner other than seeing the physician (Starr, 1982). Society has also granted to physicians exclusive or near-exclusive rights to prescribe medications, order medical services such as MRIs and physical therapy, bill insurance for services rendered to patients, and to serve as the final arbiter for which types of services are appropriate and reimbursable. These rights bestow on physicians control over medical decision making, giving them a significant power advantage over the patients they serve.

For a long time, physician power over patients manifested itself in a paternalistic approach that emphasized the caring doctor to whom the patient must listen and comply. This approach limited conflict and tension in the relationship, as patients were expected to obey the physician's orders and question less. However, this type of relationship and the one-sided nature of the power and influence implied in it have been increasingly criticized

as unnecessary and a source of lower health care quality and patient satisfaction (Wachter and Shojana, 2004).

Although the physician continues to maintain a clear and significant knowledge advantage over patients, some believe that information and knowledge asymmetries between doctor and patient are lessening with the advent of new information technologies, such as the Internet, which give patients the ability to access and absorb quick, easy-to-understand medical information (Pew Internet and American Life Project, 2002). Another reason for a shift in the balance of power between doctor and patient may stem from increasing patient distrust of health care institutions, reflected in lower confidence in our health care system, a growing health care consumer movement, and sustained emphasis on consumer-driven issues such as patient safety (Armstrong et al., 2006; Hoff, 2017).

The physician–nurse relationship is also fraught with the use of power and influence. Physicians depend greatly on the skills of nursing staff in order to perform their work effectively. However, this dependence does not translate into equal power for nurses vis-à-vis physicians since the medical profession retains control over key cultural and knowledge-based power sources. This control allows them to maintain legal privileges and exert direct influence over nursing work, pay, and employment status. For example, registered nurses (RNs) and licensed practical nurses (LPNs) are neither allowed to prescribe their own medications for patients nor diagnose and treat patients. Training for these occupational groups is limited largely to preparing them for work roles where they assist physicians in their clinical work. The pay and prestige of nursing as a field also lags behind physicians' salaries and prestige.

As a result of this relationship, which is based on mutual dependence but asymmetrical power, the physician–nurse relationship has been characterized historically by high degrees of tension. More recently, however, because of workforce shortages in medical fields such as primary care, the nursing profession has advanced a new occupational subgroup, nurse practitioners (NPs), which puts them more on a par with certain groups of physicians such as family doctors and pediatricians. In some states, NPs have independent prescribing power and can diagnose and treat patients without physician oversight (National Association of Nurse Practitioners, 2017). Recent studies show that NPs may provide care on a similar quality level as their physician counterparts (Stanik-Hutt et al., 2013). Over time, if a subgroup such as NPs can demonstrate equality in work performance in areas traditionally the purview of physicians, they will provide nursing with an opportunity to acquire new sources of power for themselves that allow them greater self-determination as an occupational group.

• • • IN PRACTICE: Artificial Intelligence and Physician Power

There is no potentially more profound development that may shift the balance of power and influence from physician to organization than the introduction of sophisticated artificial intelligence (AI) algorithms that can perform population health management, more accurately predict the onset of disease, and develop a deeper set of treatment options for certain patient conditions. IBM's Watson supercomputer is one example of the AI application in health care. As this supercomputer continues to absorb medical knowledge, and as it gains experience giving predictions or analyses, it begins to acquire a certain legitimacy that enables those using AI to wield greater influence within the system. Organizations and even managers then begin to be seen as sources for knowledge-based power that is relevant for helping the system run better. Patients may also see AI as more accurate than the individual physician, which can shift the power dynamic as well. Population health management, particularly in the area of chronic disease, may become an example of this power shift in action. If the use of AI can identify deeper patterns of morbidity and service use embedded in a group of diabetic patients, for example, and use that information to create treatment recommendations for those patients who are more robust, targeted, and likely to work, third-party payers will start to rely on machine learning assessments of care delivery more so than the individual primary care doctor. They may shift more of their payment systems toward rewarding the assessments made by AI algorithms. This will weaken doctor influence and increase the influence of the larger systems within which these doctors are embedded.

• • • IN PRACTICE: Patient Empowerment in the Internet Age

Some argue that the advent of the Internet and advanced forms of health information technology such as the electronic medical record (EMR) affords patients an opportunity to rebalance the power inequities in their relationship with physicians. There is no doubt that patients have become more consumer-oriented in their health care interactions. Anecdotes abound about the manner in which patients may now come to a physician's office armed with knowledge gained from their smartphone about symptoms and conditions they may think they have, and the ensuing confusion that can result from the physician trying to explain to the patient why the patient's self-diagnosis is inaccurate or incomplete. In a key sense, though, these anecdotes miss the main point: that the ability of patients to investigate and consume medical information prior to their interactions with the health care system inevitably creates a more proactive, inquisitive, engaged, and thus powerful health care consumer—a consumer that has to be more respected and addressed in a different, less paternalistic manner.

There are a variety of report cards, rating systems, and performance measures now available online for specific physicians, hospitals, insurance companies, and others doing the business of health care. If one requires cardiac surgery in New York State, for example, there is an easily accessed comparison of morbidity and mortality for all the cardiac surgery programs operating in New York State that helps in deciding which programs are of the highest quality. In turn, these report cards mean that cardiac surgery programs must openly compete on the basis of providing the highest quality outcome to patients, giving patients more power to help determine the direction such programs take in the way of clinical process improvements, resource investment, marketing, and customer relations.

Whether the types of patient empowerment created by the Internet and health information technology generally give patients more power in their interactions with health professionals or merely create the perception of additional power, the fact remains that much health care performance is now more transparent and available for consumers to use in comparison shopping. This "information marketplace" levels the playing field, if only in a small way, between health care consumers and producers, aiding in the transformation of an entire industry long built on "knowing what is best for the patient." However, as medical science grows increasingly complex, it may be far-fetched to presume that the availability of more information for consumers empowers as opposed to confuses them. This confusion, along with the information overload that accompanies a fully transparent health care delivery endeavor, may provide physicians and hospitals additional future opportunities to gain back any power loss from the consumer-oriented movement occurring in health care over the past decade.

The physician–administrator relationship is also one characterized by the acquisition and use of power. As noted in the "In Practice: The Pursuit of Power among Managers and Physicians" discussion, physicians and management tend to derive their power and influence from different sources, setting up an ongoing competition for power acquisition that may fester and go unnoticed for some time within the organization. In addition, the continued presence of dual hierarchies in places like hospitals creates tension between these groups because it legitimizes the claim to power for both groups simultaneously, while being less specific about where and when one group should have more authority than the other. Finally, physicians and administrators often have performance-related interests that differ, giving rise to sustained attempts by each to use power across a variety of situations to gain a specific preferred outcome.

For example, physicians may remain largely concerned with their individual patients, how they as clinicians or their immediate departments deliver care, and thus they maintain less concern about the overall performance of their peers or that of the organization as a whole. On the other hand, administrators (even physicians who become administrators) are hired directly by the organization to help ensure effective performance at a macro level, whether that is defined by work unit, department, function, or the entire organization. It is a manager's job not to overemphasize individual performance assessment but instead examine performance from an aggregate or group level. It should be noted that these different perspectives do not represent bad and good perspectives. Rather, the important point is that difference in responsibility itself sets up differences in how appropriate performance should be viewed, and this may lead to conflict and the use of power and negotiation in attempts to reconcile.

The modern-day quality movement in health care, payment reform, and the increased emphasis on high-cost, high-tech specialty care are recent examples of trends that have exacerbated power battles between physicians and administrators. For example, differing from a decade ago, these two groups now come into contact frequently in a health care system that seeks greater and more formalized performance variety, transparency, and measurement. This has led health plans, hospitals, and practices to build formal administrative systems, using managers to run them, that provide the resources and authority not only to evaluate how clinicians perform but also to make that information available for patients and the rest of the organization to view.

Related to changes in how health care quality is defined and measured is the shift in how health care services are reimbursed. Examples of this shift include elaborate pay-for-performance programs that provide financial incentives for clinicians to perform higher-quality care, standardized "bundles" of care delivery for specific conditions that require things done in the same manner all the time, and payment made on the basis of showing "value" in care delivery as defined by a complex mix of efficiency and quality metrics (Centers for Medicare and Medicaid Services, 2017). The shift from performance "as defined by the individual physician" to performance based on global, transparent standards has been profound. It may threaten physicians' source of power because it involves transferring knowledge traditionally controlled and disseminated by the medical profession to the health care organization as a whole, and also to patients. In addition, as payment systems are controlled more by health care insurers and government programs like Medicare, it is more these payers and less the providers who may acquire more legitimate sources of power within the health care sphere.

THE POLITICAL NATURE OF POWER

Power in organizations is often created, maintained, and transferred through a political process. **Organizational politics** has been defined as an ongoing process of "managing influence" (Mayes and Allen, 1977), in which different coalitions of interests or influence vie for the opportunity to achieve their desired goals. This process of managing influence often involves the use of nonlegitimate strategies and tactics, one of which is the exertion of power (Mayes and Allen, 1977). This definition is consistent with others that see politics as a process of using dynamics like power to gain desired ends (Eisenhart and Bourgeois, 1988). These definitions point to organizational politics as a key crucible in which power use is amplified and gains greater momentum. For example, the presence of a highly politicized work atmosphere both denotes and encourages the use of power, because it gives stakeholders greater freedom to assert their rights to control work, each other, and decisions.

The use of politics is characterized by its hidden nature; i.e., it involves strategies and tactics that are not transparent to everyone (Eisenhart and Bourgeois, 1988). This hidden nature also facilitates power use, especially in situations that are high stakes, are high risk, or involve activities not immediately sanctioned by the organization and its workers. An example of one of these situations is when a company in financial crisis decides it must lay off workers to help reverse its fortunes. While the layoff decision may be known at all levels of the organization, different departments and units will likely engage in a political process designed to minimize the layoff impact on their own workers. This process may include a department or unit making veiled or overt threats to management about the negative outcomes for the organization of the department or unit being included too heavily in the layoff decision, moving to get key decision makers to support their specific department or unit cause, and undermining the cases made by other departments or units to top management.

This process can be hidden from view and often involves only the most senior managers within each department and unit and top management. The process itself will likely involve a wide range of power demonstrations and attempts to control decision making. For instance, the nursing department in a hospital may threaten to walk off the job, especially if they are unionized, if too many layoffs are aimed at them, or they have concerns about proper staffing. Physicians may side with them and work on their behalf with administrators to address the issues, in part because a shortage of nurses might impact physician performance and potentially undermine their own sources of power with patients. Nurses may attempt to use their own power through a political process of trying to convince administration to impose fewer layoffs. Physician may also appeal directly to "one of their own," such as the hospital medical director or physician members on the board, and craft arguments geared to what they feel would resonate most with another physician.

To shift the example to another hospital unit, the QI department may allude to the breakdown in hospital functioning that would occur should too many of their workers be fired. That department may attempt to use its influence to demonstrate using quality data how the hospital would be impacted by too many layoffs or specific staffing ratios. Or, alternatively, the QI department might view reduction in nursing staff as an opportunity to gain greater influence throughout the hospital, by having access to the types of data needed to assess the relative care delivery impact of different staffing ratios. In this way, the QI department may end up helping or hurting the nurses' attempts to use their own influence to stop layoffs. The notion of organizations as negotiated orders or coalitions of different interests provides a rationale for why politics becomes a dominant mode of interaction for members. Seen in this way, conflict and struggles for influence are endemic, almost natural, in every organizational setting, in large part because it is acknowledged by everyone that melding different and often competing stakeholder interests into a single cohesive set of outcomes remains daunting. Through this lens, much organizational activity becomes preoccupied with two things: (1) determining whose interests and perspectives should rule in a given situation and (2) determining which specific organizational outcomes are preferred and how they should be attained.

Health care organizations are particularly political organizations. This is due mainly to the presence of several different, powerful stakeholder groups working alongside each other. For example, physicians, nurses, and administrators each have the ability to exert influence over their work settings, make key decisions, and gain control over resources. Much of the management imperative within health care settings revolves around trying to limit political activity that aims to exert power in dysfunctional ways—i.e., ways that benefit the group exerting power without clearly adding value for the organization as a whole. The use of politics can be inefficient for the organization in these situations, because it requires individuals and groups to expend valuable time and resources for self-interested ends, which often reduces the overall time and resources available to pursue collective ends related to productivity and quality (Pfeffer, 1981).

On the positive side, politics plays a critical role in organizations by encouraging groups and individuals to share power and to ally with each other, if only temporarily, to achieve common goals or outcomes. This reality can be used by the organization to mount collective efforts aimed at mutually agreed-upon goals. For example, while physicians and nurses may spend a certain portion of their collective time in conflict with one another around different issues in the workplace, or become preoccupied with exerting influence in part to gain resources at the expense of the other group, they may come together and use their political power to help the organization fulfill its accreditation requirements or to address a quality deficiency that threatens the reputation of the organization and its workers. They may also, as noted above, unite to stop the organization from doing things not in their collective interests. In pursuing these imperatives, physicians and nurses in the same setting use similar informal tactics, share information and best practices, and advocate behind the scenes for similar changes. The political activity generated by two such powerful groups working in tandem may be quite influential.

Generally, the political process creates a fluid power structure within organizations, making it more difficult to predict at a given moment which parts of the organization may exert their influence and whether or not they will be successful. The fluid nature of power within an especially political environment makes it somewhat risky for organizational leaders to attempt to manage the use and acquisition of power. Add to this the dependence of both power and politics on the type of work environment in which they are embedded, and the ability to harness political activity and the power it encapsulates remains one of the foremost management challenges in modern organization.

How Power Stratifies: Personal and Contextual Influences

Power is never equally distributed within or across organizations. **Power stratification** means that different stakeholders may have unique opportunities to access power based upon their particular characteristics or circumstances. One key source of power stratification, particularly with respect to structural sources of power, derives from the demographic qualities of stakeholder groups.

For example, historically, males have been afforded greater chances to assume top management roles in a variety of organizations compared to their female colleagues (Ragins, 1993). In U.S. medicine, the most powerful, highest-paying specialties such as surgery have long been dominated by male physicians, despite an increasing number of female physicians over the past two decades. Much academic medicine in the United States also remains populated disproportionately with male physicians, giving this demographic group inordinate power to control the educational and socialization agenda for medical students and young physicians (Hoff and Scott, 2017).

Age is another key demographic source of power stratification in health care. For example, professions such as medicine and nursing are built upon the apprenticeship model of training, where experience is the basis for seniority. In this way, individuals who have the most work experience, almost always older practitioners, retain greater influence and authority among their peers. They set the rules for professional behavior as well as impose their preferred cultural meaning systems onto the group as a whole, with sanctions applied for those choosing to deviate from their norms. Residency and fellowship programs that form the basis of professional training in health care implicitly favor age as a determining factor for which professionals deserve the access to greater power and control within their profession.

Employment status also serves as a source of power stratification in health care. For instance, salaried physicians, who work directly for their medical practices or for a health maintenance organization, generally have less individual and collective power than physicians who own their own practices. In the former situation, the physicians rely on the organization to pay them a salary, structure their workloads, and set policies that they must follow. In the latter case, the physicians may negotiate preferred rates of reimbursement with insurers and hospitals, can better self-manage their work and hours, and choose the types of patients and services they offer.

Depending on the size and type of organization in which an individual works in health care, different power opportunities may also be afforded. Being an executive in a large insurance plan that controls a majority of the market share in a geographic area provides numerous opportunities to acquire and exert power with physician practices, hospitals, and employer groups—all of whom may depend on the insurance plan heavily for the success of their business. In the same way, physicians in a particular specialty may come together within a geographic area to form a single practice organization that dominates care in that market. They may do this in part to get better payment terms for their services or to control how they deliver care. This trend has been seen increasingly in the United States, with specialists such as orthopedists, cardiologists, and urologists, among others, splitting their practices off from academic medical centers to form "super-practices" that contain significant numbers of the available specialty physicians in that geographical area.

Finally, controlling financial resources stratifies organizational power. Within any organization, the "power of the purse" means that those individuals maintaining control over the distribution of resources have additional power opportunities than individuals who do not have this control. This is being seen now in the move to "value-based" reimbursement systems that allow health insurers to tie payment more to outcomes, leaving doctors often in a reactive state (Hoff, 2017). These insurers can force providers to have to report more quality information, control costs better, and adhere to standard care guidelines—in large part because they control disbursement of the financial resources physicians need to run their businesses. Traditionally, and within the organization, departmental units such as finance and accounting retain a great deal of power within the organization because they are sanctioned to review or approve the decisions made by other units in areas such as purchasing, capital acquisition, and hiring. Very often, struggles for power within the organizational setting revolve at least in part around one group's desire for greater fiscal independence or authority over others.

THE ABUSE OF POWER IN HEALTH CARE ORGANIZATIONS

Rather than viewing power as inherently negative, it is important for managers to view the use of power as at times necessary for their organization in helping to achieve its goals in an efficient manner. Managers should, however, balance this functional view of power with a more critical perspective that views the use of power as potentially abusive to the organization's employees and external stakeholders (Hardy and Clegg, 1996). Unfortunately, there are an increasing number of examples of power abuse evident in American business and health care. **Power abuse** refers to situations where one or more organizational stakeholders use power in ways that are not generally acceptable, often involve self-interest rather than the organization's best interests, and can inflict negative outcomes on workers, customers, and supporters of the organization.

Power abuses occur within organizations for two main reasons. One reason is the advancement of personal ends at the expense of the customer, shareholder, or employee. Examples of power abuses used to pursue personal ends could involve chief executives creating boards of directors consisting solely of friends or business partners, executives directing staff to misrepresent financial and performance data to outside stakeholders, and executives using unauthorized company funds or resources to enhance personal wealth. All these examples have recently been seen in both health care and other industries.

Power can also be abused to advance organizational ends. This form of power abuse is not easy to discern, nor do all groups within the organization necessarily agree that abusing power to achieve organizational ends in a given situation has negative consequences. In fact, such abuse may be sanctioned by numerous stakeholders both within and external to the organization. Examples of power abuses by managers that are used to pursue organizational ends could include laying off employees to send positive signals to board members or shareholders, without attending to the fundamental organizational problems or bad management decisions causing poor performance, and manipulating performance measurements for the sole purpose of misrepresenting the organization vis-à-vis other competitors in the marketplace. In this vein, potential power abuses can also be tied to company founder attempts to push a certain image of their organization in the marketplace or motivate the workforce in particular ways thought to be necessary for ensuring company success. Recent news stories on companies such as Amazon and Uber demonstrate this dynamic (Isaac, 2017; Kantor and Streitfeld, 2015).

Regardless of the ends pursued, the abuse of power by managers or leaders elevates the potential for negative fallout to occur in the organization. Perhaps most important is the crisis of trust that can occur when managers or executives abuse power. This trust crisis is expressed in two primary ways: (1) loss of faith by customers and external stakeholders (e.g., regulators, shareholders, funders) in the organization (see the case of Uber for an example of this) and (2) loss of faith by employees in management. Both crises continue to be prevalent in light of corporate scandals in health care and other industries, as well as in the U.S. financial industry crisis that helped to produce a severe economic recession a decade ago.

Loss of faith by customers and other external stakeholders can meaningfully affect organizational performance and survival, in the form of lost business for the organization, reduced financial capital, stricter regulatory scrutiny, and the development of a negative reputation that allows other competitors to gain a long-term edge over the organization (Fukuyama, 1995; Sitkin and Stickel, 1996).

Loss of trust by employees toward managers when power is abused reduces the potential for positive dynamics within the organization to enhance performance. Examples of positive dynamics negatively affected by power abuse include teamwork, cooperative behavior,

communication quality, citizenship behavior, and job satisfaction (Axelrod, 1984; Blau, 1964; Hoff, 2003; Whitener et al., 1998). Other negative fallout that may occur includes increased organizational complacency, decreased work effort or "shirking" on the part of employees, slower organizational adaptation to change, high turnover, and decreased quality of services or products (Burawoy, 1979; Kantor and Streitfeld, 2015). While not a certainty, the abuse of power can seriously impact organizational performance, lead to lost business, and, in some cases, facilitate collapse in the form of bankruptcy or dissolution. Examples of these outcomes are found in recent American corporate history, including Enron, Bear Stearns, Countrywide, and Tyco.

Several conditions facilitate the abuse of power within organizations. These include high uncertainty regarding how to achieve goals or desired output; an overly centralized decision-making structure; the scarcity of rival coalitions both internal and external to the organization, a lack of reliance by key organizational stakeholders on each other; an existing culture of organizational complacency; and existing pressure to make quick decisions within the organization (Brass, Burkhardt, and Marlene, 1993; Crozier, 1964; Mintzberg, 1983; Perrow, 1989; Weber, 1978). Ironically, many of the conditions that create the potential for power abuse derive in large part from the same general conditions that give rise to power use. This highlights the paradoxical nature of power within organizations, in that the factors that allow power to grow and be used effectively are also those that, when manipulated in certain ways or taken to extremes, provide fertile conditions for power abuse. Given this reality, a key managerial task is to institutionalize a structural framework and culture within the organization that limits the probability that power use conditions are manipulated.

For example, the ability to create dependencies in relationships on the basis of resources like knowledge or funding is a potential source of organizational power within organizations. However, too much of an imbalance in terms of the extent to which a dependency relationship favors one group over another creates the potential for power abuse (Brass, Burkhardt, and Marlene, 1993). This situation is exacerbated when the resources in question are scarce, essential, and nonsubstitutable.

Control over information through structural advantages such as network centrality is another legitimate source of organizational power that, when taken to extremes, often results in power abuse. As discussed, individuals or groups who position themselves at the center of communication and information networks within the organization are in a position to exercise power. Information is a resource that allows individuals to set decision-making premises within the organization and control uncertainty (Crozier, 1964; Perrow, 1989). However, to the extent that managers or others within the organization gain exclusive control over information—i.e., to the extent that specific individuals or groups can create gaps or ambiguities in understanding within the organization that only they can fill—a foundation for power abuse is created.

The building of coalitions and alliances is a source of organizational power. However, an organizational environment in which there is a single dominant coalition or alliance provides a foundation for power abuse. Any leader-centered coalition that does not adhere to a diversity of viewpoints and perspectives can create an autocratic situation in which the leader's will and preferences become those of the larger group (Mintzberg, 1983). This leads to negative outcomes such as groupthink. The absence of rival coalitions within the organization creates a situation for power abuse, mainly by lessening the capacity for creative tension and ideas to compete with each other on the basis of their informational, logical, and strategic merits. This decreased capacity encourages the dominant coalition to introduce mechanisms by which to minimize deviation from the preferred status quo (Salancik and Pfeffer, 1977). This may hurt the organization in terms of performance and ability to adapt to changing demands in the environment.

The Role of Trust, Fairness, and Transparency in Preventing Power Abuse

Managers can take several steps to guard against the abuse of power within their organizations. These steps include structuring communication networks to create greater transparency in terms of organizational decision making, implementation, and evaluation; using boards of directors and advisory groups as counterbalances to managerial authority; creating a strong code of ethics within the organization; designing appropriate appraisal systems; and emphasizing personal integrity in the hiring function (Alford, 2001; Hoff, 2003; Thibodeaux and Powell, 1985; Westheafer, 2000).

• • • IN PRACTICE: Abusing Power at the Top Levels of the Organization

There have been instances in business and health care over the years in which top managers, a chief executive officer (CEO), a company founder, or a board of directors have abused their power through the creation and maintenance of a single dominant coalition within the organization that controls decisions and discourages dissenting viewpoints. For example, if a CEO desires to have more influence over the organization, she or he may create a board of directors that consists of close friends, business partners, or individuals who share a similar strategic viewpoint. In the extreme, these types of boards become "rubber stamps" that may fail to carry out their fiduciary responsibility as counterbalances to executive control within the organization. They also reduce the quality of strategic decision making because they abdicate their role of critiquing management decisions. In the final analysis, this allows executives to make decisions that potentially benefit their own ends at the expense of customer, employee, or shareholder interests.

Imagine a CEO of a hospital who helps place on its board of directors a banker with whom the CEO used to work, a lawyer who frequents the same country club to which the CEO belongs, the head of a local construction company that has helped perform work on the hospital, and an old college friend who still goes on fishing trips with the CEO and is one of the top cardiologists in the community. The prior and existing relationships between the CEO and these individuals, forged through other work and personal circumstances, may taint the ability of the group as a whole to generate the creative tension and independent thought needed for developing hospital strategy and evaluating the CEO's decision making. For instance, one or more of the board members, because they trust the CEO from other walks of life, may come to rely on the CEO's "version of the world" and align their thinking with the CEO's, leading to unquestioning support for the CEO's actions and take on the world. By owing the CEO for their seats on the board, some directors may be remiss to challenge or disagree with the CEO. Other directors may perceive that if they help the CEO "get his way," there is the possibility of additional rewards for themselves. Still others may simply like the CEO, be friends with him, and so be less likely to contradict his desires or decisions.

Having directors who know the CEO from prior walks of life, or who feel indebted to a CEO for their position, increases the chances that the CEO may abuse his own power, especially if he wishes to make certain decisions or impose a particular strategic decision on the organization. Friendship is important in life, but in the case of a CEO and his board, it may foster a singular alliance of interests at the very top of an organization that crowds out alternative viewpoints and critical debate, producing a leadership group that becomes insular, self-interested, and disconnected from true organizational realities. It is these attributes that can then facilitate power abuse within the group.

Creating transparency involves making the sharing of information a "public good" within organizations. This means, for example, allowing access to performance data at all levels of the organization so that everyone from line employees to the chief executive appreciates the logic by which specific decisions are made. In establishing greater internal transparency, managers end up becoming more accessible to employees. This enhances trust within the organization, and while it does not preclude the use of power as a necessary dynamic, it is likely to identify instances of abuse in a timely manner. External transparency also limits power abuse. Providing key constituents such as shareholders, regulators, and customers with complete, accurate, and timely performance data prevents executives and boards of directors from making decisions that are not rooted in strategic logic but instead derive more from the manipulation of circumstances on the part of individuals or groups in the organization.

Many recent corporate scandals that involved managerial abuse of power could have been prevented through the use of independent oversight mechanisms in the form of boards of directors and external auditors. Many boards are laden with members who are connected to the organization in some manner that makes them reluctant to enact their oversight role (see the "In Practice: Abusing Power at the Top Levels of the Organization" example). Such characteristics make boards less useful for controlling power abuse in organizations. Organizations that staff boards of directors with individuals who have the time to fulfill the oversight role, and who have no personal stake involved in the results of that oversight, place themselves in the best position to allow the use, but not abuse, of power by managers.

Creating a strong code of ethics and institutionalizing it into the organization's culture also limits power abuse (Hatcher, 2002). Recent examples of power abuses within organizations have been found to result in part from the presence of work environments that tolerated and even promoted unethical (not necessarily illegal) behavior in relation to the use of power. Establishing a code of ethics gives managers and employees formal guidance as to how to act across different situations where power may be exercised. This limits individual discretion in using power. It also conveys a sense that there are risks or potential sanctions to using power in an abusive way (Thibodeaux and Powell, 1985). Key to the success of a code of ethics is the overt dedication of top management to it.

Designing performance appraisal and hiring systems that emphasize and reward ethical behavior also limit the potential for power abuse within organizations. For example, power abuse by managers toward employees through the use of formal position in the hierarchy is minimized when appraisal systems exist that judge employee performance across a range of objective performance dimensions. Considering personal values and ethical behavior as important factors in the hiring and evaluation of managers

and employees heightens the probability that the organizational workforce consists of individuals who are less likely to take advantage of any power at their disposal. Over time, it creates an organizational culture in which a negative view toward power abuse becomes a shared norm.

POWER AS A KEY SOURCE OF CONFLICT

The use of power within organizational settings, along with the political activity that helps manifest it, can give rise to conflict. Conflict associated with power and politics derives from two primary organizational circumstances. First, conflict can occur when two or more parties have different perspectives, ideas, or agendas; they intend to move them forward in the organization; and each party is willing to behave in ways that require some form of resolution to avert a suboptimal or dysfunctional organizational outcome. Conflict in organizations can also arise when two or more interdependent parties draw upon different sources for their power or have unequal access to power opportunities in the organization. This second circumstance is most endemic to health care settings, where different groups have their work highly coordinated and must rely meaningfully upon each other to deliver services to patients. In these instances—high mutual dependence among two or more parties that have different power sources—the key conflict-generating dynamic involves parties trying to figure out who (and therefore also which power source) is more influential or controlling in a given situation.

One such instance of this second source of conflict occurs when there is a specific organizational goal that the interdependent parties are expected to pursue jointly. For example, physicians and nurses working in a hospital may be asked to help reduce the incidence of medical errors occurring to patients during their hospital stays. To accomplish this goal, each group may want the same resource—more staff positions, technology, or decision-making autonomy—and the conflict becomes centered on each group attempting to claim that resource for themselves. This is the type of conflict we generally think about.

However, conflict often occurs at a second, deeper level in this circumstance. This conflict involves disagreements about which power source to rely upon in order to solve the first-level conflict of who should claim the desired resources. When multiple sources of power exist in an organization, ideas for how to resolve conflict are not necessarily shared by all parties. For instance, those who possess a knowledge advantage might think knowledge-based power is most relevant, while those who are in supervisory or high-level positions and who have structurally derived power might think relying on administrative mechanisms like formal policies is most appropriate (Ashforth and Johnson, 2001).

A related issue is the choice of which conflict management technique to use in a given situation. For example, in the physician–nurse relationship or the physician–patient relationship, the physician has culturally derived power from his or her advanced standing in the medical profession. That power gives the physician authority over the nurse or the patient. When conflict arises between the physician and nurse or the physician and patient, that physician has to decide whether or not to employ the use of power. The physician may draw on that culturally derived power to say "I'm the physician, you are the nurse or patient, and I know better" as an influence attempt, or the physician can take a different approach that relies less on formal power use and more on less coercive means of influence. Effective conflict management is based on appreciating the sources of power for each party involved and knowing how and when a particular power source could be used.

DEBATE TIME

For those who possess some level of professional or organizational power, it can be difficult to know when and how to use that power in situations that might benefit the organization's customers. As the chapter notes, not all power use is bad. In fact, the use of power is necessary and productive in situations where the customer stands to benefit in the form of a higher-quality or more efficient service provided to them. Often, the carefully planned use of power can help overcome organizational inertia regarding the best decision to implement, move needed change forward, resolve infighting between internal stakeholders that may hold up appropriate decision making, and produce key decisions quickly in situations where time is of the essence. However, knowing the precise moment and manner in which to begin using one's power, regardless of the reason for it, is a challenging task for any health care manager or professional.

When would you use power within an organization? Several considerations should likely guide your decision making. First, consider the type of outcome toward which your use of power would contribute. Is it ethical? Does it benefit the organization as a whole? Would it help produce an outcome that improves the efficiency or quality of services provided, or directly benefit the customer in some meaningful way? Can it be done in a manner that does not undermine other important organizational goals or objectives? The answers to these types of questions are critical for establishing the prerequisite rationale for using power, a rationale that, at some point, others in the organization or external stakeholders may need to hear. Once these questions have been answered, the second consideration is to assess the type of actions required for using power and how disruptive or potentially detrimental such actions might be for the rest of the organization. For example, using power in a strictly covert, highly political manner that masks its true nature as a control or influence mechanism may not be appropriate, regardless of the type of outcome such a use of power is aiming to achieve. In short, this step requires understanding the right ways to exercise one's power. What should be the level of transparency in using power? Should everyone know that the use of power is guiding organizational action in the given situation? Are certain actions "out of bounds" with respect to how power will be used?

A third consideration involves assessing the potential unintended negative consequences the use of power might cause within an organization. Such consequences may result even if power use is determined to be necessary and the actions taken to use power are appropriate. These types of unintended consequences are important. They may include workforce effects like decreased job satisfaction, productivity, morale, and turnover; organizational outcomes like decreased profitability or client dissatisfaction; increased short-term conflict between different organizational stakeholders or constituencies; and cultural shifts within the organization that might undermine worker or management cohesiveness. Predicting which types of negative consequences might occur is not easy. However, it is imperative to at least discuss openly the probability that some of these could happen and what could be done to limit the damage done to the organization.

Finally, the use of power, even in an appropriate, required circumstance should be short-lived. Clear consideration must be given to the time frame within which power use will occur, when it is no longer appropriate to use power in a given situation, and agreement on the boundaries within which power will be used and when it will no longer be used, regardless of whether or not all the desired outcomes are achieved. This consideration is important precisely because the use of power takes a toll on the organization, and on the individuals within it, especially the longer its use occurs. Therefore, this dynamic must be used sparingly, strategically, and with careful attention paid to whether or not it is working effectively.

With these things in mind, power may be exercised by individuals and groups within organizations as well as by organizations themselves. This notion moves us beyond the idea that all power is bad, that its use is immoral, and that the organization never benefits from its employment as a tactical device to achieve particular outcomes. That said, it remains a higher-risk, more unpredictable approach to managing and must always be assessed within that regard.

The **study of conflict management** concerns how parties approach, deal with, and resolve conflict and which personal, social, and environmental factors affect that process. The focus here is on one conflict management tool—negotiation—which is presented as a direct way to resolve conflict. Other strategies to resolve conflict could include avoidance, whereby one or more parties refuse to deal with the conflict, or accommodation, where one party simply concedes to the other(s). While avoidance may work in a situation where emotions are high and time is needed to prepare for negotiation, and accommodation may work in a situation where the outcome is not of great importance, negotiation is a viable process when there is a vested interest in the outcome and when each party wishes to manage the situation as effectively as possible for themselves and their interests.

TYPES OF CONFLICT

There are generally thought to be two types of conflict that occur in groups: conflict related to ideas concerning the task at hand and conflict related to social factors in the team (Jehn, 1997). The first type of conflict, known as **task conflict**, reflects differences between parties in understanding and carrying out tasks. This type of conflict, while detrimental to overall performance or decision making in the team or group, is seen to be the "better" type of conflict in that it is less personal and somewhat easier to accommodate. Task conflict on its own can result in better decision making in a health care situation. For example, a doctor and a nurse may have differing opinions on a course of treatment due to their different interactions with the patient—in an attempt to resolve this conflict, they may discover that each has unique expertise that should come to bear in making the treatment decision.

Interdependent parties struggle in terms of both performance and satisfaction when **relationship conflict**, or conflict regarding some inherent characteristic of the other party, is present. The causes of relationship conflict can be related to interpersonal styles, personality, political preference, or other difference beyond the task at hand (De Dreu and Weingart, 2003). Relationship conflict is particularly difficult to deal with because judgments are being made about the characteristics of someone else—e.g., "I don't like them" or "I can't work with them." Even when there is a shared understanding regarding how to solve the task, those groups experiencing conflict rooted in the relationship itself possess heightened negative emotions and perceive a dislike of the other party.

If the conflict is primarily task-based, the challenge is in understanding the viewpoints and perspectives of all of those at the table. If the conflict is more relationship-based, the challenge is how to navigate around the heightened emotions and perceptions in the group, which can interfere with the mutual pursuit of a negotiated outcome. Task conflict can also lead to relationship conflict. For example, if we acknowledge that two different parties can have two different sources of power, such as with a physician and an administrator, the knowledge-based power possessed by the physician might create task conflict with the administrator, who has control over resources. In this case, each thinks they know the best way to solve the conflict, which represents conflict over the task at hand. However, if they fail to see the conflict from the other side's point of view, that task conflict can escalate into relationship conflict. Once this happens, not only do they hold different views regarding how to solve the task, but they now also may be judging each other's values and character, which can lessen mutual trust and respect. This lack of trust means they do not have a solid relational base from which to work, which makes the resolution of conflict more difficult.

The Negative Side of Emotions

The threat rigidity effect states that when individuals feel threatened, their thinking becomes rigid or inflexible (Staw, Sandelands, and Dutton, 1981). When conflict results in an individual feeling like his or her resources are threatened, or that his or her ego is threatened, threat rigidity results. These heightened emotions produce a decreased ability to cognitively process information, ideas, and possible solutions. The brain goes into "protection" mode instead of "exploration" mode, and consequently the negotiators become preoccupied with protecting their own viewpoint rather than trying to come to a creative solution with others. Threat also need not be actually experienced, as even the expectation of threat can impact individuals. Carnevale and Probst (1998) found that when participants expected a hostile situation with high conflict, they showed less cognitive flexibility and creative thinking than if expecting a collaborative situation.

Not only do heightened emotions shut down cognitive processing, but emotions can be socially contagious (Barsade, 2002). The process of **emotional contagion** occurs when emotions are transmitted from one party to another. If one individual becomes angry, others can "catch" that anger, and a negative spiral ensues where they then transfer that anger to others. Individuals experiencing conflict who travel through this negative emotional spiral may find themselves with very few options that would result in a positive negotiated resolution to the conflict at hand. This is why individuals experiencing conflict in general, and relationship conflict in particular, need to be acutely aware of the emotional state of the group.

• • • IN PRACTICE: A Negative Emotional Spiral in Hospital Human Resources

In the following example of Mary and her boss Ryan, we can see emotional contagion in action. Mary, an HR benefits administrator in the hospital, has been experiencing a bit of frustration with her career progress. While she started out in patient advocacy and later moved into advocacy training, her current job has taken her away from patient contact completely. She feels that her boss, Ryan, has taken advantage of her willingness to work "any task" and forced her away from her passion. Ryan, as her boss, has been quite pleased with Mary's performance and counts her among his top performers. She is conscientious with all assigned tasks and seems willing to do whatever he asks. This is precisely why he approached her about moving into a benefits position.

Mary has just had lunch with a colleague who was asking about her career, a conversation in which Mary "realizes" that she is not happy about her position. Without thinking through the conflict, she is placing the blame largely on Ryan and has decided to approach Ryan about this conflict:

Mary (already upset): "Ryan, I'd like to talk with you right now about my position."

Ryan: "Sure, Mary, what's the problem?"

Mary: "Why have you put me into this dead-end job?"

Ryan: "What are you talking about? You are one of my best performers!"

Mary: "You know exactly what I'm talking about—no one else wanted to do benefits and you knew that I wouldn't say no to you."

Ryan: "If you think accusing me of something is going to get you what you want, you are sorely mistaken. I've done nothing but try to help you."

Mary: "I want out of this job and a move back to patient advocacy. If I don't get that, I'm moving to another hospital."

Ryan: "If that's your attitude, then my answer is no."

In this case, the negative emotions that Mary harbors when resolving this conflict has not only clouded her ability to negotiate effectively, but they have transferred to Ryan. Her anger has become contagious in this discussion. The effect of this is that Ryan, who may have been happy to calmly discuss Mary's issues, is now unwilling to work with Mary. We can detect this here by noticing that they do not talk about Mary's passion—having direct patient contact. If this were discussed, it is possible that Ryan would agree to try to get her back to what she loves, especially considering she is a high performer. Good negotiators realize that the actions and emotions they portray will be mimicked or reciprocated by the other party.

NEGOTIATION AS A CONFLICT MANAGEMENT TOOL

Individuals are faced with conflict on a day-to-day basis, and they need a language for how to resolve those conflicts with the people with which they are interdependent. This is where negotiation comes in. Negotiation is not a skill to be reserved for special occasions like major purchases or career transitions, although it is helpful in those situations. Negotiation knowledge represents understanding that can help us in any aspect of managing conflict with coworkers, supervisors, clients, patients, kids, spouses, parents, you name it. Think about all the current or potential conflict in your life— each of those situations can be resolved from the perspective of negotiation.

One can think of negotiation potential as the degree to which a conflict might be resolved effectively through negotiation. Negotiation is effective when one gets more or loses less than they would have if they did not negotiate - and getting more of what one wants is always the objective when negotiating. The formal definition of negotiation is "a process of potentially opportunistic interaction by which two or more parties, with some apparent conflict, seek to do better through jointly decided action than they could otherwise" (Lax and Sebenius, 1986). If we simplify this definition, we can say that the basic conditions where negotiation might be possible are the following:

- There is more than one person (two or more parties).
- The people or parties want, or seem to want, different things (apparent conflict).
- The people or parties have to deal with each other in order to get what they want (joint action).

As seen in the negotiation between Mary and Ryan ("In Practice: A Negative Emotional Spiral in Hospital Human Resources"), there are actually a wide variety of situations that fit these criteria, many that we typically don't see as "negotiation." Mary is not "buying from" or "selling to" Ryan. These are just two individuals who have conflict and, more importantly, have a vested interest in resolving that conflict while also maintaining their relationship. Thus, when we think about situations that have negotiation potential we need to include any situation that involves multiple parties, apparent conflict, and joint action or interdependence.

COMMON MISTAKES IN MANAGING CONFLICT VIA NEGOTIATION

Perhaps the most significant error negotiators make when approaching conflict, and one easily seen with Mary in the "In Practice: A Negative Emotional Spiral in Hospital Human Resources" example, is failing to plan or think through the conflict before attempting to deal with it. Failing to plan is more likely to result in a haphazard approach to negotiation marked by an over-reliance on techniques most familiar to the negotiator, while planning beforehand is more likely to result in a methodical and well-thought-out approach marked by negotiation tactics more effective in resolving the conflict. An effective plan for each party to a negotiation will include a description of one's own interests or underlying needs, possible positions or offers that can satisfy those interests, goals regarding specific positions for the negotiation, and possible tactics to use in reaching the goals. If there is uncertainty regarding the interests and positions of the other party, a plan should also include a listing of questions to ask, as questions will help gain understanding about the interests and positions of the other side.

Interests, rather than positions, help a negotiator focus on what is most important, opening up possibilities for creative problem solving through the consideration of multiple positions (see Thompson, 2005). Goals are critical as they increase motivation on the part of the negotiator (Locke and Latham, 1990). When negotiators have clear goals, they are influenced to keep working toward reaching those goals, which can increase persistence and effort toward conflict resolution. Finally, planning before dealing with the conflict will give each party multiple options for how to resolve the conflict. This will help the negotiators avoid coming to an impasse or failure to reach agreement.

A negotiation plan includes a description of the logistics of the negotiation. Where will the negotiation take place? For how long? Who will be at the table? Who are the influential stakeholders not present at the table? What are the issues to be discussed? The logistics are important for various reasons. First, there must be

enough time to resolve the conflict without a sense of urgency, as a sense of urgency usually results in parties using compromise—or splitting the difference—as a strategy, which is not ideal. Second, the environment can facilitate information sharing if all parties are comfortable and relaxed. Even the ambient level of noise is important, as a quiet environment will decrease the likelihood of miscommunication. Third, as much information as possible about the parties and issues should be known beforehand so that each negotiator knows what to expect. Finally, meeting in one's own office instead of another's conveys power and comfort. Meeting at a location and time convenient to another may be seen as a gesture of good faith.

When negotiators fail to plan, they can fall victim to **functional fixedness**, which occurs when a negotiator bases his or her strategy on familiar, rather than the most effective, methods (Adamson and Taylor, 1954). For example, imagine that a particular physician has had a long, contentious relationship with one hospital administrator. Every time they have to negotiate or solve a problem, the interaction becomes emotional, and each party behaves aggressively toward the other side. Needless to say, this creates tension for them and for those around them, and it results in less-than-effective negotiated agreements—neither side is ever happy. Now imagine that the administrator is replaced by someone new. Given his or her past experiences, that physician immediately begins to rely on those same contentious behaviors with the new administrator—he or she is fixated on those types of behaviors as being the way to negotiate with all administrators. Thus, even though the new administrator may be willing to negotiate in a different way, the physician never uncovers that possibility because he or she reverts to those familiar tactics. A negotiation plan, in this case, could help the physician realize that he or she knows very little about the new administrator and should rely on asking probing questions and building a rapport with him or her before any competitive behaviors are even considered.

Another hindrance to effective negotiation is the inevitability of cognitive biases, the mental shortcuts we use automatically in daily life. Cognitive biases impede effective information gathering and synthesis—abilities central to negotiating the most effective outcomes. Each party must seek to understand not only what his or her interests are but also the interests of the other parties involved in the negotiation. One bias particularly relevant to negotiators is the **confirming evidence bias**, which is the tendency for people to seek out and pay attention only to information that confirms prior beliefs (Eagly and Chaiken, 1993). The confirming evidence bias shuts down the learning process as individuals are no longer attending to information that could potentially help them work through multiple possible offers.

Consider a job negotiation, this time focusing on a hiring manager who has "fallen in love" with an applicant based only on his or her resume. This preexisting belief will severely impair the ability of that manager to negotiate effectively with the hiring committee because he or she will pay more attention to information that confirms the preexisting belief and may ignore or under value information contradicting that belief. A negotiator who falls victim to the confirming evidence bias will not want to ask questions of the other side, will be hesitant to add issues, and will not pay attention to information suggesting the company is not satisfying their interests. While this may be a peaceful negotiation without much conflict, it raises the potential for the **winner's curse**, or the feeling of unhappiness after a negotiated outcome (e.g., "We should've hired someone else!").

One of the biggest errors made when approaching conflict management is assuming that anything won in the agreement costs the other side just as much—that is, the assumption there is a "fixed pie" in the negotiation. This is called the zero-sum assumption or the **fixed-pie bias**. The fixed-pie bias is the tendency to believe that the benefits to one side are equal to the costs paid by the other side—and when combined they always sum to zero. This bias makes the negotiation a battle for the biggest share of that pie, which in turn makes negotiation harder to resolve and likely to limit the value people get. In reality, some of the best tactics to solve conflict problems involve expanding the pie, which refers to efforts by one or more parties in the negotiation to add value to what is being negotiated. If an employee wants to telework one day a week and wants to negotiate only about telework with the manager, the negotiation could very well be zero-sum. One side wins, one side loses. However, the manager (or employee) could *add value* to the negotiation by adding the issue of new responsibilities for the employee. Essentially, the manager gets what is most important to her—the employee

taking on more responsibility—and the employee gets what is most important to him—getting to telework one day a week. By expanding the pie, these negotiators have overcome the fixed-pie bias and have found a solution via collaborating that works for both sides.

Many negotiators, especially when negotiating early in their careers or negotiating without much experience, tend to focus primarily on their own needs. Negotiators focused primarily on their own needs are self-serving, which in the context of negotiation is self-defeating. This is because negotiation requires the *other person to say yes*. If negotiators neglect this basic tenet of negotiation, they remain overly focused on their own positions and interests, creating an environment in which it is difficult to resolve conflict. They ignore the power of **reciprocity**, which is the tendency for others to exchange equal levels of goods and services (Cialdini, 2001). Reciprocity is powerful in situations of uncertainty, as negotiators are looking for cues regarding how to behave toward the other party. If one side gives a small concession, gives up some information, or behaves competitively, usually the other side will do the same (Weingart et al., 2007). Through reciprocity, the parties in the negotiation can build trust with one another. Thus, it is a mistake in negotiation is when one side ignores the needs of the other party and yet wants something in return. It is this behavior that is often reciprocated—the result being two self-focused individuals who will reach impasse.

Finally, failing to identify reasons to trust the other party is another mistake that can severely hamper effective conflict resolution. Deepak Malhotra and colleagues have investigated the importance of trust towards another party in reaching beneficial negotiated outcomes (Malhotra, 2004; Weber, Malhotra, and Murnighan, 2005). This is an important topic as most negotiators find it very hard to trust others, even when they know there is no good reason

• • • IN PRACTICE: ER Nurse Contract Negotiation and Planning to Negotiate

Joanne is a nurse who just moved to Springfield with her husband and is going in to negotiate her job at County General Hospital. This hospital happens to be her number-one choice due to the departmental opening (the emergency room) and proximity to her new house. She will be negotiating with Chandra, who is in charge of hiring nurses.

Chandra: "Joanne, we are really excited to have you on board at County General, I think you'll be a great addition to the ER department."

Joanne: "Thank you so much."

Chandra: "I know salary conversations can be touchy, and I definitely want to be fair to you as well as to the hospital. So I thought maybe we could start by discussing what you were making at your last job. That will give us a baseline from which to work."

Joanne: "But I want to make more than I was at my last job."

Chandra: "Well, I'd like to pay you fairly based on your experience and thought that your prior salary would be a piece of information we could use to figure out the right number."

• • • IN PRACTICE: ER Nurse Contract Negotiation and Planning to Negotiate
(Continued)

Joanne: "I'm not comfortable with that."

Chandra: "Why not? I thought you were excited about joining us? Do you think I'm trying to take advantage of you?"

Joanne has made both the mistake of failing to plan and the mistake of failing to trust. She has no reason to distrust Chandra and yet is unwilling to give up any information. She reciprocates with denial, instead of either giving the information or reframing the discussion. An alternative would be if the final part of the scenario had gone like this:

Chandra: ". . . That will give us a baseline from which to work."

Joanne: "I appreciate that you would like to know that information and I will provide it, but I was hoping we could focus our discussion around my skills and experience in comparison with the other nurses here as a way to figure out my salary. I've actually done quite a bit of thinking and research on this and would like to share that information with you. Is that okay?"

Chandra: "Absolutely."

Joanne: "I'd also like to discuss the shifts I might be working as well as my vacation. Those items are also very important to me as I have a toddler at home."

Chandra: "Of course. We actually have quite a bit of flexibility on hours as there are two open positions and you are the first offer we've made."

Joanne: "Excellent, let's start there . . ."

By talking about her interests instead of getting defensive with Chandra, she preserves the relationship and provides a solid base for not only discussing salary but also discussing any issue. This negotiation has gone from potentially emotional and contentious to being a comfortable problem-solving environment.

to believe the other side will take advantage of them. Negotiators often protect information and are hesitant to give even the smallest of concessions, because they worry that the other side will use the information against them and that it will be seen by the other as a sign of weakness. What these negotiators fail to realize is that the act of withholding information communicates to the other party that there is no trust between them. This then creates a **self-fulfilling prophecy**, which describes the process by which one party's beliefs cause another party to behave in such a way that supports that belief (Merton, 1968). What Bazerman and Gillespie (1999) found was that partial trust in others—or giving some information—was the worst strategy a negotiator could take. The reason is that while full trust induces positive reciprocal behaviors, and no trust protects information and other resources, partial trust sacrifices resources without invoking reciprocity.

NEGOTIATION STRATEGIES AND TACTICS

When a conflict arises that is important enough to the parties involved to address it, they engage in strategies to solve the conflict. Each of these strategies is marked

by a different approach to **value in negotiation**, defined as the combined benefits among all the parties in the negotiated agreement. The three most common strategies when individuals engage another party and seek resolution (i.e., not avoid the situation) are **compromising, competing, and collaborating** (Pruitt and Rubin, 1986).

Compromising: A negotiation strategy where the parties in the negotiation divide value and find a solution that partially satisfies everyone. This is often a "split-the-difference" solution to a problem whereby no one wins but also no one loses.

Example: *I'm going to struggle to cover my Thursday shift this week. If I take the first four hours, can you take the second four hours?*

The main benefit of taking a compromising approach is that it is timely and efficient. If a manager knows that half of his staff want the department meeting at 8:00 a.m. and half would like it at 8:30 a.m., a compromise solution would suggest that the meeting be held at 8:15 a.m. There is little need to try to find a different solution. In cases, then, where the importance of the outcome is of low or modest importance to the parties negotiating, compromise is an effective strategy. The danger with compromise solutions is that negotiators often compromise when they should not—when the importance of the problem is high and they are unable to figure out any other way to solve the problem. The downside to compromising in this situation is that this strategy *prevents* the creation of creative alternatives, which could lead to a more beneficial outcome for all parties.

Competing: A negotiation strategy where one party tries to get as much value for themselves as possible with little, if any, concern for the other party.
    Example: *I'm going to struggle to cover my Thursday shift this week. You should cover my shift for me because I have two little kids at home who are sick and am in a really tough rotation right now.*

A competitive strategy is beneficial when either (1) there is no concern for a lasting relationship with the other party or (2) there is reason not to trust the other party. In this case, the physician, rather than trying to collaborate with the other party, is trying to change the perspective of the other side—to get them to say yes without giving up very much or anything. We call this claiming value because they are trying to capture as many of the benefits contained in the agreement for themselves.

Collaborating: A negotiation strategy where parties try to help each other get what they want and in the process maximize the value created in the negotiation.
    Example: *I'm going to struggle to cover my Thursday shift this week. I know you need consecutive days off to go visit your parents—if I cover your shift next week, when you need the days off, can you cover my shift this week?*

Collaboration should be used when there is high concern for both the other party and high concern for the outcome of the negotiation. When adopting a collaborative strategy, negotiators are focused not only on pursuing self-interest but also on the needs of the other side. This is why this perspective is so powerful—by showing concern for the other party, negotiators can invoke reciprocity. This force of reciprocity leads the other party to show concern as well, opening up not just dialogue but also previously uncovered possible solutions to the problem. The negotiators become teammates rather than *adversaries*. The most important benefit of collaboration is that, in contrast to instinct, if a collaborative approach is chosen, the parties involved end up with much, much more value in the end. In general, this is the most effective negotiation strategy, especially in the context of lasting relationships (Fisher and Ury, 1983).

Tactics to Acquire More Information

There are three main categories of tactics negotiators can use for pursuing various goals: tactics to acquire more information, tactics to find a better solution, and tactics

to influence the other party. The first category focuses on doing research and asking questions both before and during the negotiation. The second category focuses on creating value in negotiation through creative problem solving. The third category, which also tends to be the one most thought of in the context of negotiation, involves changing the perspective of the other side.

Do Research

Gathering information before negotiation allows an individual to manage power when resolving conflict. While research can come in several forms, the most influential research that can be done to prepare for negotiation is gathering objective data, as objective data facilitate using knowledge-based sources of power to influence. Examples of objective data gathering when negotiating the compensation for a job in health care could be the following: (1) what others in your specialty or subspecialty are making, (2) what others in your city or region are making, (3) what others with your experience are making, (4) what others who graduated from your medical or nursing school or who have your same graduate degree are making, (5) what others in your new (or old) hospital, private practice, or company are making, (6) what certifications, degrees, or experience you have relative to what these others are making, and (7) what the cost of living is in your area compared to what you were making in your previous location. These are all objective sources of data because they are based on fact (rather than opinion) and are not easily refuted. This data can be researched either online, through personal networks, or through print publications.

Ask Questions

Asking questions of the other side is a specific way to uncover information in a negotiation. As negotiators often go into negotiations with little if any knowledge about what the other side's interests are, asking questions can help accomplish this part of the research-gathering process. Besides acquiring information, asking questions also communicates to the other party that there is concern for their interests. This invokes reciprocity, which, as described previously, is the tendency for individuals to treat others like they are being treated. However, not all questions are created equally. While some questions are designed to acquire information (e.g., "What are your interests?"), other questions can be insulting (e.g., "Why are you acting this way?"), imply threats (e.g., "Are you sure you want to take that position?"), or simply be poorly worded (e.g., "Would you be willing to share your underlying needs because right now I can't figure out what you are talking about?"). Questions likely to lead to the most relevant information are nonthreatening and are perceived by the other side as conveying genuine interest.

• • • IN PRACTICE: Nursing Union Negotiation

Many nurses are unionized, and nurses' unions regularly have to negotiate new contracts with their employers, such as hospitals and health care systems. In recent years, two of the more important collective bargaining issues for nurses and their employers have been economic issues like pensions and work-related issues like staffing levels. These issues can often get contentious. For example, nurses' unions may take the position that they are most interested in good patient care and therefore want a required ratio of patients to nurses at all times, while employers like hospitals may advocate for head nurses to be able to set staffing levels depending on patient need at the time, for quality and financial reasons. Regarding the pension issue, employers may seek to decrease or limit the pension contribution in order to make the system more "economically feasible." Both sides may posture by stating that they want the other side to come back to the table and begin negotiating "in good faith."

The difficulty in union negotiations, as highlighted in this brief summary, is that it tends to be largely position-based and not interest-based. This makes both sides entrenched in their positions and inhibits any potential for a creative solution. In instances like these, the union may take a public position on staffing that states that they want "a required ratio," while the hospital may take a public position on staffing that states that they want a system where "the head nurse dictates."

One reason for this type of stance in union negotiations is that those who are negotiating might have different interests than those whom they represent. The negotiators, in addition to satisfying their constituents, want to "look good." So what often happens is that they make public statements reflecting positions (e.g., "I want a required ratio") to fire up and garner support from their members. But we know that in negotiations, using positions is ultimately defeating—when both sides use positions (what they want) rather than interests (why they want it) to negotiate, there will ultimately be one winner and one loser—or worse, two losers, depending on how things play out.

So what happens? Because positions have been stated publicly, to give in would be to lose face in the negotiation, which is not something that the negotiators on either side wish to do. This is the hallmark of a competitive strategy, with neither side willing to budge. Of course, the potential to create value is largely destroyed, as the sides are not willing to communicate, much less work with each other. The endgame, then, is determined by power. If the company feels that it has more power, it will let the workers (in this case, nurses) strike until the workers cannot financially maintain the strike. If the workers feel they have more power, they will threaten to strike and hope the company gives in. However, what often happens is that you have two groups who, because they are mired in conflict, each become convinced that they have more power to determine the outcome and, in the process, each fails to see how they can reach out to the other side and bring them back to the table in such a way as would allow them to save face. This produces a longer negotiation process, and one that may not make either side satisfied in the end.

Find Common Ground

One of the main goals when asking questions is to get the other side to be honest about their interests. This is part of a larger tactic called "finding common ground," which is any behavior that helps multiple parties find shared goals or interests. While this could be accomplished through asking questions, it can also be accomplished through sharing similar experiences or talking about what the parties have in common, which has the effect of making negotiations go more smoothly and amicably (Fisher and Ury, 1983). While common ground could reflect mutual interests in the negotiation (e.g., the employer and employee both want the employee to start on the same day), common ground can also reflect common pastimes (e.g., we both like playing golf), common background (e.g., we both graduated from the same university), or common goals for the negotiation (e.g., we both want the process to be fair). When negotiators find common ground with each other,

they are more likely to share information with each other (Cramton, 2001).

Tactics to Find a Better Solution
Add Issues

Adding issues—items to be negotiated—is one of the simplest tactics negotiators have at their disposal and means exactly what it says—adding issues to the negotiating table. For example, in a job negotiation, if an applicant inquires of his or her new manager about possibly having a new laptop as a part of the job package in addition to salary, they are adding the issue of having a laptop to the discussion to the focal or central issue of salary. When issues are added, both sides gain the opportunity to state whether or not that issue is important to them, which facilitates logrolling, described later. It also may help find common ground as discussed above. Adding issues might also create value in the negotiation.

Let's assume that in the above example the laptop (the added issue) is worth $1,500 in value to the individual as that is what it would cost him or her to go out and buy one. Let's further assume that that the company bought the laptop for $1,200 (due to a bulk discount), and that because the manager splits technology acquisitions evenly with the information technology (IT) department, it is worth only $600 off the manager's bottom line. So when the issue of the laptop is added, it is +$1,500 for the individual and –$600 for the manager = $900 of value has been created in the negotiation.

Nonspecific Compensation

Nonspecific compensation is a negotiation tactic that involves adding issues that are not tied to money or compensation. These issues are important to consider as individuals care about more in the world than just money. For a billing specialist, getting the chance to telecommute one day a week (nonspecific compensation) might be more important than getting a 3 percent raise.

Fractioning Issues

Fractioning is a negotiation tactic that involves separating out the various components of a specific issue. While we use the tactic of adding issues to refer to situations where completely different issues are added to the table, the fractioning of issues refers to situations where current issues are split into component parts to find better solutions. For instance, in the job negotiation example, "compensation" is typically thought of as salary. However, compensation can be fractioned into the component issues of starting salary and bonus (obvious) but also tuition reimbursement and when the employee will get their next raise (less obvious). All four of these directly impact the amount of money the new employee will take home in his or her paycheck. As with adding issues, fractioning issues help to identify additional issues for discussion, and it facilitates logrolling.

Logrolling

Logrolling is a negotiation tactic that involves trading off on issues that are of different value to each party. This involves four steps. The first step is to "add issues to the table." The second step is to negotiate these issues at the same time. The third step is to realize that each party prefers one issue more than another. The fourth step is to negotiate a tradeoff, where each party receives his or her preferred position on a specific issue. In order to understand logrolling, we can take, for example, a negotiation between a manager and employee over an upcoming mundane financial reporting task assignment. A nonlogrolling solution would be the manager telling the employee to take on the assignment, which would effectively end the conflict. A logrolling solution would be that they would first talk about future task assignments in addition to this pending task assignment (Steps 1 and 2). The employee may state that their most important interest is to work more on compliance issues instead of financial reporting, while the manager states that their most important interest is getting this financial reporting task done (Step 3). Manager and employee then agree that the employee will complete this task as soon as possible, which satisfies the manager's interest, but that the manager will try to assign to the employee only compliance tasks in the future, satisfying the employee's interest (Step 4).

Making a Packaged Offer

This tactic involves making an offer with multiple issues. While logrolling is always making a packaged offer, a packaged offer does not necessarily involve logrolling. The value of making a packaged offer and thus keeping all issues on the table tentative until agreement is that it gives all negotiators a chance to see where the possibilities lie for adding further issues, fractioning issues, and logrolling issues. This helps negotiators avoid impasses, keeping everything tentative, allowing the parties to go back and try different combinations of alternatives on the various issues. This is in contrast to an issue-by-issue negotiation, where issues are dropped from discussion as soon as agreement is reached. This issue-by-issue approach lends itself to compromising on each issue.

Contingent Contracts

This tactic involves negotiators making a "bet" on the future in order to resolve a potentially difficult issue facing them in the current negotiation (Bazerman and Gillespie, 1999). That is, what one side gives to the other side is contingent on some future event. A classic example of this involves hospital department revenue. Let's say the ER department and the hospital cannot agree on the appropriate resource level for the department. The department wants to be able to hire five new personnel, and the hospital wants to allocate only enough funds to hire three. At the heart of this debate is the discrepancy in the beliefs about the number of patients who are going to be serviced by the ER department in the future, especially given that another community-based emergency care facility is about to downsize, increasing demand for the hospital ER in question. Of course, neither side knows for sure what that number is going to be—the ER department believes that it will have 63,000 patient discharges the following year (with 20,000 in the next three months) while the hospital thinks this number will be closer to 50,000 (with 15,000 in the next three months).

To resolve this conflict, the hospital might commit to hiring two personnel right away and then allocate future resources **contingent** on how many patients actually show up in the following three months. If the number of patients has been fewer than 15,000, no additional personnel are hired; if the number of patients is greater than 20,000, three additional personnel are hired; and if the number is in between, they can hire personnel on a sliding scale. The reason contingent contracts help negotiators find better solutions is that if 20,000 patients show up, the hospital is more amenable to hiring the additional personnel, and if the patients do not show up, the department probably did not really need the extra resources. Contingent contracts, in the heat of the negotiation, allow negotiators to believe that their interests will be satisfied in the future, helping to resolve potential impasses (e.g., endless arguing about how many patients the ER is going to service). This is why performance-based bonuses are so popular—if the individual achieves the benchmark (the contingency), the company is more amenable to paying the employee.

Tactics to Influence the Other Party

A Strong Opening Offer

Many negotiations have central or key issues that must be discussed in detail and which take a central role in the negotiation (e.g., salary in a job negotiation). Whether or not to make an opening offer on one of these central issues involves a two-part process of deciding whether to open and what the opening offer should be. If the negotiator has objective data on what the opening offer should be, it has been shown that there is in fact a benefit from making a strong opening offer (Galinsky, 2004). The reason a strong opening offer is beneficial in negotiations is because of the **anchoring bias**. Anchoring is a psychological effect whereby one piece of information—an initial offer in negotiation—tends to influence subsequent thinking. As with any cognitive bias, this is most influential when there is uncertainty in the thinking of one party. The anchor becomes a key piece of information that frames the negotiation and influences how much one party thinks they can get or what the other party is willing to give (Tversky and Kahneman, 1974). If there is no good information or a solid objective justification for the opening offer, it is best not to make one, as an uninformed opening offer has a chance of being either too low, thereby shortchanging themselves, or too high, angering the individual on the other side.

Using Objective Criteria

From the Merriam-Webster dictionary, "objective" is defined as "involving or deriving from sense perception or experience with actual objects, conditions, or phenomena" (2009). Notice the word "actual" in the definition—using objective criteria means using *actual* data when presenting arguments. Actual data could be facts, figures, and statistics, anything that is defendable

with nonbiased information. This is in contrast to subjective arguments, which reside only within one person's mind and are based on one's perceptions. Objective arguments are more effective than subjective arguments because they are rooted in logic, not perception, and are therefore more difficult to refute. Here are some examples:

Subjective: This task is really tough.

Subjective: My work is better than hers.

Subjective: But I'm worth more than that.

Objective: We have the lowest patient cost of any department in the hospital.

Objective: I have been able to clear 90 percent of the accounts due at the practice in the last three weeks.

Objective: I saw 73 patients last week, which is a 20 percent increase over the same week last year.

Forming a Coalition

Coalitions represent a limited-term alliance among individuals or groups that is formed in order to strengthen the power of each party and further their respective interests. The power of coalitions was discussed previously in this chapter in reference to using power in situations of mutual interest, in order to manage organizational politics. Coalitions work when parties, who have compatible interests, align themselves in order to negotiate with another party. They can present a unified front against the authority and are much more likely to influence that party because they will have increased their power. For example, when negotiating individually, each member of the staff of a physician practice may have very little power with respect to the physician in charge. However, if particular staff band together to negotiate the hours of the practice, they immediately have much more power and are able to influence the physician. In a more severe situation, those staff members could enact their power by refusing to work in order to get the concession they desire.

Using BATNA/Power of Walk-Away

BATNA stands for "Best Alternative to a Negotiated Agreement." The BATNA represents one's best option remaining if the current negotiation fails and an agreement cannot be reached. The strength of one's BATNA is an indicator of the power they have in the negotiation. If a doctor is negotiating with a health system for extra resources and office space in order to expand, his or her power in that negotiation is tied to whether or not there is *another* health system willing to provide such resources—the offer from the other health system is the BATNA. BATNAS work in two ways. First, having a strong BATNA gives negotiators confidence to pursue possible collaborative agreements without fear of "losing the deal"—they know they have somewhere else to go. Second, having a strong BATNA, if revealed, communicates to the other side that a better offer exists and that the person using the BATNA can walk-away. Part of the planning process is to evaluate one's BATNA and the likely BATNA of the other side; this can give an indication of the likely power dynamic between the negotiating parties.

CONCLUSION

The major themes of this chapter are the following: (1) power is an endemic force within organizations that can be managed but also abused, (2) politics is a means by which power is manifested, (3) conflict management through negotiation is one way to sort out power and conflict within organizations, and (4) negotiation is both a formal and informal process that has specific steps that can be learned and mastered. A major point is that all three dynamics—power, politics, and conflict—require taking an active role in understanding context, relationships, and the specific issues at hand. This puts the manager squarely in the center of ensuring that existing power dynamics in the organization are used for beneficial and collective outcomes. It also places responsibility on managers and leaders of organizations to identify where power can and will be used inappropriately and where the use of organizational politics may mask that inappropriate use.

Power and politics often create conflict within organizations, and that is an unavoidable fact that should not be ignored but rather addressed through the art and science of conflict management. By learning and mastering the activities associated with effective negotiation, individuals in organizations become empowered to resolve conflict in productive, organizationally beneficial ways. As repositories for a wide array of interactions and relationships, the organization is a breeding ground for the cultivation and use of power and politics. It is in recognition of this reality that we view these two dynamics as within the normal purview of a well-functioning organization, through a strategic approach that emphasizes proactive conflict management tools and techniques.

SUMMARY AND MANAGERIAL GUIDELINES

1. Understand where power comes from in health care organizations. It is important when attempting to understand or manage the use of power to know its particular sources. This not only helps to understand better the nature of how individuals or groups assert their power in the workplace but also provides information by which to consider targeted management strategies to offset and limit dysfunctional power use.

2. Creating new structural sources for power is perhaps the most efficient way to change the existing power distribution within the organization. In particular, establishing new resource dependencies for different stakeholders can quickly shift who has greater influence over decision making. In situations where there is a high potential for power abuse from a single stakeholder source, making that source suddenly more dependent on others in the organization for their status or resources that help them function can be an effective way to prevent the abuse from occurring.

3. Individual sources of power, particularly power deriving from expertise or knowledge, are common in the health care industry given the levels of uncertainty and variability in care delivery. This gives clinicians especially an advantage in securing and using power within health care organizations.

4. Always identify and assess organizational situations in which it appears that one or more parties are attempting to exert control over another party in a given situation. By studying different control attempts occurring within a setting, you can gain a better sense of who is attempting to exert their power and influence. This enables quicker development of effective strategies to manage the use of that power.

5. All power is relational. So to truly understand power, one must know the different types of relationships that define the organization and, more importantly, how these relationships manifest themselves. This involves observing the relationships as they play out under normal everyday circumstances.

6. Try to view and manage organizations as places filled with shifting coalitions of individuals and groups that come together or oppose each other based on the current issues at hand, or issues particularly important to one or more of them. This view makes the management job a highly daunting political challenge in the sense of trying to maintain order among the different interests. But it provides a realistic perspective that can help managers understand the barriers to change as well as how to cultivate issue-specific coalitions to move issues of importance to the organization forward in productive ways.

7. Never assume everyone is the same in terms of power just because they are in the same occupation. Not all physicians or nurses, for example, have equal access to power development and use. Some physicians and nurses have greater influence than others, and knowing how power stratifies within such occupations provides a more accurate read of work situations where both power and politics may be at work.

8. Power abuse can be avoided proactively by pursuing principles such as transparency, fairness, and trust within organizations. These principles can be translated into specific types of actions and value systems that all employees can learn about, buy into, and use to help create an ethical organizational climate, and one in which the abuse of power remains something rarer and less destructive for the organization as a whole.

9. Do not assume that just because you have a lot of experience negotiating, you are an expert negotiator. Most individuals have a hindsight bias whereby they evaluate past outcomes more favorably than they actually were. Realize that there are multiple ways to solve conflict—not just in the manner or fashion to which you are accustomed.

10. Resist the urge to use authority just because you have it. In the context of conflict management, resist using formal sources of power and a competitive strategy, which may not be the best option or lead to the most effective solution. This is especially problematic for first-time managers.

11. Think about implementation when you are working on an agreement. In other words, how is this agreement going to affect you one week, one month, and one year down the road in your relationship with the other party? If you know that there is no way you or others are going to work to carry out the agreement, solve that problem before you leave the table.

12. If you reach an impasse, take a break and reevaluate. Emotionally laden negotiations can not only hinder creative thinking and problem solving, but they can also damage relationships and hurt your confidence in future negotiations. Be thinking about this as you approach the impasse and ask the other side if it is okay to take a break and think things over.

13. Get advice from others when solving conflict. Usually when one is involved in a conflict, it is difficult to view that situation objectively from all sides. This is because we are biased creatures—we automatically think that we are right, simply because we have a position that we are trying to achieve. Having a third party, whether it is a mentor or friend outside the negotiation or a mediator in the negotiation, can help you work through the negotiation process and come up with creative solutions.

14. Remember that you have to give the other side enough in the negotiation for them to say "yes" to the deal, because getting them to say "yes" will ultimately get you what you want. When you focus only on your interests and possible positions to satisfy those interests, you ignore the interests of the other side, which may inhibit your ability to get them to agree.

DISCUSSION QUESTIONS

1. How can managers best use the principles of effective negotiation and conflict management to resolve power struggles within health care settings? What types of power struggles in health care settings do you believe are most amenable to using negotiation and conflict management techniques?

2. What are specific ways to limit the potential for power abuse in health care organizations? What specific human resource strategies and transparency mechanisms could be created within hospitals or physician practices, for example, that would help prevent any stakeholder, particularly the top leaders of an organization, from pursuing self-interested goals in suspect ways?

3. What would be the situations in which a collaborative or a competitive strategy might be most beneficial when managing conflict in health care organizations? What issues unique to health care organizations would be particularly difficult to negotiate using each of these strategic approaches?

4. In thinking about the power relationships unique to health care organizations (e.g., physician–patient), what might be some of the challenges to effective negotiation? Think about these challenges in the context of the common mistakes made when thinking about conflict and when managing relationships.

CASE

To Open or Not to Open—That Is the Question

James had eight years experience in health care human resources and wanted to move up into an administrative position. So he decided to go back to school part time for three more years and get a master of business administration (MBA) degree. As James was approaching the completion of his MBA, his boss, Jayne, knew that he was looking for a new position with a new salary. Before they sat down to talk, neither of them knew exactly what the new salary should be. James was making $63,000 currently and Jayne had no idea what James could make on the open market—three percent more, five percent more, ten percent more? She wants to be fair, but she also needs to keep her budget under control. James decided to use this uncertainty to his advantage, so he did research and decided to make a strong opening offer.

James: "Jayne, I really appreciate you meeting with me."

Jayne: "No problem. I'm really proud of you finishing your MBA. Congratulations!"

James: "Thank you. I of course do not want there to be any tension between us, so in anticipation for our meeting, I've tried to do quite a bit of research on what a fair salary increase would be. Is it okay if I present you with this information?"

Jayne: "Sure."

James: "Okay, so the first thing I did was look at the average starting salaries for everyone graduating from my MBA program. This is based on 330 graduates over the last three years and the number was $91,000. Of course not all of those are based in health care, so the next thing I did was look at those in health care with 10–15 years experience and an advanced degree. It's not easy to get this information, but from three people in this company and three others I know, the salaries ranged from $75,000 to $97,000 with an average of $88,000. Finally, I looked at the last person in my position to get an advanced degree, and she received a 20 percent raise, which for me would be $12,600 and take me to $75,600. So in averaging $75,600, $88,000, and $91,000, I came up with about $85,000. I was hoping we could start the discussion around there."

Jayne: "That's really impressive research and I respect that. We probably can't go that high but let me see what I can do."

The impetus is now on Jayne to negotiate James off his number, which is $85,000. This creates a much different negotiation than if Jayne opened with a 5 percent raise, which would have anchored the negotiation around $66,000. The impact is that the $85,000, along with the justification, changes the way Jayne is thinking about the negotiation. She might realize that they need to go to $80,000 to keep James now, whereas perhaps before the negotiation, she might have had $75,000 in her mind as the high number.

Questions

1. Where do you think this negotiation will end up?
2. What would you have done if you were James?
3. When dealing with conflict, do you think about how to begin?
4. What are other types of opening "offers" that have nothing to do with money but that still set the tone for the negotiation?
5. How can you use various types of openings to your advantage?

REFERENCES

Adamson, R. E., & Taylor, D. W. (1954). Functional fixedness as related to elapsed time and to set. *Journal of Experimental Psychology, 47*(2), 122–126.

Alford, C. F. (2001). *Broken lives and organizational power.* Ithaca, NY: Cornell University Press.

Armstrong, K. A., Rose, A., Peters N., et al. (2006). Distrust of the health care system and self-reported health in the United States. *Journal of General Internal Medicine, 21*(4), 292–297.

Ashforth, B. E., & Johnson, S. A. (2001). Which hat to wear? The relative salience of multiple identities in organizational contexts. In M. A. Hogg & D. J. Terry (Eds.), *Social identity processes in organizational contexts* (pp. 31–48). Philadelphia, PA: Psychology Press.

Axelrod, R. (1984). *The evolution of cooperation.* New York: Basic Books.

Barsade, S. G. (2002). The ripple effect: Emotional contagion and its influence on group behavior. *Administrative Science Quarterly, 47,* 644–675.

Bazerman, M. H., & Gillespie, J. J. (1999). Betting on the future: The virtues of contingent contracts. *Harvard Business Review, 77*, 155–160.

Blau, P. M. (1964). *Exchange and power in social life.* New York: John Wiley.

Brass, D. J., Burkhardt, M. E., & Marlene, E. (1993). Potential power and power use: An investigation of structure and behavior. *Academy of Management Journal, 36*(3), 441–471.

Burawoy, M. (1979). *Manufacturing consent.* Chicago, IL: University of Chicago Press.

Carnevale, P. J., & Probst, T. M. (1998). Social values and social conflict in creative problem solving and categorization. *Journal of Personality and Social Psychology, 74*, 1300–1309.

Centers for Medicare and Medicaid Services. (2017). MACRA. Retrieved October 10, 2017, from https://www.cms.gov/Medicare/Quality-Initiatives-Patient-Assessment-Instruments/Value-Based-Programs/MACRA-MIPS-and-APMs/MACRA-MIPS-and-APMs.html.

Cialdini, R. B. (2001). The science of persuasion. *Scientific American, 284*(2), 143–148.

Cramton, C. D. (2001). The mutual knowledge problem and its consequences for dispersed collaboration. *Organization Science, 12*, 346–371.

Crozier, M. (1964). *The bureaucratic phenomenon.* Chicago, IL: University of Chicago Press.

Dahl, R. A. (1957). The concept of power. *Behavioral Science, 2*, 201–215.

De Dreu, C. K. W., & Weingart, L. R. (2003). Task versus relationship conflict, team performance, and team member satisfaction: A meta-analysis. *Journal of Applied Psychology, 88*, 741–749.

Eagly, A. H., & Chaiken, S. (1993). *The psychology of attitudes.* Orlando, FL: Harcourt Brace Jovanovich.

Eisenhart, K. M., & Bourgeois, L. J. (1988). Politics of strategic decision making in high-velocity environments: Toward a midrange theory. *Academy of Management Journal, 31*(4), 737–770.

Finkelstein, S. (1992). Power in top management teams: Dimensions, measurement, and validation. *Academy of Management Journal, 35*(3), 505–538.

Fisher, R., & Ury, W. L. (1983). *Getting to yes: Negotiating agreement without giving in.* New York: Penguin Books.

Freidson, E. 1970. *Profession of medicine.* Chicago, IL: University of Chicago Press.

French, J., & Raven, B. (1959). The bases of social power. In D. Cartwright (Ed.), *Studies in social power* (pp. 150–167). Ann Arbor, MI: Institute for Social Research.

Fukuyama, F. (1995). Trust: The social virtues and the creation of prosperity. New York: Free Press.

Galinsky, A. D. (2004). Should you make your first offer? *Negotiation Journal, 7*, 1–4.

Gerstner, L. (2002). *Who says elephants can't dance?* New York: HarperBusiness.

Hardy, C., & Clegg, S. R. (1996). Some dare call it power. In S. Clegg, C. Hardy, & W. Nord (Eds.), *Handbook of organizational studies* (pp. 622–640). Thousand Oaks, CA: Sage Publications.

Hart, P., & Saunders, C. (1997). Power and trust: Critical factors in the adoption and use of electronic data interchange. *Organization Science, 8*(1), 23–42.

Hatcher, T. (2002). Ethics and HRD: A new approach to leading responsible organizations. Cambridge, MA: Perseus Publishing.

Hickson, D. J., Hinings, C. R., Lee, C. A., et al. (1971). A strategic contingencies theory of intraorganizational power. *Administrative Science Quarterly, 16*(2), 216–229.

Hoff, T. J. (2003). *The power of frontline workers in transforming government: The Upstate New York Veterans Healthcare Network.* Washington, DC: IBM Endowment for the Business of Government.

Hoff, T. J. (2017). *Next in line: Lowered care expectations in the age of retail- and value-based health.* New York: Oxford University Press.

Hoff, T. J., & Scott, S. (2017). The gendered realities and talent management imperatives of women physicians. *Health Care Management Review, 41*(3), 189–199.

Ibarra, H., & Andrews, S. B. (1993). Power, social influence, and sense making: Effects of network centrality and proximity on employee perceptions. *Administrative Science Quarterly, 38*(2), 277–303.

Isaac, M. (2017). Inside Uber's aggressive, unrestrained workplace culture. *New York Times*, February 22. Retrieved October 7, 2017, from https://www.nytimes.com/2017/02/22/technology/uber-workplace-culture.html.

Jehn, K. (1997). Affective and cognitive conflict in work groups: Increasing performance through value-based intragroup conflict. In C. K. W. De Dreu & E. Van de Vliert (Eds.), *Using conflict in organizations* (pp. 87–100). London: Sage.

Kantor, J., & Streitfeld, D. (2015). Inside Amazon: Wrestling big ideas in a bruising workplace. *New York Times*, August 15. Retrieved October 9, 2017 from https://www.nytimes.com/2015/08/16/technology/inside-amazon-wrestling-big-ideas-in-a-bruising-workplace.html.

Lax, D. A., & Sebenius, J. K. (1986). *The manager as negotiator: Bargaining for cooperation and competitive gain.* New York: Free Press, 1986.

Locke, E. A., & Latham, G. P. (1990). *A theory of goal setting & task performance.* Englewood Cliffs, NJ: Prentice Hall.

Malhotra, D. (2004). Trust and reciprocity decisions: The differing perspectives of trustors and trusted parties. *Organizational Behavior and Human Decision Processes, 94*, 61–73.

Martin, J. (1992). *Cultures in organizations: Three perspectives.* New York: Oxford University Press.

Mayes, B. T., & Allen, R. W. (1977). Toward a definition of organizational politics. *Academy of Management Review, 2*(4), 672–678.

McEvily, B., Perrone, V., & Zaheer, A. (2003). Trust as an organizing principle. *Organization Science, 14*(1), 91–103.

Merton, R. K. (1968). *Social theory and social structure.* New York: Free Press.

Mintzberg, H. (1983). *Power in and around organizations.* Englewood Cliffs, NJ: Prentice Hall.

Mintzberg, H., Raisinghani, D., & Theoret, A. (1976). The structure of "unstructured" decision processes. *Administrative Science Quarterly, 21*(2), 246–275.

National Association of Nurse Practitioners. (2017). State practice environment. Retrieved October 2, 2018, from https://www.aanp.org/legislation-regulation/state-legislation/state-practice-environment.

"Objective." (2009). In *Merriam-Webster Online Dictionary*. Retrieved November 15, 2009, from http://www.merriam-webster.com/dictionary/objective.

Perrow, C. (1989). *Complex organizations: A critical essay*. New York: McGraw-Hill.

Pew Internet and American Life Project. (2002). *Counting on the Internet: Most find the information they seek, expect*. Washington, DC.

Pfeffer, J. (1981). *Power in organizations*. Boston, MA: Pitman Publishing.

Pfeffer, J., & Salancik, G. R. (1978). *The external control of organizations: A resource dependence perspective*. New York: Harper and Row.

Pruitt, D. G., & Rubin, J. Z. (1986). *Social conflict: Escalation, stalemate, and settlement*. New York: Random House.

Ragins, B. R. (1993). Gender gap in the executive suite: CEOs and female executives report on breaking the glass ceiling. *Academy of Management Executive, 12*(1), 28–42.

Salancik, G. R., & Pfeffer, J. (1977). Who gets power—and how they hold on to it: A strategic contingency model of power. *Organizational Dynamics, 5*(3), 3–21.

Schein, E. H. (1992). *Organizational culture and leadership*. San Francisco, CA: Jossey-Bass.

Sitkin, S. B., & Stickel, D. (1996). The road to hell: The dynamics of distrust in an era of quality. In R. M. Kramer & T. R. Tyler (Eds.), *Trust in organizations (pp. 195–215)*. Englewood Cliffs, NJ: Prentice Hall.

Slater, R. (1999). *Jack Welch and the GE way*. New York: McGraw-Hill.

Stanik-Hutt, J., Newhouse, R. P., White, K. M., et al. (2013). The quality and effectiveness of care provided by nurse practitioners. *Journal for Nurse Practitioners, 9*(8), 492–500.

Starr, P. (1982). *The social transformation of American medicine*. New York: Basic Books.

Staw, B. M., Sandelands, L. E., & Dutton, J. E. (1981). Threat-rigidity effects in organizational behavior: A multilevel analysis. *Administrative Science Quarterly, 26*, 501–524.

Thibodeaux, M. S., & Powell, J. D. (Spring, 1985). Exploitations: Ethical problems of organizational power. *SAM Advanced Management Journal, 50*(2), 42–44.

Thompson, L. L. (2005). *The mind and the heart of the negotiator* (3rd ed.). Upper Saddle River, NJ: Prentice Hall.

Tversky, A., & Kahneman, D. (1974). Judgment under uncertainty: Heuristics and biases. *Science, 185*, 1124–1131.

Wachter, R. M., & Shojana, K. G. (2004). *Internal bleeding*. New York: Rugged Land.

Weber, J. M., Malhotra, D., and Murnighan, J. K. (2005). Normal acts of irrational trust, motivated attributions, and the process of trust development. In B. M. Staw & R. M. Kramer (Eds.), *Research in organizational behavior* (Vol. 26, pp. 75–102). New York: Elsevier.

Weber, M. (1978). *Economy and society: An outline of interpretive sociology* (2 vols.) (G. Roth & C. Wittich, Eds.). Berkeley: University of California Press.

Weingart, L. R., Brett, J. M., Olekalns, M., et al. (2007). Conflicting social motives in negotiating groups. *Journal of Personality and Social Psychology, 93*, 994–1010.

Westheafer, C. (2000). Integrating perspectives within a framework: Taming the dark side. *Organizational Development Journal, 18*(3), 63–74.

Whitener, E. M., Brodt, S. E., Korsgaard, M. A., et al. (1998). Managers as initiators of trust: An exchange relationship framework for understanding managerial trustworthy behavior. *Academy of Management Review, 23*(3), 513–530.

Wilson, J. Q. (1989). *Bureaucracy: What government agencies do and why they do it*. New York: Basic Books.

Chapter 8

Complexity, Learning, and Innovation

Bryan J. Weiner, Christian D. Helfrich, and Ann Nguyen

CHAPTER OUTLINE

- Health Care Organizations as Complex Systems
- Complexity and Feedback: A Closer Look
- Organizational Learning
- Innovation and Learning
- Managing Complexity, Learning, and Innovation

LEARNING OBJECTIVES

After completing this chapter, the reader should be able to:

1. Identify the characteristics that make health care organizations complex systems
2. Describe the five disciplines that promote organizational learning
3. Explain why organizational learning often proves difficult in practice
4. Describe how new-to-the-world innovations develop
5. Identify common myths and misconceptions about innovation
6. Discuss strategies for promoting organizational learning and innovation

KEY TERMS

Adaptive Learning

Balancing Feedback Loops

Combinatorial Complexity

Complex Systems

Detail Complexity

Discovery

Double-Loop Learning

Dynamic Complexity

Emergence

Generative Learning

Innovation

Learning

Learning Organization

Mental Models

Organizational Learning

Personal Mastery

Policy Resistance

Reinforcing Feedback Loops

Shared Vision

Single-Loop Learning

Systems Thinking

Team Learning

Testing

• • • IN PRACTICE: Learning from Mistakes: Problems Created by an Access Initiative Turn into Solutions in a Patient-Centered Medical Home

In 2002, Group Health Cooperative launched an ambitious plan to improve access and efficiency in primary care. Group Health (now Kaiser Permanente Washington) is a mixed-model health maintenance organization (HMO) headquartered in Seattle, Washington, serving approximately a half million members in Washington State and northern Idaho. In the late 1990s, the HMO saw its enrollment decline by 16 percent while the proportion of insured citizens remained stable. Facing declining enrollment and revenues (Robert Wood Johnson Foundation, 2008), Group Health responded with the Access Initiative: five major categories of changes based on the Institute of Medicine's principles of patient-centered care, including Web-based secure messaging with providers, redesigning the primary-care teams, instituting a new productivity-based compensation system for physicians, and allowing members direct access to specialists. Group Health realized several of the expected benefits from its Access Initiative: (1) higher overall patient satisfaction; (2) higher patient satisfaction with specific dimensions of access, such as being able to see the doctor when needed and minimizing time spent scheduling an appointment (Ralston et al., 2009); and (3) improved efficiency, both in terms of relative value units per full-time equivalent employee (i.e., a measure of the complexity of care being delivered by the clinical staff) and in terms of per-patient, per-quarter costs (Conrad et al., 2008).

However, the Access Initiative also brought increases in provider workload and troubling decreases in provider satisfaction. Providers reported routinely serving 12- to 15-hour days and feeling acute emotional burnout. Related consequences included not keeping up with the medical literature and putting information into medical records that they deemed clinically unhelpful but administratively required (Tufano, Ralston, and Martin, 2008). Equally serious, Group Health observed declines in quality of care indicators and increases in patient utilization in "downstream" services, such as specialty care, emergency care, and inpatient days (Reid et al., 2009; Robert Wood Johnson Foundation, 2008).

Because of these unexpected, undesired outcomes (i.e., mistakes), Group Health launched a pilot program to elevate some of the ideals of primary care that the Access Initiative had subordinated in the pursuit of access and efficiency (Ralston et al., 2009). Most notably, the pilot program reversed two Access Initiative components: (1) it radically decreased the providers' panel sizes, and (2) it exempted providers from the performance-based pay incentives. The pilot also made changes in patient outreach (e.g., systematic follow-up after emergency room visits), point-of-care processes (e.g., pairing of a physician with a medical assistant), organizational structure (e.g., collocation of primary team members), and management process (e.g., daily team huddles). This involved a significant up-front investment by the HMO: increases of 15 percent in physician staffing, 17 percent in medical assistants, and 72 percent in clinical pharmacists. They also had to reassign 25 percent of the clinics' patients to new providers to accommodate the smaller panel sizes and increased visit length (Reid et al., 2009).

Results proved encouraging. Compared to control clinics (which were Access Initiative sites), the pilot clinic saw improvements on six out of seven patient satisfaction indicators, 10 percent of providers reporting high emotional burnout versus 30 percent in the control clinics, and improvements in quality-of-care indicators. Group Health also saw a decline in emergency department visits of sufficient size to recoup both the cost of staffing increases and the cost of an unexpected increase in specialty visits, so at the end of 12 months the pilot intervention had paid for itself.

The Commonwealth Fund (McCarthy, Mueller, and Tillmann, 2009) and others have touted this pilot program as a possible national model for a patient-centered medical home, but the story does not end here. The pilot program was, after all, only a pilot program. The rollout of the medical home concept in Group Health Cooperative's remaining 19 clinics is ongoing. Experience tells us that the medical home will bring some new problems—for example, the pilot program already observed an unexpected increase in specialty-care visits. The challenge facing Group Health is not to avoid mistakes in the future; it is to look for those new problems as opportunities to learn and further innovate.

CHAPTER PURPOSE

The experience of Group Health Cooperative with the Access Initiative, and their subsequent pilot of a patient-centered medical home (see "In Practice: Learning from Mistakes"), illustrates three major themes of this chapter: (1) health care organizations are complex systems that respond to stimuli in expected *and* unexpected ways, (2) organizational learning becomes essential to managing complex systems, and (3) mistakes *and* unexpected outcomes can serve as the basis for novelty and innovation—provided that learning from mistakes occurs.

For managers, one of the most perplexing features of health care organizations is that they frequently exhibit counterintuitive behavior. Health maintenance organizations (HMOs) begin requiring physicians to choose less expensive generic drugs, only to find that pharmaceutical costs rise rather than fall due to unintended changes in physicians' prescribing behavior. Hospitals implement quality management tools and practices that have been proven effective in manufacturing settings, only to find that quality of care worsens rather than improves. A physician group practice introduces electronic medical records and medical errors decrease, but only for a few months, after which they rise to levels even higher than before. A department manager introduces a flexible work schedule to improve job satisfaction and job retention, only to see morale plummet and turnover increase as nurses find themselves working longer hours with less predictability in assignments.

Social systems rarely behave the way we want them to, or even the way that we predict they will. Due to unanticipated consequences, yesterday's solutions become today's problems. Our efforts to introduce change provoke opposition by those who seek to maintain the status quo. We apply solutions that worked well before or work for others, only to find that they do not work again or do not work for us. So, we try harder, applying them with even greater fervor, but the problem only gets worse. Or the solution works but introduces such deleterious side effects that the cure seems worse than the disease.

To understand and mitigate such counterintuitive dynamics, health care leaders need to rethink their views of how organizations work and how they can be improved and changed. In this chapter, we introduce a perspective of health care organizations as complex systems whose future states are unpredictable. Moreover, we regard innovation and change not as rational, controllable processes, but instead as complex, uncertain, nonlinear sequences of events and activities, often driven by actors' perceptions that are necessarily limited and flawed. Bridging these perspectives and integrating them is the notion of the **learning organization**, where innovation and change (and for that matter, mistakes) are seen as routine and as inputs for further learning (deBurca, 2000; Garvin, Edmondson, and Gino, 2008; McGill and Slocum, 1993; Schilling et al., 2011; Senge, 2014). The chapter concludes with guidelines for managing complexity, learning, and innovation.

HEALTH CARE ORGANIZATIONS AS COMPLEX SYSTEMS

Management theories reflect the "governing ideas" of their time. At the turn of the last century, management theories embraced a mechanistic view of social systems inspired by Newtonian physics (see Chapter 1). In the 1960s and 1970s, management theories took an organic view of social systems, reflecting developments in biology, ecology, and evolutionary theory. Since the 1990s, new management ideas have appeared as scholars and practitioners absorb the new science of complexity emerging in meteorology, biology, physics, chemistry, and mathematics (Arndt and Bigelow, 2000; Begun, 1994; Boulton, Allen, and Bowman, 2015; Burnes, 2005; Lemak and Goodrick, 2003; McDaniel, Driebe, and Lanham, 2013; Mowles, 2011; Plsek and Greenhalgh, 2001; Senge, 2010; Stacey, 1995; Wheatley, 2006). According to this view, organizations are dynamic, nonlinear systems that operate "at the edge of chaos," constantly changing, never quite settling into a predictable pattern, yet displaying complex forms of order within boundary conditions.

What do weather systems, ant colonies, human economies, and health care organizations have in common? They are all **complex systems**: arrangements of interacting, interdependent parts that produce emergent behavior. That is, collective behavior that cannot be predicted based on the behavior of individual parts. It is important to remember that not all systems are complex systems. Complex systems exhibit three defining characteristics. First, complex systems are richly interconnected (Miller et al., 2010). System elements are connected in many different ways, and these connections vary in levels of responsiveness. Some connections respond rapidly and strongly, some slowly and weakly, and some moderately in terms of timeliness and intensity. Management theories have long recognized that organizations are comprised of numerous, diverse, interdependent parts. Complexity theory suggests that organizations are more than simply open systems; they are "massively entangled" systems (Begun, Zimmerman, and Dooley, 2003; Holland, 2014).

Second, complex systems are nonlinear (Byrne and Callaghan, 2013; Sturmberg, Martin, and Katerndahl, 2014). In *linear* systems, output is directly proportional to its input, where small causes have small effects and big causes have big effects. By contrast, in *nonlinear* systems, output is not always directly proportional to its input. Small changes can produce big effects, small effects, or no effects at all, depending on the complex chain of cause-and-effect loops operating in the system. Nonlinearity, combined with dense interconnectedness, makes the behavior of complex systems impossible to predict reliably, especially over the long term.

Third, complex systems are dynamic. Not only do systems have the capacity to change, but prior states can influence present events (Meadow and Wright, 2008). Management theories are often criticized as discounting the importance of time and history (Pettigrew, 1985), however complexity theory suggests that a system's history cannot be ignored (McDaniel, Driebe, and Lanham, 2013).

The set of decisions one faces for any given circumstance is limited by the decisions one has made in the past, even when those past circumstances no longer exist.

These characteristics—interconnectedness, nonlinearity, and dynamism—make complex systems unpredictable and challenging to manage. Managers can be caught off guard when seemingly small, incremental, local changes in one part of the organization quickly produce large, undesirable effects in other parts of the organization. Modest changes in the standard operating procedures of the intensive care unit, for example, can quickly cascade into bed shortages in general nursing wards and disruptions in operating room schedules. Likewise, minor "technical" fixes in information systems to address patient registration problems can lead to hundreds of thousands of dollars in lost billing. Contrary to our usual thinking, effects are not always proportional to causes, nor are causes and effects always closely linked in time and space.

Likewise, in complex systems, small differences in initial conditions can send these systems down different developmental pathways. Two community health centers with comparable levels of financial resources, management support, and technical assistance trying to implement the same diabetes registry can follow very different trajectories and experience radically different outcomes due to seemingly small differences in how the physician champion frames the change effort for other providers and staff. Given the sensitivity of complex systems to initial conditions, complexity science warns that programs, processes, or practices that work well in one health care organization may work poorly (or not at all) in another health care organization even when faithfully implemented (McDaniel, Driebe, and Lanham, 2013; Wheatley, 2006).

Finally, complex systems can adjust to a wide variety of environmental conditions. In the language of complexity theory, they are robust, meaning that they resist perturbation or invasion by other systems (Sturmberg, Martin, and Katerndahl, 2014). Health care organizations have exhibited a remarkable ability to adjust to policy and market shocks (e.g., prospective payment and managed care) and slower, cumulative changes in operating conditions (Begun and Luke, 2001). While admirable, such resiliency gives rise to policy resistance: the tendency for interventions to be delayed, diluted, or defeated by the response of the system to the intervention itself (Sterman, 2000). Much to the consternation of policy makers, managers, clinicians, and patients, health care organizations often respond in ways that confound our understanding and thwart our intentions, as evidenced, for example, by the uneven and piece-meal adoption of electronic medical records (DesRoches et al., 2013).

Paradoxically, the same features that make complex systems perplexing and seemingly unmanageable also create endless potential for innovation, creativity, and novelty. Although complex systems behave unpredictably, they do not behave randomly. Rather, they exhibit a complex form of order that Ralph Stacey (1995) calls "bounded instability." In this state, a complex system's behavior follows an inherently unpredictable path, but it does so within limits (Byrne and Callaghan, 2013). While we cannot predict the specific course of the system's behavior over time, we can discern a pattern to its long-term behavior, and we can make somewhat accurate predictions about its short-term behavior. To use a meteorological example, we cannot make accurate predictions of what the weather will be three weeks from now, but we can make reasonably accurate predictions of what the weather will be tomorrow or the day after tomorrow. Moreover, we can see recognizable patterns of temperature, precipitation, and humidity over the long term, even if we cannot predict precisely the weather pattern more than a few days hence.

Complexity-oriented management scholars contend that organizations also exhibit bounded instability (Hock and VISA International, 1999; Scarpino, 2013). That is, organizations never quite settle into a stable equilibrium, but they generally do not fall apart, either. Between order (stability) and chaos (instability), there is an intermediate zone that some scholars poetically call "the edge of chaos" (Hock and VISA International, 1999). When organizations operate at the edge of chaos, new ideas, products, practices, and relationships can spontaneously emerge that are neither predicted nor anticipated by participants or observers. Complexity theorists refer to this phenomenon as emergence. The challenge for managers, complexity-oriented management scholars say, is not to give in to the pull of either order (stability) or chaos (anything goes) but rather to sustain organization at the edge of chaos, where continuous innovation and adaptability are possible. So, where does complexity science leave the health care manager? How do you manage, let alone lead, a complex system? No new management theory has emerged from complexity science, but scholars and practitioners see two implications for management. First, if we embrace the notion of health care organizations as complex systems, then we need new concepts and new tools to inform our thinking about how innovation, performance, and change occur in health care organizations (McDaniel, Driebe, and Lanham, 2013; Senge, 2010). In particular, we need to look closely at our ideas about complexity and feedback and, perhaps, employ systems dynamics and other modeling approaches to simulate the implications of the decisions we make. Second, viewing health care organizations as complex systems entails a fundamental shift in thinking about the role of management (Boulton, Allen, and Bowman, 2015; McDaniel, Driebe, and Lanham, 2013; Mowles, 2011). Complexity science draws attention to the limits of managerial control and the ease with which policy resistance occurs

DEBATE TIME: How to Manage Complex Systems

Is there still a role in complex systems for the classical management tasks of planning, organizing, deciding, and controlling? Some management scholars and practitioners argue that organizational survival depends on managers giving up their "obsession with control, knowing what is going on, and seeking stability" (Berquist, 1993; McDaniel, 1997; Vaill, 1989; Wheatley, 1992). Others contend that classical management tasks still have a place in complex systems. For instance, Stacey (1995) proposes that, in complex systems, selecting the appropriate management or leadership approaches depends on two factors: the amount of certainty about cause-and-effect linkages ("If we do X, then Y occurs") and the amount of agreement about an issue or decision ("What should we do?"). When high certainty and high agreement exist, then classical management tasks work well. Plsek and Greenhalgh (2001) observe, for instance, that a surgical team doing a routine gallbladder surgery exhibits high certainty about the surgical procedures that lead to successful outcomes and high agreement about how to do the work together. Managing such situations calls for using data from the past to predict the future, planning paths of action to achieve outcomes, and monitoring actual versus expected outcomes in order to reduce variation. When uncertainty is high and disagreement reigns, chaos and anarchy often result. In such situations, few management or leadership approaches work. When only modest levels of certainty and agreement exist, organizations enter the "zone of complexity," or the "edge of chaos," where high levels of creativity and innovation become possible. In this zone, managers cannot hope to understand what a complex system will do or how to optimize it. Hence, traditional management approaches lose their effectiveness. Instead, managers should lead by setting a few simple rules, establishing a "good enough" vision, and creating a wide space for innovation.

• • • IN PRACTICE: Adaptive Reserve in Primary Care Practices

Primary care practices are buffeted simultaneously by changes in health care financing, organization, and delivery. How is it that some primary care practices are better able than others to weather turbulent change? Drawing on complexity theory and organizational learning theory, and their own experience working with practices transforming into patient-centered medical homes, William Miller and his colleagues (2010) identified seven features of primary care practices that not only make them resilient in the face of external change but also define their ability to make and sustain internal change. These seven features, which they name adaptive reserve, include the following:

* *Trust: belief in the dependability of others and willingness to be vulnerable with others*
* *Mindfulness: openness to new ideas and different perspectives*
* *Heedfulness: interaction where individuals are sensitive to how their role and others' roles fit into the larger group and its goals.*
* *Respect: honest, tactful, mutually valuing interactions*
* *Diversity: complementary differences in mental models and perspectives*
* *Channel effectiveness: appropriate use and mix of rich (e.g., face-to-face) and lean (e.g., e-mail) communications*
* *Social/task relatedness: appropriate blend of work-related and non-work-related interactions*

These features often operate in the background (hence the term "reserve") but are called forth when practices experience or initiate change. Adaptive reserve gives rise to effective sense making, teamwork, and improvisation—emergent properties that not only promote both adaptive and generative learning but also buffer practice members from the stress and burden associated with unrelenting, arduous change. In a test of these ideas, Paul Nutting et al. (2010a) observed that practices with greater adaptive reserve implemented more elements of the patient-centered medical home in a fast-moving, two-year demonstration project. In contrast, practices with less adaptive reserve experienced "change fatigue," the symptoms of which included unresolved tension and conflict, burnout and turnover, and both passive and active resistance to further change (Nutting et al., 2010b). Similarly, Shin-Ping Tu et al. (2015) found that federally qualified health centers with greater adaptive reserve implemented more best practices for colorectal cancer (CRC) screening. These best practices included daily huddles, huddle sheets, or checklists to go over scheduled patients who need CRC screening; standing CRC screening orders or orders prepared by nurses or medical assistants and signed by providers; and tracking of patients who had CRC screening orders. So, can practices increase their adaptive reserve? Evidence suggests they can through practice-development interventions like practice facilitation (see the textbox "Practice Facilitation Supports Organizational Learning in Primary Care").

because of, not in spite of, our efforts to impose change in complex systems. From a complexity science perspective, managing involves seeing systems as "wholes," looking for leverage points that turn small changes into large effects, and creating conditions for organizational members to learn and improvise in real time (Dickens, 2013; Senge, 2010). In the sections that follow, we explore these two implications of complexity science in the context of innovation and learning.

COMPLEXITY AND FEEDBACK: A CLOSER LOOK

Like other complex systems, health care organizations exhibit two forms of complexity. **Combinatorial complexity**, or **detail complexity**, arises from the number of constituent elements of a system or the number of interrelationships that might exist among them (Senge, 2010). For instance, the problem of optimally scheduling a suite of operating rooms in a hospital is highly complex. However, the problem's complexity lies in finding the best solution out of an astronomical number of possibilities.

Dynamic complexity, or nonlinearity, arises from the operation of feedback loops. There are two basic types of feedback loops. **Reinforcing feedback loops** amplify or intensify whatever is happening in a system. In everyday language, we refer to reinforcing feedback loops as self-fulfilling prophecies, or the "Pygmalion Effect." For instance, a physician group practice that delivers high-quality care develops a positive reputation, which, through positive word of mouth, generates more referrals. More referrals, in turn, generate more resources that could be invested to further increase quality of care. **Balancing feedback loops** counteract or oppose whatever is happening in a system. For example, when the physicians in a group practice see more patients than they can realistically manage, patient satisfaction and possibly quality of care begin to suffer. Over time, negative word of mouth leads to fewer referrals and lighter schedules. Whereas reinforcing feedback loops drive a system toward disequilibrium and constitute the engines of accelerating growth or accelerating decline, balancing feedback loops drive a system toward equilibrium and constitute the engines of steady states or goal-oriented behavior. It is important to emphasize that reinforcing feedback loops can produce desirable or undesirable consequences. So, too, can balancing feedback loops.

Although combinatorial or "detail" complexity is important, dynamic complexity is critical to understanding the behavior of complex systems. When dynamic complexity exists (that is, when feedback loops operate), the same action can have different effects in the short term and the long term. Likewise, actions can have one consequence locally and a different consequence elsewhere in the system. Policy resistance itself signals the presence of dynamic complexity. What makes dynamic complexity "complex" is that feedback loops often contain delays—or interruptions between actions and consequences—that are poorly understood and often ignored. People have difficulty grasping system dynamics when cause and effect are distant from one another in space or time. In addition, most complex systems possess dozens or even hundreds of interlocking feedback loops. People can sometimes infer correctly the dynamics of systems possessing isolated loops; however, a system possessing multiple, interlocking loops quickly exceeds human perceptual and cognitive limitations (Marshall et al., 2015).

Dynamic simulation modeling can be a useful method for overcoming these limitations and gaining insight into the behavior of complex systems. Dynamic simulation models are mathematical representations of the structures and processes of complex systems that allow stakeholders in the system to experiment with and test interventions or scenarios and observe their positive and negative, intended and unintended, short-term and long-term consequences (Sturmberg, Martin, and Katerndahl, 2014). Just as airlines use flight simulators to help pilots, managers can use dynamic simulation models to develop "management simulators" that help them understand dynamic complexity, gain insight into sources of policy resistance, and explore implications of managerial decisions. In the field of health policy, dynamic simulation models have been used to assess the impact of supply-side interventions to reduce state psychiatric hospital admissions delays (La et al., 2016), examine the perils and promises of chronic disease management strategies (Homer et al., 2004; Homer, Hirsch, and Milstein, 2007), and explore options for efficiently managing emergency medical services in communities (Kergosien et al., 2015). In the field of health care management, dynamic simulation models have been used to assess the impact of interventions to reduce postponements in elective pediatric cardiac procedures (Day et al., 2015), to explore the uses of information technology to improve care (Goldsmith and Siegel, 2012), and to examine strategies for improving stroke care in the U.S. Veterans Health Administration (Lich et al., 2014).

Dynamic simulation models have several virtues (Sterman, 2000). First, they permit controlled experimentation, enabling managers to test strategies and learn more rapidly than the real world permits. In simulations, time can be compressed in order to reduce delays between cause and effect, acts can be reversed entirely or repeated under different conditions, and action can be stopped to permit reflection and dialogue. Second, simulations relax the performance pressures of the real world, creating a safe environment for managers to explore "what if" scenarios involving high-risk strategies or implausible situations. Finally, simulations can provide managers with "perfect, immediate, undistorted, and complete outcome feedback" (Sterman, 2000). Such high-quality outcome feedback allows managers to see the underlying structure of the complex system that they manage—and, importantly, to examine their own mental representations of it—in ways that the real world rarely, if ever, provides.

Systems dynamics models are not forecasting tools. Their value lies not in the prediction of some future state of the world but rather in the creation of *low-cost laboratories* for learning in complex systems. Effective simulation models as learning laboratories, however, require systems thinking and other "disciplines" that support organizational learning.

ORGANIZATIONAL LEARNING

Learning involves the acquisition of knowledge or skills through study, instruction, or experience. Learning is essentially a feedback process. We take action, we gather information about the effects of our action, and then we revise our understanding of our world and ourselves. In its simplest form, learning resembles a balancing feedback loop in which we compare a desired (or anticipated) state of affairs with the actual results of our conduct, and then act in ways that we believe or hope will close the gap (Cyert and March, 1992). Argyris and Schon (1978) refer to this type of learning as **single-loop learning**, a relatively simple error-and-correction process whereby problem solvers look for solutions within an organization's policies, plans, values, and rules. A more complex form of learning, **double-loop learning**, occurs when problem solvers attempt to close the gap between desired and actual states of affairs by questioning and modifying those organization's policies, plans, values, and rules that frame organizational problems and guide organizational action (Argyris and Schon, 1978). Changes in underlying values and assumptions, in turn, prompt changes in action strategies (see Figure 8.1).

Both single-loop and double-loop learning are necessary and useful for health care organizations. Single-loop learning promotes **adaptive learning**, in which problem solvers adjust their behavior and work processes in response to changing events or trends.

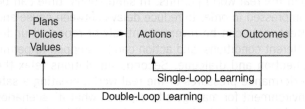

Figure 8.1 Single-Loop versus Double-Loop Learning.

For instance, a quality improvement team might invoke the Plan-Do-Study-Act (PDSA) cycle—a form of single-loop learning—to test the effectiveness of putting hand sanitizer dispensers in hallways and patient rooms to reduce hospital-acquired infections and thereby shorten lengths of stay. Double-loop learning promotes **generative learning**, in which problem solvers attempt to eliminate problems by changing the underlying structure of the system. This underlying structure includes the "operating policies" of the decision makers and actors in the system (i.e., their values and assumptions). For instance, a quality improvement team seeking to reduce handoffs among clinical professionals and thereby increase quality and safety might begin questioning deeply held assumptions about the value of staff specialization. On the basis of such questioning, they may redesign the care delivery system to employ multiskilled employees working in small, empowered work teams (Leander, 1996; Wermers et al., 1996).

We often think of learning as an individual process. However, learning, much like leadership (see Chapter 2), is a not solitary activity. Learning is a social enterprise that involves the creation, retention, and transfer of knowledge at individual, group, and organizational levels. In organizations, learning exhibits a circular dynamic where knowledge flows from the individual level to the group level to the organizational level, and back again (Argote, 1999; Chuang, Ginsburg, and Berta, 2007). As Chuang and colleagues (2007) explain,

> When an individual's learning processes are shared with other members of a workgroup, individual learning is recombined with the learning, experience, and interpretation of other group members to share learning at the group level. Through this process, group members may develop mutual understandings of one another's experiences and perspectives, which in turn modify the practices that are collectively perceived to be effective or ineffective. Practices that are deemed to be effective are likely to be retained in the group and transferred to other groups within an organization [Argote, 1999] . . . Then, what has already been learned feeds back from the organization to the group and individual levels, influencing, if not constraining, how individuals act and think [Crossan, Lane, and White, 1999].

Organizational learning is thus a multilevel phenomenon. Moreover, different factors influence knowledge creation, retention, and transfer within and across different levels. Individual learning is influenced, for example, by experience, feedback, and deliberate practice (i.e., focusing on techniques and understanding principles). Group learning is influenced by group member diversity, intergroup linkages, and group norms, such as psychological safety (see Chapter 5). Organizational learning is influenced by organizational leadership, culture, policies,

Practice Facilitation Supports Organizational Learning in Primary Care

Primary care practices often need support to implement new models of care (e.g., patient-centered medical homes) and other practice changes to deliver evidence-based care (e.g., cancer screening, diabetes care, and immunization). Clinicians often lack the time, expertise, and experience to implement practice change; taking care of patients is what they do best. Practice facilitation, in which a trained quality improvement specialist works with clinicians and staff members to implement change, has proven to be an effective strategy for increasing preventive service delivery, improving chronic disease management, and supporting practice transformation in primary care settings (Baskerville, Liddy, and Hogg, 2012; Dickinson et al., 2014; Due et al., 2014; Grunfeld et al., 2013; Noël et al., 2014; Parchman et al., 2013). But, what is practice facilitation and how does it work? Drawing on organizational learning theory, Berta et al. (2015) define practice facilitation as "a goal-oriented, context-dependent social process for implementing new knowledge into practice or organizational routines." Practice facilitation is goal-oriented in that it aims to engage, empower, and assist clinicians and staff members to implement practice changes that improve specific patient outcomes. With regard to colorectal cancer screening, for example, practices changes include visit planning, visit-based physician or nurse reminders, patient education tools, decision aids, and patient navigation. Practice facilitation is context-dependent in that the facilitator provides implementation support tailored to local needs and circumstances. As a social process, practice facilitation involves frequent communication, interactive problem solving, and relationship building. Berta and her colleagues argue that practice facilitation supports practice change by stimulating higher-order learning in organizations; it does so by "enacting micro-processes and activities that access, capitalize upon, and build on the organization's learning capacity, or absorptive capacity." For example, practice facilitation contributes to variation in organizational routines through microprocesses and activities such as assessing current practice, identifying performance gaps, introducing new ideas, and enhancing staff receptivity to change. Likewise, primary care practices can implement and retain new organizational routines through microprocesses and activities such as facilitating small tests of change, monitoring progress, and providing feedback support. Practice facilitation also supports increased delivery of evidence-based care by changing individuals' ways of thinking and working, by reconfiguring how clinic staff work together, and by embedding evidence-based practices into clinic routines (i.e., implementing practice changes).

and routines. Although the factors that facilitate or stymie learning at various levels are intertwined, we focus below on five management practices that characterize a learning organization.

Learning Disciplines

While scholars and theorists have discussed organizational learning for some time, Peter Senge's 1990 book *The Fifth Discipline* popularized the term "learning organization." In poetic terms, he described learning organizations as places where "people continually expand their capacity to create the results they truly desire, where new and expansive patterns of thinking are nurtured, where collective aspiration is set free, and where people are continually learning to learn together" (Senge, 1990). Others, in more prosaic language, define a learning organization as "an organization skilled at creating, acquiring, and transferring knowledge, and at modifying its behavior to reflect new knowledge and insights" (Garvin, 1993).

Senge (2010) describes five disciplines that, when combined, produce an organization capable of "expanding its capacity to create its future." He refers to these organizational practices as disciplines because each involves a body of theory and techniques that must be practiced in order for mastery to develop. The five disciplines are systems thinking, personal mastery, mental models, shared vision, and team learning.

- **Systems thinking** refers to the discipline of seeing wholes, perceiving the structures that underlie dynamically complex systems, and identifying high-leverage change opportunities. Systems thinking involves not only the recognition of the properties of complex systems but also the skilled application of "systems archetypes" to illuminate the deeper structures that shape everyday organizational behavior and performance (see the textbox "Using Systems Archetypes to Understand Organizational Behavior"). Through training and practice, organizational members can see "where actions and changes in structures can lead to significant, enduring improvements" (Senge, 2010).

- **Personal mastery** is the discipline of individual learning, without which organizational learning cannot occur. Personal mastery involves continuously clarifying our individual sense of purpose and vision and continuously learning how to see the world as it is without distortion. The tension created by the gap between vision and reality, if tapped creatively, generates energy for exploration and growth.

Organizational members who demonstrate personal mastery are apt to exhibit greater commitment, take more initiative, learn faster, and feel greater responsibility. Fostering personal mastery requires, at a minimum, adopting Theory Y assumptions about human behavior and instituting organizational policies and practices that promote employee growth and development (see Chapter 2).

- **Mental models** refer to the discipline of constantly surfacing, testing, and improving our assumptions about how the world works. Mental models actively shape what we see and, therefore, how we act (see the textbox "Mental Models of Learning"). By training and encouraging organizational members in the dual skills of reflection and inquiry (e.g., recognizing leaps of abstraction and uncovering censored thoughts and feelings), managers can promote

organizational learning by loosening the grip of tacit, often faulty mental models (e.g., higher quality always costs more).

- **Shared vision** is the discipline of generating a common answer to the question, "What do we want to create?" Shared vision connects people through common aspiration and derives its motivational power by tapping people's personal visions. From shared vision comes the focus and energy for learning, the willingness to take risks and experiment, the mutual alignment of individual effort, and the commitment to the long-term view. Creating shared vision requires encouraging organizational members to develop and communicate personal visions, inquiring into the deeper vision that unites the diversity of expressed views, and staying the course through difficult times.

ORGANIZATIONAL LEARNING IN THE PRESENT CLIMATE

Health care organizations are experiencing pressures from all sides to improve the patient experience, improve the health of populations, and reduce costs, all while providing a better work environment. To attain the quadruple aim, some organizations are considering mergers. Others are creating learning environments. More often than not, organizations are trying to do both. So, what exactly does that look like in the present climate? Health care organizations are striving not only to become learning organizations, with unit-based teams like those at Kaiser Permanente (Schilling et al., 2011), but they furthermore want to become learning *networks*. Auerbach et al. (2014) describe the example of the Hospital Medicine Reengineering Network (HOMERuN), a collaborative of hospitals, hospitalists, and care teams founded in 2011 with the overarching goal "to improve the outcomes of hospitalized patients by creating and expanding a learning organization that can discover, disseminate, implement, and improve practices (new and existing) to make care within hospitals and after discharge safer, more effective, and less expensive." HOMERuN serves as a laboratory for testing care models to determine whether the models actually produce better patient outcomes.

Like many health care organizations, HOMERuN relies on the five disciplines of Senge (2010), and it further extends them to integrate the principles of community-based participatory research (CBPR). The eight key principles of CBPR, as defined by Barbara Israel and her colleagues, are as follows:

1. Recognize community as a unit of identity
2. Build on strengths and resources within the community
3. Facilitate collaborative partnerships in all phases of the research
4. Integrate knowledge and action for mutual benefit of all partners
5. Promote a co-learning and empowering process that attends to social inequalities
6. Involve a cyclical and iterative process
7. Address health from both positive and ecological perspectives
8. Disseminate findings and knowledge gained to all partners

In a hospital-based CBPR—which also aligns with the accountable care network model—community engagement means targeting patients as well as the health care provider teams and groups who participate in the learning process and are also potentially affected by the results. In other words, the present-day learning organization is one that spans into the outer context of the health care system, forming feedback loops between health and social services, as well as between the hospital and the community. Auerbach and colleagues note that these types of learning networks are important for quickly developing and disseminating knowledge within the network and subsequently into health systems nationwide. Sustaining such a network, however, will have its own set of challenges, requiring strong commitment and support from research funders, health systems, and payers alike.

- **Team learning** refers to the discipline of creating alignment such that team members think insightfully about complex problems, synergize their knowledge and skills, and produce coordinated action. Team learning requires an organizational climate that promotes trust and respect—where it is safe for individuals to share both strengths *and* weaknesses. Such an environment diminishes individuals' inclination toward defensiveness as a protection from embarrassment or vulnerability to threat they may perceive in exposing such weaknesses to their colleagues (see Chapter 5). This can be achieved by promoting a mastery of open-minded dialogue where each individual learns from the others, the net result being a collective, organizational search for alternative meanings and new perspectives (Isaacs, 1999).

Senge (2010) emphasizes that all five disciplines matter because each builds upon and reinforces the others. Personal mastery, for instance, facilitates the integration of reason and intuition, which, in turn, enhances one's ability to see interrelationships among seemingly discrete events. Similarly, working with mental models loosens the grip of deeply held, often tacit assumptions that hinder systems thinking, shared vision, and team learning.

Limits of Organizational Learning

Although the promise of learning organizations is exciting, managers' enthusiasm for learning organizations needs to be tempered not only by the significant challenges involved in building such organizations but also by the seemingly intractable limits of organizational learning. First, organizational members usually possess only limited information, much of which is ambiguous or inaccurate. As Sterman (2000) observes, "No one knows the current sales rate of their company, the current rate of production, or the true value of the order backlog at any given time. Instead, we receive estimates of these data based on sampled, averaged, and delayed measurements. The act of measurement introduces distortions, delays, biases, errors, and other imperfections, some known, others unknown and unknowable." In addition, expectancy gives rise to selective perception. In other words, we see or hear what we expect to see or hear, rather than what actually occurs (Bowditch, Buono, and Stewart, 2007). For instance, our mental models about what is meaningful and important inform what we choose to define, measure, and monitor with our information systems; in turn, our information systems shape the perceptions that we form (Sterman,

---

USING SYSTEMS ARCHETYPES TO UNDERSTAND ORGANIZATIONAL BEHAVIOR

System archetypes—or patterns of structure that occur again and again—represent the key tools of systems thinking. System archetypes enable people to *see* how interlocking, reinforcing and balancing feedback loops influence the behavior of social systems; by seeing these structures at play, it becomes possible to identify "high-leverage" actions that can produce lasting change. Senge (2006) describes several system archetypes, including one he calls "Limits to Growth." As illustrated below (Figure 8.2) in Limits to Growth, a reinforcing feedback loop not only generates a spiral of success but also triggers a balancing feedback loop that, after a delay, slows down the success.

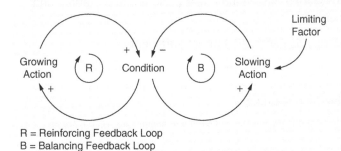

R = Reinforcing Feedback Loop
B = Balancing Feedback Loop

Figure 8.2 Limits to Growth Archetype: Generic Template.

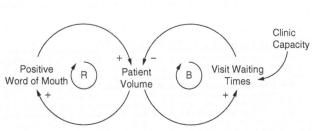

Figure 8.3 Limits to Growth Archetype: Example.

Limits to Growth structures explain that overexpansion can lead to performance decline. For example, a physician group practice that delivers high-quality care develops a positive reputation, which, through positive word of mouth, generates more referrals (Figure 8.3). More referrals, in turn, generate more resources that could be invested in high-quality care. However, if patient volumes increase more rapidly than quality-enhancing investments can be made, patient satisfaction and possible quality of care begin to suffer. Over time, negative word of mouth leads to fewer referrals and lighter schedules.

MENTAL MODELS OF LEARNING

Mental models shape not only our actions but also our capability to learn from our actions. Richard Bohmer and Amy Edmondson contend that health care managers and professionals share a widely held, yet implicit mental model that learning is an individual activity involving a linear process of repetition and error detection and correction (Bohmer and Edmondson, 2001). In this model (see Table 8.1), health professionals gain knowledge and skill through a one-way transfer of knowledge and "best practice" in their initial and continuing professional education. Through repetition, they increase their proficiency ("practice makes perfect"). On-the-job learning occurs primarily through error detection and correction, as in the case of Morbidity and Mortality conferences, or trial-and-error learning, as when a psychiatrist prescribes various antidepressants to find the one that works best for a given patient. According to Bohmer and Edmonson, this mental model of learning is incomplete. They propose an alternative model that, they argue, more fully describes what really happens in health care and that more effectively guides improvement efforts. In this model, learning is a dynamic, cyclical process in which experience gained in routine practice (i.e., knowledge-in-use) is reflected upon, reinterpreted, and refined not just by individuals but also by groups and organizations. Experience may be the best teacher, but learning from experience is not automatic. Bohmer and Edmonson observed, for example, that surgical teams with the same amount of experience, measured in terms of number of cases, exhibited varying levels of performance improvement. Team and organizational learning, they argue, does not follow inevitably from repetition and experience; rather, team and organizational learning processes must be managed. Moreover, as their research on psychological safety shows (see Chapter 5), effective team and organizational learning involves both single-loop and double-loop learning.

How can managers nurture organizational learning? The first step is to recognize that the prevailing, but largely implicit mental model of learning contains faulty, or at least incomplete, assumptions that limit collective learning capability. By examining this mental model through reflection and dialogue, managers can loosen the grip of these assumptions on their own and others' perceptions, attributions, and actions. Without a change in people's mental models, efforts to increase organizational learning through quality improvement methods, computer simulations, debriefing sessions, and other strategies do not "make sense" and therefore get little support from those who hold an individualistic, linear, single-loop model of learning.

Table 8.1 Mental Models of Learning

How We Think Learning Happens	How Learning Really Happens
Learning is an individual activity	Learning is an individual, group, and organizational activity
Learning is a linear process involving a one-way transfer of knowledge and "best practice"	Learning is a cyclical process involving knowledge interpretation, application, feedback, reinterpretation, and refinement
Repetition is the path to best practice	Repetition is necessary but not sufficient
Learning occurs through error detection and correction (single-loop learning)	Learning occurs through error detection and correction, and through diagnosis of systems and policies (single- and double-loop learning)

SOURCE: Adapted from Bohmer, R. M., & Edmonson, A. C. (2001, March/April). Organizational learning in health care. *Health Forum Journal, 44*(2), 32–35.

2000). In this sense, we "enact" the environment in which we live (Weick, 1979).

Second, even with perfect and complete information, organizational members routinely engage in unscientific reasoning due to judgment errors and biases (Dvorsky, 2013). The human mind relies upon unconscious routines, called heuristics, to cope with complexity and uncertainty (Kahneman, Slovic, and Tversky, 1982).

These heuristics, while efficient, often distort reasoning and judgment. The five learning disciplines can dampen the effects of recall bias, overconfidence, and other judgment errors, but they cannot eliminate them or the poor learning that they produce.

Finally, organizational learning often bumps up against practical problems and competing priorities. For instance, many decisions and programs experience implementation delays or alterations as they encounter technical obstacles, resource constraints, or political resistance. Imperfect implementation hinders learning, especially when long time spans are involved. In addition, as Sterman (2000) observes, "In the real world of irreversible actions and high stakes, the need to maintain performance often overrides the need to learn by suppressing new strategies for fear that they would cause present harm even though they might yield great insight and prevent future harm."

• • • IN PRACTICE: Failing to Learn from Failure

Health care managers and professionals often ask, "Why do we keep solving the same problems time after time?" Organizational learning is frequently inhibited by the system dynamic called "Fixes that Fail." This archetype describes a pattern wherein people act expediently to solve an immediate problem. The quick fix works, but it triggers unintended consequences that make the problem reappear after some delay, often worse than before.

Anita Tucker and Amy Edmondson's study of nursing care processes illustrates how the "Fixes that Fail" dynamic prevents hospitals from learning from failure (see Figure 8.4) (Tucker and Edmondson, 2003). They observed that nurses often encounter workflow problems like missing or broken equipment or missing or incorrect information. Nurses overwhelmingly engaged in first-order problem solving (i.e., single-loop learning) to address such problems. That is, they used short-term fixes that allowed them to return quickly to patient care. They did not try to address the underlying causes of the problem through second-order problem solving (i.e., double-loop learning). For example, when an oncology floor nurse working the night shift ran out of clean linens for patients' beds, she went to a unit that had linen in stock and took from that supply. She did not communicate to the person or department responsible for the problem, or bring the problem to managers' attention, or share with others ideas about how to prevent this problem from recurring. She solved the immediate problem, but no organizational learning occurred.

Why did these nurses rely so heavily on first-order problem solving? Tucker and Edmonson suggest four reasons. First, industry norms encourage nurses and other health professionals to take personal responsibility to solve problems. Counterintuitively, norms promoting personal responsibility prompted nurses to take decisive, independent action to solve immediate problems without considering the systemic causes of the problem or the systemic consequences of their short-term fixes. Second, nursing units seek to maximize individual unit efficiency through lean staffing. Nurses often have little time to resolve the underlying causes of the problems they face in their daily work. Short-term fixes are efficient solutions, even if they are not effective in the long term. Third, for a host of reasons, nurse managers are typically less involved in the daily work activities of those whom they supervise. This makes it more difficult for overburdened frontline staff to tackle problems that cross organizational boundaries. Finally, Tucker and Edmonson observed that the nurses found it personally gratifying to overcome problems on their own; they reported a sense of satisfaction knowing that they did everything they could for their patients.

One of the lessons of systems dynamics is that the cure is often worse than the disease. First-order problem solving works but only in the short term. Systemic causes go unaddressed, things get worse but only after a delay. For nurses, frustration and exhaustion build over time as they confront the same problems again and again, ultimately resulting in burnout and the nurse leaving the organization and possibly the profession—representing the loss of a very expensive knowledge asset. Taken to the extreme, first-order problem solving can also actually precipitate catastrophic failure of the system it is meant to support. This is because the consequences of some chronic problems accumulate like a toxin. Paul Levy wrote about the Nut Island sewage treatment plant in Boston Harbor, where employees took pride in first-order problem solving in dealing with facility maintenance (Levy, 2001). They went to heroic lengths to keep the plant operating without bothering their superiors, which resulted in failure to complete critical strategic maintenance and upgrades. Ultimately, the plant experienced catastrophic failures resulting in billions of gallons of raw sewage being dumped into the harbor.

What can managers do to escape the "Fixes that Fail" dynamic like that depicted in this situation? Managers can look for leverage points that promote second-order problem solving. Tucker and Edmondson highlight two such leverage points: (1) increasing managerial support by increasing managers' availability for at least part of all shifts, providing assistance to frontline problem-solving efforts, and acting as a role model for second-order problem solving; and (2) creating an environment where frontline staff feel safe to speak up about workflow problems without fear of embarrassment or punishment.

• • • IN PRACTICE: Failing to Learn from Failure *(Continued)*

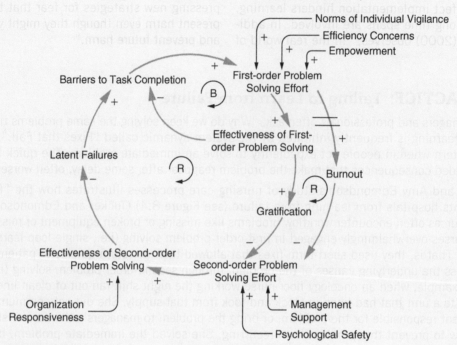

Figure 8.4 First-Order and Second-Order Problem-Solving Behavior.

SOURCE: Copyright 2003 by The Regents of the University of California. Reprinted from the *California Management Review*. Vol. 45, No. 2. By permission of The Regents.

ORGANIZATIONAL LEARNING AND UNLEARNING

The notion of "learning" organizations (i.e., organizations that continuously transform themselves through policies and structures to help their members systematically learn new knowledge, technologies, and practices) has been around for decades, popularized by Peter Senge's Fifth Discipline. As has the notion that change entails discarding old practices, for example, in Lewin's model of change as an "unfreezing" of an old mode of performance before instituting a change. However, some organizational behavior and psychology scholars have suggested that unlearning represents a distinct process with identifiable steps, and that these steps contain an inherent paradox that may help us understand why institutional-level unlearning—or deimplementation—of practices is uniquely challenging.

Fiol and O'Connor argue that organizational unlearning happens in three steps. The first step is destabilization, in which the old practice causes dissonance, creating the opportunity to reconsider it. They argue that organizational abandonment of an entrenched practice occurs only when that practice is demonstrated to be a problem. They illustrate their model using a case study of Beta Heart, a pseudonymous cardiovascular service in one of the largest physician groups in the United States. In the case of Beta Heart, destabilization occurred when its parent company mandated a reorganization from functional groups to centers of excellence that provided the full continuum of care for a given disease or condition. The development of centers of excellence was advocated by administrators who were alarmed at wide practice variation and outcomes and anticipated they could see losses in profit due to declining reimbursements and payment incentives linked to clinical outcomes. A key part of the consolidation was an emphasis on specialization and best practices. For example, a physician who provided general cardiology services would no longer also be allowed to perform procedures, and all electrophysiologists had to dress the surgical site for implanted devices the same way when dressings had previously been performed as many as eight different ways. Destabilization is inherently negative and stressful, and the shift to centers of excellence at Beta Heart was disruptive.

ORGANIZATIONAL LEARNING AND UNLEARNING (*Continued*)

However, Fiol and O'Connor also argue that sustained change from the old practice occurs only when experimentation happens and the organization explores new practices (displacement). This is the second step. The paradox is that this process of experimentation is most effective—may only be effective—when employees feel a high level of psychological safety and optimism; fear tends to curtail creative problem solving. This is a problem with the burning-platform metaphor of organizational change that Chip and Dan Heath have raised in their book *Switch*: using an existential threat may motivate employees to action, but fear narrows peoples' focus, inhibiting the creativity and innovation necessary for successful experimentation. Without the opportunity to experiment, say Fiol and O'Connor, inertia leads the organization back to the old practice. The challenge for the organizational leader is to allow the destabilization to occur, creating the opportunity for change, and simultaneously to create a sense of confidence and freedom to experiment. In the case of Beta Heart, the CEO of the parent company gave the Beta Heart leadership the prerogative to revamp the delivery of care. Some physicians came to share the concerns of administrators that practice variation represented inferior quality, and they began tracking data and running pilots of new ways of delivering care. Some were failures and some were successful.

With experimentation and the discovery of a solution by the members who must institute it, Fiol and O'Connor argue that employees (over time) see the fruits of success, release their old understandings, and embrace new understandings that come out of experimentation. This is the third step. The new practice demonstrates benefits and creates a self-reinforcing cycle. Beta Heart went through multiple cycles where new clinical pathways were adopted, then relapsed to old practices, and then renewed efforts with the new clinical pathways. They could demonstrate numerous wins, in terms of the advantages of a more integrated care model, and over time this model was increasingly accepted by the physicians. The challenge for the leaders was to create both a sense of crisis and a sense of opportunity.

INNOVATION AND LEARNING

Learning lies at the heart of innovation. When we innovate, we introduce something new into a setting for the first time, or as if for the first time. Learning—the acquisition of knowledge or skills—occurs throughout the innovation "journey" of discovery, exploration, experimentation, and reflection. Not all learning involves innovation, but all innovation involves learning.

It is important to recognize that innovation is both a noun and a verb. Researchers, consultants, managers, and policy makers often talk past one another because they forget this simple fact. As a noun, **innovation** refers to an "idea, practice, or object that is perceived as new by an individual or other unit adopting it" (Rogers, 2003). Although an innovation can be something that is "new to the world," it does not have to be so for this definition to apply. All that is necessary is that the idea, practice, or object be new, or perceived as new, to the individual, group, organization, community, or other social entity that decides to put that idea, practice, or object into use. For example, we could refer to the patient-centered medical home as an innovation for U.S. Veterans Health Administration when it first began implementing this model of care in 2010 (Helfrich et al., 2016). One of the central concerns for those who think about innovation as a noun is the following: How do new ideas, practices, or objects diffuse through a social system over time?

Other concerns include the following: What factors influence individual or organizational decisions to adopt an innovation? Why do some individuals or organizations adopt innovations more quickly than others do? How can individuals and organizations implement innovations more effectively and sustain innovation use?

As a verb, innovation refers to the act (or process) of introducing something new into an environment or setting. In other words, innovation is something that one does rather than some "thing" that one adopts. In a landmark study, Van de Ven et al. (1999) defined innovation as "a purposeful, concentrated effort to develop and implement a novel idea." They observed that innovation often involves collective effort by many people for a considerable amount of time, frequently under conditions of substantial technical, organizational, and market uncertainty. Moreover, the effort usually requires more resources to complete than those who undertake it possess. One of the central concerns for those who think about innovation as a verb is the following: How exactly do organizations create something new? Other concerns include the following: Why are some organizations more innovative (i.e., innovation-generating) than others? How can organizations innovate more quickly, efficiently, and effectively? How can less innovative organizations become more innovative?

Hundreds of studies have examined the adoption, implementation, and diffusion of new ideas, technologies, programs, practices, and services (for reviews, see Greenhalgh et al., 2004; Lau et al., 2015; Rogers, 2003). By comparison, few studies have examined the generative process through which new ideas, technologies, programs, practices, and services develop. Instead, much of what we know, or think we know, about the process of innovation comes from the anecdotes, reflections, and reports of current and former executives, management consultants, and popular business publications. Although conventional wisdom contains useful insights, it also contains misconceptions, biases, and myths that do not withstand empirical scrutiny. Here, we mention three.

"Innovation Is Good"

A strong cultural presumption exists, especially in the United States, that innovations are economically and socially valuable and, further, that innovating is desirable and admirable. Researchers call this presumption the "pro-innovation bias" (Gripenberg, Sveiby, and Segercrantz, 2012). Not all innovations are economically or socially beneficial (e.g., crack cocaine). Some have harmful unanticipated consequences, even when used correctly (e.g., Vioxx). Others have disastrous unintended consequences, especially when overly diffused or improperly used (e.g., financial derivatives). For example, the cost of innovating to treat a myocardial infarction now outweighs their incremental improvements to health, producing a lot of waste (Skinner, Staiger, and Fisher, 2006). The process of innovation itself is disruptive and fraught with risk for organizations and managers alike. Although some companies innovate themselves into prosperity, others innovate themselves into insolvency (Pfeffer and Sutton, 2006; Rosenzweig, 2007; Van de Ven et al., 1999); the failure rate of new products (i.e., failure to ever return a profit) appears to be on the order of 30–60 percent and is higher for new start-ups (Pfeffer and Sutton, 2006). Successful innovation journeys can enhance managers' careers; unsuccessful innovation journeys can lead to stigmatization, demotion, or termination (Van de Ven et al., 1999).

"There's a Formula"

Popular management books often promise spectacular results from simple formulae, such as "stick to your knitting" (Peters and Waterman, 1982) or "set audacious goals" (Collins and Porras, 1994). Yet, empirical studies indicate that the innovation journey, even when successful, is a complex, messy affair that cannot be easily summarized, let alone reduced to a dictum (Van de Ven et al., 1999). Rosenzweig (2007) suggests that the pervasive belief that organizational innovativeness can be attributed to simple formulae arises from a form of observational bias called the *halo effect*: the tendency to infer specific characteristics of a person or organization

from our overall impressions or feelings about that person or organization. Much of what we know, or think we know, about innovation comes from studies of successful cases: businesses that have done exceptionally well (Collins, 2001; Collins and Porras, 1994; Peters and Waterman, 1982). Management experts first identify successful companies and then try to reconstruct what these companies did to set themselves apart from their less-accomplished peers. The problem with this sort of retrospective analysis is that management experts interpret what they see in the glow (i.e., the halo) of what they already know about the companies' performance. The halo that surrounds these companies can lead experts to accept uncritically the simple formula or rules of thumb that executives use to describe the secrets of the company's success. Unfortunately, many of the companies from which management experts derive simple formulae subsequently *underperform* the rest of the market in the years *after* they are profiled (Rosenzweig, 2007).

"Innovation Is Linear"

The most pervasive misconception of the innovation journey is that it follows a logical, predictable sequence of stages or phases of activity. In the typical stage model, innovation begins with needs assessment or problem identification and proceeds from basic or applied research, to development, and then to commercialization (Rogers, 2003; Van de Ven et al., 1999). These stages are seen as a linear progression: one stage follows another in a predictable, orderly fashion. Stage models can be useful as heuristics for talking about the innovation journey. But, the simplicity, clarity, and predictability of linear stage models belie the complex, uncertain, and indeterminate nature of the innovation journey revealed by empirical research (Greenhalgh et al., 2004; Van de Ven et al., 1989).

What, then, does the innovation journey look like? Over the course of 17 years, Andrew Van de Ven and a group of management scholars at the University of Minnesota sought to answer this question by studying 14 new-to-the-world innovations, including the development of cochlear implants at 3M, the formation of multihospital systems in the 1980s, and the creation of new programs in schools. The Minnesota Innovation Research Project (MIRP) was conducted prospectively, meaning the researchers began collecting data at the beginning of the innovation journey. MIRP researchers thus avoided the twin problems that Rosenzweig (2007) cites as the main culprits in falling victim to the halo effect: selecting your case studies based on outcomes and collecting data that are not independent from the outcome. To foreshadow the discussion below, MIRP results suggest that the innovation is neither predictable nor random. Instead, the journey reflects the nonlinear dynamics of a complex system. MIRP researchers identified 12 patterns, which they categorized according to three broad phases of activity (Van de Ven et al., 1999). These categories lend these disparate, nonlinear patterns a degree of narrative coherence. But importantly, in every case, the essential pieces of the innovation story changed radically over time: the people involved in the effort, the objectives of the effort, even the idea of what the innovation itself was. Finally, MIRP results reveal a more complex picture of organizational learning in the innovation journey than prior innovation and learning research suggested.

Innovation Journey

The MIRP researchers began with assumptions that managers and researchers generally held at the time and that many still hold today. They assumed that "innovation" involved a single, common idea or technology that retained its identity through the development process. While different stakeholders might hold varying or even opposing views about the innovation, they nonetheless would see the innovation as the same (identifiable) thing. A team of individuals pulled from their other duties would work primarily, if not exclusively, on innovation development; moreover, the team would remain intact through the development process. Likewise, the team's relationships with venders, suppliers, and other external stakeholders would remain stable once established. The team would shepherd the innovation through a linear progression of stages that would culminate in a definitive outcome: success or failure.

What the MIRP researchers found was quite different from what they expected. Innovation involved a proliferation of ideas, frequent reinvention, with multiple entrepreneurs engaging, disengaging, and reengaging over time. None of the 14 innovations that they studied developed in a simple, linear sequence of stages. Most produced indeterminate or ambiguous results. MIRP researchers described the complex, messy progression of events that they observed in terms of three broad phases of activity: genesis, development, and termination. Although they parsed the innovation journey into three phases for the purposes of description and reporting, they emphasized that these phases were fuzzy, incomplete, and nonlinear.

Genesis

Innovations do not arise from a single, spur-of-the-moment event. The essence of the idea develops over years, with unpredictable events setting the stage. For example, MIRP researchers studied the development of the cochlear implant, a device implanted within the cochlea (the auditory portion of the inner ear) with an external processor that would allow the profoundly deaf to hear. The 3M Corporation began development of the cochlear implant when researchers at the University of

Melbourne contacted one of 3M's Australian subsidiaries about commercializing research they had conducted on a "bionic ear." At the same time, independent of this work, another 3M division was doing similar work based on hearing aids. These research streams evolved independently but converged when university researchers initiated contact.

At some point a shock or event, often external, triggers concentrated effort to develop the innovation. The innovators submit a plan to those who control the resources needed to initiate intensive innovation development. These sponsors might be senior executives within the company or external investors such as venture capitalists. This plan marks the beginning of concerted efforts to develop the innovation, but the plan generally serves first and foremost as a "sales vehicle" to get sponsors on board. Initial plans often include vague goals, optimistic projections, and downplayed risks. For example, with the cochlear implants, initial projections of the market were based on an assumption that nearly all profoundly deaf adults would be interested in the technology, which put the potential market in excess of $100 million.

Development

Once intensive work begins, the original idea quickly proliferates into multiple, often divergent ideas and activities. There is no uniform "innovation." There is a nebula of related and evolving ideas, and it is not always clear where one draws the boundaries around this shifting cloud. Though it makes linear narrative nearly impossible, this divergence is logical given how uncertain innovation is. Pursuing multiple development paths is adaptive because innovators and managers do not know which ideas are going to pay off. In the face of such uncertainty, the best bet is to invest limited resources in a number of plausible alternatives simultaneously, in the hope of eventually shifting resources to the most promising option as uncertainty diminishes.

Innovators invariably experience setbacks, often due to unexpected changes in the external environment that alter their original ideas and assumptions. Perhaps a competing technology emerges, a new market opens up, or a financial crisis occurs and capital becomes scarce. In the case of the cochlear implant, the innovators discovered that to the profoundly deaf, "Deaf" (with a capital D) was a whole subculture and community, not a disability they hoped to escape. This type of new information can throw the original plan into disorder. At first, innovators may successfully petition their sponsors for allowances: more time, additional funds, and a change in the goals. But typically, problems continue to accumulate. The innovators may think of the original plan as an aspirational statement, to be revisited and revised as unexpected problems and opportunities arise. The sponsors, however, may think of the original plan as a contract, and, as time passes, seek to hold the innovators accountable to it. For example, as it became clear that the market for the cochlear implant among the profoundly deaf was not sufficient to support the innovation, the 3M innovation managers began exploring options for adapting the technology for hearing aids.

The goals of innovation evolve over time. Sponsors and innovators change the criteria by which they judge innovation a success or failure, often diverging and sometimes fighting over these criteria. Likewise, the people themselves—the innovators and their teams—fluctuate over time, becoming involved and subsequently leaving, and in some cases coming back again. These shifting criteria and turnover in staff inhibit learning. It is difficult to understand if planned strategy leads to the desired goals when the goals change repeatedly and unpredictably. Likewise, much of learning that occurs in the innovation journey is tacit: held by individuals and hard to express in words or images. Tacit knowledge is susceptible to loss when individuals leave or are reassigned.

Sponsors (investors and top managers) are frequently involved throughout the process of innovation development, often serving a variety of changing and conflicting roles. Van de Ven and colleagues concluded in their MIRP work that no significant innovation problems were solved without the direct involvement of sponsors. Power dynamics between innovators and sponsors changed over the course of the innovation development processes (see the textbox "The Role of Management in the Innovation Journey"). Initially, the sponsors held the essential power as innovators negotiated for support to develop their innovations. After the sponsors had invested significant resources into the innovation, the investment translated into greater influence for the innovators, as sponsors were reluctant to do anything that jeopardized their investment. Innovators developed relationships with other organizations, and these relationships locked the innovators into certain courses of action, curtailing others, often with consequences they could not foresee. Innovation occurs within an ecosystem of competitors, trade associations, regulators, legislators, and others, all of whom contribute to a common infrastructure that supports or inhibits the innovation. Thus, the innovation does not evolve just as a function of what the innovators do but also as a function of the support and inhibition provided by the broader ecosystem.

Termination

The innovation continues to evolve as users integrate it and adapt it to local situations. Eventually, the innovation ceases. Either it is "implemented" and is no longer an innovation or the innovators exhaust their resources and cease work on the innovation. However, even when work ceases due to exhaustion of resources, it could resume if some new confluence of events triggers interest.

At some point, sponsors draw conclusions about innovation success or failure and assign credit or blame. The greater the consequences of failure, the greater the tendency to attribute failure to the innovation team. In many cases, MIRP researchers found that the attribution of credit or blame was misdirected, but even invalid attributions had important implications for the ultimate fate of the innovation (in cases where the innovation persists) and the innovator's careers. This was particularly striking, because many of the companies that the MIRP researchers studied explicitly or implicitly espoused a culture of risk-taking, where employees ostensibly are not punished for taking reasonable risks and failing.

In lieu of a simple stage-model diagram of the innovation journey, the MIRP researchers captured the nonlinear, dynamic nature of the process in a figure they call the "fireworks" diagram (so named for the branching lines, which evoke the shower of sparks as from a Roman candle—though it could equally allude to the drama that marked nearly every case they studied). Overall, the cases studied by Van de Ven and colleagues demonstrated that the process cannot be reduced to stages or phases. Instead, the process is a cycle of divergent and convergent activities operating at multiple organizational levels, and it continues for as long as there are resources to sustain it.

Learning in the Innovation Journey

When we think about innovation, we imagine a process that involves a great deal of trial-and-error learning. Indeed, innovation conjures the popular image of an inventor tinkering in his or her workshop, experimenting with materials and processes to find the right combination that will realize his or her idea. Thomas Edison's comment that "invention is one percent inspiration and 99 percent perspiration" reinforces the notion that innovation is essentially an extended process of single-loop (or adaptive) learning. The inventor acts, compares the results of his or her actions to some goal, and then acts in ways that he or she believes will close the gap between desired outcomes and actual results. The MIRP researchers observed that the innovation journey did feature single-loop (or adaptive) learning, which they termed **testing**. Through testing, innovators learn about action–outcome relationships; in particular, they learn through successive experimentation which actions reliably produce desired outcomes. However, MIRP researchers also observed that learning by testing did not occur until relatively late in the innovation journey. Learning by testing requires some prior knowledge about the tasks to be performed. In particular, learners must first know what courses of action are possible, what goals or outcomes are preferable, and what rules, resources, and other contextual factors are relevant to the learning process. For the first several months and

THE ROLE OF MANAGEMENT IN THE INNOVATION JOURNEY

One of the lessons from the MIRP studies was that multiple managers, at multiple hierarchical levels, played multiple roles in bringing along every innovation. Managers alternately served as sponsor, mentor, critic, and institutional leader, with different managers serving different roles at different times. In doing so, they served as checks and balances to each other. As sponsors, managers advocated for the innovation and the innovation team when investment decisions and other issues were considered. As mentors, managers coached, counseled, and served as role models. As critics, managers played "devil's advocate," taking a "hard-nosed" view of innovation goals, progress, and prospects. As institutional leaders, managers sought to balance these opposing roles by establishing structure and settling disputes. MIRP researchers observed that these management roles were reciprocally related to one another and counterbalanced each other over time through self-correcting cycles (i.e., balancing feedback loops). They also noted the importance of balance and timing in the performance of these roles.

in some cases years of the innovation journey, the conditions necessary for learning by testing did not exist. That did not mean, however, that no learning occurred during the developmental period. Instead, a different kind of learning took place, which MIRP researchers termed **discovery**. Through discovery, innovators learn about possible action alternatives, outcome preferences, and contextual factors. Learning by discovery resembles double-loop (or generative) learning in that it opens up and investigates possibilities. Whereas testing involves a process of error detection and correction, discovery involves a process of exploration. Pathways multiply and diverge rather than winnow and converge.

The MIRP studies further indicate that learning by discovery is a precondition to learning by testing. Innovation typically begins with a high degree of uncertainty. To illustrate, Van de Ven et al. (1999) described the innovation journey of two new-to-the-world biomedical innovations as follows:

> The initial plans contained vague but optimistic proposals to develop and commercialize new technologies that were believed to have the potential to sustain the organizations' businesses in the next generation [Van de Ven et al., 1989]. The plans indicated that the starting conditions were highly ambiguous; they focused on possibilities and opportunities, not specific project goals, objectives, or outcome criteria. The action plans were also highly uncertain; they emphasized exploratory research and discovery, not testing or evaluation, because the innovations represented novel undertakings for the organizations.

Before innovators can test which actions lead to which outcomes, they first have to discover what courses of action are possible, what outcome goals and criteria they and others prefer, and in what kind of environmental

context they are expected to work. It is during this time of learning by discovery that the initial idea for the innovation proliferates to many ideas and the actions that innovators take proceed in many different directions at once. While this expansive, divergent period of activity seems random and unproductive, Van de Ven et al. (1999) write, this chaotic process of learning by discovery is necessary before innovators can "converge into the still confusing, but better defined period of trial-and-error learning."

The MIRP studies also shed light on how and when transitions occur from learning by discovery to learning by testing. MIRP researchers noted that innovation efforts must import energy and resources from the organization itself and from outside sources in order to continue. Start-up companies, for example, require a constant flow of venture capital to sustain product development. Similarly, innovation efforts within established organizations require a constant flow of internal "venture capital" in the form of human resources, managerial support, and budgetary allocation. Moreover, innovation efforts occur within a context of institutional rules that shape the timing, pace, content, and process of innovation efforts. Drug development, for example, is strongly affected by U.S. Food and Drug Administration rules, regulations, and procedures. Management directives, institutional rules, and resource flows can trigger transitions from discovery to testing by constraining the freedom of innovation efforts to move along multiple, diverse developmental pathways. For example, managers can impose specific goals for the innovation effort or impose a set of outcome criteria judging the success of the innovation effort. Requiring a tighter linkage between actions and outcomes focuses attention on testing which action alternatives optimally produce a chosen outcome or goal. Likewise, looming deadlines imposed by resource holders and institutional rule makers can shift innovation efforts from exploring action alternatives and possible outcomes to finding the best linear combination of feasible actions and desired outcomes. MIRP researchers contend that learning in the innovation journey does not simply progress in a one-way direction from discovery to testing. While the search for a tighter coupling of actions and outcomes narrows the focus of attention, it also opens new questions and issues that require exploration and resolution. Thus, the innovation journey involves repeatable, but not predictable, cycles of learning by discovery and learning by testing. As noted earlier, the cycles continue until the innovation effort succeeds or runs out of resources.

Finally, the MIRP studies indicated that the innovation journey is characterized by a long delay between actions and outcomes, sometimes lasting years. "During the developmental period, intensive investments and efforts are required to transform a vague inventive idea into a concrete reality without having any objective information that is useful for narrowing developmental activities toward specific outcomes" (Van de Ven et al., 1999). Indeed, the most definitive information about outcomes does not become available until the innovation is launched into the market or implemented by an adopting organization. This long delay in the feedback loop between action and outcomes explains why adaptive, single-loop, trial-and-error learning often occurs late in the innovation journey. In the absence of concrete goals and timely feedback on outcomes, action persistence appears to be the prevailing and preferred strategy for narrowing the complexity of innovation efforts to manageable proportions. In other words, when faced with ambiguity about goals, means, and performance, the best and perhaps only strategy available is to pick what seems like the best course of action and stick to it. As a prominent organizational scientist notes, action persistence is psychologically satisfying. "Commitment marshals forces that destroy the plausibility of alternatives and remove their ability to inhibit action" (Weick, 1993). MIRP researchers agreed that there is some value in treating probabilistic information as if it were deterministic information and regarding beliefs that are only relatively true as if they were absolutely true. However, such action persistence underscores a key feature of complex systems: sensitivity to initial conditions. If one persists in certain courses of action in the absence of any feedback that might signal the need for correction, then small differences in starting points can take an innovation journey in very different directions. Persisting in "veering left" at every fork in the road could ultimately lead one to a desired destination, or not. It all depends on the starting point. As MIRP researchers pointed out, if the innovation journey is successful, action persistence creates heroes. If the journey is not successful, action persistence creates tragedies and scapegoats.

MANAGING COMPLEXITY, LEARNING, AND INNOVATION

Complexity-oriented management scholars tell us that continuous innovation and learning occur when organizations operate at the "edge of chaos," that intermediate zone between stability and instability where new ideas, products, practices, and relationships spontaneously emerge that are neither predicted nor anticipated. However, keeping organizations poised at the edge of chaos is challenging. It requires constant managerial vigilance to avoid falling into too much structure (order) or too little (chaos). Complexity-oriented management scholars contend that when it comes to fostering innovation and learning, managers should neither impose order by adopting top-down, command-and-control approaches, nor should they neglect order by adopting freewheeling, "anything goes" approaches. Instead, they should create conditions in which order can emerge in a spontaneous, creative, and self-organizing fashion. Since managerial thinking, writing, and research typically focus on creating and maintaining order, we focus below on how managers can promote innovation and learning through nurturing foresight, fostering improvisation, maximizing serendipity, and learning from mistakes.

Nurturing Foresight

Managers can sustain continuous innovation even in the face of rapidly changing, highly competitive environments by nurturing foresight—that is, by developing organizational capabilities and processes to "spot developments before they become trends and to grasp the relevant features of social currents that are likely to shape the direction of future events" (Tsoukas and Shepherd, 2004). Consistent with the principles of complexity science, nurturing foresight is not about developing comprehensive strategic plans or investing in any one vision of the future. Rather, it is about probing possible futures, exploring weak or ambiguous signals, and developing viable options. Specific practices for nurturing foresight include (1) promoting rapid experimentation using prototypes, pilot programs, and computer simulations to accelerate learning (Andriopoulos and Gotsi, 2006); (2) knowledge brokering—making connections between ideas from different industries, business units, or projects—to identify disruptive trends (Choi and Lee, 2015); and (3) using simulations, scenarios, and other tools to promote thoughtful dialogue about implausible, unthinkable, and "forbidden" futures (Sarpong and Maclean, 2014). Practices for nurturing foresight allow organizations to avoid the rigidity of planning with as well as the chaos of reactivity. These practices also promote rapid learning by discovery—that double-loop, generative process whereby innovators gain knowledge of possible action alternatives, outcome preferences, and contextual factors.

Fostering Improvisation

Improvisation can be another important source of innovation and learning. Improvisation fuses planning and execution in the moment in response to unexpected events (Cunha, Clegg, and Mendonça, 2010). Although improvisation involves "making it up as you go along" (Moorman and Miner, 1998), it is not the same as "anything goes." In jazz music, for example, individual expression and mutual adjustment occur within a few specific rules (e.g., order of soloing, valid chord sequences). In fact, the adherence to a few simple rules makes improvisation possible; if everyone "did their own thing," the result would be cacophony. Improvisation is a fact of life in organizations, given the inevitable limitations of planning and anticipation in the face of intractable and unpredictable events. Improvisation takes many forms. Some improvisations occur in the "underlife" of organizations as individuals act creatively and in unplanned ways to acquire resources or solve problems in the face of rigid rules and organizational constraints. For example, improvisation occurs routinely in the emergency department as clinicians grapple with patient variability that formal protocols do not recognize or accommodate (Batista et al., 2016). Although not officially sanctioned, such improvisation can serve organizational interests so long as it remains hidden from view. Other forms of improvisation can be nurtured by managers seeking to subvert the status quo and challenge the organization. At IBM, for example, a "gang of unlikely rebels" transformed IBM with a subversive change initiative that they developed and launched from the bottom up in a "skunkworks" that operated backstage and out of sight (Hamel, 2000). Although by definition, improvisation is an emergent phenomenon, managers can facilitate improvisation by creating semi-structures (Cunha et al., 2015). Consistent with the principles of complexity science, which emphasize the value of minimum specifications, semi-structures combine well-defined managerial responsibilities and clear-cut project priorities with loosely specified development processes. Frequent formal and informal communication within and across project teams complement these semi-structures, fostering spontaneous, unexpected idea sharing and problem solving. Semi-structures keep the organization at the edge of chaos in that ambiguous, fluid, and messy space depicted by the MIRP studies where ingenuity, creativity, and innovation occur.

Maximizing Serendipity

Discoveries occur when we find things we did not know we were looking for, and when we see unexpected connections among seemingly unrelated events, objects, or facts. Discovery, by definition, involves an element of surprise. The discovery of penicillin, for example, was a fortunate accident. So too was the discovery of vaccinations, X-rays, anesthesia, coronary catheterization, Viagra, lithium, Valium, insulin, quinine, antibiotics, antidepressants, and cancer therapies. In almost every case, scientists were looking for and expecting one thing but found something completely different and unanticipated. Serendipity, or the accidental discovery of something that turns out to be valuable, depends in no small part on luck, chance, and happenstance, common features of organizational life that never disappear yet receive little attention among managers or researchers (Lindsay, 2013). While serendipity is an emergent phenomenon, managers can facilitate its emergence by creating the conditions in which it is likely to occur (Cunha et al., 2015). Louis Pasteur famously remarked, "In fields of observation, chance favors the prepared mind." Indeed, chance favors inquisitive, venturesome, persistent people. Hiring and nurturing people with these qualities, putting them in physical proximity to one another, and encouraging informal interaction, especially among people with different types of knowledge, create fertile ground for unexpected discovery and learning to occur. The crucial element in serendipity, though, the element that distinguishes it from improvisation or creativity, is bisociation, or the combining of previously unrelated ideas or information in an original way (Cunha, Clegg, and Mendonça, 2010). While managers cannot engineer luck, chance, or happenstance, they can promote them through hiring, training, and rewarding the analogical or metaphorical thinking that underlies bisociation. Minimal structuring through the use of clear priorities and tight deadlines, coupled with loosely specified development processes, can also facilitate surprising discovery (Brown and Eisenhardt, 1997).

Learning from Mistakes

Mistakes and failures can be valuable and unexpected opportunities for organizational learning (Lapre and Nembhard, 2011). Unfortunately, such opportunities for learning are often missed. For example, studies suggest that despite the increased focus in recent years on medical errors and investigation, hospitals have not gotten safer (Landrigan et al., 2010). In health care and other fields, there is an ingrained attitude that all mistakes and failure are bad and a common response is to "blame and shame" the individuals who commit them. Such

MOVING BEYOND EXPERIENCE TO DELIBERATE PRACTICE

A popular proverb holds that experience is the best teacher. But, is it always? In his bestseller *Outliers*, Malcolm Gladwell (2008) introduces the "10,000-hour rule," the idea that across a range of professions—from music to physics to chess—those who become highly accomplished have almost always amassed 10,000 or more hours of practice at the activity. As it turns out, Gladwell got some of this research wrong (e.g., these were high-performing violin students the study he cited, not concertmasters of major orchestras, and 10,000 hours were the average practice times for these students, not the minimum practice hours). But more importantly, Gladwell missed half the story: repetition may lead to automaticity (i.e., the ability to accomplish a task without conscious effort), but it does not inevitably lead to excellence. Most performers, including in medicine, achieve competence where they complete a task without having to concentrate on it. At that point, their performance plateaus, and they cease to improve.

Experts achieving the highest levels of excellence, on the contrary, continue to focus consciously on the task, engaging in *deliberate practice*. The hallmarks of deliberate practice are breaking a task into discrete components that can be learned sequentially, engaging in tasks of increasing difficulty in order to stress existing capacity and ultimately expand it, and having a mechanism for monitoring and correcting performance. As a consequence, these experts continue to improve (Ericsson, 2006, 2015).

Though it is often perilous to apply lessons from individual behavior to the collective, the hallmarks of deliberate practice have clear parallels for organizations. For example, one of the tenants of systems engineering is to map an organizational process, breaking it into discrete components that can be assessed for opportunities to improve (Anderson and Johnson, 1997). In health care, we can create opportunities for teams to practice through simulations (Ericsson, 2015). Likewise, managers can use "stretch goals," i.e., setting a goal well beyond current performance such that it cannot reasonably be met by existing processes and requiring teams to find new ways of doing things (Wright et al., 1993).

Perhaps the most important lesson from deliberate practice relates to the third point, the use of feedback mechanisms. While performance measures such as the Healthcare Effectiveness Data and Information Set (HEDIS) and Joint Commission measures abound in health care, these are largely summative; they are reported long after the care processes occur and are frequently linked to incentives. Implicitly, performance measures become more tools of motivation and less tools of instruction. Managers can use other techniques to provide their teams with monitoring mechanisms that put the emphasis on learning and improving rather than proving that they are performing well. Two underused techniques are team debriefs and huddles. Team debriefs are meetings after a specific event or encounter to walk back through what occurred and identify potential areas for improvement. Team huddles are regular, brief meetings to confer and identify issues as they occur.

The important point to remember with all three of these hallmarks is that the objective is to keep teams from falling into a pattern of operating by rote, without opportunity to intentionally evaluate the work and how it is accomplished.

attitudes and responses deter people from admitting and reporting mistakes and failures, a critical precondition for examining and addressing their root causes. Importantly, such attitudes and responses ignore the fact that mistakes and failures occur for a variety of reasons, ranging from deliberate deviation, attentional lapses, poor training, error-prone processes, situational uncertainty, and thoughtful experimentation (Edmondson, 2011). With the exception, perhaps, of deliberate deviation from prescribed processes or standards, something valuable can be learned from most mistakes and failures, but only if organizational leaders make it psychologically safe for employees to identify, report, analyze, discuss, and address mistakes and failures. Organizational

leaders can build a psychologically safe environment by (a) acknowledging that mistakes and failures are inevitable in routine, complex operations and represent opportunities to learn and improve; (b) embracing messengers by celebrating the value of the news and focusing on what happened and how to fix it rather than who did it; (c) leading by example by being open about what you do not know, what mistakes you have made, and what cannot get done without help from others; and (d) holding people accountable for specific behaviors, such as conscious violation of standards, reckless conduct, and failing to ask for help when situations demand it (Edmondson, 2011). Creating a psychologically safe environment could play a critical role in overcoming the paradox of failure: Individuals learn from the failures of others but not their own failures. In a study of 10 years of data from 71 cardiothoracic surgeons who completed more than 6,500 procedures using a new technology for cardiac surgery, Diwas, Staats, and Gino (2013) observed that surgeons learned more from their own successes than from their own failures, but they learned more from the failures of others than from others' successes. However, they also found that surgeons' prior success and others' failures could help individuals overcome their inability to learn from their own failures. The opportunity to learn from others' failures depends in no small part in making it psychologically safe for people to admit and discuss their own mistakes and failures and those of others.

SUMMARY AND MANAGERIAL GUIDELINES

1. Health care organizations exhibit three characteristics of complex systems: interdependence, nonlinearity, and dynamism. There are no hard and fast rules for managing learning and innovation in complex systems, though management scholars propose a range of ideas for balancing between too much structure (order) or too little (chaos). These include (1) relying on a few simple rules rather than detailed planning and (2) thinking about the effects on the whole system when setting goals and allocating resources.

2. Organizational learning is a feedback-loop process. Single-loop learning (adaptive learning) occurs when problem solvers compare desired states of affairs with actual results and seek to close the gap. Double-loop learning (generative learning) occurs when problem solvers attempt to close the gap between desired and actual states of affairs by questioning and modifying the underlying conditions that contribute to the actual state, such as an organization's policies, plans, values, and the rules that frame organizational problems.

3. Five "disciplines" promote organizational learning: (1) systems thinking, (2) personal mastery, (3) mental models, (4) shared vision, and (5) team learning. A powerful way to spread the discipline of systems thinking is to encourage organizational members to learn and make use of systems archetypes.

4. Organizational learning is constrained by (1) the availability of limited information, often ambiguous or inaccurate; (2) human errors of judgment and biases, often related to the heuristics we rely on to cope with complexity and uncertainty; and (3) competing priorities, resource constraints, and broader political considerations. Systems dynamics models can help people overcome these "learning disabilities" by helping people grasp the underlying structure of the organization as a complex system, surfacing people's mental models about how the system "works," and allowing managerial strategies to be tested through rapid, low-cost, controlled experimentation.

5. Beware of three common myths or misconceptions about innovation: (1) innovation is good, (2) there is a formula, and (3) innovation is linear.

6. Learning in the innovation journey involves both discovery and testing. Discovery resembles double-loop (generative) learning. Testing resembles single-loop (adaptive) learning. One way to promote discovery is to encourage constant scanning for information about conditions and practices outside the organization's boundaries. Scanning promotes alertness, surfaces discrepant information, and uncovers new ideas. Scanning methods include benchmarking; ongoing contact with purchasers, suppliers, and partners; and soliciting feedback from employees, physicians, and patients.

7. The innovation journey often begins with discovery but thereafter cycles in nonpredictable ways between discovery and testing. It is important to manage expectations about the impacts of innovation. Even highly technical innovations involve major organizational challenges, such as shifting roles, prerogatives, and responsibilities. Acknowledging the challenging nature of the innovation journey up front will help mitigate frustration and keep lines of communication open.

8. Organizations can promote learning and innovation by nurturing foresight, fostering improvisation, maximizing serendipity, and learning from mistakes. Actively look for mistakes—unanticipated, unwanted consequences—from new programs. Repeatedly let your staff members know that mistakes are bound to occur, and the most essential thing is to understand how they occurred as a result and why. These mistakes may prove the most fertile ground for future innovation.

DISCUSSION QUESTIONS

1. Complexity theorists advise organizational leaders to abandon command-and-control styles of management and instead set global performance targets and establish a few simple rules. This approach can unleash creativity and innovation, but it can also promote conflict and waste. How can managers "let go of control," yet still ensure that organizational activities are coordinated with each other aligned with organizational goals? What could managers do to mitigate the potentially negative consequences of following complexity theorists' advice?

2. Organizational learning requires a climate of openness, trust, and honesty. What can managers do to establish and maintain such a climate?

3. How can managers hold health professionals and employees accountable for personal and organizational performance, yet still encourage them to try new ideas and take prudent risks to improve quality, safety, and efficiency?

4. If innovation is inherently unknowable and creates unintended consequences which are often far downstream, how can managers effectively evaluate the outcomes of innovation initiatives? Is there ever a point when a manager can reliably draw a conclusion about whether an innovation has been a success?

5. The Minnesota Innovation Research Project found that innovation managers' careers were often unfairly penalized when innovations turned out poorly. Is this an important concern for senior managers? If so, what can they do to mitigate it? What, if anything, should innovation managers do to protect themselves and their teams?

6. Schoemaker and Gunther (2006) recommend making deliberate mistakes as ways of breaking out of ineffective or suboptimal strategy borne of flawed or outdated assumptions. They provide some guidelines for which kinds of mistakes to deliberately make, such as those with a limited cost versus the potential gain. Based on their criteria, can you think of a potential "mistake" you might suggest to your primary-care provider to improve his or her clinic performance? For example, you might suggest that they eliminate visit co-pays. What are the costs or harms that make this a mistake? What are the assumptions that underpin the practice? What are the potential advantages?

CASE

Innovating for Care Coordination: Does Developing a New Program Make Sense?

Alliance Health System is a large hospital chain in the Northwest that serves over 80,000 covered lives each year. Alliance has been on the leading edge of care coordination, being one of the first in its region to partner with retail clinics, greatly expanding walk-in options for its patients. More recently, Alliance launched a new program called Personal Care Navigator (PCN). The PCN program aims to reduce total cost of care by reducing patient readmissions, preventing medication errors, and decreasing duplicate testing. The program was developed by a registered nurse who also serves as the administrator of patient navigation and care coordination at Alliance. She hopes to take traditional care management and social work support from the hospital setting and apply it to patients across the care continuum.

How does the PCN program work? Patients are first screened and evaluated by nurses and social workers, who determine whether the patients' individual circumstances call for a PCN. The role of a PCN is to identify barriers that might get in the patients' way—such as transportation issues or risk of taking medications incorrectly—remove those barriers, and connect patients with the services they need, when they need them. An example of a qualifying patient profile is: elderly, lives alone, and in need of a breast cancer screening. In this case, a PCN may call or send a letter to explain the screening and how to access the service. If the patient reveals she cannot get to the clinic, the PCN would help coordinate a bus ticket or another form of transportation. As another example, the program identifies patients who use the emergency room as their main source of care. PCNs reach out to these patients to find out why they keep returning to the emergency room. Is it a chronic condition? Are they aware of other sources of care? Are they having issues with their discharge orders?

The PCN program is now a year old, with generally favorable responses externally; the marketing campaign was well-received in the community, boosting the reputation of Alliance Health System. However, the response internally has been rather mixed. The vice president (VP) of quality and safety needs to decide whether to continue the PCN program. The VP has informal discussions with several stakeholders, including the chief of the emergency department, the chief nursing officer (CNO), the head of social work, and the chief financial officer (CFO). The chief of the emergency department cites that 10 percent of patients are confused about their discharge orders and that someone needs to look at the data to see whether the PCNs are helping to reduce that number. The CNO worries that using PCNs will create another legal vulnerability. She also expresses concerns about the quality of the PCN coordinators. The head of social work is enthusiastic about expanding the reach into the community, but she worries that no matter how sophisticated the training is for PCNs, the training can never reflect the complexity of a patient's needs and behaviors outside of the hospital setting. Finally, the CFO brings up concerns about unpredictable operating costs. The program has not demonstrated any cost savings and, in fact, had large up-front costs due to marketing (e.g., television ads, billboards, and booths are community fairs) as well as the hiring and training of dedicated PCN coordinators.

In light of these concerns, the VP decides to engage in a generative or double-loop learning cycle.

Questions

1. What are the underlying assumptions that drive the VP's interest in the Personal Care Navigator (PCN) program?

2. How can she or he explore or test those assumptions? In other words, how can he or she determine if the assumptions are incorrect?

3. What environmental events could change those assumptions?

REFERENCES

Anderson, V., & Johnson, L. (1997). *Systems thinking basics: From concepts to causal loops.* Cambridge, MA: Pegasus Communication.

Andriopoulos, C., & Gotsi, M. (2006). Probing the future: Mobilising foresight in multiple-product innovation firms. *Futures, 38*(1), 50–66.

Argote, L. (1999). *Organizational learning: Creating, retaining, and transferring knowledge.* Boston, MA: Kluwer Academic.

Argyris, C., & Schon, D. A. (1978). *Organizational learning.* Reading: MA: Addison-Wesley.

Arndt, M., & Bigelow, B. (2000). Commentary: The potential of chaos theory and complexity theory for health services management. *Health Care Management Review, 25*(1), 35–38.

Auerbach, A., Patel, M., Metlay, J., et al. (2014). The Hospital Medicine Reengineering Network (HOMERuN): A learning organization focused on improving hospital care. *Academic Medicine: Journal of the Association of American Medical Colleges, 89*(3), 415–420.

Baskerville, N. B., Liddy, C., & Hogg, W. (2012). Systematic review and meta-analysis of practice facilitation within primary care settings. *Annals of Family Medicine, 10*(1), 63–74.

Batista, M. D. G., Clegg, S., Pina e Cunha, M., et al. (2016). Improvising prescription: Evidence from the emergency room. *British Journal of Management, 27*(2), 406–425.

Begun, J. W. (1994). Chaos and complexity: Frontiers of organization science. *Journal of Management Inquiry, 3*(4), 329–335.

Begun, J. W., & Luke, R. D. (2001). Factors underlying organizational change in local health care markets, 1982–1995. *Health Care Management Review, 26*(2), 62–72.

Begun, J. W., Zimmerman, B., & Dooley, K. (2003). Health care organizations as complex adaptive systems. In S. S. Mick, & M. E. Wyttenbach (Eds.), *Advances in health care organization theory* (pp. 253–288). San Francisco, CA: Jossey-Bass.

Berquist, W. (1993). *The postmodern organization: Mastering the art of irreversible change.* San Francisco, CA: Jossey-Bass.

Berta, W., Cranley, L., Dearing, J., et al. (2015). Why (we think) facilitation works: Insights from organizational learning theory. *Implementation Science, 10*(1), 141.

Bohmer, R. M., & Edmondson, A. C. (2001). Organizational learning in health care. *Health Forum Journal, 44*(2), 32–35.

Boulton, J. G., Allen, P. M., & Bowman, C. (2015). *Embracing complexity: Strategic perspectives for an age of turbulence.* Oxford, UK: Oxford University Press.

Bowditch, J. L., Buono, A. F., & Stewart, M. M. (2007). *A primer on organizational behavior* (7th ed.). New York: John Wiley & Sons.

Brown, S. L., & Eisenhardt, K. M. (1997). The art of continuous change: Linking complexity theory and time-paced evolution in relentlessly shifting organizations. *Administrative Science Quarterly, 42*(1), 1–34.

Burnes, B. (2005). Complexity theories and organizational change. *International Journal of Management Reviews, 7*(2), 73–90.

Byrne, D. S., & Callaghan, G. (2013). *Complexity theory and the social sciences: The state of the art.* London: Taylor and Francis.

Choi, C., & Lee, H. (2015). Hetero expert innovation new product development through exploitation of ideas from other industries. *Research Technology Management, 58*(2), 40–46.

Chuang, Y. T., Ginsburg, L., & Berta, W. B. (2007). Learning from preventable adverse events in health care organizations: Development of a multilevel model of learning and propositions. *Health Care Management Review, 32*(4), 330–340.

Collins, J. C. (2001). *Good to great: Why some companies make the leap—and others don't.* New York: HarperBusiness.

Collins, J.C., & Porras, J. I. (1994). *Built to last: Successful habits of visionary companies.* New York: HarperBusiness.

Conrad, D., Fishman, P., Grembowski, D., et al. (2008). Access intervention in an integrated, prepaid group practice: Effects on primary care physician productivity. *Health Services Research*, 43(5), 1888–1905.

Crossan, M. M., Lane, H. W., & White, R. E. (1999). An organizational learning framework: From intuition to institution. *Academy of Management Review*, 24(3), 522–537.

Cunha, M. P. E., Clegg, S. R., & Mendonça, S. (2010). On serendipity and organizing. *European Management Journal*, 28(5), 319–330.

Cunha, M. P. E., Rego, A., Clegg, S., et al. (2015). The dialectics of serendipity. *European Management Journal*. 2015;33(1):9–19.

Cyert, R. M., & March, J. G. (1992). *A behavioral theory of the firm* (2nd ed.). Cambridge, MA: Blackwell Business.

Day, T. E., Sarawgi, S., Perri, A., et al. (2015). Reducing postponements of elective pediatric cardiac procedures: Analysis and implementation of a discrete event simulation model. *Annals of Thoracic Surgery*, 99(4), 1386–1391.

deBurca, S. (2000). The learning health care organization. *International Journal for Quality in Health Care*, 12(6), 457–458. https://doi.org/10.1093/intqhc/12.6.457.

Desroches, C., Charles, D., Furukawa, M., et al. (2013). Adoption of electronic health records grows rapidly, but fewer than half of US hospitals had at least a basic system in 2012. *Health Affairs (Project Hope)*, 32(8), 1478–1485.

Dickens, P. M. (2013). Facilitating emergent change in a health care setting. *Healthcare Management Forum*, 26(3), 116–126.

Dickinson, W. P., Dickinson, L. M., Nutting, P. A., et al. (2014). Practice facilitation to improve diabetes care in primary care: A report from the EPIC randomized clinical trial. *Annals of Family Medicine*, 12(1), 8–16.

Diwas, K., Staats, B., & Gino, F. (2013). Learning from my success and from others' failure: Evidence from minimally invasive cardiac surgery. *Management Science*, 59(11), 2435–2449.

Due, T., Thorsen, T., Kousgaard, M., et al. (2014). The effectiveness of a semi-tailored facilitator-based intervention to optimise chronic care management in general practice: A stepped-wedge randomised controlled trial. *BMC Family Practice*, 15, 65.

Dvorsky, G. (2013). The 12 cognitive biases that prevent you from being rational. *Gizmodo i09*. Retrieved January 15, 2018, from http://io9.gizmodo.com/5974468/the-most-common-cognitive-biases-that-prevent-you-from-being-rational.

Edmondson, A. (2011). Strategies of learning from failure. *Harvard Business Review*, 89(4), 48–55, 137.

Ericsson, K. A. (2006). The influence of experience and deliberate practice on the development of superior expert performance. In K. A. Ericsson (Ed.), *The Cambridge handbook of expertise and expert performance* (pp. 683–703). Cambridge: Cambridge University Press.

Ericsson, K. A. (2015). Acquisition and maintenance of medical expertise: A perspective from the expert-performance approach with deliberate practice. *Academic Medicine*, 90(11), 1471–1486.

Garvin, D. A. (1993). Building a learning organization. *Harvard Business Review*, 74(1), 78–91.

Garvin, D. A., Edmondson, A. C., & Gino, F. (2008). Is yours a learning organization? *Harvard Business Review*, 86(3), 109–116.

Gladwell, M. (2008). *Outliers: The story of success*. New York: Little, Brown and Company.

Goldsmith, D., & Siegel, M. (2012). Improving health care management through the use of dynamic simulation modeling and health information systems. *International Journal of Information Technologies and Systems Approach*, 5(1), 19–36.

Greenhalgh, T., Robert, G., Macfarlane, F., et al. (2004). Diffusion of innovations in service organizations: Systematic review and recommendations. *Milbank Quarterly*, 82(4), 581–629.

Gripenberg, P., Sveiby, K. E., & Segercrantz, B. (2012). Challenging the innovation paradigm: The prevailing pro-innovation bias. In K. E. Sveiby, P. Gripenberg, & B. Segercrantz (Eds.), *Challenging the innovation paradigm* (pp. 1–14). New York: Routledge.

Grunfeld, E., Manca, D., Moineddin, R., et al. (2013). Improving chronic disease prevention and screening in primary care: Results of the BETTER pragmatic cluster randomized controlled trial. *BMC Family Practice*, 14, 175.

Hamel, G. (2000). Waking up IBM: How a gang of unlikely rebels transformed Big Blue. *Harvard Business Review*, 78(4), 137–140.

Helfrich, C., Sylling, P., Gale, R., et al. (2016). The facilitators and barriers associated with implementation of a patient-centered medical home in VHA. *Implementation Science*, 11, 24.

Hock, D., & VISA International. (1999). *Birth of the chaordic age*. San Francisco, CA: Berrett-Koehler.

Holland, J. (2014). *Complexity: A very short introduction* (1st ed., *very short introductions*; 392). Oxford, UK: Oxford University Press.

Homer, J., Hirsch, G., Minniti, M., & Pierson, M. (2004). Models for collaboration: How system dynamics helped a community organize cost-effective care for chronic illness. *System Dynamics Review*, 20(3), 199–222.

Homer, J., Hirsch, G., & Milstein, B. (2007). Chronic illness in a complex health economy: The perils and promises of downstream and upstream reforms. *System Dynamics Review*, 23(2–3), 313–343.

Isaacs, W. (1999). *Dialogue and the art of thinking together*. New York: Random House.

Kahneman, D., Slovic, P., & Tversky, A. (Eds.). (1982). *Judgment under uncertainty: Heuristics and biases*. Cambridge: Cambridge University Press.

Kergosien, Y., Bélanger, V., Soriano, P., et al. (2015). A generic and flexible simulation-based analysis tool for EMS management. *International Journal of Production Research*, 53(24), 7299–7316.

La, E., Lich, K., Wells, R., et al. (2016). Increasing access to state psychiatric hospital beds: Exploring supply-side solutions. *Psychiatric Services*, 67(5), 523–528.

Landrigan, C. P., Parry, G. J., Bones, C. B., et al. (2010). Temporal trends in rates of patient harm resulting from medical care. *New England Journal of Medicine*, 363(22), 2124–2134.

Lapré, M. A., & Nembhard, I. M. (2011). Inside the organizational learning curve: Understanding the organizational learning process. *Foundations and Trends in Technology, Information and Operations Management, 4*(1), 1–103.

Lau, R., Stevenson, F., Ong, B. N., et al. (2015). Achieving change in primary care—effectiveness of strategies for improving implementation of complex interventions: Systematic review of reviews. *BMJ Open, 5*(12), e009993. DOI: 10.1136/bmjopen-2015-009993.

Leander, W. J. (1996). *Patients first: Experiences of a patient-focused pioneer.* Chicago, IL: Health Administration Press.

Lemak, C. H., & Goodrick, E. (2003). Strategy as simple rules: Understanding success in a rural clinic. *Health Care Management Review, 28*(2), 179–188.

Levy, P. F. (2001). The Nut Island effect: When good teams go wrong. *Harvard Business Review, 79*(3), 51–59.

Lich, K., Tian, Y., Beadles, C., et al. (2014). Strategic planning to reduce the burden of stroke among veterans: Using simulation modeling to inform decision making. *Stroke, 45*(7), 2078–2084.

Lindsay, G. (2013). Working beyond the cube: AT&T, Zappos, and other companies are sharing office space with strangers—and not to save rent. *Fast Company,* (173), 34.

Marshall, D., Burgos-Liz, L., Ijzerman, M., et al. (2015). Applying dynamic simulation modeling methods in health care delivery research-the SIMULATE Checklist: Report of the ISPOR Simulation Modeling Emerging Good Practices Task Force. *Value in Health, 18*(2), 353.

McCarthy, D., Mueller, K., & Tillmann, I. (2009). *Group Health Cooperative: Reinventing primary care by connecting patients with a medical home.* New York: The Commonwealth Fund.

McDaniel, R. R. (1997). Strategic leadership: A view from quantum and chaos theories. *Health Care Management Review, 22*(1), 21–37.

McDaniel, R. R., Driebe, D. J., & Lanham, H. (2013). Health care organizations as complex systems: New perspectives on design and management. *Advances in Health Care Management, 15*, 3–26.

McGill, M. E., & Slocum, J. W. (1993). Unlearning the Organization. *Organizational Dynamics, 22*, 67–78.

Meadows, D., & Wright, D. (2008) *Thinking in systems: A primer.* White River Junction, VT: Chelsea Green Publishing.

Miller, W., Crabtree, B., Nutting, P., et al. (2010). Primary care practice development: A relationship-centered approach. *Annals of Family Medicine, 8*(Suppl. 1), S68–S79.

Moorman, C., & Miner, A. S. (1998). Organizational improvisation and organizational memory. *Academy of Management Review, 23*(4), 698–723.

Mowles, C. (2011). *Rethinking management: Radical insights from the complexity sciences.* New York: Gower Publishing.

Noël, P. H., Robertson, M. L., Romero, R., et al. (2014). Key activities used by community based primary care practices to improve the quality of diabetes care in response to practice facilitation. *Quality in Primary Care, 22*(4), 211–219.

Nutting, P. A., Crabtree, B. F., Stewart, E. E., et al. (2010a). Effect of facilitation on practice outcomes in the National Demonstration Project Model of the patient-centered medical home. *Annals of Family Medicine, 8*(Suppl. 1), S33–S44, S92.

Nutting, P. A., Crabtree, B. F., Miller, W. L., et al. (2010b). Journey to the patient-centered medical home: A qualitative analysis of the experiences of practices in the National

Demonstration Project. *Annals of Family Medicine, 8*(Suppl. 1), S45–S56, S92.

Parchman, M., Noel, P., Culler, S., et al. (2013). A randomized trial of practice facilitation to improve the delivery of chronic illness care in primary care: Initial and sustained effects. *Implementation Science, 8*, 93.

Peters, T. J., & Waterman, R. H. (1982). *In search of excellence: Lessons from America's best-run companies.* New York: Harper & Row.

Pettigrew, A. M. (1985). *The awakening giant: Continuity and change in imperial chemical industries.* Oxford: Blackwell.

Pfeffer, J., & Sutton, R. I. (2006). *Hard facts, dangerous half-truths, and total nonsense: Profiting from evidence-based management.* Boston, MA: Harvard Business School Press.

Plsek, P. E., & Greenhalgh, T. (2001). Complexity science: The challenge of complexity in health care. *British Medical Journal, 323*(7313), 625–628.

Ralston, J. D., Martin, D. P., Anderson, M.L., et al. (2009). Group Health Cooperative's transformation toward patient-centered access. *Medical Care Research and Review, 66*(6), 703–724.

Reid, R. J., et al. (2009). Patient-centered medical home demonstration: A prospective, quasi-experimental, before and after evaluation. *American Journal of Managed Care, 15*(9), E71–E87.

Robert Wood Johnson Foundation. (2008). *Improving access to improve quality: Evaluation of an organizational innovation.* Washington, DC: AcademyHealth.

Rogers, E. M. (2003). *The diffusion of innovations* (5th ed.). New York: Free Press.

Rosenzweig, P. M. (2007). *The halo effect and the eight other business delusions that deceive managers.* New York: Free Press.

Sarpong, D., & Maclean, M. (2014). Unpacking strategic foresight: A practice approach. *Scandinavian Journal of Management, 30*(1), 16–26.

Scarpino, G. (2013). *The rise and fall of faith-based hospitals: The Allegheny County story.* Bloomington, IN: AuthorHouse.

Schilling, L., Dearing, J. W., Staley, P., et al. (2011). How Kaiser Permanente became a continuous learning organization (Press Release). Retrieved March 7, 2018, from https://share.kaiserpermanente.org/article/how-kaiser-permanente-became-a-continuous-learning-organization/.

Schoemaker, P. J. H., & Gunther, R. E. (2006). The wisdom of deliberate mistakes. *Harvard Business Review, 84*(6), 108–115.

Senge, P. M. (1990). *The fifth discipline: The art and practice of the learning organization.* New York: Currency Doubleday.

Senge, P. M. (2006). *The fifth discipline: The art and practice of the learning organization* (rev. and updated ed.). New York: Doubleday/Currency.

Senge, P. (2010). *The fifth discipline: The art & practice of the learning organization.* New York: Doubleday.

Senge, P. M. (2014). *The fifth discipline fieldbook: Strategies and tools for building a learning organization.* New York: Crown Publishing Group.

Skinner, J., Staiger, D., & Fisher, E. (2006). Is technological change in medicine always worth it? The case of acute myocardial infarction. *Health Affairs, 25*(2), W34–W47.

Stacey, R. D. (1995). The science of complexity: An alternative perspective for strategic change processes. *Strategic Management Journal, 16*(6), 477–495.

Sterman, J. D. (2000). *Business dynamics: Systems thinking and modeling for a complex world*. Boston, MA: Irwin McGraw-Hill.

Sturmberg, J., Martin, C., & Katerndahl, D. (2014). Systems and complexity thinking in the general practice literature: An integrative, historical narrative review. *Annals of Family Medicine, 12*(1), 66–74.

Tsoukas, H., & Shepherd, J. (2004). Coping with the future: Developing organizational foresightfulness—introduction. *Futures, 36*(2), 137–144.

Tu, S. P., Young, V., Coombs, L. J., et al. (2015). Practice adaptive reserve and colorectal cancer screening best practices at community health center clinics in seven states. *Cancer, 121*(8), 1241–1248.

Tucker, A. L., & Edmondson, A. C. (2003). Why hospitals don't learn from failures: Organizational and psychological dynamics that inhibit system change. *California Management Review, 45*(2), 55–72.

Tufano, J. T., Ralston, J. D., & Martin, D. P. (2008). Providers' experience with an organizational redesign initiative to promote patient-centered access: A qualitative study. *Journal of General Internal Medicine, 23*(11), 1778–1783.

Vaill, P. B. (1989). *Managing as a performing art: New ideas for a world of chaotic change*. San Francisco, CA: Jossey-Bass.

Van de Ven, A. H., Polley, D. E., Garud, R., et al. (1999). *The innovation journey*. New York: Oxford University Press.

Van de Ven, A. H., Venkataraman, S., Polley, D., et al. (1989). Processes of new business creation in different organizational settings. In A. H. Van de Ven, H. L. Angle, & M. S. Poole (Eds.), *Research on the management of innovation: The Minnesota studies* (pp. 221–298). New York: Ballinger/Harper & Row.

Weick, K. (1979). *The social psychology of organizing*. Reading, MA: Addison-Wesley.

Weick, K. E. (1993). Sensemaking in organizations: Small structures with large consequences. In J. K. Murningham (Ed.), *Social psychology in organizations: Advances in theory and research* (pp. 10–37). Englewood Cliffs, NJ: Prentice Hall.

Wermers, M. A., Dagnillo, R., Glenn, R., et al. (1996). Planning and assessing a cross-training initiative with multiskilled employees. *Joint Commission Journal on Quality Improvement, 22*(6), 412–426.

Wheatley, M. J. (2006). *Leadership and the new science: Discovering order in a chaotic world* (3rd ed.). San Francisco, CA: Berrett-Koehler.

Wheatley, M. J. (1992). *Leadership and the new science: Learning about organization from an orderly universe*. San Francisco, CA: Berrett-Koehler.

Wright, P. M., George, J. M., Farnsworth, S. R., et al. (1993). Productivity and extra-role behavior—the effects of goals and incentives on spontaneous helping. *Journal of Applied Psychology, 78*(3), 374–381.

Chapter 9

Improving Quality in Health Care Organizations (HCOs)

Jennifer L. Hefner and Ann Scheck McAlearney

CHAPTER OUTLINE

- Quality Improvement in Health Care
- Approaches to Quality Improvement
- Performance Measurement in Quality Improvement
- Getting to Higher Quality and Quality Improvement
- Applying Quality Improvement Frameworks

LEARNING OBJECTIVES

After completing this chapter, the reader should be able to:

1. Explain the importance of quality improvement (QI) in health care
2. Define quality and performance measures for organizations
3. Differentiate the important issues in using quality and performance measures
4. Identify the challenges of undertaking QI and implementing QI in health care organizations (HCOs)
5. Distinguish among QI frameworks
6. Describe opportunities to apply QI tactics and strategies to support QI in HCOs
7. Assess conditions for QI change
8. Justify the need to manage for QI in health care
9. Explain the importance of people and focusing on people issues in QI efforts
10. Describe management roles to create high-performance, quality-focused organizations

KEY TERMS

Access

Benchmarking

Clinical Practice Guidelines

Continuous Quality Improvement (CQI)

High-Performance Work Practices (HPWPs)

Implementation

Lean

Outcome Measures of Performance

Patient Experience Measures

Performance Improvement

Performance Measures

Plan–Do–Study–Act (PDSA) Method

Process Measures of Performance

Quality Improvement (QI)

Quality Improvement (QI) Interventions

Six Sigma

Structural Measures of Performance

Transactional Leadership

Transformational Leadership

• • • IN PRACTICE: Sharp HealthCare and Its Quality Improvement Journey

Sharp HealthCare is a large, not-for-profit health system based in San Diego, California. With over 14,000 employees and 2,600 physician affiliates, the system is comprised of four acute-care hospitals, three specialty hospitals, and two medical groups, and includes a wide range of other facilities and services. Given its location in a highly regulated state, Sharp faces particular challenges associated with corporate practice of medicine laws and the laws regulating nurse-staff ratios as they impact Sharp's abilities to employ and deploy health care professionals throughout their organization. Yet despite these challenges, Sharp HealthCare has received increased attention over the past decade as it has received national recognition for Magnet designation for nursing excellence at two of its acute-care hospitals, national designation as a Planetree hospital at another acute-care hospital, and the prestigious 2007 Malcolm Baldrige Award for Quality for the system as a whole.

Sharp's self-described quality improvement "journey" has been multifaceted and has touched the entire health system. In the late 1990s, Sharp had a solid reputation in the San Diego area, and patient satisfaction scores collected by the organization were high, indicating that there was not much to worry about. A change in system leadership, however, created an opportunity to focus on quality and quality improvement in a new way.

Curious about how they were doing, Sharp decided to convene some focus groups to find out how patients felt about their health care experience. Much to the surprise and chagrin of health system leaders, Sharp's patients told them the experience was not all that good, and health care in general left much to be desired from a customer perspective. Instead of confirming their belief that Sharp was well regarded by satisfied patients, these focus groups indicated many opportunities for improvement. The health system began to benchmark data against other health systems and contracted with Press Ganey for patient satisfaction measurement. Patient satisfaction scores as measured by the new scale were in the lowest quartile.

Sharp's leaders used these data to spark employee interest in quality and performance improvement and to motivate employees to address needed changes. Over the course of the next decade, Sharp made a substantial investment in **Lean** and Six Sigma methods as its selected approaches to **performance improvement** and built a QI focus into the culture of the organization. In addition, as an organizing framework for the QI journey, Sharp designed The Sharp Experience as a performance improvement initiative designed to help Sharp realize its mission-driven goal to be *the best place to work, the best place to practice medicine, and the best place to receive care*. Sharp's receipt of the coveted Baldrige Award for Quality in 2007 provided public recognition of Sharp's success in its QI journey. Now beyond Baldrige, Sharp continues to capitalize on opportunities for QI and is currently driving improvements in patient safety, including "just culture," transparency, team training, standardized communication processes, handoff standardization, and design change to improve quality of care and patient safety throughout the health system. Most recently, Sharp HealthCare was recognized as "Most Wired" in 2016, was ranked 16th Best Employer in America by Forbes out of 500 large employers, and was recognized as a 2017 World's Most Ethical Company.

SOURCE: Nancy G. Pratt, RN, MS, Senior Vice President, Clinical Effectiveness, Sharp HealthCare; Sharp HealthCare website (http://www.sharp.com)

CHAPTER PURPOSE

With the release of the Institute of Medicine's (IOM's) report, *To Err Is Human: Building a Safer Health System* (2000), quality and patient safety reemerged as sentinel issues in health care delivery. The Institute's report prompted renewed effort to identify and implement **quality improvement (QI) interventions**, interventions designed to decrease medical errors and enhance patient safety. It also rekindled attempts to hold health care organizations (HCOs) accountable for quality. Government agencies, accrediting bodies, employer groups, and other organizations have developed an ever-growing number of performance measures and patient safety goals against which they intend to measure a health care organization's quality performance and improvement over time. Table 9.1 presents a sample of two types of these metrics—organizational measures and clinical measures. One five-hospital Academic Medical Center recently claimed that it reports 1,600 unique measures to 49 different sources (Murray et al., 2017). In many cases these measures are publicly reported, on websites such as the Centers for Medicare and Medicaid Services (CMS) Hospital Compare, and they are also used by groups such as Healthgrades, Leapfrog, and *U.S. News and World Report* to rank top performers on domains such as clinical processes, patient outcomes, and patient experience ratings. This chapter outlines how HCOs can

Table 9.1 Examples of Quality Measures

Organizational Metrics	Clinical Metrics (Institute of Medicine's Aims for Improvement—IOM 2001)
Quality of Work Life • Perceptions of work–life balance • Often derived from organizational survey	*Safe* • Standardized mortality rate for unit, for organization • Adverse drug events per doses (1,000) administered
Employee Satisfaction with the Organization • Willingness to refer a friend or relative to the organization • Willingness to seek care within the organization • Employee turnover rates	*Effective* • Lost days of work per employee • Growth in market share for organization • Statistics related to patient safety • Perceptions about quality of care within organizational culture
Financial Metrics • Margins, etc. • Bed days per 1,000 • Market share	*Patient-Centered* • Patient satisfaction with unit, with organization • Drill down into patient education statistics
Patient Satisfaction • With care, safety, providers • Willingness to refer friend/relative for care	*Timely* • Access to care as measured by waiting times, other process measures • Measurement of delays in care
Achievement of Strategic Goals • Alignment with balanced scorecard goals • Achievement of national patient safety goals • Participation in Institute for Healthcare Improvement (IHI) campaigns	*Efficient* • Cost per adjusted hospital admission • Operating margin as measured by cash from operations *Equitable* • Disparities in care access • Disparities in utilization • Disparities in referrals made

improve quality and patient safety through QI efforts and describes the challenges and strategies for changing organizational systems to ensure that QI is an accepted part of organizational behavior.

QUALITY IMPROVEMENT IN HEALTH CARE

Almost everyone agrees that high quality is an important and desirable characteristic of health care services. However, quality can be a difficult concept to define. Donabedian (2005) observed that although quality can be very broadly defined, it usually reflects the values and goals of the current medical system and of the larger society of which it is a part. According to Donabedian (1988), there are three major elements of quality: structure, process, and outcomes. *Structure* pertains to having the necessary resources to provide adequate health care; *process* focuses on how care is provided, delivered, and managed; and *outcomes* refers to changes in a patient's health status as a result of medical care.

Another definition of quality that is commonly used and widely accepted in health care is contained in the influential report from the Institute of Medicine (IOM), *Crossing the Quality Chasm: A New Health System for the 21st Century*. This report defined quality as "the degree to which health services for individuals and populations increase the likelihood of desired health outcomes and are consistent with current professional knowledge" (Institute of Medicine Committee on Quality of Health Care, 2001). The report also discussed the six major aims for improvement in health care, which emphasize the need for care to be *safe, effective, patient-centered, timely, efficient,* and *equitable*. HCOs, then, are challenged to provide care, or support the microsystems that deliver care, in a manner that achieves these aims (Berwick, Nolan, and Whittington, 2008).

The current consensus in the scientific literature is that quality is a multidimensional concept including both patient experiences of care as well as clinical quality measures such as readmission and adverse events (Lehrman et al., 2010; Price et al., 2014). The CMS acknowledges this by linking value-based purchasing penalties to a variety of performance measures across these dimensions. Measures include Donabedian's elements of structure, process, and outcomes. Recently, there has been a move toward public reporting of these measures and ranking hospitals to identify top performers. However, there is a lack of consensus around how to define quality in order to achieve this goal. Healthgrades, the Leapfrog Group, *U.S. News and World Report*, Press Ganey, and CMS Hospital Compare all publish a yearly list of top performers in which they score hospitals using different methodologies and, by extension, different definitions of quality. Pressure from this public reporting, as well as given the spread of payer reimbursement incentives and penalties, is driving HCOs to focus on improving their scores across measures and dimensions of quality. The key to success in this effort is quality improvement.

Quality Improvement

Quality improvement (QI) is an organized approach to planning and implementing processes driving continuous improvement in performance. QI emphasizes continuous examination and improvement of work processes by teams of organizational members trained in basic statistical techniques and problem-solving tools, and who are empowered to make decisions based on their analysis of the data. Typically, QI efforts are strongly rooted in evidence-based procedures and rely extensively on data collected about the processes and outcomes experienced by patients in organizations. Table 9.2 presents a glossary of common terms and programs associated with QI in Health Care.

Similar to other systems-based approaches, QI stresses that quality depends foremost on the processes by which services are designed and delivered. The systemic focus of QI complements a growing recognition in the field that the quality of the care delivered by clinicians depends substantially on the performance capability of the organizational systems in which they work. While individual clinician competence remains important, many increasingly see that the capability of organizational systems to prevent errors, to coordinate care among settings and practitioners, and to ensure that relevant, accurate information is available when needed is critical in providing high-quality care (Elder et al., 2008). This systems-based perspective on QI emphasizes organization-wide commitment and involvement because most, if not all, vital work processes span many individuals, disciplines, and departments in all clinical settings.

Table 9.2 Glossary of Common Terms and Programs Associated with QI in Health Care

AIDET: A communication tool espoused by the Studer Group, designed to help clinicians establish trust with patients in order to improve compliance and clinical outcomes. AIDET is an acronym that stands for Acknowledge, Introduce, Duration, Explanation, and Thank You (http://www.studergroup.com/dotCMS/detailProduct?inode=110454).

Baldrige Award: A prestigious national award to companies in several categories, including health care that recognizes demonstrated excellence in seven categories: leadership; strategic planning; customer and market focus; measurement, analysis, and knowledge management; workforce focus; process management; and results. Applications are reviewed by an independent Board of Examiners (http://www.baldrige.nist.gov/).

Benchmarking: A key feature of many QI approaches, benchmarking is the process of comparing an organization's performance metrics (e.g., quality, cost, operational efficiency) to those of other "best practice" or peer organizations.

Business Process Reengineering (BPR): Term used to describe efforts to radically review and reorganize existing work processes, or adopt new and innovative work processes, designed to improve customer value, organizational efficiency, and market competitiveness. A key to BPR is the development of organizational and management structures to effectively support the redesign (e.g., information technology) (see Hammer, 1990).

Clinical Practice Guidelines: Typically developed by expert panels, clinical practice guidelines synthesize evidence from the literature and make recommendations regarding treatment for specific clinical conditions (see IOM, 2001). The National Guideline Clearinghouse (http://www.guideline.gov) is a publicly available resource for evidence-based guidelines covering a full range of clinical conditions.

Continuous Quality Improvement (CQI): A participative, systematic approach to planning and implementing a continuous organizational improvement process.

Table 9.2 Glossary of Common Terms and Programs Associated with QI in Health Care *(Continued)*

Crew Resource Management (CRM): A technique from the aviation field that addresses errors resulting from communication and decision making in dynamic environments, such as teams, that has been adopted in the health care field to improve patient safety. CRM is among the evidence-based safety practices included in the Agency for Healthcare Research and Quality's document entitled "Making Health Care Safer: A Critical Analysis of Patient Safety Practices Evidence Report/Technology Assessment, No. 43." (http://www.ncbi.nlm.nih.gov/ bookshelf/br.fcgi?book=erta43&part=A64100).

Crucial Conversations: Refers to concepts and techniques articulated in Patterson et al. (2002).

Fortune "Best Places to Work": *Fortune* magazine's annual ranking of U.S. companies with greater than 1,000 FTEs that have been nominated as a "great place to work." Awards are based on results of employee surveys (in 2009, 81,000 employees surveyed across 353 companies) and a "culture audit" conducted in each company (http://www.greatplacetowork.com/).

High-Reliability Organizations: High-reliability organizations (HROs) are those that have incorporated a culture and processes to "radically reduce system failures and effectively respond when failures occur" (http://www.ahrq.gov/ qual/hroadvice/hroadviceexecsum.htm).

High-Performance Work Practices (HPWPs): Workforce or human resource practices that have been shown to improve an organization's capacity to effectively attract, select, hire, develop, and retain high-performing employees.

Just Culture/Just Safety Culture: Term used to describe an organizational culture that encourages open dialogue to facilitate patient safety practices; often described in contrast to a "blame" culture (that focus on individuals, rather than systems, as the source of safety infractions). A just culture gives some "leeway to individuals, but is still premised on . . . accountability and bureaucratic control." More recently, scholars are advocating that just culture focus on organizational learning in the areas of quality and safety (Khatri, Brown, and Hicks, 2009).

Lean: A management and operations improvement approach, often described as a "transformation" that focuses on eliminating waste across "value streams" that flow horizontally across technologies, assets, and departments (as opposed to improving within each). The intent of a Lean approach is cost-effectiveness, error reduction, and improved service to customers. The term "Lean" was originally coined by Jim Womack, PhD, to describe innovations in Toyota's manufacturing processes (http://www.lean.org).

Magnet Status: A prestigious external designation from the "Magnet" program, this status recognizes hospitals that demonstrate 14 characteristics that comprise an excellent working environment for nurses (e.g., nursing leadership, quality of patient care, level of nursing autonomy, staffing ratios, professional development) (http://www.nursecredentialing.org/Magnet).

Pay-for-Performance (P4P): Reimbursement for health care services which is designed to link payment incentives to quality and performance outcomes. Demonstration programs to test various approaches have been under way through the Centers for Medicare and Medicaid Services (see IOM, 2007).

Pebble Project: An initiative through the Center for Health Design, which works with partners to develop facilities that incorporate "evidence-based design" features that have been demonstrated to reduce errors, improve quality and efficiency, and improve work experience (https://www.healthdesign.org/research-services/pebble-project).

Performance Improvement International: A consulting company that espouses a system-oriented, engineering-based performance improvement methodology, which uses performance indicators and root cause analysis to reduce errors and improve performance (http://www.errorfree.com).

Planetree: The Planetree Institute has developed a model of care that is a "patient-centered, holistic approach to healthcare, promoting mental, emotional, spiritual, social, and physical healing. It empowers patients and families through the exchange of information and encourages healing partnerships with caregivers. It seeks to maximize positive healthcare outcomes by integrating optimal medical therapies and incorporating art and nature into the healing environment." Planetree partners adapt the model to fit their unique circumstances (http://www .planetree.org/).

Table 9.2 Glossary of Common Terms and Programs Associated with QI in Health Care *(Continued)*

Quality Improvement Organization (QIO): The Centers for Medicare and Medicaid Services contracts with QIOs in each state to monitor, report on, and facilitate improvements in the appropriateness, effectiveness, and quality of care provided to Medicare beneficiaries (http://www.cms.gov/QualityImprovementOrgs/).

Six Sigma: A data-driven methodology for eliminating defects in any process by applying a consistent framework of DMAIC (define, measure, analyze, improve, control) to minimize variation and improve processes. Six Sigma was started at Motorola and has been widely adopted at other companies, including General Electric (http://www.isixsigma.com).

Studer Group: A health care consulting organization "devoted to teaching evidence-based tools and processes that organizations can immediately use to create and sustain outcomes in service and operational excellence." Additional ideas and methods are available from leader Quint Studer (e.g., Studer, 2003) through Web-based resources, a newsletter, and organizational consulting engagements (http://www.studergroup.com).

Total Quality Management (TQM): A participative, systematic approach to planning and implementing QI in quality.

QI Interventions

QI interventions vary widely (Chassin and Loeb, 2011). *Externally developed* QI involves looking outside the organization for new or redesigned practices—often evidence-based—to bring into the organization. The emphasis of the intervention is on the desired new practice. Many efforts to bring research into practice, such as guideline implementation, fall into this category. By contrast, in *locally developed* QI, the improvement process begins with a problem, but participants do not know what the improved practices will look like; solutions evolve through analysis and experimentation. In this case, the emphasis is on changing the process by which a service or product is produced. Still other QI interventions are broadly predefined but allow for considerable flexibility and local tailoring.

In practice, QI interventions can also be described in organizational terms. Interventions can be described (1) by the *levels of organization* at which the intervention is targeted (e.g., individual level; microsystem level such as teams, work units or departments; or at the macrosystem level of the full organization) and (2) by the *scale of the intervention* (e.g., single medical center or clinic, multiple sites, or national rollout). Specifying the level and scale of QI interventions can help organizational members better understand the nature of the QI goals as well as the potential reach and impact of the QI intervention.

Quality Improvement Interventions

Within the QI frameworks discussed above, a variety of interventions can be employed to alter the behavior of health care providers within an organization. Common interventions include audit and feedback, reminders, pay-for-performance (P4P), continuing medical education, clinical decision support (CDS), practice facilitation, and incident reporting systems. Table 9.3 presents a summary of the effectiveness of each of these interventions based on findings from systematic reviews available in the scientific literature.

Most of these QI efforts show small to modest improvements in adherence to evidence-based clinical practice. However, there is less evidence linking these improvement strategies to patient outcomes. When aiming to change clinical processes to meet performance metrics, HCO managers should select the intervention strategy that best fits with the target metrics and is most widely supported by a multidisciplinary QI team of "frontline" staff and clinicians. For example, if the goal is to increase adherence to asthma guidelines, then continuing medical education may be an appropriate first intervention, followed by CDS if the HCO has resources to incorporate CDS into its electronic health record (EHR) system. If EHR resources are scarce but managerial engagement is high, audit and feedback of individual providers or units may be an effective alternative strategy.

Table 9.3 Quality Improvement Interventions and Evidence for Their Effects

QI Interventions	Effect	Systematic Review Citation
Audit and Feedback	Small improvements in professional practice	Ivers N., Jamtvedt G., Flottorp S., et al. (2012). Audit and feedback: Effects on professional practice and healthcare outcomes. *Cochrane Database of Systematic Reviews, 6*, CD000259.
Reminders	Modest improvements in professional practice	Cheung A., Weir M., Mayhew A., Kozloff N., Brown K., & Grimshaw J. (2012). Overview of systematic reviews of the effectiveness of reminders in improving healthcare professional behavior. *Systematic Review, 1*, 36.
Pay for Performance (P4P)	a) Varying improvements in professional practice; best outcomes when adapted to hospital characteristics b) No widespread effect on health outcomes c) Varying effectiveness in professional practice and insufficient evidence on effect of patient outcomes	a) Stavropoulou C., Doherty C., & Tosey P. (2015). How effective are incident-reporting systems for improving patient safety? A systematic literature review. *Milbank Quarterly, 93*(4), 826–866. b) Mendelson A., Kondo K., Damberg C., et al. (2017). The effects of pay-for-performance programs on health, health care use, and processes of care: A systematic review. *Annals of Internal Medicine, 166*(5), 341–353. c) Flodgren G., Eccles M. P., Shepperd S., Scott A., Parmelli E., & Beyer F. R. (2011). An overview of reviews evaluating the effectiveness of financial incentives in changing healthcare professional behaviours and patient outcomes. *Cochrane Database of Systematic Reviews, 7*, CD009255.
Continuing Medical Education	Small improvements in professional practice	Forsetlund L., Bjorndal A., Rashidian A., et al. (2009). Continuing education meetings and workshops: Effects on professional practice and health care outcomes. *Cochrane Database of Systematic Reviews, 2*, CD003030.
Practice Facilitation	Moderately robust effect on evidence-based guideline adoption within primary care	Baskerville N. B., Liddy C., & Hogg W. (2012). Systematic review and meta-analysis of practice facilitation within primary care settings. *Annals of Family Medicine, 10*(1), 63–74.
Clinical Decision Support	Improvement in preventive services, appropriate care, and clinical and cost outcomes with strong evidence for clinical decision support system (CDSS) effectiveness in process measures	Murphy E. V. (2014). Clinical decision support: Effectiveness in improving quality processes and clinical outcomes and factors that may influence success. *Yale Journal of Biology and Medicine, 87*(2), 187–197
Incident-Reporting Systems	Evidence indicates that improved definitions of "incident" and management at the clinical team versus organizational level would improve effectiveness	Stavropoulou C., Doherty C., & Tosey P. How effective are incident-reporting systems for improving patient safety? A systematic literature review. *Milbank Quarterly 93*(4), 826–866.

• • • IN PRACTICE: Million Hearts Initiative

Heart disease and stroke are responsible for over 800,000 deaths annually in the United States and contribute an estimated $316.6 billion in health care costs and loss of productivity (Department of Health and Human Services, 2017). To address both human and monetary costs, the Department of Health and Human Services (DHHS) and other governmental and private sector partners launched the "Million Hearts Initiative" in 2011 (U.S. Centers for Medicare & Medicaid Services, 2017). This initiative was developed to provide standardized guidance on clinical and community interventions that could be implemented to prevent one million heart attacks and strokes by 2017.

The program is based on the "ABCS" (appropriate aspirin use, blood pressure control, cholesterol management, and smoking cessation) of cardiovascular management. Tools were developed to help practices understand and implement a standard practice for screening and managing patients with cardiovascular disease.

In 2015, the DHHS announced additional programming, the "Million Hearts: CVD Risk Reduction Model." This is a value-based payment model that awards payments to providers who successfully reduce their patients' risk of heart disease. Outcomes of the program are only beginning to be published, but there are initial reports of its effectiveness. Ritchey et al. (2017) estimated a reduction in 115,000 heart attack and strokes between 2012 and 2013. They suggest that while the Million Hearts Initiative cannot be the sole factor reducing these events, there is evidence to indicate suggest that efforts being made throughout the country as part of this initiative have positively impacted the risk of death by cardiovascular disease.

Additional evidence of the program's success is found in the California Medicaid program (Implementing a Quality Improvement Collaborative to Improve Hypertension Control and Advance Million Hearts among Low-Income Californians, 2014–2015). The organization partnered with nine managed-care programs to improve hypertension management in its patient population using Million Hearts Initiative guidelines. This programming was associated with a significant improvement of blood pressure control in seven of the nine managed care programs.

The effectiveness of the Million Hearts Initiative in preventing one million heart attacks and strokes has yet to be determined. However, it does appear that providing standardized practice guidelines to providers can have a population-level impact on health care outcomes.

APPROACHES TO QUALITY IMPROVEMENT

All forms of QI share certain principles. QI approaches focus on making improvements that are systematic, guided by data, and efficient (Lynn et al., 2007). Key elements of QI approaches include continuous improvement, customer focus, structured processes, and organization-wide participation (Shortell et al., 1995). These approaches are often based on experiential learning, view improvement as part of the work process, and involve deliberate steps that are expected to improve care (Lynn et al., 2007). Often, an organization employs multiple QI approaches together.

Continuous Quality Improvement

Continuous quality improvement (CQI) is a QI approach that originated in the mid-1980s. The CQI movement focuses on improving organizational processes, which in turn creates better quality. Through CQI, one applies scientific work processes using effective, straightforward techniques. As opposed to QI approaches, such as clinical practice guidelines, CQI focuses on the use of generic analytic techniques that facilitate improvement of both clinical and nonclinical processes. CQI is also characterized by its encouragement of managerial reforms that are designed to bring about organizational change. Such reforms include the need to empower employees to learn and participate in the continuous improvement process. Due to these elements, CQI is often described as a cultural mindset. Two prominent CQI approaches are **Six Sigma** and the **Plan–Do–Study–Act (PDSA) Method**. In the following sections, we outline these two approaches, describe the steps, and present commonly used tools.

Six Sigma

Six Sigma is a QI approach invented by Motorola in the mid-1980s. "Sigma" is a term used in statistics that indicates variation. The premise for the Six Sigma strategy is that if you can measure the number of defects that occur in a process, you can systematically work to eliminate them, getting as close to zero defects as possible. The goal is to reduce variation by employing the DMAIC (define, measure, analyze, improve, control) system to improve processes (Adams et al., 2004). Although Six Sigma was first applied to manufacturing, it is relevant to the health care field as well. In health care, the number of defects might be the number of diabetes patients who do not receive an annual eye exam, per million diabetes patients. Six Sigma is known as a data-driven approach to QI. As such there are a number of tools associated with this method, commonly referred to as the Six Sigma Toolkit. In the Define and Measure stages, tools such as the process flowchart, a tree diagram, and a value stream map can be used to collect data about the processes under study. In the Analyze phase, a cause and effect matrix (fishbone diagram) is a tool that can be used to identify the root causes of a problem. In the Improve and Control phases, there are additional sets of tools that can be used to implement and measure improvement.

Plan-Do-Study-Act

The Institute for Healthcare Improvement (IHI) model employs the PDSA methodology to guide QI interventions. The steps of this methodology are to establish aims, define the problem, identify success metrics, and systematically implement a QI intervention in short, rapid cycles. The IHI model emphasizes that the PDSA cycle is for action-oriented learning. The cycle is meant to test a change on a small scale, reevaluate the process, and then test on a broader scale. This model can be applied to small QI interventions implemented by one physician in her own practice and to large-scale changes in health care process on the level of a health care system.

The field of program evaluation is one place where the PDSA cycle features prominently as a methodology. A program evaluation focuses on determining the success of a program according to predefined goals to determine the need for adjustments to future programming. QI is framed as an important element in the program evaluation process. The PDSA cycle can be employed in this context to plan the evaluation of a program, implement the program, study the effects based on the predefined performance metrics, and act upon findings to improve the program. Run charts are a tool that can be used to determine if a

PDSA cycle has resulted in improvements to the program or process. Though the analysis and interpretation of a run chart can be complicated, the chart itself is a simple plotting of a performance metric over time.

The different QI approaches are not mutually exclusive. The PDSA framework can be used to achieve small, quick wins on projects, and can be used in concert with a Six Sigma focus on data analytics. Lean is another QI approach that focuses on improving operational efficiency through reducing waste and creating value. Lean is often used in concert with Six Sigma. The Health Information Technology Research Center (HITRC)—funded by a consortium of U.S. Health and Human Services Agencies and tasked with improving health care through health information technology (HIT)—recommends focusing on a culture of CQI and utilizing a combination of these approaches to achieve quality goals.

PERFORMANCE MEASUREMENT IN QUALITY IMPROVEMENT

In order for organizations to focus on quality and QI in health care, they must understand how quality is measured and monitored. Similar to how QI interventions can be measured, performance can be measured at various levels of the organization, including across an organization, at a single clinic, or for a single provider. The level of measurement guides the scope of the QI intervention as well as the evaluation goal. The following sections describe metrics and measurement of quality and discuss some of the issues related to the definition and use of different performance measures to drive QI efforts in HCOs, and Table 9.4 summarizes this information and presents examples of both the metrics and data sources for those measures.

Table 9.4 Performance Measure Domains, Example Metrics, and Data Sources

Performance Measure Category	Examples	Potential Sources
Structure	Nurse/patient ratios, EHR meaningful use stage, certification and accreditation	Administrative data
Access	Wait time for a specialty referral, emergency department wait time	Administrative data, medical records
Process	Rate of preventive services, rate of controlled blood pressure or diabetes, compliance with safety protocols	Administrative data, medical records
Outcomes	30-day readmission rate, health care-associated infections, mortality rate	Administrative data, medical records
Patient Experience	Patient satisfaction, cleanliness, provider communication	Patient surveys, patient interviews

Performance Measures

Based on Donabedian's (1966) definition of quality in health care, three basic domains of **performance measures** have been specified: structural, process, and outcome measures. First, **structural measures of performance** are defined as those based on aspects of an organization or an individual's actions that could impact overall quality or organizational performance. From a business operations standpoint these structural measures are associated with the capacity of an organization to promote effective work. Examples of structural measures of quality in health care are numerous and include indicators such as the number and type of beds in a given organization, the ownership model, and the existence of an EHR system. Even the presence of certain organizational certifications or accolades can be used as structural measures of performance, including accreditation by the Joint Commission or receipt of Magnet status in nursing.

Access is another quality domain often placed under the structural measure category. Measures of access are considered to be under the control of health care managers and are therefore becoming more commonly used as measures of quality. Access refers to the ability of patients to get the care they need at the time they need it. Access metrics are often used in the ambulatory setting and include measures such as the "on hold" time when a patient calls a clinic, the percentage of patients who are scheduled for a new patient visit by a certain time frame (e.g., within 30 days), and waiting times for scheduled appointments. Access measures can also be used in the hospital, including the wait-time for an ED bed or referral time to see a doctor at a specialty clinic.

Next, **process measures of performance** refer to indicators of the activities involved in carrying out work in an organization. Activities such as reviewing medical records to ensure completion of patient education, monitoring physician and nurse compliance with organizational standards for cleanliness, or evaluating the use of central lines are all examples of process metrics. Process measures are often favored over structural measures because they are perceived to be more closely linked to clinical care quality, and because they are viewed as firmly within the span of control managers have to influence and improve work processes (Grossbart and Agrawal, 2012).

Third, **outcome measures of performance** are metrics based on the results of work performed. In many ways, outcome measures can be considered measures, of work process outputs. Examples of outcome measures in health care are numerous and include metrics, such as readmission rates, patient safety incidents, and mortality. Patient-reported outcomes (PROs) are a class of outcome measures that incorporate the patient voice into the collection of quality of care information. A PRO is directly reported by the patient and refers to the patient's service satisfaction, functional status, or quality of life. PROs related to service satisfaction are referred to as **patient experience measures**, a subdomain of outcomes that is typically considered a separate class of measures for reporting and QI purposes.

Sources of Data for Performance Measures

Data for performance measures can come from a variety of sources including administrative data, patient medical records, patient surveys, and patient interviews. Administrative data, sometimes called claims data, are used both to pay bills and to manage care at the population level. The limitations to using this type of data for performance measurement include the bias inherent in the initial purpose of reimbursement and an associated lack of clinical precision. Patient medical records offer more precise clinical documentation but the process of pulling data from individual medical charts can be laborious. The proliferation of EHRs has facilitated the use of medical records for research and QI. However, there are barriers to using EHR data, including the need for sophisticated data warehousing and capabilities for report generation at the institution level.

Patient surveys are a data source for PROs. The Hospital Consumer Assessment of Healthcare Providers and Systems (HCAHPS) survey is a patient satisfaction survey required by CMS for all hospitals in the United States. In addition to reporting the results of this survey to CMS, health care managers can use the various metrics in the survey—provider communication, cleanliness, and hospital rating—as data sources for QI interventions. PROMs (patient-reported outcome measures) turn PROs into a numerical score. The most widely known source of PROMS is PROMIS. Through PROMIS (patient-reported outcomes measurement information system), the National Institutes of Health (NIH) supported the creation of an item bank of rigorously developed and validated measures of patient-reported health, well-being, and functioning. The final source of data to mention is comments from individual patients, either from open-ended survey questions, in person interviews, or post-discharge telephone calls. This type of performance data can be used to provide context to quantitative metrics when evaluating QI interventions.

Using Performance Measures for QI

The performance measures discussed in the above sections are used by HCOs in public reporting, accreditation/licensure, payment models, and to conduct QI interventions. A key foundation of any QI effort is the ability to accurately measure quality and use those measures to identify problems, monitor progress, and formulate strategies to improve quality of care. A 2012 study of 70 large, prominent HCOs found that 69 percent reported using a variety of performance measures in their QI efforts (Damberg et al., 2012). The National Quality Forum (NQF), a nonprofit organization that establishes consensus standards for measuring performance, has endorsed more than 700 measures that can be found on the NQF website in a searchable directory categorized by measure type, measure steward (entity that designed and maintains the measures), or care settings.

Given the large number of available measures, there is a need to balance using a concise number of performance measures with the flexibility to choose measures that fit the QI goals of specific projects. This is true at the policy level for CMS and insurance companies when developing reimbursement models and incentive programs, and it is true for managers of HCOs and hospital quality departments. Measures that an HCO reports to external entities for payment, public reporting, or accreditation may not be applicable to QI interventions at the unit or clinic level due to small numbers. Scholars have stressed the need to seek less variability in performance measures while simultaneously allowing for flexibility to meet the needs of specific innovations and populations (Higgins, Veselovskiy, and McKown, 2013).

Limitations of Using Performance Measures for QI

A problem that prevents widespread use of performance measures is the nature of the measures themselves. The validity and attribution of many outcomes-based quality measures are vigorously debated. There are three CMS P4P programs that rely on various performance measures: the Hospital Readmission Reduction Program (HRRP), the Hospital Value-Based Purchasing (VBP) Program, and the Hospital-Acquired Condition Reduction (HACR) Program. Across these three programs, large hospitals, major teaching, and safety-net hospitals were far more likely to be penalized, potentially due not to differing quality but to differences in patient case mix (Figueroa, Wang, and Jha, 2016).

Given this, some performance measures are rejected because they are seen to be affected by factors other than the care provided by the organization or its members. For instance, a patient's responsiveness to a particular treatment for heart failure will likely depend upon whether the prescribed treatment actually works (based upon the patient's genetics and biology), what other (comorbid) conditions that patient has, and whether the patient is compliant with the prescribed treatment. Thus, while the care provided could have been evaluated as successful based on structural or process measures (e.g., the physician was board-certified, the bed was available without

delay, the medications were available and prescribed appropriately), the outcome measure might indicate poor quality of care if the patient suffered a heart attack or died while in the hospital.

Attempts to "standardize" for such extraneous factors often take the form of debates around risk adjustment in quality metrics such as hospital mortality rates. In this case, simply counting the number of in-hospital deaths would inaccurately reflect the quality of the institution unless this rate were adjusted for the complexity and severity of cases treated by the hospital, the ages of the patients, and other risk-related factors. From a managerial perspective, this makes performance measures much more difficult than, say, financial indicators to motivate change in behavior.

GETTING TO HIGHER QUALITY AND QUALITY IMPROVEMENT

The Challenge of Implementation

Although QI holds promise for improving quality of care, HCOs that adopt QI interventions often struggle with implementation. Implementation is the critical gateway between the decision to adopt the QI intervention and its integration into routine practice. For example, implementation of a QI mindset occurs when clinical and nonclinical staff apply QI approaches and interventions routinely to improve clinical care processes. There are three general classes of success or failure in QI interventions: (1) widespread or unit-/role-specific avoidance of the QI intervention (nonuse), (2) meager and unenthusiastic use (compliant use), and (3) skilled, enthusiastic, and consistent use (committed use) (Klein and Sorra, 1996). The frequency of the first two categories is disturbingly high. Recent studies show that the rate of evidence-based practices has not increased in the last decade despite the focus on evidence-based medicine (Levine, Linder, and Landon, 2016; Willis et al., 2017).

Why is the success of QI interventions so variable? In a general sense, implementation of most new, innovative practices is demanding on both individuals and organizations. It requires a complex mix of sustained leadership, extensive training and support, robust measurement and data systems, realigned incentives and human resource practices, and an organizational culture receptive to change. Further, QI efforts are often complex interventions that, by definition, evolve over time. Assuming that the intervention will immediately function exactly as planned is both unrealistic and impractical. Finally, the context in which improvement initiatives are implemented (i.e., the structures, processes, and culture of the larger organization and environment) can exert a powerful influence

Table 9.5 Health Care Organization Features, Implications, and Principles for QI Implementation Effectiveness

Industry Feature	Contribution to Implementation Failure	Key Principle for Implementation Success
Nature of work • High uncertainty • Risk of customer fatality • Hinges on clinician discretion	• Workforce aversion to the experimentation required for successful implementation	• Create opportunities for nonthreatening workforce experimentation and adaptation of innovation
Workforce • Interprofessional interactions governed by an established hierarchy • Strong professional identification, weak organizational identification	• Workforce aversion to the collaborative learning required for mastering increasingly interdisciplinary innovations • Little workforce interest in participating in organizational improvement efforts	• Frame implementation as a learning challenge • Increase the attractiveness of the perceived organizational identity and construed external image to generate interest in organizational citizenship behavior
Leader–workforce relations • Transactional exchanges are prevalent • Perceived conflict of goals between leaders and workforce	• Leaders and workforce unable to place collective goal (i.e., innovation implementation) above self-interest	• Incorporate transformational leadership processes for innovation implementation
Performance measurement and control systems • Underdeveloped • Performance/implementation not rewarded • Founded on calculus-based trust, not relational trust	• Difficult to detect implementation problems and thus make adjustments • Incentives do not favor implementation	• Involve workforce in development of system • Measure and reward implementation efforts

SOURCE: Adapted from Nembhard et al. (2009).

DEBATE TIME: Which Quality Improvement Strategy?

Health care systems are being challenged to increase value through both improvements in care quality and reductions in service delivery costs. Many different strategies can be deployed to address these issues, such as the process improvement techniques outlined by Six Sigma, Lean, and PDSA, among others. For an organization deciding among the various alternatives, what should be considered? How much do you think it matters which QI approach is selected? What other factors could affect the success of a QI approach?

---

on the success of a QI intervention, independent of the intervention itself (Kaplan et al., 2010). Table 9.5 lists features of a HCO and how each can contribute to implementation failure alongside key principles for success.

Context Matters

Researchers have suggested that the context of a QI intervention is integral to its success (Kaplan et al., 2012; Leonard, Graham, and Bonacum, 2004; McAlearney et al., 2015; Weaver et al., 2013). Above sections of this chapter have discussed the importance of

a culture of continuous quality improvement. Yet, context is characterized as broader than culture, and includes management approaches and strategies, external factors, and the availability of implementation and management tools (Kaplan et al., 2010). A 2010 systematic review of the effect of context on QI interventions identified specific factors such as leadership from top management, data infrastructure and information systems, and years involved in QI (Kaplan et al., 2010). This research led to the development of a model for studying the impact of culture on QI efforts: the Model for Understanding Success in Quality (MUSIQ) (Kaplan et al., 2012).

• • • IN PRACTICE: Contextual Factors in Reducing Central Line-Associated Bloodstream Infections

Central Line-Associated Bloodstream Infection (CLABSI)-Reduction Efforts. Evidence has shown that implementing a "bundle" of five clinical practices can significantly reduce CLABSI rates (Pronovost et al., 2006). This clinical bundle, combined with dedicated line insertion and maintenance teams, checklists to ensure practice consistency, and practitioner education, has led hospital ICUs to see significant and sustained CLABSI rate reductions over the past 15 years. However, while some hospitals have virtually eliminated CLABSIs in their ICUs, others struggle to attain and/or sustain near-zero rates. In an attempt to address this variation, the Comprehensive Unit-Based Safety Program (CUSP)—a formal model for translating CLABSI-reduction evidence into practice—was developed at Johns Hopkins University and disseminated by the Agency for Healthcare Research and Quality (AHRQ) (Pronovost et al., 2006). CUSP helps hospital units assemble a multidisciplinary team of frontline providers, supported by senior executives, to identify why CLABSIs occur in their unit, and to generate solutions. By 2013, the overall rate of CLABSI infections among hospitals implementing CUSP dropped by 41 percent (AHRQ, 2013). Additionally, 68 percent of units reported zero CLABSIs for at least one quarter, up from 30 percent at baseline. While these statistics support program efficacy and the feasibility of achieving "zero," variability across participating ICUs remains, raising questions about what hospitals can do to improve their likelihood of success and sustain success over time.

This model identifies 25 contextual factors and proposes that factors within the microsystem of an HCO (QI leadership, supportive culture, motivation to change), and specifically factors within the QI team (team leadership, prior QI experience), directly influence QI success while factors in the broader organization and the external environment affect success indirectly. These findings are supported by a 2015 study applying the MUSIQ model to a review of systematic reviews of QI interventions (Kringos et al., 2015). However, the authors also report that while they found that contextual factors were significantly associated with success, these factors were rarely included in published reports. The success of QI efforts within HCOs could be significantly improved by the consideration and measurement of contextual factors throughout the implementation and evaluation process.

Context Is Important across Prevention Efforts

While patient safety culture is critical, differences in management strategies and practices are also part of the implementation context and may explain variability in efforts to reduce CLABSIs and other health care-associated infections (HAIs). Recently, research conducted by this chapter's authors sought to open the metaphorical "black box" of management practices to better understand the specific strategies that can influence HAI prevention. Using an exploratory, qualitative approach, eight hospitals from the first wave of AHRQ's CUSP initiative were classified as higher- versus lower-performing on the basis of success with CLABSI-reduction efforts. Interviews were conducted with administrative leaders, clinical leaders, professional staff, and frontline physicians and nurses to examine perspectives about CLABSI-reduction efforts. The resulting analysis characterized contrasts between higher- and lower-performing hospitals to improve our understanding of factors that contribute to variable

performance in CLABSI-reduction efforts (McAlearney et al., 2015).

Six management strategies were almost exclusively present in the hospitals classified as higher-performing and absent or appreciably different in the lower-performing hospitals: (1) aggressive goal setting and support, (2) strategic alignment/communication and information sharing, (3) systematic education, (4) interprofessional collaboration, (5) meaningful use of data, and (6) recognition for success. For instance, one of the main management strategies that differentiated higher- from lower-performing hospitals was aggressive framing of the goal of "getting to zero" infections. While all sites reported establishing infection rate reduction goals, at the higher-performing sites the goal of zero infections was explicitly stated, widely embraced, and aggressively pursued through specific activities. In contrast, at lower-performing hospitals, the goal of "getting to zero" was more of an aspiration, with a notable absence of corresponding strategic actions as part of the hospitals' efforts to prevent CLABSIs. Further, in exploring these differences, it was noted that culture was not enough; higher-performing hospitals pursued a wide array of activities linked to these six management strategies in support of their CLABSI-prevention efforts (McAlearney et al., 2015).

MUSIQ Domains and Implementation Challenges

The MUSIQ domains provide a framework to guide discussion of the contextual factors affecting the success of well-coordinated QI interventions. Below potential contextual factors and implementation challenges are discussed within the four MUSIQ domains of *organization*, *quality improvement support and capacity*, *microsystem*, and *QI team*.

Organization

Culture Supportive of QI

Culture comprises the fundamental values, assumptions, and beliefs held in common by members of an organization. It is often treated as if it is stable, socially constructed, and subconscious. Employees impart the organizational culture to new members, and culture influences in large measure how employees relate to one another and the manner in which they approach their "work." Although nearly all QI efforts are targeted at "objective" aspects of an organization, such as work tasks, structures, and processes, many of these initiatives fail because there is no corresponding change in organizational culture (Carman et al., 2010). In other words, these changes often do not stick because they are inconsistent with prevailing values, understandings, and unspoken "rules" in the organizations.

Governance Leadership

Governing boards have an important role to play in overseeing QI efforts and patient safety initiatives because they are the organizational entity legally accountable for quality of care. Beyond fulfilling their oversight responsibilities, boards can potentially play a leadership role by establishing quality and safety as organizational priorities, allocating resources to support QI efforts and patient safety initiatives, revising executive compensation and performance evaluation criteria, and fostering a corporate culture that values quality and safety. In HCOs, the governing board responsibility for quality is clearly delineated in statutory law, regulatory requirements, and accreditation standards.

Although boards have a potentially valuable role to play, several features of board composition, structure, process, and context must be addressed to ensure the board's fulfillment of its responsibility for quality (Jha and Epstein, 2010; Joshi and Hines, 2006). For instance, few board members possess health care backgrounds or clinical expertise. Board members are often selected on the basis of their business experience, professional skills (e.g., legal, marketing, finance), community ties, personal values, time availability, or a combination of these factors. In addition, many boards do not possess adequate governance information systems—that is, information systems designed to support governance work. Board members receive either too much information or too little to monitor quality effectively. Moreover, they do not receive information in a format that makes it easy to discern what action they should take to rectify a quality problem or improve quality.

Quality Improvement Support and Capacity

Resource Availability

Developing robust information systems and reorganizing around clinical processes require significant financial resources (Cummings et al., 2007; Greenhalgh et al., 2004). Allocation of resources to QI efforts represents a key indicator of organizational commitment (Alexander et al., 2006). The support of QI with resources may differentiate those organizations that are serious about QI from those that are simply mimicking the latest trend. Hence, beyond the organization's general financial health, its specific investment in QI may be an important feature of a supportive organizational context. Although financial support is a key aspect of QI infrastructure, other resources, such as training, education, physical space, and even time have been positively associated with QI interventions (Kaplan et al., 2010). For example, organizations that have "slack resources" that allow people to "squeeze" time to experiment with a new QI intervention without disrupting existing routines may lead to higher rates of implementation (Damschroder et al., 2009).

Data Infrastructure

A sophisticated data infrastructure is necessary to support the information needs of a successful QI intervention (Alexander et al., 2006; Kaplan et al., 2010). HCOs can utilize data from a variety of data sources—claims data, administrative data, EHR data, etc. However, appropriate use of this data for problem identification and success measurement requires not only a sophisticated data infrastructure but also employees with strong clinical informatics skills to navigate through all the HCO data and prepare useful metrics for QI, research, and public reporting. Developing the informatics staff and data infrastructure requires a significant financial commitment in addition to the allocation of clinical and administrative staff resources to QI efforts discussed in the above section.

Microsystem

QI Leadership from Middle Managers

Leadership refers to leaders at all levels of an organization who have a direct or indirect influence on QI efforts. In addition to high-level leaders, middle managers are important because of their ability to network and negotiate for resources and because they are often in a position to assign greater (or lesser) priority to QI relative to other organizational demands (Birken et al., 2013). Commitment, involvement, and accountability of leaders and managers can all have a significant impact on the success of QI efforts. Management support in terms of commitment and active interest leads to a stronger implementation climate that is in turn related to implementation effectiveness. Managers can be important conduits as they can help persuade stakeholders via interpersonal channels and by modeling norms associated with implementing an intervention. Managerial patience (taking a long-term view rather than a short-term view) allows time for the often-inevitable reduction in productivity that occurs until the intervention takes hold; this patience is also more likely to

MANAGING THE DISNEY WAY

The importance of quality and QI is not limited to health care. Even though other industries are concerned with different products and services, those in the health care industry can still learn valuable lessons by studying other companies and management techniques.

In his book, *If Disney Ran Your Hospital: 9½ Things You Would Do Differently* (2004), Fred Lee shares insights from his experience working for a short time as a Disney cast member. Lee develops his perspective by examining Disney and the Disney culture based on comparisons with his experiences in the health care industry, and specifically drawing on his perspective as senior vice president at Florida Hospital in Orlando.

Lee ties together his list of things hospitals could do differently by focusing on the importance of culture in organizations. Rather than emphasizing service, he notes that a focus on cultural excellence can tie together an organization and its employees' pursuit of common, valued goals. Disney's four areas of "quality focus" are prioritized: (1) safety, (2) courtesy, (3) show (i.e., the areas of Disney that create a "sensory impression"), and (4) efficiency. By clearly delineating these strategic priorities, employees have an accessible map by which to guide their actions.

The 9½ things Lee highlights as opportunities for hospitals to learn from Disney include the following:

1. Redefining the competition
2. Emphasizing courtesy over efficiency
3. Reducing reliance on patient satisfaction as a metric
4. Focusing on measurement for improvement
5. Decentralizing authority
6. Changing the concept of work
7. Harnessing the power of employees' imaginations to motivate them
8. Creating a climate of dissatisfaction
9. Ending the use of competitive monetary rewards as a means of motivating employees
10. Closing the gap between knowledge and action

Lee acknowledges that being a manager in a hospital is considerably more challenging than being a manager at Disney, where customers want to be and where the lower-risk environment presents situations that can be standardized. Yet despite the obvious differences, Lee's list and accompanying discussion present intriguing QI opportunities that those working in the health care industry may wish to consider.

SOURCE: Lee (2004).

lead to implementation success. However, if the decision to adopt and implement is made by leaders higher in the hierarchy who mandate change with little user input in the decision to implement an intervention, then implementation is more likely to fail. Middle managers are more likely to support implementation if they believe that doing so will promote their own organizational goals and if they feel involved in discussions about the implementation.

Learning Climate

Developing a climate that promotes learning is a "core property" that HCOs need for ongoing QI. Similar to culture, a positive learning climate creates a receptive context for change. Specifically, a learning climate is one with a set of interrelated practices and beliefs that support and enable employee and organizational skill development, learning, and growth (Damschroder et al., 2009). Key characteristics of a learning climate that promotes

QI efforts are that (1) a compelling and inspiring reason for QI intervention use is clearly articulated, (2) leaders express their own fallibility and need for team members' assistance and input, and (3) leaders communicate to team members that they are essential, valued, and knowledgeable partners in the change process. Having the time and space for reflective thinking and evaluation is another important characteristic because it promotes learning from past successes and failures to inform future QI efforts. It is important to note that learning "climates" often vary across subgroups, and unit- or team-based expressions of these attributes may have a stronger influence than overall organizational learning.

Quality Improvement Team

Team Tenure and Diversity. Burgeoning medical knowledge and the complexity of health care delivery have resulted in increasing specialization in the health care

MANAGEMENT LESSONS FROM MAYO CLINIC

Mayo Clinic is known worldwide for excellence in both quality of care and service. Founded in Rochester, Minnesota, over 140 years ago, Mayo Clinic has expanded to include additional hospitals in Rochester and new Mayo Clinic facilities in Jacksonville, Florida, and Scottsdale, Arizona. Leonard Berry and Kent Seltman, in an effort to learn more about the success behind this "100-Year Brand," undertook a study of Mayo Clinic's service culture and systems through interviews and observations of clinician–patient interactions. Their book, *Management Lessons from Mayo Clinic* (2008), describes their findings.

Throughout the book, Berry and Seltman provide multiple examples of the important roles of culture, teamwork, learning, communication, and professional integration in providing excellent care and succeeding with efforts to implement improvement interventions that can ensure quality and service. With respect to quality and QI, for instance, at Mayo Clinic, "quality is defined by clinical outcomes, safety, and service" (p. 229). While Mayo Clinic is consistently listed among the best when ranked by objective metrics assessing quality of care, the clinic continues to strive for improvement. As explained by one leading Mayo Clinic physician, "No one is better positioned to break away from the rest of the leaders in clinical reliability than an integrated group practice that values teamwork, understands the dividends of a more horizontal, cross-functional team of nurses, technicians, doctors, pharmacists, and administrators, and has a century-long history of patient-centered care facilitated by a large contingent of systems engineers" (p. 229). With an attitude that "we can do better," physicians and administrators at Mayo Clinic work together in a learning environment, united by the Mayo Clinic core value of "the needs of the patient come first" that is embedded in the organization's culture.

SOURCE: Berry and Seltman (2008).

workforce. For example, physicians specialize in 1 of 120 disciplines including internal medicine, cardiology, adult cardiothoracic anesthesiology, hand surgery, pediatric endocrinology, and abdominal radiology. Other specialized health care professionals include nurses, therapists, nutritionists, phlebotomists, pharmacists, and so forth.

The high degree of specialization in health care means that each professional brings only part of the knowledge needed to care for patients. In practice, the expertise of over 20 health professionals must be integrated to provide care for a single patient in a hospital. There is increasing recognition that these professionals must collaborate to be effective. Yet despite the imperative for collaboration, it is often missing from professional interactions, and its absence is a leading cause of quality problems (Hughes, 2008). At a children's hospital in Boston, a five-year-old boy died from a seizure because he received no treatment. An investigation later revealed that his physicians had never communicated with each other about who was in charge of his care. Instead, each assumed another had taken charge, and each therefore removed himself from the boy's care, leaving no one to provide treatment.

Team Decision Making and Collaboration Skills

Collaboration problems in the health care workforce result largely from the hierarchical, individualistic culture of medicine, which is deeply rooted in the socialization process for health professionals (Horwitz, Horwitz, and Barshes, 2011). Health professionals are socialized before employment through their specialty training programs, which often span a period of 10 or more years—a

period longer than is required in most service industries. During training, professionals learn not only how to treat patients but also how to view themselves and how to interact with others inside and outside of their profession. Physicians, for example, learn to be independent, authoritarian, autonomous, competitive, conservative, reactive, quick, and detached actors. They learn to treat others in their discipline with respect and in high regard. They learn to treat individuals in other professions in accordance with the established medical professional hierarchy. In this professional hierarchy, specialists rank higher than primary care physicians, who rank higher than nurses, who rank higher than therapists, and so on. The lower an individual's professional rank, the less consideration is given to that individual in clinical decision making. In practice, all individuals are mindful of the hierarchy and feel a strong sense of professional identification—characteristics that affect not only quality of care but also efforts to improve quality of care through QI, which depend fundamentally on team-based approaches to change rather than top-down control (Nembhard et al., 2009).

Team Norms

Health care QI increasingly requires interdisciplinary teamwork, meaning its implementation cannot succeed without professionals from multiple disciplines collaborating both to develop new approaches to care and to learn to use them. Unfortunately, HCOs' hierarchical culture can stifle organizational members' willingness to participate in the collaborative learning that is necessary for QI success (Carman et al., 2010). Collaborative learning is the iterative process of individuals or groups of individuals *working together* to improve their actions by incorporating new knowledge and understanding. It involves jointly analyzing information, openly discussing concerns, and consciously sharing decision making and coordinating experimentation. In turn, individuals must be willing to challenge others' views, acknowledge their own errors, and openly discuss failed experiments. These behaviors are interpersonally risky because they create the possibility for an individual to appear incompetent or belligerent and thereby potentially diminish that individual's reputation among colleagues (Nembhard et al., 2009).

Individuals take such risks only when they perceive a psychologically safe work climate. Unfortunately, the medical professional hierarchy has undermined the psychological safety of individuals whose professions fall lower in the hierarchy. Nurses frequently report that "it is difficult to speak up" and "nurse input is not well received." Moreover, they report negative consequences (e.g., punishment, rejection, embarrassment) of voicing concerns and suggestions to individuals of higher status and of participating in failed experiments. Hence, they shy away from collaborative learning situations such as QI efforts.

Factors influencing "speaking up" include perceived safety versus "costs" of reporting incidents, perceived efficacy versus utility, individual staff factors, such as communication skills and job satisfaction, and contextual factors, such as attitudes of leaders and hospital policy (Okuyama, Wagner, and Bijnen, 2014). A 2014 systematic review of the literature determined that research on "speaking up" has shown training to be effective at enhancing team communication across the

• • • IN PRACTICE: Research on High-Performance Work Practices in Health Care Organizations

Critical in providing high-quality care is the presence of a competent and capable workforce. Outside health care, a breadth of research suggests that innovative human resource (HR) practices (or **high-performance work practices [HPWPs]**) can be an important element of efforts to improve quality and performance. These HPWPs include activities such as systematic personnel selection, incentive compensation, and the widespread use of teams, and they can help organizations in their efforts to attract and retain highly qualified employees.

Within health care, the question was raised as to whether the use of HPWPs could have a similarly important effect on quality of care and organizational performance. Subsequently, a research team funded by the Agency for Healthcare Research and Quality (AHRQ) designed a project to investigate the use of HPWPs, with particular interest in exploring potential links between the use of HPWPs and factors related to quality of care and patient safety in U.S. HCOs.

The team's first task was to undertake an extensive review and synthesis of the literature available—both academic and "gray" literature, such as reports and publications available outside peer-reviewed journals. Next, the team developed a preliminary model that outlined four key subsystems (or "bundles") of HPWPs and delineated the relations among these subsystems as well as their potential organizational effects. Then, the team performed five case studies of U.S. HCOs that had been selected based on the HCOs' known success with HPWP implementation. The team conducted site visits in 2009, where they performed 71 interviews with key organizational and clinical informants and collected organizational documents related to the HPWPs that were in use. All the key informant interviews were recorded and transcribed for further analysis.

The team found that all four of the HPWP subsystems they had previously characterized as directly relevant to health care (organizational engagement, staff acquisition/development, frontline empowerment, and leadership alignment/development) were emphasized in the five case study organizations. They found substantial variation in what HPWPs were selected and also noted innovative applications in the HCOs. The group also found evidence of links between the use of HPWPs and employee outcomes (e.g., turnover, higher satisfaction/engagement). While the team was unable to collect hard data, they noted that the key informants consistently reported believing that HPWPs made important contributions to both care system and organization-level outcomes (e.g., fewer "never events," innovation adoption, lower agency costs, and lower turnover costs), some of which were directly related to quality of care.

The results of this research provide preliminary evidence and examples of ways that HPWPs can be used to improve operations in HCOs. The results also suggest that HPWPs have promise with respect to their ability to impact quality and safety. The team concluded that HPWPs should be considered when addressing the challenges of performance improvement in health care and suggested the need for further research to investigate which HPWP practices and combinations might have the greatest potential for health care QI.

SOURCE: McAlearney et al. (2011).

hierarchy (Okuyama, Wagner, and Bijnen, 2014). By targeting trainings to address the above factors, managers of HCOs can influence the team dynamic and the climate and culture of their organization.

Building a Patient Safety Culture

Patient safety is an area of health care where culture has been highlighted as integral to successful QI; patient safety culture has been defined as a product of group values, attitudes, and patterns of behavior that influence an organization's health and safety activities (AHRQ, 2016). Building a strong patient safety culture has been the a key priority of many U.S. health care systems since the IOM's report in 2000 on the number of errors, adverse events, and near misses that happen each year in U.S. hospitals (Kohn, Corrigan, and Donaldson, 2000). Research has shown that perceptions of strong patient safety cultures do appear to be associated with fewer adverse events or other indicators of potential harm.

Given this link between culture and outcomes, a variety of strategies have been used to improve patient safety culture. One widely adopted strategy is a focus on improving teamwork in high-intensity health care settings and developing standardized processes to implement in this enhanced teamwork framework. Crew resource management (CRM) is a systematic approach for training teams in interpersonal communication, leadership, and decision-making practices, which allows teams to function effectively under even the most demanding, unpredictable situations (Maynard, Marshall, and Dean, 2012). Adapted from the airline industry, CRM and related approaches such as TeamSTEPPS (Clancy and Tornberg, 2007) have been linked to improved perceptions of patient safety culture (Pettker et al., 2011; Weaver et al., 2010), increased adherence to clinical guidelines (Tapson, Karcher, and Weeks, 2011), improved team performance (Lisbon et al., 2016; Mayer et al., 2011), reductions in surgical mortality (Neily et al., 2010) and adverse events (Moffatt-Bruce et al., 2015; Starmer et al., 2014).

Also in promoting the importance of a patient safety culture, the AHRQ has developed a survey to measure transformation toward a safety culture. Called the Hospital Survey on Patient Safety Culture (HSOPS), this publicly available survey tool is composed of 42 items addressing 12 dimensions of safety culture: teamwork within units, supervisor expectations/actions promoting patient safety, organizational learning, management support for patient safety, overall perceptions of patient safety, feedback and communication about error, communication openness, frequency of events reported, teamwork across units, staffing, and nonpunitive response to errors. This tool has been used extensively to measure cultural transformation and has been fielded in hospitals across the United States and internationally,

with moderate-to-strong validity and reliability across dimensions (Blegen et al., 2009). Given that culture change may be one of the most difficult tasks facing HCO managers implementing QI interventions, effective change programs, such as TeamStepps and CRM, as well as publicly available culture surveys can be utilized and adapted to a variety of contexts.

APPLYING QUALITY IMPROVEMENT FRAMEWORKS

QI Tactics and Strategies

Create Opportunities for Staff Experimentation and QI Adaptation

HCOs' members' reluctance to participate in QI efforts may be addressed by creating opportunities for them to experiment with QI innovations in nonthreatening ways. Nonthreatening opportunities (e.g., training, pilot projects, dry runs) create low-risk settings where failures have little or no consequence for patients. They enable staff to gain familiarity with the innovation, experience its benefits, and develop user competence. As a result, staff members in such settings are less likely to view the innovation as posing high risks, and thus are less likely to resist its implementation.

When staff are not resistant, implementation success is more likely. For example, staff having time to train with a QI intervention is a positive predictor of implementation success. Similarly, units that used activities such as dry runs (with a dummy serving as the patient in clinical procedures) and pilot projects to implement innovative practices experienced greater implementation success (Tucker et al., 2008). Use of these activities facilitates implementation success not only by reducing resistance to the intervention but also by fostering "attitudinal commitment," or commitment that generates active involvement of staff in QI efforts.

Frame QI as a Learning Challenge

To counter the negative psychological and behavioral effects of the hierarchical culture of medicine with respect to implementation, QI efforts must be appropriately framed. Framing is the process of providing a lens through which to interpret a situation. Challenges can be framed in terms of performance or learning. Individuals or groups that adopt a performance frame view a new task as similar to current practice, while those that adopt a learning frame see the task as different, and therefore an opportunity to explore new actions and relationships. Consequently, the behavior that follows from adoption of each frame differs. Teams whose leaders explicitly framed implementation as learning rather than as a performance

STAGES OF GRIEF IN EHR IMPLEMENTATION

The transition from paper medical records to electronic health records (EHRs) has created significant disruption in the workflow of medical professionals. Interviews with primary care physicians across six U.S. health care organizations—identified because of purported success with EHR implementation—revealed that physicians' perceptions of the change guided their reactions (McAlearney et al., 2014). Many physicians perceived the EHR transition as a loss, and the authors of this study proposed that the Kubler-Ross five stages of grief model could be mapped onto physicians' reactions to this loss. The five stages—denial, anger, bargaining, depression, and acceptance—can be articulated as required phases of personal change for physicians adopting and integrating an EHR system.

Loss as a part of change is often overlooked. Addressing it directly and compassionately can potentially facilitate the success of QI implementation efforts. Combining insights from both individual (e.g., Kubler-Ross and Kessler, 2014) and organizational change management (e.g., Kotter, 2012), the investigators further note that managers can employ 10 strategies to facilitate change through perception management:

(1) Manage expectations

(2) Make the case for quality

(3) Recruit champions

(4) Communicate

(5) Acknowledge that it is a painful transition

(6) Provide good training

(7) Improve functionality, when possible

(8) Acknowledge competing priorities

(9) Allow time to adapt to the new system

(10) Promote a better, but changed, future

While these strategies were articulated in the context of EHR implementation (McAlearney et al., 2014), they can be applied to perception management across QI change efforts.

---

challenge were more likely to abandon existing interpersonal routines, including those premised on hierarchical interactions, and were more likely to adopt collaborative learning behaviors (Edmondson, 2003). Moreover, members of these teams (regardless of professional rank) felt psychologically safe and excited about offering their input.

Promote Organizational Identification

While professional identification may often conflict with the need for organizational identification associated with successful QI implementation in health care, such conflict is not necessary (Dukerich, Golden, and Shortell, 2002). There are at least two strategies for fostering the organizational identification needed for implementation success in HCOs: (1) increase the attractiveness of the organizational identity and (2) increase the attractiveness of the external image of the organization (i.e., the image held by those outside of the organization) (Dukerich, Golden, and Shortell, 2002). The former strategy builds on the research finding that physicians feel stronger organizational identification when they perceive alignment between their goals and values and those of the

organization. The second strategy reflects the finding that physicians' feelings about organizations with which they are affiliated are influenced by how outsiders view those organizations. Thus, the challenge for HCOs is to find ways to highlight the similarities between their goals and their workforce's values. They must also showcase their positive attributes (e.g., pro bono work, awards, new facilities) in order to enhance their external image and their affiliates' perceptions of them.

Applying these principles helped the Royal Devon and Exeter NHS Foundation Trust in England dramatically shift from weak to strong organizational identification (Bate, Mendel, and Robert, 2008). Until the late 1990s, identification with the Trust had been so weak that professionals refused to implement innovations that the Trust desired. Moreover, the Trust had a negative reputation due to high turnover in management and the perception that some physicians were "difficult." The turning point came shortly after a devastating incident in which 82 patients were given incorrect diagnoses, with 11 of them dying. At that point, the CEO decided to make organizational identification a priority and took actions to build identification without tampering with professional identity. For example, she instituted meetings between the executive team and the clinical directors to discuss issues of mutual interest, used quarterly reviews to link individuals across the organization who were working on similar issues, invited the staff to develop its own improvement projects, stressed the importance of interprofessional dialogue, and used "the incident" as a story that exemplified the need to unify as an organization. The Trust now has a positive reputation for organizational identification and QI.

Use Transformational Leadership Processes

Transformational leadership is defined as influencing followers by "broadening and elevating followers' goals and providing them with confidence to perform beyond the expectations specified in the implicit or explicit exchange agreement" (Bass, 1990). Transformational leaders provide vision and a sense of mission, communicate high expectations, promote intelligence, and provide personal attention to employees.

In contrast, **transactional leadership** is based on transactions between managers and employees, such as managers initiating and organizing work and providing recognition and advancement to employees who perform well while penalizing those who do not (Bass, 1990). Transactional leaders provide rewards for effort and good performance, watch for deviations from rules and standards or intervene only if standards are not met, and avoid making decisions (Bass, 1990).

With respect to QI efforts, transformational leaders use processes that effectively shift the focus of organizational members from their individual goals to collective goals such as QI interventions. By being intellectually stimulating, transformational leaders motivate the workforce to consider how individual goals overlap with collective goals. By being charismatic, they elicit positive feelings in organizational members, which lead members to commit to the leader's and the organization's goals. By modeling collaborative behavior, transformational leaders inspire organizational members to work as a collective. By being individually considerate, they ensure that individuals' developmental needs are fulfilled while working on organizational goals. The workforce often responds to this goodwill by working diligently toward the organization's goals, including implementation (Gilmartin and D'Aunno, 2007).

The workforce also responds to the support for implementation that transformational leaders provide to them (e.g., allocating needed resources, removing organizational barriers such as existing institutional policies, soliciting and addressing feedback, and championing the work of members). This support greatly facilitates implementation success through legitimation, further motivating organizational members' commitment to

implementation. Moreover, it cultivates a climate in which the workforce feels comfortable offering feedback to leaders about how to improve QI implementation. Last, leadership support helps maintain the momentum for change in the face of setbacks and performance declines, which are common in implementation efforts.

Given the demonstrated effectiveness of transformational leaders at eliciting targeted organizational members' commitment to organizational change goals, such as QI efforts, HCOs are advised to use transformational leadership processes (Spinelli, 2006). The inclusion of this behavior does not necessitate the exclusion of transactional behaviors. Indeed, the transactional and transformational leadership styles are complementary, coexist well, and are equally needed to manage the dual challenges of QI implementation and addressing current organizational needs.

There are at least two strategies for increasing transformational leadership in HCOs. One strategy is to hire leaders who innately use transformational processes or who are equally strong users of transformational and transactional processes. Children's Hospitals and Clinics in Minnesota took this approach in hiring Julie Morath, who, during her interviews for the position of chief operating officer, explicitly talked about how she would create a culture of teamwork and safety at Children's (Edmondson et al., 2005). In Morath's case, her reputation preceded her, and the change platform she presented in her job interviews reinforced her reputation as a transformational leader.

A second strategy is to train current leaders in the appropriate use of transformational leadership processes via leadership development programs. Many have debated whether individuals can be trained to be effective leaders and whether leader development programs truly improve the leadership capabilities of individuals. However, management research increasingly affirms the value of such training, especially for HCO leaders, including improvement in leadership style and communication skills in physician leaders (Spinelli, 2006). Leaders at all levels within the HCO should learn to use transformational leadership processes adeptly. Use of these skills at the senior level is important because transformational behavior cascades down the organization (see the preceding discussion of governance leadership). Staff tend to adopt the behavior and suggested behaviors of senior leaders with this style. When senior leaders with transformational styles commit to QI implementation, organizational members are likely to commit to this collective purpose as well (Aarons et al., 2016). However, to enlist organizational members' sustained commitment to implementation, the implementation message must also come from transformational leaders who are closer to them in the hierarchy. These leaders' actions are even more salient and motivating.

• • • IN PRACTICE: The Role of Leadership Development in Quality Improvement

Expanded use of leadership development programs in HCOs has been relatively recent, particularly in comparison with the use of leadership development programs in other industries (McAlearney, 2010). However, formal leadership development programs are increasingly viewed as a means of helping HCOs to focus on organizational priorities such as quality of care and patient safety (McAlearney, 2010).

Study of leadership development activities in HCOs has highlighted several important opportunities for these programs to improve quality and patient safety in health care (McAlearney, 2008, 2010). First, leadership development programs are typically developed to increase the caliber of the health care workforce. By including education and training in QI approaches, these programs can help ensure that employees can understand and participate in QI interventions deployed by the organization. Further, this attention paid to developing leaders who will be able to lead QI interventions can help HCOs accelerate the QI process within the organization.

Second, leadership development programs can be used to focus organizational attention on strategic priorities. When quality and QI are included in the organization's strategic priorities, alignment of leadership development goals with organizational objectives can help ensure consistency of communication and clarity of organizational messages about quality as a priority. Through leadership development programs, emerging leaders learn how to emphasize organizational messages about quality in their management and leadership practices.

Finally, leadership development programs can be specifically designed to emphasize and reinforce an organization's culture, particularly cultures that value care quality. Mission, vision, and values are public indicators of what organizations find important, and weaving quality into those statements creates an opportunity to focus on quality, since it is embedded in the culture. Leadership development programs can provide specific and focused opportunities to highlight the importance of quality as it fits into the HCO's culture. Further, under those circumstances when increasing the amount of attention paid to quality-of-care issues involves a change in organizational culture, leadership development programs can be a particularly important component of the culture change effort.

Build Evidence for QI

QI Intervention Source

Perceptions of key stakeholders about whether the QI intervention is externally or internally developed may influence the success of QI implementation (Damschroder et al., 2009). The QI intervention may enter into the organization through an external source such as through information from a formal research entity; as a market, system, or governmental mandate; or through another external source. Alternatively, a QI intervention may have been internally developed as a good idea, a solution to a problem, or from a grassroots effort. For example, using coated catheters to prevent infections may have been formally studied and reported in the literature, and a nurse may have decided that her organization needs to use these devices to help decrease infection rates. Stakeholders within the organization may regard this QI intervention as external (e.g., the literature for the Centers for Disease Control and Prevention strongly recommends using them) or as an internally developed QI intervention (e.g., the IV nurse team believes these offer the best solution to the problem). However, selection of an externally developed QI intervention coupled with a lack of transparency in the decision-making process about implementation of that QI intervention may lead to implementation failure (Damschroder et al., 2009). On the other hand, key ideas that come from outside the organization that are tailored to the particular organization more often result in successful implementation.

Reporting and Disseminating Successful Quality Improvement Interventions

The Standards for Quality Improvement Reporting (SQUIRE) provides guidelines on what and how information should be presented when discussing health care QI endeavors. These guidelines are described briefly below, but more information can be found at http://squire-statement.org/.

First, in developing a paper reporting QI results, the title of the paper should clearly identify what topic is being covered in the manuscript and how it relates to health care. The abstract should follow the journal guidelines for word count and topics covered. Abstracts should consolidate all of the major sections included in the manuscript, and provide an overview of the study and key findings.

• • • IN PRACTICE: Building Evidence Through Practice-Based Health Services Research

As emphasized in this chapter, increasing evidence suggests that success in achieving QI goals depends on implementation processes and contexts and not only on the nature of the QI intervention. Hence, to advance QI, additional research is needed to study what types of QI interventions work, including considerations about where, when, and how they work. Researchers gain this understanding when they learn about the effects of introducing QI interventions in different practice contexts, as well as the effects of using different implementation strategies, thus contributing to the evidence base supporting future QI efforts.

Evidence of this sort typically comes from practice-based research. Federal programs fostering this type of research include the Quality Enhancement Research Initiative (QUERI) of the Veterans Administration (http://www.queri.research.va.gov) as well as the Accelerating Change in Transforming Networks (ACTION, http://www.ahrq.gov/research/ACTION.htm) and the Practice Based Research Networks (PBRNs, https://pbrn.ahrq.gov/) funded by the Agency for Healthcare Research and Quality. Managers and policymakers alike can use the results of these research projects to inform decisions about QI interventions, helping to maximize the likelihood of QI success.

The Introduction section is comprised of the problem statement and existing knowledge on the topic covered. Answer why the problem is significant and where the literature succeeds and fails to provide valuable insight. Introductions should also include the rationale for why the selected approach/intervention(s) is appropriate for the stated problem. Last in this section, the Specific Aims should clearly communicate the purpose of the project.

Methods sections should include a description of the intervention(s) at a level that allows for reproducibility by others and a justification for why the selected intervention(s) is appropriate. Additionally, the key people involved in the study should be described in detail. For example, "our team included a unit nurse manager, chief quality officer, an administrative intern, and an epidemiology intern."

Measures used in studying the effects of the intervention should be described in detail as well as including a justification for their use. The Analysis section should include the methods used to assess and understand the data and should be appropriate given the selected measures. Study Results should review the association between the intervention and the measured outcomes. Include description of any missing data, the impact of contextual factors on the outcomes (e.g., is there any other explanation for the findings outside of the intervention(s)?), and any unanticipated benefits, challenges, or barriers with implementing the intervention(s).

The Discussion section outlines the findings and how these relate to outcomes as well as how they compare to similar studies. Describe how the intervention affected the organization and if there were any identified differences between observed and expected outcomes. Additionally, limitations of the study need to be identified and communicated. Include descriptions of efforts undertaken to mitigate these limitations how they affect the generalizability of the work. Finally, the Conclusions section should describe practice implications, the sustainability of the intervention(s), and next steps given the outcomes of the study.

DEBATE TIME: Focusing Quality Improvement Efforts

When considering QI, some people believe that major opportunities for improvement can be realized by increasing clinicians' skills and competence. However, others believe that more opportunities for improvement can result from changes made to the organization and management of clinical care units. A third group believes that quality of care is tied to technology availability or to participation in teaching activities. What do you think? Where do you think the most emphasis should be put? In considering these questions, what conditions, factors, or variables might influence your decision?

SOURCE: Adapted from Shortell and Kaluzny (2005).

SUMMARY AND MANAGERIAL GUIDELINES

1. HCOs have strong imperatives to initiate and support efforts to improve quality of care and patient safety. QI interventions can be designed and implemented to address many of these two issues. Address quality issues proactively by looking for opportunities to improve quality by detecting and preventing potential problems in processes of care delivery. Quality measures must be defined so that organizations striving to improve quality have a basis on which to evaluate improvement or identify problems. The development and deployment of such measures can affect how QI success is defined. Managers must recognize the problems and tradeoffs associated with different definitions of quality measures and different approaches to quality measurement.

2. Undertaking QI efforts within an HCO can be challenging due to the uncertain nature of work in health care as well as the professional makeup of the health care workforce. Set high standards by establishing "best practices" in one's own organization as well as using benchmarking to make comparisons with competitors and industry leaders.

3. The selection of performance measurement and control systems can affect how QI efforts proceed and how achievement of improvements in quality is measured. Select such systems based on accurate and timely data, and develop incentives to improve quality based on work activities under the control of organizational members.

4. Specific implementation policies and procedures will directly affect the use of QI interventions in HCOs. Factors such as organizational structure, financial support, organizational culture, leadership and management support and engagement, governance, leadership, and a learning climate are all critical elements of organizational context that will affect the implementation of QI. Focus energy on working smarter, and consider these factors when developing implementation policies and procedures.

5. Seven QI approaches and strategies hold particular promise for QI implementation efforts in HCOs: (1) creating opportunities for staff experimentation, (2) framing QI as a learning challenge, (3) promoting organizational identification, (4) using transformational leadership processes, (5) involving the workforce in performance measurement and control system development, (6) measuring and rewarding QI implementation efforts, and (7) building evidence for QI. Apply these tactics in combination when undertaking QI interventions in HCOs in order to maximize the likelihood of success in QI interventions.

6. Focusing on the "people" processes associated with QI can help HCOs become high-performance organizations. Strive to develop a participative, team-oriented organizational culture that encourages input from professionals and other workers from all levels of the organization, and seek opportunities to cross-train staff to gain greater flexibility.

7. A crucial element of QI is focusing on organizational change issues and the management of participants' perceptions. If the reasons for QI are understood, if it does not threaten security, if it has involved those affected by it, if it follows a series of successful changes, if it is inaugurated after the previous change has been assimilated, and if it has been planned, there will be a much higher likelihood of successful QI within an HCO. Involve organizational members, particularly professionals, in the development, implementation, and monitoring of QI interventions.

DISCUSSION QUESTIONS

1. Take the perspective of the CEO of a large health care system that owns its own health plan. Describe three major ways that you could improve the quality of health care in your organization. Critique your solutions regarding the extent to which your solution may cause other problems to surface (what kind?) and the extent to which you as the CEO should have the responsibility and power to implement these changes.

2. Using an HCO that you know well, provide three examples each of possible structural, process, and outcome measures of care quality. Would you expect these measures to be highly associated? Why or why not?

3. Consider a community hospital, a major teaching hospital, and a hospital in a large for-profit system. For each, list the major stakeholder groups (both internal and external). Indicate what kinds of quality criteria each group would be most likely to promote.

4. Hospital A and Hospital B both have set as their major goal for this year to implement a QI intervention. Hospital A hired a consultant firm and sent its top managers to a program to learn how to change the corporate culture and to set up quality teams to investigate problems. They formed teams to plan strategies for meaningful QI in two specific areas: billing and use of the emergency room. Hospital B, lacking funds, tried to have study groups and use self-teaching but involved everyone from the CEO to the janitor. Which hospital do you think will succeed in implementing QI? Why?

5. Health System Q is located in the same geographic area as Health System P, its main competitor. While Health System Q touts its status as a community-based integrated delivery system, Health System P leverages its role as a research-intensive academic medical center. Both health systems have achieved Magnet designation for nursing, both have been listed among the "Most Wired" by HIMSS, and both have centers of excellence (or service lines) in the areas of cardiology, cancer, and women's health. You have heard that community members seem to favor Health System Q for most conditions but appreciate having a local academic health system if they have problems that are out of the ordinary. You are considering a job with one of these health systems in the area of QI and are trying to decide where your expertise will have the most impact. What factors would you consider in trying to evaluate which place might be better positioned to leverage your skills and move forward with QI efforts?

CASE

Moving beyond Data Access to QI Action

After a considerable investment of both money and time, executives at Northrop Healthcare were delighted that the new incident-reporting system at Northrop was now fully operational. The incident-reporting system had been deployed across the health care system; frontline and management staff as well as physicians in both inpatient and ambulatory settings had been trained and were able to use the incident-reporting system to access patient information, document adverse events, and report as required to senior management, risk management, and the QI department.

However, even with full system deployment, QI interventions across the health system had not changed. The QI department had full access to the data warehouse that housed data collected through the incident-reporting system as well as data from the EHR and other information systems, yet QI staff members were apparently not using these data. Instead, QI interventions continued to follow historical patterns involving laborious efforts to develop queries and reports rather than use the new system's immediate reporting capabilities to supply information for managers and to drive process improvement projects both locally and across the hospital system.

Similarly, the potential for clinicians to use the newly accessible data was not being realized. Physicians were reluctantly compliant with requirements to use the incident-reporting system for documentation and reporting events, but the general consensus seemed to be that the system was just a way to point fingers at the medical staff. Despite efforts from the senior management team to work individually with clinicians to educate and explain the importance of error and near-miss reporting that would provide information to reduce errors, these physicians continued to view the incident-reporting system as a punitive tool, not as an opportunity for them to explore ways to improve their work.

Questions

1. Given this situation, what are the apparent barriers to using incident-reporting systems for QI?
2. How can these barriers be overcome?
3. What steps would you propose to engage both clinicians and QI staff in enhanced QI interventions?

REFERENCES

Aarons, G. A., Green, A. E., Trott, E., et al. (2016). The roles of system and organizational leadership in system-wide evidence-based intervention sustainment: A mixed-method study. *Administration and Policy in Mental Health and Mental Health Services Research, 43*(6), 991–1008.

Adams, R., Warner, P., Hubbard, B., et al. (2004). Decreasing turnaround time between general surgery cases: A six sigma initiative. *Journal of Nursing Administration, 34*(3), 140–148.

AHRQ. (2013). *Eliminating CLABSI, a national patient safety imperative: Final report.* Retrieved October 2, 2018, from https://www.ahrq.gov/professionals/quality-patient-safety/cusp/clabsi-final-companion/index.html.

AHRQ. (2016). Hospital survey on patient safety culture. Retrieved October 2, 2018, from http://www.ahrq.gov/professionals/quality-patient-safety/patientsafetyculture/hospital/index.html.

Alexander, J. A., Weiner, B. J., Shortell, S. M., et al. (2006). The role of organizational infrastructure in implementation of hospitals' quality improvement. *Hospital Topics, 84*(1), 11–21.

Bass, B. M. (1990). From transactional to transformational leadership: Learning to share the vision. *Organizational dynamics, 18*(3), 19–31.

Bate, P., Mendel, P., & Robert, G. (2008). *Organizing for quality: The improvement journeys of leading hospitals in Europe and the United States*. Oxford: Radcliffe Publishing.

Berwick, D. M., Nolan, T. W., & Whittington, J. (2008). The triple aim: Care, health, and cost. *Health Affairs (Millwood), 27*(3), 759–769. doi:10.1377/hlthaff.27.3.759.

Birken, S. A., Lee, S.-Y. D., Weiner, B. J., et al. (2013). Improving the effectiveness of health care innovation implementation: Middle managers as change agents. *Medical Care Research and Review, 70*(1), 29–45.

Blegen, M. A., Gearhart, S., O'Brien, R., et al. (2009). AHRQ's hospital survey on patient safety culture: Psychometric analyses. *Journal of Patient Safety, 5*(3), 139–144. doi:10.1097/PTS.0b013e3181b53f6e.

Carman, J. M., Shortell, S. M., Foster, R. W., et al. (2010). Keys for successful implementation of total quality management in hospitals. *Health Care Management Review, 35*(4), 283–293.

Chassin, M. R., & Loeb, J. M. (2011). The ongoing quality improvement journey: Next stop, high reliability. *Health Affairs (Millwood), 30*(4), 559–568.

Clancy, C. M., & Tornberg, D. N. (2007). TeamSTEPPS: Assuring optimal teamwork in clinical settings. *American Journal of Medical Quality, 22*(3), 214–217. doi:10.1177/1062860607300616.

Cummings, G. G., Estabrooks, C. A., Midodzi, W. K., et al. (2007). Influence of organizational characteristics and context on research utilization. *Nursing Research, 56*(Suppl. 4), S24–S39. doi: 10.1097/01.NNR.0000280629.63654.95.

Damberg, C. L., Sorbero, M. E., Lovejoy, S. L., et al.. (2012). An evaluation of the use of performance measures in health care. *Rand Health Quarterly, 1*(4), 3.

Damschroder, L. J., Aron, D. C., Keith, R. E., et al. (2009). Fostering implementation of health services research findings into practice: A consolidated framework for advancing implementation science. *Implementation Science, 4*, 50-5908-5904-5950. doi:10.1186/1748-5908-4-50; 10.1186/1748-5908-4-50.

Department of Health and Human Services. (2017). Million Hearts: Costs & Consequences. Retrieved October 2, 2018, from https://millionhearts.hhs.gov/learn-prevent/cost-consequences.html.

Donabedian, A. (1966). Evaluating the quality of medical care. *Milbank Memorial Fund Quarterly, 44*(Suppl. 3), 166–206.

Donabedian, A. (1988). The quality of care. How can it be assessed? *Journal of American Medical Association, 260*(12), 1743–1748.

Donabedian, A. (2005). Evaluating the quality of medical care. *Milbank Quarterly, 83*(4), 691–729. doi:10.1111/j.1468-0009.2005.00397.x.

Dukerich, J. M., Golden, B. R., & Shortell, S. M. (2002). Beauty is in the eye of the beholder: The impact of organizational identification identity and image on the cooperative behaviors of physicians. *Administrative Science Quarterly, 47*(3), 507–533. doi:10.2307/3094849.

Edmondson, A. (2003). Speaking up in the operating room: How team leaders promote learning in interdisciplinary action teams. *Journal of Management Studies, 40*(6), 1419–1452. doi:10.1111/1467-6486.00386.

Edmondson, A. C., Roberto, M. A., Bohmer, R. M., et al. (2005). The recovery window: Organizational learning following ambiguous threats. In William H. Starbuck, & Moshe Farjoun (Eds.), *Organization at the limit: Lessons from the Columbia disaster* (pp. 220–245). Malden, MA: Blackwell.

Elder, N., McEwan, T., Flach, J., et al. (2008). Advances in patient safety: New directions and alternative approaches (vol. 2: culture and redesign). In K. Henriksen, J. B. Battles, M. A. Keyes, & M. L. Grady (Eds.), *Creating safety in the testing process in primary care offices*. Rockville, MS: Agency for Healthcare Research and Quality.

Figueroa, J. F., Wang, D. E., & Jha, A. K. (2016). Characteristics of hospitals receiving the largest penalties by US pay-for-performance programmes. *BMJ Quality & Safety, 25*(11), 898–900.

Gilmartin, M. J., & D'Aunno, T. A. (2007). 8 leadership research in healthcare: A review and roadmap. *Academy of Management Annals, 1*(1), 387–438.

Greenhalgh, T., Robert, G., Macfarlane, F., et al. (2004). Diffusion of innovations in service organizations: Systematic review and recommendations. *Milbank Quarterly, 82*(4), 581–629. doi:10.1111/j.0887-378X.2004.00325.x.

Grossbart, S., & Agrawal, J. (2012). Conceptualization and definitions of quality. *Health care quality: The clinician's primer. ACPE, Sydney Olympic Park Google Scholar*.

Hammer, M. (1990). Reengineering work: Don't automate, obliterate. *Harvard Business Review, 68*(4), 104–112.

Higgins, A., Veselovskiy, G., & McKown, L. (2013). Provider performance measures in private and public programs: Achieving meaningful alignment with flexibility to innovate. *Health Affairs (Millwood), 32*(8), 1453–1461. doi:10.1377/hlthaff.2013.0007.

Horwitz, S. K., Horwitz, I. B., & Barshes, N. R. (2011). Addressing dysfunctional relations among healthcare teams: Improving team cooperation through applied organizational theories. *Advances in Health Care Management, 10*, 173–197.

Hughes, R. (2008). *Patient safety and quality: An evidence-based handbook for nurses*. Rockville, MD: Agency of Healthcare Research and Quality.

Institute of Medicine (IOM). (2007). *Rewarding provider performance: Aligning incentives in Medicare*. Washington, DC: The National Academies Press.

Institute of Medicine Committee on Quality of Health Care in America. (2001). *Crossing the quality chasm: A new health system for the 21st century*. Washington, DC: National Academies Press. Copyright 2001 by the National Academy of Sciences. All rights reserved.

Jha, A., & Epstein, A. (2010). Hospital governance and the quality of care. *Health Affairs (Millwood), 29*(1), 182–187.

Joshi, M. S., & Hines, S. C. (2006). Getting the board on board: Engaging hospital boards in quality and patient safety. *Joint Commission Journal on Quality and Patient Safety, 32*(4), 179–187.

Kaplan, H. C., Brady, P. W., Dritz, M. C., et al. (2010). The influence of context on quality improvement success in health care: A systematic review of the literature. *Milbank Quarterly, 88*(4), 500–559. doi:10.1111/j.1468-0009.2010.00611.x.

Kaplan, H. C., Froehle, C. M., Cassedy, A., et al. (2012). An exploratory analysis of the model for understanding success in quality. *Health Care Management Review, 38*(4), 325–338. doi:10.1097/HMR.0b013e3182689772.

Khatri, N., Brown, G. D., & Hicks, L. L. (2009). From a blame culture to a just culture in health care. *Health Care Management Review, 34*(4), 312–322.

Klein, K. J., & Sorra, J. S. (1996). The challenge of innovation implementation. *Academy of Management Review, 21*(4), 1055–1080.

Kohn, L. T., Corrigan, J. M., & Donaldson, M. S. (2000). *To err is human: Building a safer health system* (Vol. 6). Washington, DC: National Academies Press.

Kotter, J. P. (2012). *Leading change.* Boston, MA: Harvard Business Press.

Kringos, D. S., Sunol, R., Wagner, C., et al. (2015). The influence of context on the effectiveness of hospital quality improvement strategies: A review of systematic reviews. *BMC Health Services Research, 15*(1), 277.

Kubler-Ross, E., & Kessler D. (2014) *On grief and grieving: Finding the meaning of grief through the five stages of loss.* New York: Scribner.

Lee, Fred. (2004). "If Disney ran your hospital." Chicago: American Hospital Association.

Lehrman, W. G., Elliott, M. N., Goldstein, E., et al. (2010). Characteristics of hospitals demonstrating superior performance in patient experience and clinical process measures of care. *Medical Care Research and Review, 67*(1), 38–55. doi:10.1177/1077558709341323.

Leonard, L. B., & Kent, D. S. (2008). Management lessons from Mayo clinic. McGraw-Hill Professional Publishing.

Leonard, M., Graham, S., & Bonacum, D. (2004). The human factor: The critical importance of effective teamwork and communication in providing safe care. *Quality & Safety in Health Care, 13*(S1), i85. doi:10.1136/qshc.2004.010033.

Levine, D. M., Linder, J. A., & Landon, B. E. (2016). The quality of outpatient care delivered to adults in the United States, 2002 to 2013. *JAMA Internal Medicine, 176*(12), 1778–1790. doi:10.1001/jamainternmed.2016.6217.

Lisbon, D., Allin, D., Cleek, C., et al. (2016). Improved knowledge, attitudes, and behaviors after implementation of TeamSTEPPS training in an academic emergency department: A pilot report. *American Journal of Medical Quality, 31*(1), 86–90. doi:10.1177/1062860614545123.

Lynn, J., Baily, M. A., Bottrell, M., et al. (2007). The ethics of using quality improvement methods in health care: The ethics of using quality improvement methods in health care. *Annals of Internal Medicine, 146*(9), 666–673.

Mayer, C. M., Cluff, L., Lin, W. T., et al. (2011). Evaluating efforts to optimize TeamSTEPPS implementation in surgical

and pediatric intensive care units. *Joint Commission Journal on Quality and Patient Safety, 37*(8), 365–374.

Maynard, M. T., Marshall, D., & Dean, M. D. (2012). Crew resource management and teamwork training in health care: A review of the literature and recommendations for how to leverage such interventions to enhance patient safety. *Advances in Health Care Management, 13*, 59–91.

McAlearney A. S. (2008). Using leadership development program to improve quality and efficiency in healthcare. *Journal of Healthcare Management, 53*(5), 319–331.

McAlearney A. S. (2010). Executive leadership development in U.S. health systems. *Journal of Healthcare Management, 55*(3), 206–222.

McAlearney, A. S., Hefner, J., L, Sieck, C., J, & et al. (2014). The journey through grief: Insights from a qualitative study of electronic health record implementation. *Health Services Research, 50*(2), 462–488.

McAlearney, A. S., Garman, A. N., Song, P. H., et al. (2011). High-performance work systems in health care management, Part 2: Qualitative evidence from five case studies. *Health Care Management Review, 36*(3), 214–226. doi:10.1097/HMR.0b013e3182100dc4.

McAlearney, A. S., Hefner, J. L., Robbins, J., et al. (2015). Preventing central line-associated bloodstream infections: A qualitative study of management practices. *Infection Control & Hospital Epidemiology, 36*(5), 557–563. doi:10.1017/ice.2015.27.

Moffatt-Bruce, S. D., Hefner, J. L., Mekhjian, H., et al. (2015). What is the return on investment for implementation of a crew resource management program at an academic medical center? *American Journal of Medical Quality, 32*(1), 5–11. doi:10.1177/1062860615608938.

Murray, K. R., Hilligoss, B., Hefner, J. L., et al. (2017). The quality reporting reality at a large Academic Medical Center: Reporting 1600 unique measures to 49 different sources. *International Journal of Academic Medicine, 3*(1), 10.

Neily, J., Mills, P. D., Young-Xu, Y., et al.. (2010). Association between implementation of a medical team training program and surgical mortality. *Journal of American Medical Association, 304*(15), 1693–1700. doi:10.1001/jama.2010.1506.

Nembhard, I., Alexander, J., Hoff, T., et al. (2009). Understanding implementation failure in health care delivery: A role for organizational research and theory. *Academy of Management Perspectives, 23*(1), 1–27.

Okuyama, A., Wagner, C., & Bijnen, B. (2014). Speaking up for patient safety by hospital-based health care professionals: A literature review. *BMC Health Services Research, 14*(1), 61. doi:10.1186/1472-6963-14-61.

Patterson, K., Grenny J., McMillan, R., et al. (2002). *Crucial conversations: Tools for talking when stakes are high.* New York: McGraw-Hill.

Pettker, C. M., Thung, S. F., Raab, C. A., et al. (2011). A comprehensive obstetrics patient safety program improves safety climate and culture. *American Journal Obstetrics & Gynecology, 204*(3), 216. e211–e216. doi:10.1016/j.ajog.2010.11.004.

Price, R. A., Elliott, M. N., Zaslavsky, A. M., et al. (2014). Examining the role of patient experience surveys in measuring health care quality. *Medical Care Research and Review, 71*(5), 522–554. doi:10.1177/1077558714541480.

Pronovost, P., Needham, D., Berenholtz, S., et al. (2006). An intervention to decrease catheter-related bloodstream infections in the ICU. *New England Journal of Medicine, 355*(26), 2725–2732.

Ritchey, M. D., Loustalot, F., Wall, H. K., et al. (2017). Million Hearts: Description of the national surveillance and modeling methodology used to monitor the number of cardiovascular events prevented during 2012–2016. *Journal of American Heart Association, 6*(5), e006021. doi:10.1161/jaha.117.006021.

Shortell, S. M., O'Brien, J. L., Carman, J. M., et al. (1995). Assessing the impact of continuous quality improvement/total quality management: Concept versus implementation. *Health Services Research, 30*(2), 377.

Shortell, S. M., & Kaluzny, A. D., (Eds.), *Health care management: Organization design and behavior* (5th ed.). Clifton Park, NY: Delmar Cengage Learning.

Spinelli, R. J. (2006). The applicability of Bass's model of transformational, transactional, and laissez-faire leadership in the hospital administrative environment. *Hospital Topics, 84*(2), 11–19.

Starmer, A. J., Spector, N. D., Srivastava, R., et al. (2014). Changes in medical errors after implementation of a handoff program. *New England Journal of Medicine, 371*(19), 1803–1812. doi:10.1056/NEJMsa1405556.

Studer, Q. (2003). *Hardwiring excellence: Purpose, worthwhile work, making a difference.* Gulf Breeze, FL: Fire Starter Publishing.

Tapson, V. F., Karcher, R. B., & Weeks, R. (2011). Crew resource management and VTE prophylaxis in surgery: A quality improvement initiative. *American Journal of Medical Quality, 26*(6), 423–432. doi:10.1177/1062860611404694.

Tucker, A. L., Singer, S. J., Hayes, J. E., & Falwell, A. (2008). Front-line staff perspectives on opportunities for improving the safety and efficiency of hospital work systems. *Health Services Research, 43*(5 part 2), 1807–1829. doi:10.1111/j.1475-6773.2008.00868.x.

U.S. Centers for Medicare & Medicaid Services. (2017). Million Hearts: Cardiovascular Disease Risk Reduction Model. Retrieved July 4, 2017, from https://innovation.cms.gov/initiatives/Million-Hearts-CVDRRM/.

Weaver, S. J., Lubomksi, L. H., Wilson, R. F., et al. (2013). Promoting a culture of safety as a patient safety strategy: A systematic review. *Annals of Internal Medicine, 158*(5 Pt 2), 369–374. doi:10.7326/0003-4819-158-5-201303051-00002

Weaver, S. J., Rosen, M. A., DiazGranados, D., et al. (2010). Does teamwork improve performance in the operating room? A multilevel evaluation. *Joint Commission Journal on Quality and Patient Safety, 36*(3), 133–142.

Willis, T. A., West, R., Rushforth, B., et al. (2017). Variations in achievement of evidence-based, high-impact quality indicators in general practice: An observational study. *PLoS One, 12*(7), e0177949. doi:10.1371/journal.pone.0177949.

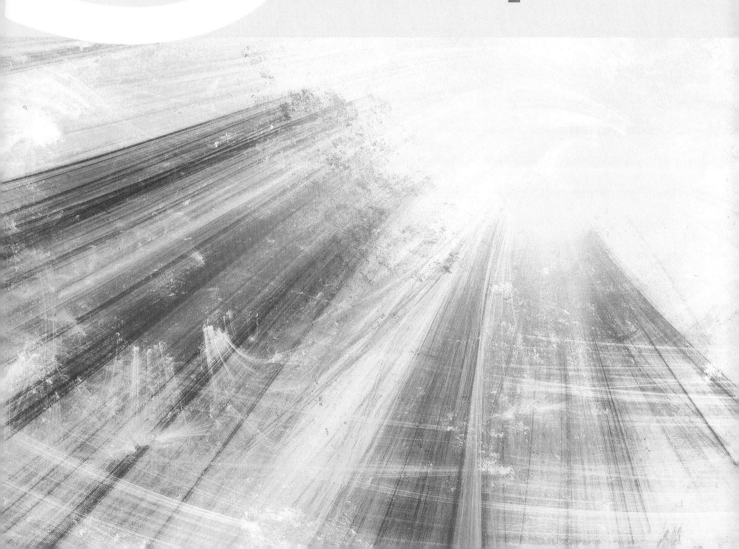

PART THREE
Macro Perspective

Chapter 10

Strategy and Achieving Mission Advantage

Stephen Walston and Ann F. Chou

CHAPTER OUTLINE

- Definition and Meaning of Strategy
- Strategic Management
- Values, Mission, and Vision
- Strategy and Health Care
- Evaluation of Organizational Environment
- Internal Resources: A Source of Competitive Advantage
- Generic Strategies

LEARNING OBJECTIVES

After completing this chapter, the reader should be able to:

1. Discuss concepts of strategy and strategic management
2. Explain the importance and the formulation of mission, vision, and values in strategy
3. Describe how strategic advantage can be different in health care
4. Explain how strategy is developed and can evolve in organizations
5. Discuss the concept and components of business models
6. Explain how to analyze the internal and external environments and the integration of these analyses into strategic planning
7. Identify different generic strategic approaches and how these may be used in health care
8. Identify various strategy evaluation methods
9. Discuss how strategy and strategic management apply to health care markets

KEY TERMS

Business Model

Buyer Power

Competitive Advantage

Differentiation

Barriers to Entry

External Environment

First Mover Advantage

Generic Strategies

Horizontal Integration

Internal Environment

Mission

Monopoly

Oligopolies

Porter's Five Forces Framework

Portfolio Analysis

Rivalry

Strategy

Strategic Group

Strategic Management

Supplier Power

Switching Costs

SWOT Analysis

Threat of Substitution

Values

Vertical Integration

Vision

DEBATE TIME: Hospital Monopolies

Monopoly power has a negative connotation, as monopolists frequently extract higher prices as the sole player in the market. Nevertheless, many hospitals in the United States are considered monopolies. Many act as a monopoly by default as the market in which they operate cannot support another facility. Many, however, have actively attempted to achieve monopoly status and some hospitals have used that status to their advantage. Norman Regional Hospital (NRH), a 288-bed facility, is the only hospital in Norman, Oklahoma, a growing suburb of Oklahoma City and the third largest city in the state with a population of 110,000. NRH's mission is to serve the community as the leader in health and wellness care. Their vision is as follows: "NRHS will be the provider of choice to improve the health and well-being of our regional communities." While the number of hospitals in other suburban communities has grown and competition is intense in the state, NRH remains the only hospital in its city. How has it maintained its monopoly position? In the 1980s, NRH worked with the city of Norman to pass legislation requiring any hospital desiring to enter the market to obtain city permission or a type of "certificate of need." With competitors unable to meet this criterion, NRH has effectively maintained its monopoly position. NRH has claimed that it can offer higher quality and lower cost medical care in the absence of competition. Why do you think NRH can make this claim? Do you agree? To judge their quality and costs, you can go to http://www.ucomparehealthcare.com and https://www.medicare.gov/hospitalcompare/search.html.

CHAPTER PURPOSE

Strategy and strategic thinking remain a critical skill for health care leaders. The concept of strategy has been the focus of study for many management scholars, which has led to hundreds of books and publications, and strategy has become a core course for almost all business programs. This chapter provides an essential overview of strategy. First, we define strategy in terms of how it evolves and its relationship to the environment. Second, our definition helps illustrate the relationship of an organization's values, mission, and vision to strategy. Successful organizations derive strategies from their missions and, as we describe, seek mission advantage in their markets by developing strategies to fulfill these missions.

Third, the chapter provides methods and means to understand, develop, and implement strategies. Business models with four interacting components are discussed for general and health care firms. Readers learn that business models change as internal and external pressures motivate organizations to adapt to be successful. Fourth, the chapter explores the impact of external and internal environments and market structures on strategies. Fifth, to better understand the competitive forces in an industry, the Five Forces Framework is introduced. The importance of internal resources and their related organizational competencies is discussed where these resources and competencies should be valuable, rare, difficult to imitate, and lacking substitutes to achieve competitive advantage. Finally, the chapter concludes

with a number of tools and concepts relating to strategy development and implementation. Examples of these tools include value chains, SWOT analysis, generic strategies, first mover advantage, product life cycle, and portfolio analysis. This chapter provides students with a broad overview of strategy and the ability to apply it to achieve mission advantage.

DEFINITION AND MEANING OF STRATEGY

Definition of Strategy

Strategy has a myriad of definitions. While strategy occurs at all levels of firms and organizations, there is little agreement on how strategy is defined (Luke, Walston, and Plummer, 2004; Murray, Knox, and Bernstein, 1994). Some see strategy as a formal plan, and some view strategy as crafting a process or means to beat a competitor. Yet others perceive strategy as a way of doing business, positioning an organization, and gaining advantage from either a prospective or an emergent viewpoint (Mintzberg, Ahlstrand, and Lampel, 2005; Porter, 1980). Strategy can also be considered a guide for future action, a pattern of past behaviors, and the fundamental way in which an organization operates (Mintzberg, Ahlstrand, and Lampel, 2005). Michael Porter (1980) defines strategy as developing a broad formula for how a business is going to compete and collaborate, what goals should be, and what policies are needed to carry out those goals to achieve the organization's mission. This perspective of strategy as deliberate, purposeful behavior allows a firm to plan decisions that maximize opportunities while minimizing threats. Thus, strategy allows for conscious action to take advantage of external opportunities with a firm's own internal capabilities. Strategies are developed to guide future behaviors and achieve organizational goals.

Although we recognize that a firm's actual strategy can evolve through many different methods, we analyze strategy in a practical manner to provide students and health care managers with the knowledge and skills to improve their understanding and practice of strategy through intentional and cognitive decisions. Overall, at its essence, strategy is about efficiently organizing information to improve decision making and allocating resources accordingly. Leaders are faced with many critical choices: where to invest, whom to hire, what services to offer, etc. Leaders who develop strategic skills make better decisions. Strategies assist organizations to choose wisely among the many available options.

An organization's mission and **vision** statements should drive its strategy formulation. An organization should identify which business it is in (and will be in) and then set strategic goals and objectives to achieve its mission and vision. The strategic plan becomes a company's plan to address how a company will:

- Grow and develop its business lines
- Determine the level and extent of competition and collaboration with other organizations
- Integrate and coordinate its functional components
- Choose the services and programs it will emphasize and toward which to allocate greater resources
- Form and develop its culture (Walston, 2017)

Strategy does not create a blueprint for future decisions. The specific actions and paths to follow cannot be a detailed map, since the future is uncertain. Strategy must be flexible enough to allow for changing circumstances. However, strategic actions often commit resources that may be difficult to recover. For example, construction of health care facilities can take three to five years to complete and systems invest millions anticipating future returns. In South Florida, Hospital Corporation of America (HCA) planned to spend $449 million on hospital and health care facilities in 2017 (Hurtibise, 2016). Whether or not this strategy focusing on capital investment would benefit HC remains to be seen. However, successful strategies must balance committed resources with the need for flexibility and the advantage of being first in a market. These are decisions that leaders must make after careful consideration of their situation and environment. Strategic planning must be flexible to allow for changing environments and conditions and yet disciplined enough to sustain competitive advantage. Within these choices, strategy provides a unifying theme that provides coherence and direction to the actions and decisions of the organization.

• • • IN PRACTICE: How Strategies Evolved

Strategy literally means "the art of the general" (from the Greek *strategos*) and originally signified the planning of a military campaign. This concept of strategy has been discussed for thousands of years. Strategy, along with the concept of organizational structure, was refined and articulated to further military purposes. Military campaigns motivated the training of leaders to obtain competitive advantage on the battlefield. Generals often recorded their experiences and wisdom to improve their armies' prospects. Some of the first records emerged between 500 BCE and 700 ACE in China, where a number of significant treatises on warfare emerged, the most familiar being Sun Tzu's *Art of War* (Sawyer, 2007).

This military perspective continued until the advent of the Industrial Revolution when the size of companies grew to a point that required more coordination and direction. In the twentieth century, the need for explicit strategy was initially emphasized by executives of large corporations, such as Alfred Sloan of General Motors and Chester Barnard of New Jersey Bell. During this time, eminent economists also sought to answer questions related to the purpose of firms and the relationship between resource allocation and business success (Ghemawat, 2001).

Today, strategy and strategic management have become widely accepted. Courses about strategy are widespread in business schools, and strategic management is an integral part of leadership training. Yet, given its diverse nature, teaching strategy is a difficult task that involves instructing how to craft future-directed plans, while developing an intuitive insight and the ability to learn, adapt, and change (Burns, 2002). The concept and importance of strategy has proliferated widely in business. A recent search for "business strategy" on Google yielded over 34.5 million search results and 429,000 books (search May 2017). Overall, the nature of strategy remains very complex but widely accepted.

• • • IN PRACTICE: How Strategies Evolved (Continued)

Strategy has two very important functions. First, as mentioned previously, good strategies should improve decisions that allocate finite resources today for a more prosperous and successful tomorrow. Leaders, faced with multiple projects, must determine which ones receive personnel, materials, and other resources.

Another important function of a strategy is to challenge existing assumptions and open our eyes to new possibilities. For example, many hold on to old, often false assumptions that the elderly cannot surf the Internet and men make most of the financial decisions for families (Weinstein Organization, 2017). Both have proven to be false. Moreover, assumptions that were correct a decade ago may not hold true today. Good strategic thinking challenges existing assumptions and awakens leaders to new realities. Those that do not adjust to new realities and see changes will make decisions based on outdated or even erroneous information, which can lead to poor results.

Oftentimes, these assumptions may be based upon incorrect information. Take a look at Figure 10.1 below. When asked if Lima, Peru, is west or east of Miami, Florida, most people would believe that Lima is further west than Miami, when in fact Miami is west of Lima. In the late 1980s and early 1990s, most assumed that health maintenance organizations (HMOs) would be the dominant model for health care delivery. Based upon this assumption, many health care leaders rapidly purchased physician practices and formed insurance products to create integrated delivery systems. Some hospitals went so far as to alter their mission statements to become integrated systems. Yet, by the late 1990s, it was apparent that HMOs' growth had dissipated and preferred provider organizations (PPOs) began to dominate the health care market. Many health care systems that pursued integrated delivery systems, based on this assumption, made significant strategic blunders and generally failed to achieve their strategic goals (Burns and Pauly, 2002). Strategic thinking thus requires not only challenging assumptions but also the data on which they are based.

UNDERSTANDING AND DISCOVERING OUR BIASES

When asked which city is farther west, Miami, Florida, or Lima, Peru, almost all would choose Lima. However, on a map or comparing the degrees of longitude, one would find that Miami, Florida, is actually further west than Lima, Peru. Miami, Florida, has a longitude of $-80° 11' 37''$, while Lima, Peru's longitude is only $-77° 3' 0''$.

Why do most individuals have this inaccurate knowledge? Generally, people perceive South America directly below North America, an incorrect fact. South America actually protrudes to the east of North America.

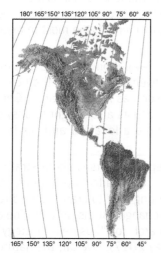

Figure 10.1 The Americas.

STRATEGIC MANAGEMENT

Steps in the strategic management process may include (1) goal formation, (2) environmental scanning, (3) strategy formulation, (4) strategy evaluation, (5) implementation, and (6) strategic control. **Strategic management** requires both internal and external management functions to facilitate this process. Internally, strategic management involves the participation of everyone in the organization, especially the leadership. Organizational leadership and management play key roles in (a) formulating strategies and integrating them into the organization's mission, visions, and goals; (b) leveraging organizational mechanisms, cultures, and resources to support the strategic implementation; and (c) conducting analyses and evaluation. Externally, strategic management enhances organizational success by anticipating possible changes in the environment in which the organization operates and enabling organizations to change and maintain their **competitive advantage** against their rivals. Both external analyses and internal mechanisms are thus important in the strategic management process (Ginter, Swayne, and Duncan, 2002; Luke, Walston, and Plummer, 2004; Mintzberg, Lampel, and Ahlstrand, 2005; Schendel, 1994).

Environment

No organization is immune to influences from its external environment. Strategic management identifies and positions a firm to respond appropriately to external threats and opportunities. As an industry, health care is particularly sensitive to its external environment, which has continually experienced demographic, societal/cultural, economic, technological, political/legal, and global changes (Fahey, 1999; Moseley, 2018; Walter and Priem, 1999). For the most part, health care organizations cannot directly control these external factors but must develop strategies to effectively respond to these changes.

Demographic changes (e.g., population size, age distribution, geographic variation, racial/ethnic mix, and income levels) affect health care across the globe (Fahey and Narayanan, 1986). Populations across the world are getting older and in industrialized countries the birth rate has fallen dramatically (Altergott, 2016). The U.S. Census Bureau estimates that about 20 percent of the U.S. population will be older than age 65 by 2050. The U.S. population will also become more racially and ethnically diverse. As summarized in Figure 10.2, the minority population is rapidly growing in the United States. Roughly 43 percent of millennials today are nonwhite; by 2050, no racial or ethnic group will make up the majority.

The increased diversity of the population will prompt health care organizations to develop strategies that address changes in the cultural and demographic needs of their constituents. Culture, race, ethnicity, and primary language significantly dictate how health care is accessed and what prevention and treatment strategies are effective. A more diverse society requires more diverse and multicultural strategies. Professional organizations, like the American Hospital Association, have encouraged their members to take the lead and proactively adopt recommendations to address these needs (http://www.aha.org/content/00-10/09elim-disp-essentials.pdf, accessed May 17, 2017).

Along with an aging population, life-style changes have increased the prevalence of obesity and chronic conditions, leading to greater patient complexity. As patients become more difficult to manage clinically, the health care industry faces a continuing shortage of both clinicians and allied health workers (DesRoches et al., 2015). The industry also needs new models of delivery and care coordination to address its complex needs.

Technological advancements have also contributed to escalating health care costs that, in turn, spur broader insurance coverage to finance them. Increasingly, this financing role has shifted from the private to the public sector. In the United States, the federal and state governments pay for over 37 percent of health care costs through the Medicare and Medicaid programs in 2015 (CMS, 2017). As a result, they can mandate rules and regulations that require compliance in exchange for reimbursement. As a result, the health care industry is particularly susceptible to political and legal influences because the government has a complicated relationship with the industry as a provider, regulator, and payer.

The health care industry thus operates in a very large, dynamic, complex, and challenging external environment with many opportunities as well as threats. Health care organizations must craft strategies to deal with an aging and diverse customer base, increased competition, technological innovation, and pressures to improve quality while lowering costs ("value").

Achieving Strategic Success

In turn, successful strategies require direction, resources, and institutionalized processes. Too often, organizations believe that strategy is accomplished when direction is

---

1. There is more racial and ethnic diversity in the United States, where by 2050, no single racial or ethnic majority will exist in the United States.

2. Asia is supplying the highest number of immigrants to the United States.

3. Millennials are more racially diverse, with 43 percent identified as nonwhite.

4. There is a continuing increase of women in labor force, with over 40 percent of women working as the primary or sole household provider.

5. The percentage of Americans living in middle-class households decreased to under 50 percent.

6. Increasing population is not affiliated with any religion, which in itself has become the second largest group in most nations.

Figure 10.2 Demographic Changes Shaping the United States and World.

SOURCE: Cohn and Caumont (2016).

formulated. This, however, is only the first step in taking strategic action. As Scott Becker, CEO of Conemaugh Health System in Johnstown, Pennsylvania, said, "Everybody has a great strategic plan. The organizations that are successful are the ones that effectively operationalize it" (Rodak, 2013). Operationalizing strategy involves allocating responsibilities, authority, resources, and expected outcomes (key performance indicators) to measure progress. For example, one large international hospital that was established to primarily provide tertiary services identified as one of its strategic priorities to improve its service capacity. This was subdivided into project areas to (1) reduce the nontertiary patient load, (2) increase the efficiency and throughput of patients, (3) expand existing facilities, (4) better coordinate patient care with other institutions, and (5) expand off-site patient care services. Each of these was further segmented into specific goals that had assigned responsibilities, key performance indicators, and reporting time frames.

Experience suggests that most strategies fail as a result of improper or inattentive implementation (Dye and Sibony, 2007). The best strategic plan, if poorly implemented with inadequate follow-up, is just another poor plan. Too often, there is only motion without concrete action. In fact, developing strategies without implementation can create many organizational problems.

This is oftentimes the most difficult aspect of strategic action. Organizations often spend an incredible amount of time and resources developing strategic plans. Yet, many of these plans do not get implemented, as surveys have shown that almost half of companies having strategic plans do not track the outcomes of their strategic initiatives, resulting in little actual strategic accomplishments (Dye and Sibony, 2007). This waste of resources is caused by an inward focus on the planning process and not making strategic activities outcome-oriented. If the plan is poorly developed, the organization will fail to improve its competitive position and attain its mission and vision.

To facilitate implementation, health care organizations should seek to:

- Identify responsibility and outcomes with definite time lines and key performance indicators: This should include managerial responsibility and related budgets necessary to accomplish targeted strategic objectives.
- Establish a monitoring and evaluation process: This process should facilitate communication of the progress and challenges in implementing the strategies.
- Develop and promote policies that facilitate strategic action: Organizations should establish policies that encourage innovation and aid in change.
- Appropriately use information and operating systems to drive the strategies: Health care organizations generally have far too much data and lack good

synthesis of these data to drive strategic decisions. Strategic thinking requires accurate, timely information delivered to the decision maker.

- Tie rewards to the achievement of strategic action: Successful strategic-oriented firms are results-oriented and motivate and celebrate achievement of strategic outcomes.
- Link budgets to strategies: Strategic plans are too often divorced from organizational budgets. Strategies need to be integrated into annual budgets and be used to drive strategic action.
- Incorporate strategic action into annual evaluations: Annual employee evaluations should be mapped to organizational goals. In particular, organizational values should be directly reflected in each evaluation. Employees and managers should determine how closely the employee is living the values in his or her work.

The Strategic Action Cycle

Strategic management includes a strategic action cycle that begins with development of a plan, identification of values, formulation of the mission and vision, strategic objectives, strategic analyses to identify corporate and then operational plans, followed by implementation (Figure 10.3). Implementation integrates budgeting, monitoring, and evaluation. Efforts and resources must be assigned to each of these tasks. Performance standards are established, measured, and monitored, which inform the next round of strategic planning.

It is important to recognize that strategic planning is not a "one-time event" but part of a strategic action cycle that should continue for the life of the business. While corporate/business strategic plans should lay out the future directions for the organization, progress should be reviewed annually and strategies updated accordingly. Performance targets and key strategies for at least three to five years should be a part of the time line.

VALUES, MISSION, AND VISION

Organizations can be effective with radically different strategies. Even similar organizations in geographic proximity may have different strategies that each produces spectacular results. There is not one right, optimal, or "one-size-fits-all" strategy. Effective strategies are created by matching internal abilities and resources to the external environment to meet the purpose for the organization's existence. Since organizations exist for many reasons, an effective and successful outcome may be different for different organizations. For example, a

The Strategic Action Cycle

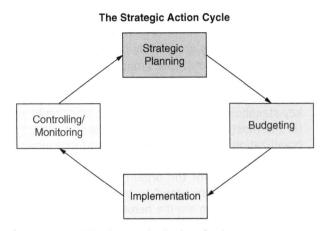

Figure 10.3 The Strategic Action Cycle.
SOURCE: Adapted from Walston (2017).

for-profit hospital may seek high financial returns to satisfy its stakeholders, while a church clinic might define success by the greater number of patients it serves.

The definition of success is based upon the important values and purposes of an organization. Each organization may have different values and external influences that will influence its objectives and how it would define its success. Different business models will also be associated with different statements of values, mission, and vision, as well as with differences in their approaches to strategy. This is especially the case in the health care sector, where strategies often differ significantly across for-profit versus not-for-profit organizations, academic medical centers versus community hospitals, rural versus urban facilities, multimarket systems versus single market hospitals, and so on.

Organizations should seek "mission advantage" by strategically positioning themselves to best achieve their established mission (Walston, 2017). The basis of all successful strategies should originate with the organization's mission, vision, and values. Too often, however, these statements end up as a written document sitting on a shelf or a plaque hanging on the wall and are disconnected from the strategic formulation and implementation. Strategy experts suggest that in many organizations, few know the elements of their strategies, including their executives (Collis and Rukstad, 2008). When this disconnect occurs, organizations frequently find themselves in trouble with their stakeholders. For example, HealthSouth, HCA, and Tenet (among many others) experienced indictments, significant fines, lower stock prices, and tarnished public reputation as a result of their fraudulent actions that contradicted their stated mission, vision, and values. HCA paid almost $1.7 billion in criminal fines, civil restitution, and penalties in 2000 and 2003 to resolve fraudulent actions that violated the very visible mission and values statements that have been ubiquitously displayed in their hospitals (http://www.usdoj.gov/opa/pr/2003/June/03_civ_386.htm).

Values

What are values and why are they important? **Values** are the expression of ethics that should guide employees' actions. They define what behaviors are both acceptable and unacceptable and should constrain how the mission and vision are accomplished. Certain behaviors, no matter how they accomplish the organizational mission, are unacceptable; even if the mission is accomplished, if the values have been violated, the organization has failed.

Unfortunately, many organizations fail to engrain values into their culture. Frequently, values are used only as marketing slogans, as organizations ignore them and fixate on financial results and profits (Walston, 2017). Often, organizations survey employees to ascertain compliance with their values, as in general, employees may be in the best position to observe whether or not an organization's expressed values have been incorporated into its culture. In many ways, employees are the best judge to determine if an organization's value statements are mere gestures or if they are connected to their strategic behaviors.

Is it valuable for organizations to articulate their values? Written organizational values are important for a number of reasons. For one, they serve as an ethical compass, the absence of which could leave an organization without a viable rudder to direct its strategies. Particularly during times of stress, an organization lacking such a compass might feel pressures to deviate from standards and take decisions contrary to normal ethical practices. Pressure to achieve goals may also generate personality conflicts that could induce inappropriate and unethical behaviors. Written values serve as visible reminders of the organization's commitment to basic beliefs.

Moreover, written values assist in grounding organizational ethics over time. Values and ethics should endure and not fluctuate based on current encounters or challenges. Strategies will (and should) change over time. However, values should not. Thomas Watson, Jr., former chairman of IBM, expressed the need for common beliefs upon which a business should be founded: "I believe that any organization, in order to survive and achieve success, must have a sound set of beliefs on which it premises all of its policies and actions" (Watson, 1963, p. 3).

In theory, organizational values represent the sum total of individual values held by each person affiliated with an organization—i.e., the stakeholders. In practice, however, the values of top executives almost always exert the greatest influence on an organization's prevailing tone and practices. More generally, it is the role of the CEO, other top executives, and the board of directors to formulate an organization's values and to assure that they are lived throughout the organization. As a consultant once said, "Values should not be just written on a wall, but to be effective they must be written on the hearts of employees."

Expressed values can also be the means by which an organization shapes attitudes of its members toward selected categories of stakeholders. This is especially important in health care, given the diversity and importance of different stakeholders. A good example of this can be found in the value statements offered by All Saints Healthcare System, a hospital system based in Racine, Wisconsin. All Saints is a member of the Wheaton Franciscan System, a Catholic multihospital system. Three of their expressed values include the following:

- *Respect*: We value each person as sacred, created in the image and likeness of God, which gives worth and meaning to each person's life.

- *Excellence*: We value superior performance in our work and service.

- *Stewardship*: We value our responsibility to use human, financial, and natural resources entrusted to us for the common good, with special concern for those who are poor.

Note how these values craft expected behaviors toward patients and the poor. Assuming that these values are inculcated within the system's culture, one should expect the provision of excellent care and that the poor are treated with dignity by this system. Furthermore, the location of their facilities and financial policies should reflect these values. One might expect one's hospitals to be located near lower socioeconomic areas and to provide generous discounts from billed charges to the poor.

How Should Values Be Established and Evaluated?

Values should be established and evaluated based on core beliefs, values, and expectations of key shareholders.

- *Understand key stakeholder expectations for the organization*. In some organizations, the owners might be the only group truly deemed to be important. For others, multiple groups including owners, customers, employees, and suppliers might all have influenced a search for values. One way to identify key stakeholders is to identify those who would suffer the most if the organization ceases to exist. The organization can conduct surveys and interviews to see what values are believed to be important. For what do they want the organization to be known? What makes them proud to be affiliated with the organization? Who are the heroes of the organization and why?

- *Compile common values among stakeholders*. Commonly expressed values should be identified and related values merged to express the ethical base of the organization's purpose. An organization should seek to identify those values that set it apart and make it distinctive.

- *Make values visible*. Organizational values must be visible and tied to performance. The values should be clearly incorporated into employees' (including the CEO's) evaluations, and the appraisal should be based on how well they are living the values. The organization should also link values to measurable strategic outcomes, as reflected in satisfaction scores, error rates, quality indicators, etc.

- *Establish memorable values*. Values should be in terms that stakeholders will understand and can remember. As a general rule, there should be no more than five to seven values.

• • • IN PRACTICE: How Values Dictate Actions and Outcomes: The Mongol and Arab Conquests

The values an organization holds can directly influence its behavior and outcomes. Two different peoples conquered huge swaths of the known world across different centuries with different outcomes. The Arab or Muslim armies emerged in 632 CE, as the Arab Peninsula was unified. By 732 CE, the Muslims controlled land from Spain to India. The Muslims were skilled warriors but held deeply rooted values that dictated how war was to be conducted. Muslims felt a deep need to share Islam with others, and travelers and traders peacefully spread it into Africa, China, Malaysia, and Indonesia. However, even during conflicts, the sharing of Islam was a primary mission of the Arab armies. Thus, their values and actions reflected their mission.

War was strongly discouraged (see Al-Baqarah 2:190 in the Quran) but necessary against oppressive nations and for self-defense. Muslims, when engaged in war, were never to fight against noncombatants, especially women and children. Trees were not to be harmed. Justice was to be highly valued, as during peace. Medical assistance was to be available to all, irrespective of religion or creed, even enemies. Captives were to be shown mercy, be fed, and allowed to gain their freedom through ransom, labor, or on their word. When people were conquered, they were allowed to choose their religion and, generally, had more freedoms and opportunities. As a result, most of their conquered populations freely converted to Islam over time, achieving their primary mission (DeWeese, 1994).

• • • IN PRACTICE: How Values Dictate Actions and Outcomes: The Mongol and Arab Conquests (Continued)

In contrast to the Muslim Expansion, the Mongol Empire arose during the thirteenth and fourteenth centuries. At its height, the empire covered lands from China, Russia, and India to the Middle East. The Mongols lacked a religious motive but were a warlike people who enjoyed hunting and conquest. The original Mongol leader, Genghis Khan, was reputed to once have asked and then answered himself, "What is the greatest joy in life?" He said, "The greatest joy a man can know is to conquer his enemies and drive them before him, ride their horses and take away their possessions, see the faces who were dear to them bedewed with tears, and to clasp their wives and daughters in his arms" (Prawdin and Chaliand, 2005, p. 60).

Yet, the Mongols had a strict sense of honor and loyalty. The Mongol "mission" was to conquer and obtain gains. They were very intelligent and used superb tactics and strategies. They gained accurate knowledge of their enemies prior to attacking, used superior technology and tactics, and were highly mobile. The Mongols were extremely ruthless in battle but also displayed extraordinary military discipline. Resistance was met by ruthless annihilation. Captured enemies might be killed, enslaved, or used as a human shield in subsequent battles. Cooperative territories received relatively benevolent rule that included religious tolerance. When a Mongol army first approached a city, it would most often give the city an opportunity to surrender and pay tribute. If rejected, the city would be ransacked and destroyed. Everyone and everything was likely to be attacked, including armies, animals, women, and children. For instance, Bagdad, the capital of the then existing Muslim empire, was destroyed in 1257 CE. As many as a million people were estimated to have been killed (Frazier, 2005, p. 4). Total destruction occurred to many cities including Kiev and Moscow. The Mongols expanded their empire to the gates of Vienna, Austria, but the empire began to unravel in less than two centuries. Ironically, most of the Mongol-controlled areas eventually converted to Islam.

For both, values can readily dictate actions and outcomes.

Mission

A mission should be the foundation for strategic direction. The existence and enactment of the organization's mission is critical to its success. A mission keeps management focused on its primary purpose. A mission should be an enduring statement of core organizational purpose that distinguishes it from other organizations and identifies the scope of its operations in terms of products and markets (Business Dictionary, 2016). It is a key indicator of how the organization views its stakeholders. As such, it should germinate from the organization's values. A mission provides the reason for the organization's existence and forms the basis for strategy. It should guide the organization to focus its energies and frame its choices of strategy and commitments of resources. A mission should be the solid base upon which strategic direction is established that drives investments and resource allocation.

What should be included in a mission? Most successful statements have measurable, definable, and actionable items. They contain as well an emotional appeal that all recognize and can act upon. Key components should include the definition of product or service, the standards employed, and the population or segment served by the organization. A mission should describe what the organization does or its scope. What does it do? What are the boundaries beyond which it will not venture? They should also reflect the organization's values through expressed standards and objectives. Such standards may include providing "world-class services" or "setting the community's quality standards." This segment is the essence of the organization's competitive advantage. What will your business do differently or better than others? The customer base should also be identified. Organizations may state in their missions that they serve a demographic segment, like women or children, or a nation or region.

Missions are expressed in many ways. Some are short and others lengthy. Collis and Rukstad (2008) suggest no more than 35 words. However, organizations establish many different kinds of missions. HealthTrust, Inc., a company formed in 1987 from Hospital Corporation of America, used a generic mission that it was the "Hospital Company." While, this two-word mission reflected HealthTrust's exclusive focus on hospital care, mission statements in general should have more than a simple phrase in order to differentiate and guide the organization.

Missions should be distinctive and guide an organization's strategies but short enough that employees can comprehend and apply. If a mission statement is too long, it cannot be readily communicated and internalized by everyone in the organization, which in turn cannot be effectively used to drive strategies. As demonstrated by Primary Children's Hospital (see below), missions can be short enough to be a mantra that employees can easily remember and use in their work.

DEBATE TIME: Missions

Missions can be written in many different ways. Which of the following could you, as an employee, understand and use in your work? What could be done to improve each? What is the value of a long versus a short mission? Examine the mission for different types of organizations: an academic medical center, hospitals owned by a religious order, and a major pharmaceutical firm. How do their missions reflect the types of organizations that they are?

1. At [name], our mission is leading health care.
2. Through our exceptional health care services, we reveal the healing presence of God.
3. As a Christian health center, our mission is to improve the health of the people in the communities we serve.
4. We, the management and employees, are striving for entrepreneurial success. Entrepreneurial success starts with people. Our goal is to operate a worldwide business that produces meaningful benefits for consumers, our market partners, and our community. Through efficient research and development, production, and marketing of pharmaceutical and chemical specialties, we want to extend opportunities to our customers. To achieve this, we focus our endeavors on business areas where we can achieve a competitive advantage through the excellent quality of our products, systems, and services. Our objective is to establish permanent business relationships and not merely short-term success.

On the basis of these principles, we operate as an independent and profit-oriented enterprise. We expect a high level of performance from each other and reward this accordingly. We wish to secure an acceptable return on capital for our investors.

We respect the cultural distinctions and national interests of all countries in which we operate. We strive to achieve positive recognition for our company within the community. We attach particular importance to its responsibility for safety. We have an obligation to respect the environment.

We will deal honestly and constructively with one another. We regard open communication, both internal and external, as a fundamental prerequisite for reaching an understanding of our common goals and for giving meaning to what we do. We shall not be constrained by borders between business areas or countries. All employees, male or female, have equal opportunities to develop their careers. All of us make a personal contribution to the company's entrepreneurial success through our mutual initiative, creativity, and sense of responsibility.

Too often, companies use "cookie cutter" mission statements that fail to inspire (Persico, 2016). Businesses should avoid using nondescript, generic statements like "providing the highest quality of care for the lowest possible cost" or "maximizing shareholder wealth by exceeding customer expectations," which in some derivation often appear in many mission statements. Buzz words should be avoided. A hospital stating that its mission is "to provide the highest possible quality" is virtually meaningless. Other examples include a large health care system's mission to "remain at the forefront of health care delivery." What does this mean? Is it at the forefront of clinical technology, market share, quality, or innovation?

Missions should also be crafted to express the core function and purpose of the organization's existence. Although missions among successful organizations vary, in general, missions should contain the following:

1. Services or products offered
2. Values and standards that distinguish the organization from others
3. Market(s) in which the organization operates (Walston, 2017).

For example, a large health care organization had at first stated its mission to be the following:

> Center provides medical services of a highly specialized nature and promotes medical research and education programs, including postgraduate education training, as well as contributes to the prevention of disease.

After extensive discussion, the leadership agreed that the main purpose for the medical center was to provide highly specialized health care and that education and research would support the delivery of specialized care. As a result, they altered their mission to this:

> Center provides the highest quality specialized health care in an integrated education and research setting.

Although the differences may seem subtle, they are important. The hospital's primary purpose and the reason for its existence were to provide tertiary and quaternary care to its service population. In the context of their strategic development, education and research were to be instituted chiefly to support the primary mission and not to be developed in an isolated, self-supporting manner that had occurred before.

A mission should also not be too restrictive. During the early 1900s, the railroads in the United States fell on hard times because they had narrowly defined their mission as providing rail service rather than being in the transportation business in a larger sense. The railroad companies remained committed to transportation on two rails, while much transportation shifted to roads and air. Likewise, hospitals that narrowly define their mission to be in the acute care business might encounter competitive difficulties in markets in which more integrated services are demanded.

In contrast to railroads, Xerox has defined itself as "The Document Company" and its mission as "to help people find better ways to do great work—by constantly leading in document technologies, products and services that improve our customers' work processes and business results." Note that Xerox does not portray itself as a copier company but expands and widens its purpose to be a "document company." As such, it can provide both electronic and hard-copy documents that serve to improve its customers' business.

To be useful, a mission must also "call employees to action." To do this, it must motivate employees emotionally to act. It must be easily understood and short enough to be remembered. It should be measurable and reasonably attainable. It must be reviewed periodically to ensure relevance. A mission may need to change as the organizational external environment and internal resources evolve.

In summary, a mission should direct the organization to focus its energies on certain products, standards, and market/geographic segments. The mission statement should express why the organization exists and motivate employees to action. The organizational mission should both constrain and guide strategies and tactical actions.

Vision

A vision is a statement about what the organization wants to become. It focuses on the future. The vision should resonate with members of the organization and help them feel proud, excited, and part of something much bigger to come. A vision should challenge and stretch the organization's capabilities and image of itself. It gives shape and direction to the organization's future. Better vision statements describe outcomes that organizations would like to see that may be 5 to 10 years in the future, or further. Leaders and managers should possess competencies to structure the strategic vision, develop short- and long-term plans, and communicate them efficiently to employees so that the employees are empowered to act toward achieving the vision (Vainieri et al., 2017).

Mission and vision go hand in hand. A vision should describe the desired future state of the organization while the mission provides a description of the existing purpose and practice of the organization. For a vision to be effective, it should align with the organizational values, have understandable language, describe a desirable future, be clear, realistic, and concisely written.

Actions also need to be undertaken to move toward realizing the vision. For example, one large, international hospital set its vision to "become a world-leading institution of excellence and innovation in health care." This required that it benchmarks against the industry leaders, designates key services centers of excellence, and assures that necessary resources would be allocated to these services. Another example shows the vision statement of an academic medical center in the Southern United States, where the center seeks to "be recognized as a leading medical center in [the state] and one of the best in the nation. We will be at the forefront of

• • • IN PRACTICE: Primary Children's Hospital Mission

The Primary Children's Hospital is a tax-exempt, academic pediatric center of excellence serving five states in the intermountain region of the west. When Joseph Horton became its CEO, the mission statement was several sentences long and, while being factually correct, was rather ordinary and did not reflect the deep passion and powerful commitment to children that so many of the employees and physicians of the hospital felt. No one referred to the mission statement to explain why they made decisions.

The new CEO sought a powerful, short, and memorable mission statement to inspire the hearts and minds of those who served it. He wanted more of a "mission mantra" rather than a mission statement. The new mission was simply "The Child First and Always." It was carved into the granite wall of the entrance to the new hospital building that replaced the old one in 1990. While simple, history has shown the aligning power of these five words.

Twenty-five years after this simple mission was adopted by the hospital, a branding firm was asked to assess the hospital's brand. The firm found a high degree of unity among constituents and stakeholders. The consultants reported not only that there was incredible agreement among constituents but also that over 90 percent of them used the exact same words to describe it: "The Child First and Always."

clinical services, medical research and education. With our physician and university partners, we will create, teach, and deliver tomorrow's breakthroughs in medical science." In this case, the medical center articulated its intended actions to achieve this vision.

Compare these two vision statements from a health care system located on the East Coast and a hospital on the West Coast:

> To create a new standard of community health care, one that combines the personalized, caring environment of the finest community hospital with a commitment to providing the most advanced medical technology and capabilities available to it.
>
> To be the premier regional health care provider to the residents of its service area within . . .

The first might be too long to be impactful and contain unrealizable outcomes, while the second is more succinct and defines a geographic area to where that vision applies.

Vision statements often are more important in not-for-profit organizations. Lacking a primary bottom-line focus, an effective vision can guide not-for-profits to meet the challenges of their environment (Kilpatrick and Silverman, 2005). A concise vision written in clear language can provide specific, meaningful ideas to bring together an organization's goals and direction.

In summary, a vision should motivate and direct an organization. Vision and mission should be the foundation of all strategic plans. Leaders should seek to only craft strategies that help fulfill them. These two items should be the first and last discussion items of every strategic thinking process. This process should begin with a review of mission and vision, an environmental scan, followed by strategy formulation, and conclude with leaders confirming that the work aligns and promotes the organizational vision and mission.

STRATEGY AND HEALTH CARE

Competitive Advantage versus Mission Advantage

The concept of competitive advantage is widely used in strategy and has been conceptualized as the "Holy Grail" for businesses (Chiquan, 2007). This concept is defined by an increase in market power as a result of its actions (Luke, Walston, and Plummer, 2004), outperforming and distinguishing a company from its competitors (Porter, 1980), and the implementation of a value-creating strategy not simultaneously implemented by current or potential players (Barney, 1991). Each suggests a

---

DEBATE TIME: Missions, Visions, and Values

Here is an example of a home health service using its mission, vision, and values to drive its organizational direction and strategies. Is this organization effective in conveying why it exists, what it wants to be, and how it should behave and act?

Mission:

> To assist all New Brunswickers, who wish to remain in their homes, with the activities of daily living and or home health care necessary for them to do so for as long as they desire by providing them with the highest quality, most reliable services available

Vision:

> To be the provider of choice to all who require home health care and the employer of choice for all who wish to provide home health care services

Values:

> QUALITY—To provide the highest quality of service from the initial contact to the cessation of service
>
> CONTINUITY—To quickly establish regular caregivers at the beginning of service and within our power to ensure the same caregivers continue to provide service throughout
>
> COMMUNICATIONS—To keep the client and their circle of care up to date and aware of all aspects of their care
>
> RELIABILITY—To be dependable and trusted in all our dealings with clients, employees, and customers
>
> INTEGRITY—To act with the highest moral principles and professional standards in everything we do

competitive business environment of winners and losers in which organizations struggle to gain an advantage over their market competitors. Markets reward winners for superior service, pricing, and product innovation that provide consumers greater value. Organizations do this by exploiting their internal strengths to take advantage of environmental opportunities. Therefore, the sources of competitive advantage often come from external positioning (Porter, 1980) and/or organizational resources and capabilities (Barney, 1991).

While competitive advantage may generally apply to for-profit firms, it is not necessarily relevant for all health care organizations. Competitive advantage works well for those whose strategies are based on a "win–lose" perspective and whose success depends on finishing ahead of competitors in terms of market share, earnings, or other comparative metrics. However, health care organizations, especially those that are not-for-profit and/or whose mission involves service to vulnerable or disadvantaged populations, may consider that gaining strategic advantage over competitors is not an organizational priority or even inappropriate. Rather than promoting competitive advantage (which does not apply to many organization types such as nongovernmental organizations, not-for-profits, socially conscious firms, etc.), stressing mission advantage strengthens the applicability and alignment of mission statements and strategic focus to a wider variety of measures beyond the solely financial. Mission advantage focuses on achieving an organizational mission that can include profitability but also takes into account customer, community, and employee-desired benefits. A mission advantage focus allows companies to better tie core values and other mission-directed goals to drive organization's strategies.

Financial objectives of players in the health care sector have evolved over time. Hospitals, nursing homes, and health insurance plans were mostly established for charitable purposes. Studies suggest that health care organizations in the United States focus more on competition for patients compared to health care systems in other countries. Another marked difference is that collaboration and sharing responsibilities appear to be the norm among health care providers in other nations (Commonwealth Fund, 2004), creating greater efficiency in provision of care. There are various arguments for and against fostering health care competition (Hansen, 2008; Muscalus, 2008; Mutter, Wong, and Goldfarb, 2008). Although all organizations must generate sufficient income to survive, seeking competitive advantage may not be as effective in health care, where it is difficult to eliminate competition. Intense competition may just lower everyone's profits without improving service (Brandenburger and Nalebuff, 1997, p. 37).

Actions taken by one hospital, if proven successful, are frequently imitated by competitors, regularly leading to service overcapacity and increased aggressiveness.

In Indianapolis, for example, no hospital dedicated to heart disease existed prior to the year 2002. Soon after one hospital announced the construction of a freestanding heart facility, all other competitors began development of their own heart hospitals, resulting in three freestanding heart hospitals and one inhospital heart hospital. Building a specialty hospital is not an inimitable strategy. The intensity in competition in the Indianapolis market ensured lower profit margins for all players. The division of market shares and resulting lower patient volume may have prevented quality improvement based on sufficient volume and learning.

Evolving Strategies

Strategies often evolve and change according to environmental pressures. Turbulent or uncertain environments may force an organization to consider strategic change. Factors that create uncertainty include the following:

1. Political/legislative changes
2. Technological innovation
3. Changing customer demand

The pace of change and uncertainty in health care has been spurred on by the numerous legislative proposals that have been considered in the past two decades. As U.S. governmental sources fund nearly half (46 percent in 2015) of health care, and as ongoing health reform efforts increase this share, the strong political influence in health care will surely continue. In addition, the U.S. health care system is one of its most regulated sectors; almost every aspect of it is under federal or state scrutiny (Field, 2007). Recently, fundamental philosophical differences between two major political parties in the United States are creating uncertainties as they seek radically different outcomes.

The pace of change is also often dictated by the rate of introduction of new technology. The speed of innovation is extremely rapid for some products and slower for others. Personal computers and cell phones are two products that have continued to experience rapid product innovation. Some predict that the integration of smartphones into health care delivery will radically change how we receive care in the future (Topol, 2015). Health care has also seen continuing progress in new pharmaceutical drugs, medical devices, and diagnostic equipment. According to the Centers for Disease Control and Prevention (CDC), genetic tests have been developed for thousands of diseases (https://www.cdc.gov/genomics/gtesting/), which can be integral in treating heritable disorders, especially cancers.

In addition, changing consumer demand introduces uncertainty and requires better aligned strategies. These changes may occur as a result of general economic conditions, population demographics, and cultural values.

When financial uncertainty arises for families due to loss of employment or insurance coverage, individuals often cut back on medications, preventive care, and visits to their doctor (Kaiser Family Foundation, 2015). Health care spending also varies significantly by age, race, and gender with those over age 65 spending 3.6 times more on health care than those between the ages of 19 and 44 (CMS, 2014).

Finally, a clearer strategy needs to be defined for adaptation to the changing marketplace and regulatory pressures. In health care, the marketplace is changing in both the government and the private sector, shifting from providing episodic care to managing health for the population (Caldararo and Nash, 2017). The federal government continues to exert pressure on health care organizations to move toward managing populations as a whole during the entire care delivery continuum. Private payers are also beginning to follow suit as risk-based payer contracts and bundled payment models have become more popular (Caldararo and Nash, 2017). As patients, providers, payers, and other stakeholders also demand high-quality and cost-effective care, new programs and organizational structures have been emerging as a response to these changes. For example, some health care organizations have signed onto Comprehensive Primary Care Plus (CPC+), a national advanced primary care medical home model that aims to strengthen primary care through regionally based multipayer payment reform, as a strategy to transform their care delivery. Accountable care organizations (ACOs) represent another example that promotes the quality agenda (Chukmaitov et al., 2017; Lewis et al., 2017). ACOs and similar reforms aim to achieve quality through improving coordination among health care providers. However, successful coordination requires health care organizations to think "outside of the box" and form strategic alliances and partnerships across organizational boundaries (Lewis et al., 2017; see also Chapter 11).

Business Models

A **business model** is a helpful way to see how an organization is organized, creates value, generates revenues, and compares with its competitors. Many have called for fundamental changes in the business model of health care (Crean, 2010; Lin, 2008; Perkins, 2010). The way health care is organized and funded (its business model) is predicted to change dramatically in the future (Jackson, 2008). Health care organizations face the challenge to identify when new technology or other factors make conditions right for newer, more efficient ways of providing value, and to modify their business models accordingly.

Business models contain four components, each continuing to influence one another as the organization begins, evolves, and progresses:

1. Customer value: Meeting customer needs in terms of product differentiation, cost, and/or access/availability
2. Inputs: The combination of resources used to provide the product and/or service
3. Processes: The sequence of steps taken to deliver the product and/or service
4. Profitability: The financial mechanism to recover enough revenue to sustain the provision of the product and/or service

Figure 10.4 illustrates the interrelated components of a business model that constantly interact to produce services and products. Each of these components may be altered over time to address new challenges and environmental pressures.

Customer Value

Different business models provide different forms of value to customers. Customers have differing desires and needs. Some value ease of access and availability, others want low cost, while others seek higher quality. An innovative business model will seek to address those unmet needs. This is usually the first component that is addressed in developing a new business model. For example, generic drugs offer lower prices, home health provides convenience, and retail clinics offer both.

Inputs

The combination and mix of resources used significantly affect the business model. Resources include personnel, materials, and equipment/machines. Organizations choose how much and what type of each that will be used. New technology that supplants human labor is often incorporated into a new business model for the delivery of the product or service. Personnel may be a mix of licenses and skill sets that may complement or substitute for one another. For example, clinics may use nurse practitioners or family practitioners, anesthesia may be administered by nurse anesthetists or anesthesiologists, and inpatient care may be delivered by hospitalists and intensivists rather than the admitting physician.

Processes

A process is a series of steps that ultimately transforms inputs into customer-valued products and services (Walston, 2017). An organization is composed of many different processes that are ordered to simplify decision making and increase efficiency. These include admitting, financial, and service processes, among many others. Processes can vary. Some hospitals will admit patients directly to their inpatient or outpatient room and use standardized protocols (also called clinical pathways) to direct how physicians should treat certain conditions.

Other hospitals traditionally make patients check in at a centralized location, transport them to their rooms, and allow physicians to treat patients as they wish.

Profitability

Any organization must generate enough revenues to sustain itself. Some mechanism, be it direct payments, insurance, donations, or other means, must be found to generate adequate revenues to cover the cost of operation. Sufficient numbers of customers must be found who garner value from the product and/or services. At the same time, the inputs and processes must cost less than the revenues generated. For example, religious organizations generate revenues from donations, governmental facilities from governmental allocations, insurance companies from premium payments, and hospitals obtain almost half their revenues from Medicare.

Business models change as both internal and external pressures cause companies to seek different ways to compete and survive. Many argue that the U.S. health care business model must move to a patient-centered, value-based, and/or population-based focus that will require greater coordination of care and a greater attention to preventive and primary care (American Hospital Association, 2016; CMS Quality Strategy, 2016; Friedman et al., 2016).

The U.S. Health Care Business Model

Traditionally, the business model of the U.S. health care system has offered fragmented treatment of acute care at the expense of primary, preventive, and chronic care (Marvasti and Stafford, 2012). Little coordination has occurred among health care providers, duplicating services and driving up costs. Hospitals are costly structures to build and, since they are central to health care provision, have promoted high-cost acute care medicine (Perkins, 2010). The United States spends more than double per capita on health care than any other country. Yet, the U.S. health care system performs relatively poorly in terms of quality, access, efficiency, equity, and health outcomes, as Americans have relatively shorter life expectancy and more chronic disease (Squires and Anderson, 2015).

Today, many feel that the traditional hospital business model dramatically overshoots the needs of the average patient, yet misses basic concerns. National reports have long raised questions about the quality of care provided in hospitals (Institute of Medicine, 2001), and rapidly escalating prices have caused many consumers to seek alternatives. As a result, new business models have sprung up to include retail health clinics located in retail stores, supermarkets, and pharmacies for uncomplicated illness, medical tourism (travel beyond international borders to obtain health care) (Vasquez, 2016), specialty hospitals, alternative medicine, and patient-centered medical homes (Berry and Mirabito, 2010; Society for Health Care Strategy and Market Development, 2008). Health care systems have also adopted structures to facilitate clinical integration that links physicians, hospitals, and services for chronic care and post-acute needs (Morrissey, 2015).

Customer Value

Traditional hospital business models originated in the early twentieth century as hospitals became the hub for clinical training, scientific research, and the repository of expensive medical technology to be used in acute-care medical treatment. Hospitals were the only medical facilities that possessed the collective technology to diagnose and treat serious illnesses. The unpredictability of

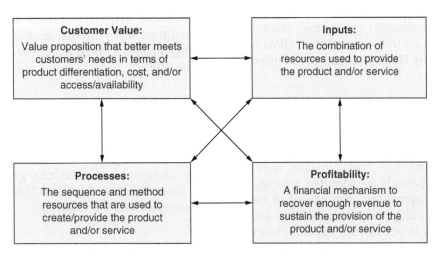

Figure 10.4 Components of a Business Model.

the medical problems dictated that hospitals needed to house many specialists to provide value to a wide variety of customers.

The three main values to be obtained in a service-related industry, like hospitals, include quality, cost, and access. Hospitals initially reorganized care by moving patient treatment from the home to the hospital. Patients obtained value by receiving sophisticated technology and higher quality of care. More recently, escalating costs and technological advances have encouraged the movement of traditional services provided in the hospital to alternative delivery settings (e.g., ambulatory surgery centers). Consumers now increasingly elect to access care through alternative models that hopefully improve population health and focus on preventive medicine and the reduction of disease (LaPenna, 2010).

Inputs

Inputs include highly professionalized health care personnel such as physicians, nurses, respiratory therapists, physical therapists, pharmacists, dieticians, laboratory technicians, and others. Hospitals also use large quantities of supplies, drugs, equipment, and support personnel. New, alternative models vary their inputs to use much less expensive manpower (e.g., nurse practitioners), settings (e.g., medical tourism), or innovative technology (e.g., telemedicine) to transmit health information. Certain health care professionals have also been given more responsibilities. For example, in some states, nurse practitioners and physician assistants can prescribe certain medications, perform physical exams, and other duties that have traditionally been provided by physicians.

Also, inputs vary by type of hospital. Community hospitals often do not have salaried medical staff but instead rely on voluntary staff or contracted providers. By contrast, academic medical centers employ the majority of their medical staff. Similarly, some types of HMOs (staff models like Kaiser Permanente) employ their physicians, while independent practitioner association (IPA) models like Hill Physicians Medical Group use contractual relationships.

Processes

Health care occupations have traditionally been segregated by professional expertise, status hierarchies, and location in the organizational chart. Similarly, work processes regarding how patients are admitted, treated, and released have been segmented. The advent of health information technology (e.g., electronic medical records) now allows providers to access the documentation of care received from other physicians, which may streamline the process to reduce duplicative testing and cut costs.

Revenue Generation

Whereas hospitals used to rely on charitable donations and insurance reimbursement, the government has become the biggest payer of hospitals. In 2015, U.S. state and federal governments collectively accounted for 37 percent of health care expenditures through the Medicare and Medicaid programs and 46 percent of spending overall (Keehan et al., 2017). Most hospitals are still mostly paid on a fee-for-service basis. Some delivery systems like Kaiser Permanente are financed by prepaid insurance premiums in which the hospital is a "cost center" and increased utilization decreases the organization's margin.

EVALUATION OF ORGANIZATIONAL ENVIRONMENT

A critical aspect of strategic planning and strategic thinking is to understand the organization's **external** and **internal environment**. It is important to understand existing and projected environments as they impact the basis of our assumptions, the subsequent allocation of resources, and strategic direction. Assumptions are propositions that are taken for granted, often with limited evidence. It is critical that our assumptions are checked and challenged, as past assumptions can be proven faulty. For example, in the past, assumptions were made that (1) hospital care would become outmoded and supplanted by outpatient services, (2) HMOs would control health insurance, and (3) only integrated health care systems could be successful. Each was shown to be false (Burns and Pauly, 2002). Organizations that clung too long to such assumptions suffered.

Organizations should periodically scan the environment to identify changing factors and challenge their assumptions. They should monitor both the external and internal environment: external market analysis should focus on competition, while internal assessment should examine the organization's own unique resources and capabilities (Burns, 2002).

External Evaluation

The nature of customers and the structure of the market directly influence how organizations must compete. Health care is highly sensitive to external variables, such as technological innovation, changing customer demand, and governmental regulation. Factors that should be evaluated include the following.

Customers

Who are they? Are there specific segments by age, gender, income, or geographic locations that use the

Table 10.1 Hospital Patient Origin by Region and Gender—Admissions

	2000				
Numbers	**Eastern Region**	**Western Region**	**Central Region**	**Other**	**TOTAL**
Female	1,299	903	5,497	2,583	10,282
Male	1,054	956	4,721	3,981	10,712
TOTAL	2,353	1,859	10,218	6,564	20,994
Percentage of Total					
Female	6.2%	4.3%	26.2%	12.3%	49.0%
Male	5.0%	4.6%	22.5%	19.0%	51.0%
TOTAL	11.2%	8.9%	48.7%	31.3%	100.0%
	2005				
Numbers	**Eastern Region**	**Western Region**	**Central Region**	**Other**	**TOTAL**
Female	1,021	744	6,310	2,444	10,519
Male	929	844	7,340	4,328	13,441
TOTAL	1,950	1,588	13,650	6,772	23,960
Percentage of Total					
Female	4.3%	3.1%	26.3%	10.2%	43.9%
Male	3.9%	3.5%	30.6%	18.1%	56.1%
TOTAL	8.1%	6.6%	57.0%	28.3%	100.0%

hospital's services? Which are increasing? Decreasing? Organizations should consider completing a customer (patient) origin study to define what geographic locations their customers come from. For example, the patient origin study in Table 10.1 shows that more than half of patients come from the Central Region, a percentage that grew from 48.7 percent in 2000 to 57 percent in 2005. The number of patients coming from the Central Region has grown as has the overall total, while the number and percentage of patients from the Eastern and Western Regions have declined significantly. Such information is strategically important to determine the impact of current strategies and inform what adjustments are needed. In this case, the strategies in the Central Region seem to be effective, while something negative is occurring in the other regions. These data may trigger other questions, such as whether other health care facilities have been opened in the other regions and/or physicians have changed their referral patterns.

Competition

Who is the competition and what is the nature of that competition? Is the competitive landscape changing? Are there new market entries? Exits? Which products and services are more competitive? Are there clusters or competitive strategic groups that compete intensely?

Other Factors

Health care organizations should also seek to identify other factors, like their key referral sources (e.g., key physician and insurance groups), consumer perceptions of their organization, facility vacancy of competitors (e.g., bed occupancy rates), and price sensitivity for different services and how they change over time. Many health care organizations will find that they rely on a small number of organizations for a large portion of their patients. The perceptions of these patients are especially critical. For hospitals, competitors who have greater idle capacity (due to falling bed occupancy) may compete most vigorously on (lower) prices.

Market Structure

Strategies vary according to the market structure. The nature of competition is directly related to the structure and degree of fragmentation of a market. Market structure is comprised of the number, concentration, and relative strength of organizations in an industry; the type of market structure influences the intensity and form of competition in the industry (Walston, 2017). As a result, organizations vary their strategies according to the structure of the market in which they exist.

As illustrated in Figure 10.4, markets can be categorized into fragmented and consolidated markets. The most fragmented market is perfect competition, which is characterized by many buyers and sellers, and many products that are similar and undifferentiated. Markets in perfect competition have few **barriers to entry**, with firms struggling to differentiate their products and compete on price. Markets for agricultural commodities (wheat, corn, soy beans, etc.) often come closest to perfect competition. Products are homogeneous, product and pricing information are known by all, and each individual seller has little or no effect on market prices and must sell at the going rate. Firms often earn only minimal profits. Generic drugs can be considered close to perfect competition. One generic drug is often seen comparable to another (of the same prescription); customer choice is frequently restricted by insurance coverage, which is dictated by price.

The next level of market fragmentation is monopolistic competition. This market structure is characterized by a large number of small firms that have similar but not identical products. There is relative free entry and exit, and knowledge of prices and technology is common. Competition is relatively vigorous, but each firm, depending on the degree of its differentiation, has some control over its prices. General examples would include restaurants and clothing stores. In the United States, physician services exemplify monopolistic competition. There are many physicians but minimal competition based on price. Physicians may be differentiated by their office locations, education, and personal relationship with their patients.

An oligopolistic market is dominated by a few large organizations. The degree of market concentration is very high with only a few firms dominating the market. Barriers to entry exist. Organizations are interdependent in that they must take into account the reactions of their competitors when they make decisions regarding pricing and resource allocation. Organizations in **oligopolies** rarely compete on price but seek to "brand" and differentiate their products on other characteristics. Air travel is an industry where oligopolies exist in both the production side (large manufacturers like Boeing and Airbus) and the commercial side (e.g., large air carriers like United, Delta, American, and Southwest). Many health care systems, medical device companies, and insurers are oligopolies and, as such, seek to differentiate themselves and compete on factors such as access, quality, and relationships with physicians.

Monopolies are fully consolidated markets with only one firm. Monopolists lack competition, as they produce goods or services for which there are no close substitutes. Monopolies often lack incentives to be efficient but maintain high prices. Much of their strategic effort goes into creating barriers to entry against potential competitors. Water and electric services are often monopolies. Likewise, in many markets, especially in rural America, hospitals are monopolies. Monopolies are often associated with higher prices because of the lack of choice. Most studies support this relationship as markets with high hospital concentration (close to monopoly conditions) have also extracted higher prices (Federal Trade Commission and Department of Justice, 2004). The high cost of branded pharmaceutical drugs in the United States is partially explained by the "monopoly rights" given through patents and regulatory approvals by governmental agencies. These monopolies give drug companies greater ability to raise prices, often many times the rate of inflation. Some drugs, like Daraprim, used to treat serious parasite infections, enjoyed price hikes of 5,000 percent in 2015 alone (Tuttle, 2016).

The Five Forces Framework

Porter's Five Forces Framework has often been employed to define the structure of a market and understand the competitive forces in industries (Figure 10.6). The forces are five common threats from the environment: (1) the threat of new entrants, (2) the threat of substitutes, (3) the bargaining power of suppliers, (4) the bargaining power of buyers, and (5) the intensity of rivalry. At the center is the intensity of rivalry or competition; rivalry is heightened by the other four forces. Taken together, these forces help define an industry's market structure. Porter suggests that firms gain competitive advantage by

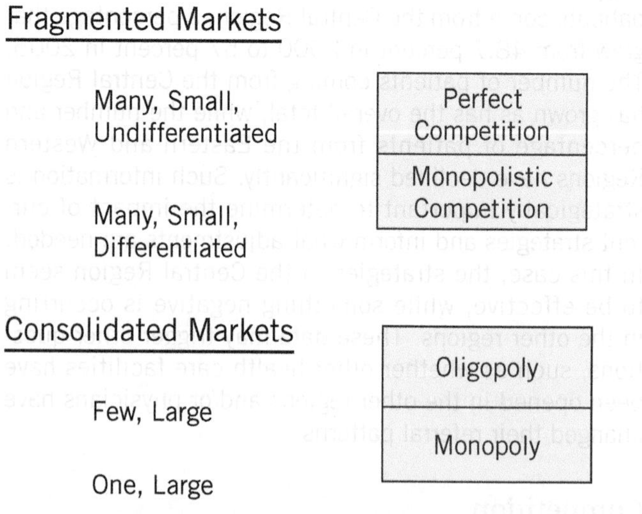

Fragmented Markets

Many, Small, Undifferentiated	Perfect Competition
	Monopolistic Competition
Many, Small, Differentiated	

Consolidated Markets

	Oligopoly
Few, Large	
	Monopoly
One, Large	

Figure 10.5 Market Structure.

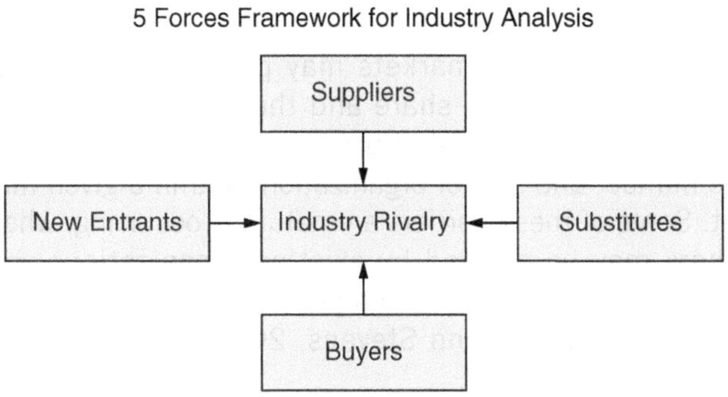

5 Forces Framework for Industry Analysis

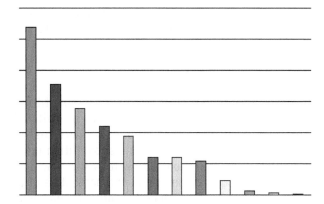

Figure 10.6 The Five Forces Model for Industry Analysis.

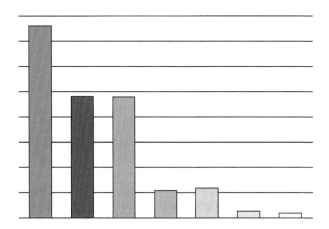

Figure 10.7 Phoenix Market Share.
SOURCE: https://www.ahd.com/

exploiting weaknesses in these five forces or by adopting strategies that modify these forces and reduce competitive pressures (Porter, 1980). As intensity of the forces increases and as the market structure approaches perfect competition, the industry environment becomes more hostile and overall industry profitability declines. On the other hand, weaker forces allow the creation of monopolist conditions, which can enhance industry profits. Each of the five forces is discussed below.

Rivalry

Rivals in a market compete for customers and market share. Such competition is based on a combination of price and product attributes. The degree of **rivalry** is influenced by many factors. One is the number of organizations in the competitive space. In an industry where new rivals can enter relatively easily, the industry is more competitive, and organizations are less likely to enjoy high average profitability. Rivalry is also likely in markets where competitors differ substantially from one another. For example, markets that have public, community, and private hospitals will create more competition due to expanded customer choice, compared to markets with only one type of hospital. Likewise, rivalry is affected by the size distribution of market firms. Competition increases as a market becomes less concentrated and/or firms control more equal shares of the market; by contrast, the existence of one (or a few) dominant organization diminishes rivalry. Hospital markets in the United States exhibit wide variations in their market structures. Many are monopolies or oligopolies (Walston, 2017). Figures 10.7 and 10.8 show two different markets, both in cities of about 1.5 million population. Figure 10.7 represents the market in Phoenix, Arizona, which has more hospital systems, greater variation in ownership due to more for-profit penetration, and less concentration. Figure 10.8 shows the market in Indianapolis, Indiana, which has fewer hospitals, is dominated by not-for-profit organizations and more concentrated. Comparing the two figures would lead to the conclusion that the Phoenix market is more competitive than Indianapolis.

Figure 10.8 Indianapolis Market Share.
SOURCE: https://www.ahd.com/

Moreover, there are nonmarket structural characteristics that affect the intensity of competition (Porter, 1980). These include the difficulty in deploying organizational assets outside the industry (asset specificity), the amount of fixed costs, and excess capacity. As each of these increases, the intensity of rivalry grows, as firms are motivated to more aggressively seek volume to augment economies of scale and asset utilization. Other product factors include the degree of product similarity or differentiation and issues of switching costs. Products not perceived differently by the consumer become price competitive. The greater the differentiation, the more a firm can charge for its product, and the higher profits that can be produced. Likewise, the less it costs to switch to another product, the greater the competition.

Finally, the nature of the sales process can influence the level of competition. If sales are based on large, infrequent orders, firms will compete more intensely.

Similarly, if sales transactions are not very observable and understandable, rivalry will be higher (Burns, 2002).

Threat of Substitution

The extent and degree of product/service substitution influences the propensity of customers to switch to alternatives. Substitutes are products or services that replace another. The strength of the substitution is tied to the customer perception of how fully the new product matches the quality and price characteristics of the old. Other factors that influence the threat of substitution by new products include the relative price performance, switching costs, and the buyer's propensity to substitute (Porter, 1980). For example, technological advances in the 1990s such as minimally invasive surgery have replaced traditional open cases for gall bladders, hernias, and appendectomies. Likewise, medications have now all but replaced surgery for treatment of peptic ulcer disease (Kotler, Shalowitz, and Stevens, 2008).

Buyer Power

An organization's buyers or customers always seek to drive down price and improve quality. Their ability to do so, known as buyer power, depends on how much they purchase, how well informed they are, and their willingness to experiment with alternatives (Mintzberg, Lampel, and Ahlstrand, 2005). As with rivalry, a buyer's bargaining power is partly dependent on market structure. If, as in the defense industry, there is only one or a few buyers for a product, the buyer(s) can exert strong influence on the firm's behavior. In health care, medical clinics will seek to contract with more than one insurer so that they do not depend on a single source for a significant portion of their business.

Supplier Power

Supplier power is the opposite of buyer power. Contrary to buyers, suppliers desire the ability to increase price and maintain the same quality. Suppliers gain power by how important their product or service is to the purchasers, when few suppliers exist, and the cost of switching to another supplier is high. Powerful suppliers can extract concessions from their buyers. Suppliers are more powerful when they are few in number and more concentrated than their buyers (Walston, 2017). For example, there are many vendors of health care information systems, but the cost to switch from one system to another is very high, which increases a supplier's power. On the other hand, some pharmaceutical companies are the only source for special drugs. As a result, they can charge very high prices. For example, Gilead Sciences' monthly price to take Sovaldi, a drug for hepatitis C, is $81,000 (Ramsy, 2016).

Threat of New Entrants

New entrants into markets may potentially decrease incumbents' market share and thereby increase price competition. The extent of barriers to entry will influence the number and size of organizations within a given market. Some of these barriers are naturally occurring, where others may be erected by existing organizations as a means to maintain and strengthen their market position (Kotler, Shalowitz, and Stevens, 2008). These barriers include the following:

- *Economies of scale and high capital requirements*: Incumbent firms might enjoy economies of scale and benefits of learning that may allow existing firms a price and production advantage over new entrants. Scale economies tend to exist in industries with significant fixed costs. As volumes increase, the high fixed costs are spread out and the average price declines; competitive success thus rests on high volume. For example, pharmaceutical wholesalers and manufacturers have very high fixed and capital costs. An organization desiring to enter such markets must have a substantial amount of financial resources and be willing to remain at competitive disadvantage until sufficient market share can be achieved. This serves as a deterrent to new entry.

- *Access to key resources or distribution channels*: In markets that have scarce critical resources or high distribution costs, lacking access to such resources or distribution channels can be a significant barrier to entry. For providers, this may be the lack of skilled, specialized personnel; for biotechnology start-ups with a new drug, it may be the lack of market access to specialists who prescribe it for their patients.

- *Legal restrictions*: Legal barriers often present barriers to entry. These can be patents, copyrights, or requirements for licensure. Government regulation might restrict entry by requiring potential entrants to gain prior government approval to offer products or service. Many states in the United States still require "certificate of need" for hospitals to obtain state approval prior to initiating a large capital expenditure. Other state laws create barriers for certain professions. In 2016, 29 states did not allow full practice authority to nurse practitioners, even though most evidence does not support these restrictions (Pohl et al., 2016).

- *Branding*: Marketing advantages are also enjoyed by incumbents as a result of their reputation. Some firms have successfully used their reputation to lower barriers to entry. For example, many U.S. providers with excellent reputations for delivering high quality of care have leveraged their "brand" to enter health care markets across state borders or even international boundaries. Harvard International, Cleveland Clinic, Johns Hopkins, and others now have a presence in the Middle East.

- *Exclusive and/or long-term agreements*: Incumbents with long-term agreements, especially those that are exclusive, create strong barriers to entry. Many managed care plans establish exclusive arrangements for the provision of psychiatric and chemical dependency problems. These agreements restrict entry of other organizations into these markets (Kotler, Shalowitz, and Stevens, 2008).

- *Current excess capacity and threat of retaliation*: If current firms have excess capacity, they are often willing to reduce price to increase volume. Even the threat of entry will frequently motivate existing firms to lower or maintain low prices. Incumbents with a credible history of aggressive retaliation will pose an additional barrier to new entrants.

Evaluation of Rival Positioning

An organization should know and understand its competitors. The concept of "strategic groups" was initially introduced by Hunt in 1972 but further developed by Porter in 1980. A **strategic group** is defined as a set of organizations within an industry that have similar business models and/or strategic orientations such that they directly compete with one another. For example, in the restaurant business, there are many different classifications of dining, from fast food to fine dining. McDonald's clearly competes with Burger King and Wendy's but does not with five-star restaurants. These groups can be distinguished, based on factors such as the following:

- Price/quality
- Geographic coverage
- Degree of vertical integration
- Product breadth
- Use of distribution channels

INTERNAL RESOURCES: A SOURCE OF COMPETITIVE ADVANTAGE

Internal resources are a key component of strategic advantage. Resources are of critical importance to ensure the successful implementation of strategies (Barney, 1991; Wernerfelt, 1984). An organization is a combination of resources, both tangible and intangible. Tangible resources include physical assets, such as equipment, buildings, and technology and financial strength. Intangible resources include intellectual property (patents, copyright), brand name, and culture.

According to Barney (1991), these resources may be further classified into three categories: (1) physical capital resources, which include technology, plant and equipment, geographic location, and access to raw materials; (2) human capital resources, which include personnel skill sets, training, experience, judgment, intelligence, relationships, and insights of all organizational participants; and (3) organizational capital resources, which include the organization's formal structure, reporting hierarchy, formal and informal processes such as planning, controlling, and coordinating systems, as well as informal relations among groups within, between, and among organizations in its environment.

To be strategically important, internal resources must offer sustained benefits in the face of competition. To do so, these resources must be valuable, rare, difficult to imitate, and lack substitutes. Obviously, a resource should be valuable to be strategic and needs to improve an organization's effectiveness and efficiency. A resource should also be rare enough to generate demand and hard to replicate. For example, for many organizations, location is the critical resource that can be rare and hard to duplicate. Finally, even if a resource is valuable, rare, and hard to imitate, it may not provide sustained strategic advantage if it can be easily substituted. Physical assets are less likely to provide sustained strategic advantage. For example, purchasing the latest imaging machine is a strategy that can be easily and quickly imitated by competitors. Human resources can also be hired away from organizations. Advantage must be found in the combination of physical, human, and organizational resources. Sustained strategic gains come when the intangible resources are combined with the tangible to create a competitive organizational culture (Mintzberg, Lampel, and Ahlstrand, 2005). Culture has been suggested as the most effective and durable barrier to imitation, as it generates unique outcomes, is difficult to discern, and is very difficult to replicate (Barney, 1986). Of course, a positive culture is the most difficult to create, but organizations that do tend to innovate more have greater patient satisfaction and are more likely to achieve their goals (Bellou, 2007).

Evaluating Organizational Capabilities

One way to evaluate the use of organizational resources and capabilities is through a value chain analysis. Organizational capabilities refer to an organization's skillset in combining resources to produce goods and services. Capabilities can range from simple tasks in daily operations to complex processes. These capabilities collectively are the activities of an organization's value chain. That is, these capabilities are organized in a chain of activities that gives the product or service more added

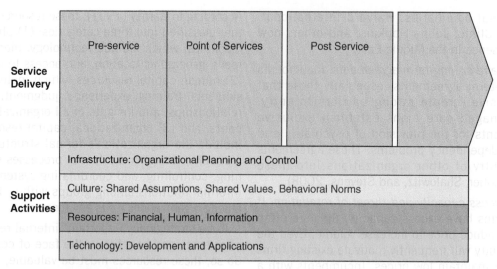

Figure 10.9 Value Chain.
SOURCE: Adapted from Ginter, Swayne, and Duncan (2002).

value. Traditionally, value chains have primary activities, which include inbound logistics, operations/production, outbound logistics, marketing and sales, and service/maintenance. In examining the use of capabilities, the costs and value drivers for each activity would also be included in the calculations.

In health care, a value chain assumes a systems approach where there are two subsystems: service delivery and support activities (Figure 10.9). The service delivery subsystem is further divided into preservice, point of service, and postservice, illustrating where the service is delivered. The support activities consist of organizational infrastructure, culture, resources, and technology. These subsystems support the service delivery system by ensuring the availability of an inviting and supportive environment as well as a service-oriented culture, sufficient resources and financing, highly qualified staff, and appropriate information technology (Ginter, Swayne, and Duncan, 2002).

Another common tool for evaluating an organization and its resources is a **SWOT analysis**. The SWOT (strengths, weakness, opportunities, and threats) analysis is a common analytical tool for evaluating organizational capabilities to enhance organizational effectiveness and strategic directions (Figure 10.10). It enables members of the organization to assess all aspects of the organization. These encompass strengths and weaknesses of the internal organization's capabilities and activities in the areas of organizational culture, structure, access to resources, staffing, operations, external relationships, information technology capacity and function, administrative processes, clinical control processes, and organizational decision making. Organizations may identify areas where they can grow based on agreed-upon opportunities and mitigate sources of major threats (Luke, Walston, and

Plummer, 2004). Based on results of internal analysis, organizations may develop strategies that would respond to the assessment of their internal strengths and weaknesses as well as the external opportunities and threats that are present. SWOT analyses are frequently used, as they are easy to initiate and involve many stakeholders. However, it is important to keep in mind some of the tool's limitations. SWOT does not provide trend information, may include erroneous information, and may not provide clear direction at its conclusion. Participants can come with singular perspectives, which may reflect their biases and misperceptions. In addition, unless a competent facilitator is used, vocal individuals may inappropriately influence the analysis, thereby leading to potentially inaccurate or biased results (Walston, 2017).

GENERIC STRATEGIES

Porter (1980) argued that a firm's competitive advantage would primarily derive from either its cost leadership or an ability to differentiate its product and/or services. The application of these strengths to either a broad or narrow market results in **generic strategies** (Figure 10.11).

Low-Cost Leadership

This generic strategy calls for being the low-cost producer in an industry for a given level of quality. Some companies are very successful as low-cost leaders. Walmart and Aldi Stores are known for their low prices and acceptable quality. They both work hard on their inputs and processes to maintain very low prices. Generic pharmaceutical companies and retail health clinics also seek to gain strategic advantage from their cost advantage. Factors that allow low cost to work include the following:

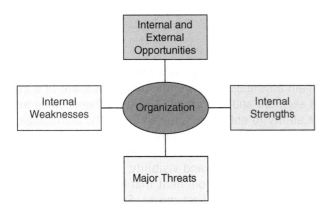

Figure 10.10 SWOT Analysis.

SOURCE: Adapted from Bourgeois, Duhaime, and Stimpert (1999).

- Vigorous price competition among rivals
- Similar products from rival sellers (products hard to differentiate)
- Most customers use product in similar ways
- Low switching costs
- High bargaining power with large buyers
- Low barriers to entry and new entries use introductory low prices to attract buyers
- Narrow product line to standardized, no-frills goods and services
- High asset turnover
- Low-cost distribution systems

A challenge for any organization in establishing a low-cost position is to assure an acceptable level of quality for its consumers. Quality preferences will vary according to the consumer's income, education, and cultural norms. However, for some products, such as health care, the quality requirements are very high for the vast majority of consumers. Health care providers that seek a low-cost position have extreme difficulty attracting desirable patients.

The challenge of a low-cost position in health care is partly due to consumers equating low cost to low quality and partly due to the insulation of many consumers from the actual cost of health care. Patients with insurance are mostly protected from high costs of care. Rather than having to pay the full charges, insured patients pay a fixed deductible and then generally a small percentage (coinsurance) on charges that have been discounted by the insurance company. However, low pricing can be an effective strategy for some services that are less likely to be covered by insurance. In areas with more price-sensitive consumers, low cost may help organizations attract patients. Consumers with high out-of-pocket costs more often compare prices, choose lower-cost health

care services, and select less expensive drugs. For example, health care organizations may set low prices for normal obstetrical deliveries, physicals, and plastic surgeries. Health care providers may seek to have low-price (cost) positions in these market segments but realize that patients are not very price-sensitive in many other services (Ungar and O'Donnell, 2015).

Differentiation

A generic strategy based on **differentiation** requires the provision of a product or service that offers unique attributes that are valued by customers and perceived by customers to be better than competitors' products. In turn, that value may allow the organization to charge a premium price for the product or service. Product differentiation may also be accomplished through its products, services, personnel, channel, and image (Kotler, Shalowitz, and Stevens, 2008). Organizations may incorporate features that raise product performance or add attributes that buyers desire, such as greater reliability, durability, ease of use, convenience, safety, and low maintenance. Some health care systems have changed their facilities to provide "healing gardens," adding additional hallways to reduce noise, and adding gourmet chefs and room service (Landro, 2007). Organizations can also differentiate products to heighten customer satisfaction in noneconomic or intangible ways. They may improve service by increasing the ease of ordering, delivery, and/or maintenance and repair. An organization's personnel can also make a difference by their competence, courtesy, reliability, and communication skills. Many health care organizations, including the Virginia Mason Medical Center in Seattle, Washington, have partnered with patients and families to initiate service excellence programs that integrate quality and services (Bodnar, 2014). Channel differentiation can also distinguish an organization. The extent of coverage, expertise, and performance can be significant advantages. Health care providers seek to set up referral clinics in key areas, pharmaceutical firms offer multimodal drug delivery, and insurance companies develop networks that offer the widest scope of providers.

Image also can be a powerful way to differentiate a product. When competing products or services are similar, buyers may obtain value based on the company's image. A favorable image takes a significant amount of time to build but can be destroyed very quickly (Armstrong and Kotler, 1999). Image in health care has also become more important. U.S. hospitals, health care systems, and clinics spent about $2.3 billion on health care advertising in 2015, 41 percent above the amount spent in 2011 (Kantar Media, 2016). Image advertising is often different from conventional marketing efforts (Rowland, 2006). If strong image and brand name exists, it can potentially be transferred to related products and businesses. For example, entities have partnered with educational institutions such as Harvard University, which has a very recognizable and strong image worldwide. It has used its name to go into related businesses of consulting and publishing with Harvard Medical International, a subsidiary of Partners Health Care System in Boston.

Focused Strategies

Focused or market niche strategies constitute another category of generic strategies. In Figure 10.11, a focused strategy can be based on either differentiation or cost. The key for a market niche (targeted to a narrow market segment) or focused strategy is that it should be based on some important characteristic, such as population, product line, geography, political boundaries, etc. Many consider specialist hospitals as an example of organizations that compete in certain market niches. These hospitals are often physician-owned (in contrast to public ownership of most general hospitals), offer somewhat limited services, and only treat one disease type. Other health care organizations pursue focused strategies by establishing luxury services to attract wealthy domestic and foreign patients. Differentiating services include uniformed valets, professional greeters, 24-hour room service, and spas (Pourat, 2016). Competitive advantage is achieved by matching an appropriate strategy to the target market and defining the focus as unique/differentiated or low cost. Broad, uniquely focused strategies should be highly differentiated; narrow and low-cost strategies should be focused on cost leadership.

Other Aspects of Strategies

First Mover Advantage

The **first mover advantage** is a recognized strategic move to gain advantage by being the initial occupant of a market segment and/or product. This advantage comes from the ability to obtain heightened visibility, technological leadership, or control of crucial resources. First movers often receive extensive free publicity and gain public name recognition and visibility. Sometimes, the first mover becomes so prominent that the product becomes associated with the first mover. For example, Kleenex has become synonymous with facial tissue and Xerox with copies. Likewise, Roger Bannister has been honored and remember in athletics as the first man to break the four-minute mile barrier in 1954, even though he placed fourth in the 1952 Olympics and his record was broken just 46 days later (Bascomb, 2005).

First movers can gain advantage from (1) breakthroughs in research and development, (2) acquisition and control of scarce assets, and (3) reputation. Sustained advantage can be obtained by moving quickly up the learning curve. Amazon and eBay, for example, have excelled in adopting new technology, making key acquisitions, and establishing solid reputations to grow their businesses. Blue Cross and Blue Shield were the first entrants into the private health insurance market during the 1930s and 1940s and continue as market leaders today. Likewise, first mover pharmaceutical and biotech companies may gain strategic advantage for their innovation through patented new drugs. If first movers can gain access to crucial resources and capabilities, they

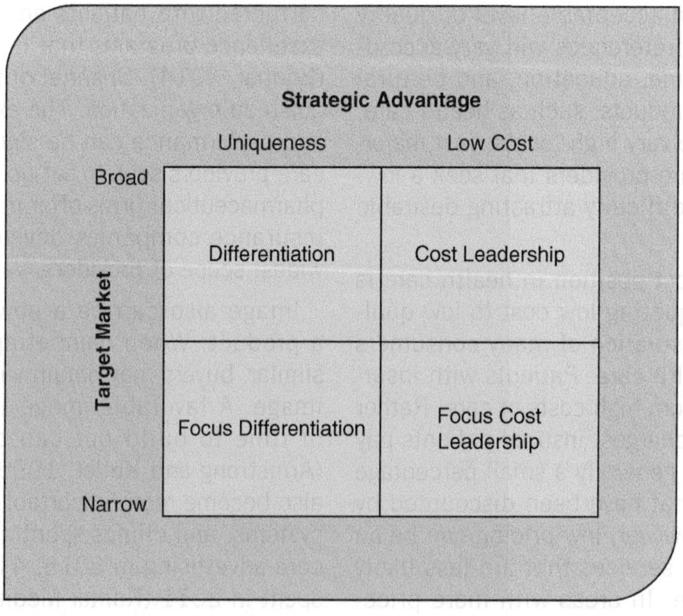

	Strategic Advantage	
	Uniqueness	Low Cost
Broad	Differentiation	Cost Leadership
Narrow	Focus Differentiation	Focus Cost Leadership

(Target Market)

Figure 10.11 Generic Strategies.
SOURCE: Adapted from Walston (2017).

can potentially block other market entrants or place them at a competitive disadvantage. Such crucial resources might be access to patents, superior physical locations, and more competent staff that can be used to solidify their position.

On the other hand, first movers may not be able to sustain their initial gains. Later entrants (second movers) may be able to imitate or gain a "free ride" on their investments. Also, late movers have the advantage of not sustaining risks of creating new markets and are able to follow set industry standards. There are many firms that moved rapidly into a new product with strong financial backing that lost to later entrants. For example, Prodigy Communications was the first mover in online shopping; Dumont led in selling televisions; Chux led in disposable diapers; and Ampex led in video recorders. All were surpassed by later movers (Shilling, 2007). Apple was not the first mover in digital music, smartphones, or tablets but used the experience of others to dominate the market in these areas (Anthony, 2012). Second movers or "fast followers" may succeed more often than first movers because of existing demand and consumer acceptance (Shankar and Carpenter, 2013).

Product Life Cycle

All products and services go through phases or life cycles that relate to the level of costs and sales, which have strategic implications. Product life cycles occur because of the inherent limited life of any product, resulting from technological advances and adapting consumer preferences. Figure 10.12 shows the four life cycle stages. In the Emerging Stage, there may be initially few organizations as the technology is developed and explored. Competition remains low, as there may be few substitutes. Sales and profits also remain low in this stage. The Growth Stage sees increasing market entry by competitors as sales grow rapidly. The product has now proven a success and customers are rapidly adopting it. The Maturity Stage tends to be the most profitable, but sales increase at a slower rate. Competing products at this stage become more similar, which increases the difficulty of differentiating individual company products. Strategically, companies seek to maintain or expand their market share. In the last stage, Declining, the volume of sales drops substantially and organizations merge to increase the market concentration, as competition pushes down profit margins.

Some believe that U.S. health care emerged in the early 1900s and underwent a growth stage in the mid-1900s aided by financing from insurance companies and significant growth in expenditures. The general health care industry now sits in the mature stage with significant competition and governmental regulation (Kepros et al., 2007).

Level of Concentration & Competition

Life Cycle Stage	Concentration	Competition
Emerging	High	Low
Growth	Decreasing	Increasing
Mature	Increasing	Moderate to High
Declining	High	High

Figure 10.12 Life Cycle.

Portfolio Analysis

In the 1970s, consulting firms developed various methods to analyze the strategic position of organizations. One very popular method is **portfolio analysis**. Various derivations of this concept still exist, such as the Boston Consulting Group's Growth-Share Matrix and the GE/McKinsey Nine-Block Matrix. The strategic purpose behind these analyses is to understand which parts of the firm should receive greater capital investment, which should be underfunded, and which perhaps divested (Ghemawat, 2001) These tools assume that scale economies, market power, and other strategic advantages are directly related to higher relative market share and that market growth provides the greatest opportunity for firm expansion. Each portfolio tool seeks to:

1. Comparatively evaluate the viability and future of the main components of an organization's business

2. Graphically depict the performance of an organization's products and services

3. Examine the balance between cash flows and growth among key business components

4. Guide strategic allocation of resources (Walston, 2017)

An organization can examine the components of its business, sometimes known as strategic business units (SBUs), by their competitive position and environmental favorability (Figure 10.13). This leads to placing the SBU into one of the four quadrants. Such placement then suggests what strategic actions should take place for each SBU.

Portfolio analysis can be beneficial, especially when funds are scarce. Health care companies have used it to evaluate and prioritize their services to help them maintain strategic direction (Bess and Bess, 1990).

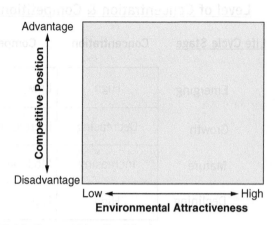

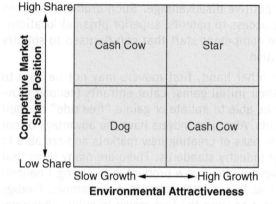

Figure 10.13 Competitive Positioning.

Common Strategies in Health Care

Health care strategies commonly focus on growth. Health care organizations frequently expand vertically to own products and services previously offered by their buyers or suppliers, grow horizontally to include similar products, or diversify by developing new products and services. Growth promises greater economies of scale, improved reputation, fast entry into markets, synergies, increased market power, higher salaries for top managers, and repositioning of the organization to take advantage of new opportunities and changing markets.

Health care strategic expansion is often referred to as **vertical** and **horizontal integration**. However, common ownership is not sufficient—true integration must occur to achieve the above benefits of growth strategies. In many cases, organizations that have been acquired are simply absorbed rather than actually integrated.

Vertical expansion happens when an organization acquires a business in its value chain that is a supplier (backward expansion) or a buyer of the organization's product(s) (forward expansion). For example, a hospital might employ physicians or have its own insurance company and create an integrated delivery system, which has been encouraged by national bodies to advance a population health focus (American Hospital Association, 2014). For example, in 2011, WellPoint, Inc., paid about $800 million to acquire CareMore, a provider of preventive services and UnitedHealth Group, Inc., bought Monarch HealthCare, an association of 2,300 physicians. Vertical integration of hospitals and physicians has become commonplace, with roughly 25 percent of physicians now working as employees. By contrast, integration with insurance companies and physicians has remained relatively rare, with only 2 percent of all primary care physicians working for insurance companies in 2016 (Herman, 2015; Matthews, 2011).

Horizontal expansion occurs when organizations producing similar products merge or are acquired. Thus, an organization grows by buying or merging with other organizations that provide comparable products. Hospitals and physician groups have used this strategy extensively and expanded horizontally to form multihospital systems and larger physician groups. In 2016, for example, 3,183 of 4,926 (65 percent) community hospitals belonged to a health care system (American Hospital Association, 2016). Health insurance companies also grew larger; in 2015, the largest 10 insurance companies controlled over half of the U.S. health care insurance market (Statista, 2016). Specialist physicians, especially cardiologists and orthopedists, are also increasingly consolidating into larger, single-specialty groups (Kash and Tan, 2016).

A third way to grow is *diversification* or acquiring organizations that offer different products or services. Organizations can diversify into either related or unrelated businesses. *Related diversification* leverages existing organizational competencies to expand its customer or product base. For instance, United Health Group has diversified into related areas such as population health management, health information technology consulting, and pharmacy care services (United Health Group, 2016). Chains, such as Walgreens, Walmart, Rite Aid, Kroger, Target, and CVS, have also diversified by opening retail clinics that offer basic medical services for minor illnesses. These clinics are often located within their store locations to provide convenient "one-stop" shopping for the customers/patients. By 2016, there were about 2,000 such clinics across the United States, reporting more than 6 million visits per year (Abelson, 2016); almost 93 percent of these retail clinics were owned by one of these chains (Hennessy, 2016; Rand Corporation, 2016)

On the other hand, unrelated diversification involves the acquisition and expansion into products and services that have little relationship with an organization's existing products and customers. For example, a hospital acquiring a hotel, sports store, mall, or restaurant represents an unrelated diversification.

The health care industry will continue to evolve and change with growth and integration strategies certainly being part of the future. Some argue that if health care financing moves back toward some form of capitation—a fixed amount per person payment—health care organizations will rapidly move to greater vertical integration (James and Poulsen, 2016). Pressures for greater efficiencies will motivate health systems, physicians, and other providers to closer collaboration and cooperation, creating greater horizontal and vertical integration. Health care systems will employ more physicians to grow and develop clinically integrated networks to promote population health and value-based models (Jacobs, 2015).

SUMMARY AND MANAGERIAL GUIDELINES

In today's market, health care organizations need strategies to manage change. Effective change strategies require preparation. This involves motivating and educating key stakeholders, building consensus within a strategic process, gathering relevant data, and identifying and challenging existing assumptions. Good organizations plan for strategic changes when they are not forced to do so. Medical staff and board members will often question the need for change and may resist moving forward, unless they understand the necessity for action. Leaders should be prepared to educate stakeholders regarding the purpose and motivation for change.

Strategic planning processes must involve the right people. However, involving key stakeholders often presents a challenge to organizations. Top executives should lead the strategic planning and exhibit their commitment by the dedication of time, resources, and intellect. Organizational boards, if appropriate, should also direct the strategic planning process and monitoring of results. In many health care organizations, the board represents the community and has responsibility to assure that management actions and direction align with its mission and vision. Frequently, the board's direct involvement with strategic planning is coordinated by the creation of a board strategic planning committee.

It is important to also identify others who should be involved and clearly define their degree of involvement and responsibilities. Employees, medical staff, and other organizations dependent upon the services of the health care organization have vested interests in the firm performing strategic planning and may be asked to participate in the planning process. The level of involvement and scope of responsibility should be plainly understood. Unclear responsibilities and involvement can lead to frustration and withdrawal of partners and key stakeholders, which will lead to greater impediments to creation and strategy implementation.

Health care organizations have used expansion strategies of vertical and horizontal integration that have created larger organizations linking stages in the industries value chain and expanding the geographic reach of health care companies. These strategies are predicted to continue, especially if the industry moves to payment through capitation. Organizational leaders should articulate for their stakeholders how these expansion strategies support the organization's missions and values and contribute to desired societal goals of higher quality, lower cost, and increased access to care.

Throughout this chapter, we see that strategy is an important and complex concept. Organizations struggle to successfully implement their strategic direction, as they wrestle with uncertainties and critical decisions. Although difficult, strategy and strategic thinking are critical in ensuring the success and survival of organizations. Organizations that understand and use these concepts to make better decisions are more likely to achieve their missions and visions. Strategic skills are increasingly important in the complicated and challenging industry of health care.

MANAGERIAL GUIDELINES

1. Understand the importance of mission and vision and their relationship to strategy and strategic management. All strategic actions and direction of an organization should be driven by its mission and vision. Leaders should seek to make their mission and vision meaningful by incorporating them into decision-making processes.

2. Establish values that are meaningful and guide actions at the organization. Values should be directly tied to performance and be reflected in annual evaluations.

3. Realize that strategy is more than creating a written plan for the future. Strategy encompasses the ability to analyze the environment, understand potential futures, and allocate resources to strategically position the organization. It involves strategically managing personnel and assets to direct the organization through uncertain times.

4. Understand that good strategies are not static but evolve over time based upon the experiences and preferences of leaders. Successful organizations must be adaptable, learn from their experiences, and have the agility to evolve.

5. See how a firm's competitive position can change with shifts in any of the four components of a business model. The concept of a business model allows leaders to understand factors that can be individually or jointly altered to improve the competitiveness of an organization. Likewise, it provides a method to analyze competitors to discern how they differ and what potential advantages they might have.

6. Managers should understand different methods for analyzing the environment in which the organization operates. Porter's Five Forces Framework and Value Chain provide two means for examining the organization's environment and those factors that affect the level of competition.

DISCUSSION QUESTIONS

1. Find the mission and values statements for four different hospitals types. Do their missions and values reconcile with your expectations for that type of organization? Look at a religious organization. Does its mission and values reflect its religious teachings and mission? Now examine a for-profit hospital. Does its mission and values include the need to increase its owners' value and maximize their earnings? Why do you think the missions and values are structured as they are?

2. Health care in the United States has been traditionally a mixture of not-for-profit and for-profit organizations. Do you think that markets where more for-profit firms exist would be inherently more competitive? Why or why not?

3. Business models describe four components of how an organization is organized. They can show comparative differences in a competitive analysis. What is the relationship of strategy and business models?

4. An important aspect of strategic planning is analyzing the internal and external environments. Recently, a large organization completed its environmental analyses using only a very extensive SWOT process. It then used the strengths, weaknesses, opportunities, and threats generated by this process as its environmental analysis. What would be the value of using this technique by itself? Should other methods also be used? How could data trends be used?

5. There are many firms that have positioned part or all of their products as low cost. Low costs are also commonly thought to equal low prices. Are low costs necessarily the same as low prices? Could an organization have low costs and still have high prices?

6. Large pharmaceutical companies have prospered by owning their discovery, production, and marketing assets and have traditionally made significant portions of their profits from a small number of "blockbuster" drugs. How are pharmaceutical companies' business model predicted to change? What are the forces that are influencing this change?

7. Porter recommends generic strategies of low cost or differentiation. Is it possible to obtain both at the same time? In health care, is low cost a reasonable strategy? If so, in what circumstances might this be an acceptable strategy?

8. To sustain a competitive advantage, an organization must have resources that are valuable, enduring over time, hard to imitate, and difficult to find substitutes for. What are some of the common resources in health care that could convey sustained competitive advantage? How do these differ for the different segments of the health care industry? For hospitals? Insurance companies? Pharmaceutical companies? Manufacturers of durable medical equipment?

9. When should competitive advantage be the premise for a health care organization? How can mission advantage and competitive advantage coexist?

CASE 1

Concierge and Direct Primary Care Medicine: Solutions or problems?

Michael West runs the Glenton Medical Clinic, which is a group of 45 multispecialty physicians in Greenwich, Connecticut. He has been in this position for almost 15 years and has seen numerous changes in the health care sector. Although the clinic has prospered, expenses have continued to rise over the past five years, while revenues have remained stagnant. This has especially been true with the 22 primary care physicians within practice.

The clinic has billed insurance and sought to collect the difference from patients. If the patients are uninsured, the clinic sets up a payment plan.

At a conference Michael attended recently, a physician presented his transition to concierge medicine. The physician noted that more and more physicians feel overworked, especially spending more time with nonclinical paperwork. This has caused many to look for practice options and alternative financial arrangements with their patients. One option is concierge medicine, where practices charge a flat fee (monthly or annually) for enhanced services and greater access. Some of these "enhanced" services consist of same day access to the doctor via cell phone and text messaging; telephone, text message, and online consultations; unlimited office visits with no co-pays; prescription refills; and preventive care services. Another option presented was direct primary care (DPC), which likewise charges a monthly or annual fee. Practices using these models derive most of their revenues from membership fees and generally experience an increase in profitability.

Proponents suggest the DPC model works well for patients with complex medical conditions needing careful monitoring and help coordinating multiple specialists. Yet, only a few studies suggest better results. One study showed patients in a DPC model had 27 percent fewer emergency department (ED) visits, 60 percent fewer hospital days, and their health care coverage cost their employers 20 percent less (Beck, 2017).

Concierge practices' average monthly fees begin at $175 a month but can be more than $5,000 per year. Most practices that transition to concierge medicine will retain only 15 percent to 35 percent of their existing patients, but the physician will end up having a patient panel of only 300 to 600 patients. On the other hand, DPC practices are somewhat less expensive with monthly fees at about $100 and, as a result, they have larger patient panels of 600 to 800 per physician. DPC services generally include basic lab tests, vaccinations, and generic drugs (Colwell, 2016).

DPCs can establish care with a more restrictive and expensive practice for higher-income families. A few very restrictive practices charge $40,000 to $80,000 per family for an extensive, immediate array of services. These practices have only 50 families on their patient panel. These high-end practices can increase a primary care physician's income from mid-$200,000 to about $600,000 (Schwartz, 2017).

In the case of Glenton Medical Clinic, its primary care physicians currently have 2,000 to 3,000 active patients. Moving to either model would mean each physician would lose over 1,000 patients or more than 22,000 for the full clinic.

The insurance market has also changed, which encourages families to consider concierge medicine. A recent survey demonstrated that over half (51 percent) of workers were insured with a health care plan that required them to pay up to $1,000 out-of-pocket costs for health care before insurance covered any of the expenses. Many complain about the long wait to be seen in physician offices and then very short physician consultation visits. In fact, an average primary care physician in a traditional practice would spent 13 to 15 minutes seeing a patient, while a physician in a DPC practice would spend 30 to 60 minutes with the patient (Ramsey, 2017).

Patients appear to like the DPC model, as it includes in the monthly fee basic checkups with same-day or next-day appointments and the right to purchase medications and lab tests at or near wholesale prices. This means that DPC comes with almost 24/7 access to a primary care doctor, which might include using FaceTime while a family is on vacation or meeting in the office for stitches after a bad fall on a Saturday night. Since DPC does not accept insurance, there are no co-pays and no costs beyond the monthly fee.

Yet, upfront, prepaid fees in both models do not qualify as medical expenses that can be reimbursable from a flexible spending account (FSA) or health savings account (HSA). Patients have to have the financial means to pay these fees directly.

Michael has recently heard that a large company from Philadelphia has entered concierge medicine and DPC across the East Coast and is seeking to enroll up to 800,000 workers in the next few years. They will soon begin to offer very high salaries to attract good primary care practitioners. Given the Glenton Medical Clinic's current business model, he cannot see how the company can keep its primary care physicians if they are given lucrative offers from this company.

Michael is concerned that switching to either model would leave more than half of their patients seeking another physician in a market that already has a shortage of primary care practices. In addition, currently the primary care physician referrals make up about 40 percent of their clinic's specialist patient load. It would appear that reducing the primary care panels would directly reduce the number of specialist referrals and subsequently impact the revenues for the clinic. However, Michael's assistant pointed out that the specialists were too busy now, had long wait times, and frequently turned down referrals from physicians from outside their clinic.

Questions

1. What are the advantages and disadvantages of the Glenton Medical Clinic moving its primary care physicians to either a concierge or DPC model?

2. Given the direction of health care, what would you recommend if you were Michael?

CASE 2

Improving Quality of HIV Care in Veterans Affairs (VA) Medical Centers

The Department of Veterans Affairs (VA) operates the largest integrated health care system in the United States, paying for and providing medical care to Veterans, with more than 1,700 hospitals, clinics, community living centers, domiciliaries, readjustment counseling centers, and other facilities. These VA facilities are organized into 1 of the 18 Veterans Integrated Services Networks (VISNs) by geographic location and each VISN has its own administrative hierarchy. Consider below the VA's mission and values (http://www.va.gov):

Mission
To fulfill President Lincoln's promise "To care for him who shall have borne the battle, and for his widow, and his orphan" by serving and honoring the men and women who are America's Veterans.

Core Values
VA's five core values underscore the obligations inherent in VA's mission: Integrity, Commitment, Advocacy, Respect, and Excellence. The core values define "who we are," our culture, and how we care for veterans and eligible beneficiaries. Our values are more than just words – they affect outcomes in our daily interactions with Veterans and eligible beneficiaries and with each other. Taking the first letter of each word—Integrity, Commitment, Advocacy, Respect, Excellence—creates a powerful acronym, "I CARE," that reminds each VA employee of the importance of their role in this Department. These core values come together as five promises we make as individuals and as an organization to those we serve.

Integrity: Act with high moral principle. Adhere to the highest professional standards. Maintain the trust and confidence of all with whom I engage.

Commitment: Work diligently to serve Veterans and other beneficiaries. Be driven by an earnest belief in VA's mission. Fulfill my individual responsibilities and organizational responsibilities.

Advocacy: Be truly Veteran-centric by identifying, fully considering, and appropriately advancing the interests of Veterans and other beneficiaries.

Respect: Treat all those I serve and with whom I work with dignity and respect. Show respect to earn it.

Excellence: Strive for the highest quality and continuous improvement. Be thoughtful and decisive in leadership, accountable for my actions, willing to admit mistakes, and rigorous in correcting them.

However, at various times, critics have expressed concerns about the substandard care provided by the VA and the resulting negative press created pressure on the VA to do better. As a response, the VA has launched transformation efforts to address its quality gaps over the last decade, with significant internal restructuring of the care delivery system, including changes in delivery models (e.g., primary care teams, service lines), adoption of new technologies (e.g., computerized patient record system [CPRS]), and management strategies (e.g., guideline implementation, performance audit/feedback) (Jha et al., 2003). The VA also created nationally centralized data repositories in quality and utilization to support these efforts (Chou et al., 2015). These organizational changes in the aggregate have demonstrated positive associations with substantial gains in VA quality over time.

Moreover, VA funded a number of research and operational projects that focused on improving care quality for certain high-cost conditions, such as cardiovascular disease, diabetes mellitus, major depressive disorder, etc. In particular, Dr. Matthew Bidwell Goetz, the Chief of Infectious Diseases at the Greater Los Angeles VA Health Care System, implemented a project to improve routine HIV screening across multiple VISNs in areas where rates of HIV were on the rise (Goetz et al., 2013, 2015). Although medical advances have significantly improved the survival and quality of life of those who are infected with HIV, the rates of infection continue to be a major problem for some regions of the United States. As recent as 2015, the Centers for Disease Control and Prevention (CDC, 2016) estimated that southern states accounted for approximately 44 percent of all people living with an HIV diagnosis, despite making up only about one-third (37 percent) of the national population (Figure 1). By region, rates of HIV diagnoses per 100,000 adults and adolescents were 16.8 in the South, 11.6 in the Northeast, 9.8 in the West, and 7.6 in the Midwest.

Research evidence has shown that identifying and treating asymptomatic HIV-infected individuals can be highly cost-effective with vast reduction in morbidity and mortality (Goetz et al., 2015). However, full treatment benefits are not being realized, as many HIV-infected persons tend to be unaware of their disease status. Both provider and patient factors factors (e.g., low prioritization, time required for counseling, and poor accountability) as well as organizational barriers (e.g., lack of leadership support, poor information sharing) may have impeded disease identification and treatment.

Within the VA, despite frequent opportunities to achieve early diagnosis, the number of VA patients with documented risk factors for HIV infection who have been tested remains lower than ideal. The VA, in fact, changed its HIV screening policy from risk-based to routine. The Multi-VISN Quality Improvement Project for HIV was launched to develop an exportable intervention for increasing HIV testing rates across a number of VISNs. To measure the effectiveness of various components of the intervention, the project set up a natural experiment to compare the amount of support/resources delivered to individual VA facilities: three sites that were supported by a national team, seven sites that were supported by their respective local teams, and four facilities that served as control sites. The national team provided assistance to the sites with (1) a context-specific, computerized clinical reminder for HIV testing of individual patients; (2) audit/feedback consisted of a retrospective summary of provider-specific HIV screening rates of at-risk patients; (3) provider activation via established academic detailing and social marketing methodology; and (4) tools and resources to facilitate organizational change to remove barriers to HIV testing. Sites supported by local teams received only audit-feedback reports. At the control sites, it was "business as usual."

Findings from the project showed significant increases in HIV testing rates following the implementation of the interventions (Figure 2). In particular, patients receiving care from facilities where resources were provided by either the national or local team reported higher likelihood of getting tested, compared to their counterparts at control facilities (Goetz et al., 2013). At the end of the study, it was demonstrated that routine HIV testing proved to be cost-effective, especially among persons younger than 65 years (Goetz et al., 2015).

Questions

1. Please review the VA mission and values. Does the Multi-VISN QI Project for HIV support VA's mission and values? If so, how? If not, why not and how can the project align better with the VA mission and values?

2. What are the factors that may have led to the results achieved by the Multi-VISN QI Project for HIV?

3. Apply one of the analytic tools to assess if the Multi-VISN Project for HIV creates mission advantage for the VA.

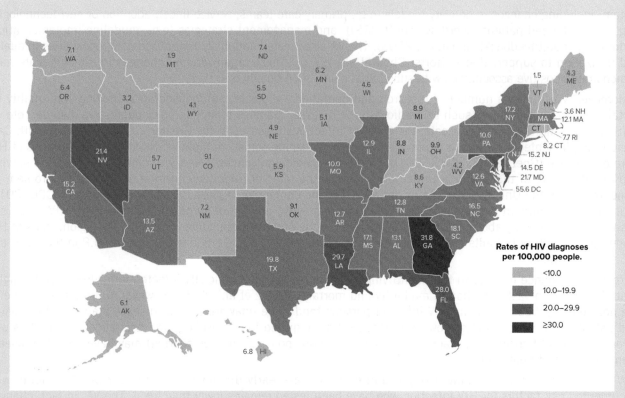

Figure 1 Rates of HIV Diagnoses per 100,000 People by State.

SOURCE: Adapted from CDC (2016). Diagnosis of HIV Infection in the United States and Dependent Areas, 2015. HIV Surveillance Report.

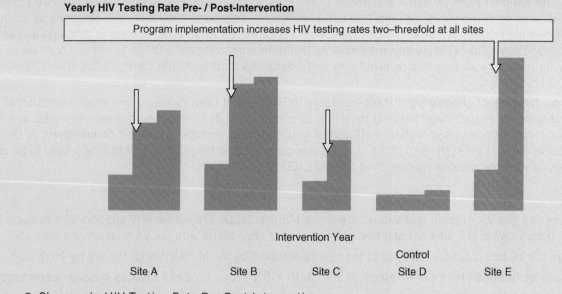

Figure 2 Changes in HIV Testing Rate Pre-Post Intervention.

REFERENCES

Abelson, R. (2016). Retail health clinics result in higher spending, survey finds. *New York Times,* March 7, 2016. Accessed October 1, 2018.

Altergott, B. (2016). US birth rate is dropping, but other countries have it worse. Retrieved October 20, 2017, from https://www.aol.com/article/news/2016/12/03/us-birth-rate-is-dropping-but-other-countries-have-it-much-wors/21619994/.

American Hospital Association. (2014). Trend watch: The value of provider integration. Retrieved October 20, 2017, from http://www.aha.org/content/14/14mar-provintegration.pdf.

American Hospital Association. (2016). AHA fast facts on US hospitals. Retrieved October 20, 2017, from http://www.aha.org/research/rc/stat-studies/fast-facts.shtml.

Anthony, S. (2012). First mover or fast follower. *Harvard Business Review*, June 14. Retrieved October 20, 2017, from https://hbr.org/2012/06/first-mover-or-fast-follower.

Armstrong, G., & Kotler, P. (1999). *Principles of marketing* (8th ed.). Upper Saddle River, NJ: Prentice Hall.

Barney, J. (1986). Organizational culture: Can it be a source of sustained competitive advantage? *Academy of Management Review, 11*(3), 565–665.

Barney, J. (1991). Firm resources and sustained competitive advantage. *Journal of Management, 17*, 99–120.

Bascomb, N. (2005). *The perfect mile: Three athletes, one goal, and less than four minutes to achieve it.* New York: Mariner Books.

Beck, M. (2017). With direct primary care, it's just doctor and patient. *Wall Street Journal*, February 27. Retrieved from https://www.wsj.com/articles/with-direct-primary-care-its-just-doctor-and-patient-1488164702.

Bellou, V. (2007). Achieving long-term customer satisfaction through organizational culture: Evidence from the health care sector. *Managing Service Quality, 17*(17), 510–522.

Berry, L., & Mirabito, A. (2010). Innovative health care delivery. *Business Horizons, 53*(2), 157.

Bess, J. L., & Bess, A. (1990). Hospital portfolio analysis. *Health Care Strategic Management, 8*(5), 10–14.

Bodnar, W. (2014), Health care's evolving role of service excellence. *Becker's Hospital Review*, April 25. Retrieved October 20, 2017, from http://www.beckershospitalreview.com/hospital-management-administration/health care-s-evolving-role-of-service-excellence.html.

Bourgeois, L. J., Duhaime, I. M., & Stimpert, J. L. (1999). *Strategic management: A managerial perspective.* Charlottesville, VA: Dryden Press.

Brandenburger, A., & Nalebuff, B. (1997). *Co-opetition.* New York: Doubleday.

Burns, L. (2002). Competitive strategy. In D. Albert (Ed.), *A physician's guide to health care management*. Malden, MA: Wiley-Blackwell, 1–240.

Burns, L., & Pauly, M. (2002). Integrated delivery networks: A detour on the road to integrated care? *Health Affairs, 21*(4), 128–143.

Business Dictionary. (2016). Retrieved October 20, 2017, from http://www.businessdictionary.com/definition/mission-statement.html.

Caldararo, K. L., & Nash, D. B. (2017). Population health research: Early description of the organizational shift toward population health management and defining a vision for leadership. *Population Health Management, 20*, 368–373. doi: 10.1089/pop.2016.0172.

CDC. (2016). Diagnoses of HIV infection in the United States and dependent areas, 2015. *HIV Surveillance Report, 27*. Retrieved June 14, 2018, from https://www.cdc.gov/hiv/library/reports/hiv-surveillance.html.

Chiquan, G. (2007). Is sustainable competitive advantage an achievable Holy Grail: The relevance gap between academia and business. *Journal of Business & Management, 13*(2), 115–126.

Chou, A. F., Rose, D. E., Farmer, M., et al. (2015, December). Organizational factors affecting the likelihood of cancer screening among VA patients. *Medical Care, 53*(12), 1040–1049. doi: 10.1097/MLR.0000000000000449. PubMed PMID: 26569643.

Chukmaitov, A. S., Harless, D. W., Bazzoli, G. J., et al. (2017). Factors associated with hospital participation in Centers for Medicare and Medicaid Services' Accountable Care Organization programs. *Health Care Management and Review*. doi: 10.1097/HMR.0000000000000182. [Epub ahead of print]. Retrieved October 11, 2018, from https://insights.ovid.com/crossref?an=00004010-900000000-99730.

CMS. (2014). Health expenditures by age and gender. Retrieved October 20, 2017, from www.cms.gov.

CMS. (2017). NHE Fact Sheet. Retrieved October 20, 2017, from https://www.cms.gov/research-statistics-data-and-systems/statistics-trends-and-reports/nationalhealthexpenddata/nhe-fact-sheet.html.

CMS Quality Strategy. (2016). Retrieved October 20, 2017, from https://www.cms.gov/Medicare/Quality-Initiatives-Patient-Assessment-Instruments/QualityInitiativesGenInfo/Downloads/CMS-Quality-Strategy.pdf.

Cohn, D., & Caumont, A. (2016). 10 demographic trends that are shaping the US and the world. Pew Research Center Fact Tank. Retrieved October 20, 2017, from http://www.pewresearch.org/fact-tank/2016/03/31/10-demographic-trends-that-are-shaping-the-u-s-and-the-world/.

Collis, D., & Rukstad, M. (2008, April). Can you say what your strategy is? *Harvard Business Review*, 82–90. Retrieved October 20, 2017, from https://eclass.aueb.gr/modules/document/file.php/DET162/Session%201/Can%20you%20say%20what%20your%20strategy%20is.pdf.

Colwell, J. (2016). Concierge medicine becomes an option in reform era. *Medical Economics*. Retrieved from http://medicaleconomics.modernmedicine.com/medical-economics/news/concierge-medicine-becomes-option-reform-era.

Crean, K. (2010). Accelerating innovation in information and communication. *Health Affairs, 29*(2), 278–284.

DesRoches, C., Buerhaus, P., Dittus, R., et al. (2015). Primary care workforce shortages and career recommendations from practicing clinicians. *Academic Medicine, 90*(5), 671–677.

DeWeese, D. (1994). *Islamization and native religion in the golden horde: Baba Tukles and conversion to Islam in historical and epic tradition*. University Park: Pennsylvania State University Press.

Dye, R., & Sibony, O. (2007). How to improve strategic planning. *McKinsey Quarterly*. Retrieved October 20, 2017, from http://www.mckinsey.com/business-functions/strategy-and-corporate-finance/our-insights/how-to-improve-strategic-planning.

Fahey, L. (1999). *Competitors*. New York: John Wiley and Sons.

Fahey, L., & Narayanan, V. K. (1986). *Macroenvironmental analysis for strategic management*. St. Paul, MN: West Publishing Company.

Federal Trade Commission and Department of Justice. (2004). Improving health care: A dose of competition. A report by the Federal Trade Commission and the Department of Justice.

Field, R. I. (2007). *Health care regulation in America: Complexity, confrontation, and compromise*. New York: Oxford University Press.

Frazier, I. (2005). Annals of history: Invaders: Destroying Bagdad. *New Yorker*, April 25.

Friedman, A., Howard, J., Shaw, E., et al. (2016). Facilitators and barriers to care coordination in patient-centered medical homes from coordinators' perspectives. *Journal of the American Board of Family Medicine, 29*(1), 90–101.

Ghemawat, P. (2001). *Strategy and the business landscape*. Upper Saddle River, NJ: Prentice Hall.

Ginter, P. M., Swayne, L. E., & Duncan, W. J. (2002). *Strategic management of health care organizations*. Oxford, UK: Blackwell Publishing.

Goetz, M. B., Hoang, T., Kan, V. L., et al. (2015, August). Rates and predictors of newly diagnosed HIV infection among veterans receiving routine once-per-lifetime HIV testing in the Veterans Health Administration. *Journal of Acquired Immune Deficiency Syndromes, 69*(5), 544–550. doi: 10.1097/QAI.0000000000000653. PubMed PMID: 25886931.

Goetz, M. B., Hoang, T., Knapp, H., et al. (2013, October). QUERI-HIV/Hepatitis Program. Central implementation strategies outperform local ones in improving HIV testing in Veterans Healthcare Administration facilities. *Journal of General Internal Medicine, 28*(10), 1311–1317. doi: 10.1007/s11606-013-2420-6. Epub 2013, Apr 19. PubMed PMID: 23605307; PubMed Central PMCID: PMC3785651.

Hansen, F. (2008). A revolution in health care. *Institute of Public Affairs Review, 59*(4), 43–46.

Hennessy, M. (2016). Will more retail clinic ownership shift to health systems? *Contemporary Clinic*. Retrieved October 20, 2017, from http://contemporaryclinic.pharmacytimes.com/journals/issue/2016/february2016/from-the-chairman-will-more-retail-clinic-ownership-shift-to-health-systems.

Herman, B. (2015). Lost appetite: The expected surge in insurers buying physician practices never materialized. *Modern Healthcare*. Retrieved October 20, 2017, from http://www.modernhealthcare.com/article/20151010/MAGAZINE/310109979.

Hunt, M. (1972). Competition in the major home appliance industry. Doctoral dissertation, Harvard University, Cambridge, MA.

Hurtibise, R. (2016). Amid growing revenues, South Florida hospitals buzz with capital improvements. *Sun Sentinel*. Retrieved October 20, 2017, from http://www.sun-sentinel.com/business/consumer/fl-hospital-market-2017-20161230-story.html.

Institute of Medicine. (2001). *Crossing the quality chasm*. Washington, DC: The National Press.

Jackson, S. (2008). Predicting changes in industry structure. *Journal of Business Strategy, 29*(2), 54–57.

Jacobs, L. (2015). Looking ahead in 2016: Top 10 trends in health care, hospitals & health networks. Retrieved October 20, 2017, from http://www.hhnmag.com/articles/6800-looking-ahead-in---top---trends-in-health-care.

James, B., & Poulsen, G. (2016). The case for capitation. *Harvard Business Review, 94*(7–8), 102–111.

Jha, A. K., Perlin, J. B., Kizer, K. W., et al. (2003). Effect of the transformation of the Veterans Affairs Health Care System on the quality of care. *New England Journal of Medicine, 348*, 2218–2227.

Kaiser Family Foundation. (2015). 2015 employer health benefits survey. Retrieved October 20, 2017, from http://kff.org/report-section/ehbs-2015-summary-of-findings/.

Kantar Media. (2016). Health care marketing. Retrieved October 20, 2017, from http://gaia.adage.com/images/bin/pdf/KantarHCwhitepaper_complete.pdf.

Kash, B., & Tan, D. (2016). Physician group practice trends: A comprehensive review. *Journal of Hospital & Medical Management, 2*(1), 1–8.

Keehan, S., Stone, D., Poisal, J., et al. (2017), National Health Expenditure Projections, 2016-25: Price Increases, Aging Push Sector to 20 Percent of Economy, *Health Affairs, 36*(3): 553–563.

Kepros, J., Mosher, B., Anderson, C., et al. (2007). The product life cycle of health care in the United States. *Internet Journal of Health care Administration, 4*(2), 1–5. Retrieved October 11, 2018, from https://print.ispub.com/api/0/ispub-article/5390.

Kilpatrick, A., & Silverman, L. (2005). The power of vision. *Strategy & Leadership, 33*(2), 24–26.

Kotler, P., Shalowitz, J., & Stevens, R. (2008). *Strategic marketing for health care organizations*. San Francisco, CA: Jossey-Bass.

LaPenna, A. M. (2010). "Alternative" health care: Access as a revenue source in a consumer-driven market. *Journal of Health Care Management, 55*(1), 7–11.

Lewis V. A., Tierney K. I., Colla C. H., et al. (2017). The new frontier of strategic alliances in health care: New partnerships under accountable care organizations. *Social Science and Medicine, 190*, 1–10.

Lin, D. (2008). Convenient care clinics: Opposition, opportunities, and the path to health system integration. *Frontiers of Health Services Management, 24*(3), 3–12.

Luke, R., Walston, S., & Plummer, P. (2004). *Health care strategy: In pursuit of competitive advantage*. Chicago, IL: Health Administration Press.

Marvasti, F., & Stafford, R. (2012). From sick care to health care—reengineering prevention into the U.S. System. *New England Journal of Medicine, 367*, 889–891.

Matthews, A. (2011). The future of U.S. health care: What is a hospital? An insurer? Even a doctor? All the lines in the industry are starting to blur. *Wall Street Journal*. Retrieved October 20, 2017, from http://online.wsj.com/article/SB1000142405297020431900457708455386999 0554.html.

Mintzberg, H., Lampel, J., & Ahlstrand, B. (2005). *Strategy safari: A guided tour through the wilds of strategic management*. New York: Free Press.

Morrissey, J. (2015). Finding a path to clinical integration. *Hospital & Health Networks*. Retrieved October 20, 2017, from http://www.hhnmag.com/articles/3746-finding-a-path-to-clinical-integration.

Moseley, G. (2018). *Managing health care business strategy* (2nd ed.). Burlington, MA: Jones & Bartlett Learning.

Murray, W., Knox, M., & Bernstein, A. (1994). *The making of strategy: Rulers, states, and war.* Cambridge, UK: Cambridge University Press.

Muscalus, R. (2008). Competition and community: Key evolving issues that require careful consideration. *Frontiers of Health Services Management, 25*(2), 25–31.

Mutter, R., Wong, H., Goldfarb, M. (2008). The effects of hospital competition on inpatient quality of care, *Inquiry—Excellus Health Plan, 45*(3), 263–280.

Perkins, B. B. (2010). Designing high-cost medicine. *American Journal of Public Health, 100*(2), 223–233.

Persico, J. (2016). Do you really need a mission statement? *Innovation Excellence*. Retrieved October 20, 2017, from http://innovationexcellence.com/blog/2011/05/14/do-you-really-need-a-mission-statement/.

Pohl, J., Thomas, A., Barksdale, D, et al. (2016). Primary care workforce: The need to remove barriers for nurse practitioners and physicians. *Health Affairs Blog*. Retrieved October 20, 2017, from http://healthaffairs.org/blog/2016/10/26/primary-care-workforce-the-need-to-remove-barriers-for-nurse-practitioners-and-physicians/.

Porter, M. (1980) *Competitive strategy*. New York: Free Press.

Pourat, N. (2016). Luxury hospital care limits care for the less affluent. *New York Times*. Retrieved October 20, 2017, from http://www.nytimes.com/roomfordebate/2016/08/22/hospitals-that-feel-like-hotels/luxury-hospital-care-limits-care-for-the-less-affluent.

Prawdin, M., & Chaliand, G. (2005). *The Mongol Empire: Its rise and legacy*. Piscataway, NJ: Transaction Publishers.

Ramsy, L. (2016). The 10 most expensive drugs in the US. *Business Insider*. Retrieved October 20, 2017, from http://www.businessinsider.com/most-expensive-drugs-in-america-2016-9/#viekira-pak-abbvie-34600-1.

Ramsey, L. (2017). A new kind of doctor's office charges a monthly fee and doesn't take insurance—and it could be the future of medicine. *Business Insider*, March 19. Retrieved from http://www.businessinsider.com/direct-primary-care-a-no-insurance-health care-model-2017-3.

Rand Corporation. (2016). The evolving role of retail clinics. Retrieved October 20, 2017, from http://www.rand.org/content/dam/rand/pubs/research_briefs/RB9400/RB9491-2/RAND_RB9491-2.pdf.

Rodak, S. (2013). Creating accountability in health care strategic plan execution. *Becker's Hospital Review*. Retrieved October 20, 2017, from http://www.beckershospitalreview.com/strategic-planning/creating-accountability-in-health care-strategic-plan-execution.html.

Rowland, C. (2006). Hospitals blitz airwaves with ad campaigns. *Boston Globe*. Retrieved October 20, 2017, from http://www.boston.com/business/health care/articles/2006/02/21/hospitals_blitz_airwaves_with_ad_campaigns/.

Sawyer, R. (2007). *The seven military classics of ancient China*. New York: Basic Books.

Schendel, D. (1994). Introduction to "competitive organizational behavior: Toward an organizationally-based theory of competitive advantage. *Strategic Management Journal, 15*(S1), 1–4.

Schwartz, N. (2017). The doctor is in. Co-pay? $40,000. *New York Times*, June 3. Retrieved from https://www.nytimes.com/2017/06/03/business/economy/high-end-medical-care.html.

Shankar, V., & Carpenter, G. (2013). The second-mover advantage. *KellogInsight*. Retrieved October 20, 2017, from http://insight.kellogg.northwestern.edu/article/the_second_mover_advantage.

Shilling, G. (2007). First mover disadvantage. *Forbes*. Retrieved October 20, 2017, from https://www.forbes.com/forbes/2007/0618/154.html.

Society for Health Care Strategy and Market Development. (2008). *FutureScan 2008: Healthcare trends and implications 2008–2013*. Chicago, IL: Health Administration Press.

Squires, D., & Anderson, C. (2015). U.S. health care from a global perspective. *The Commonwealth Fund*. Retrieved October 20, 2017, from http://www.commonwealthfund.org/publications/issue-briefs/2015/oct/us-health-care-from-a-global-perspective.

Statista. (2016). Market share of leading health insurance companies in the United States in 2016, by direct premiums written. Retrieved October 20, 2017, from https://www.statista.com/statistics/216518/leading-us-health-insurance-groups-in-the-us/.

The Commonwealth Fund. (2004). A 5-nation hospital survey: Commonalities, differences, and discontinuities. Retrieved October 20, 2017, from https://www.commonwealthfund.org/sites/default/files/documents/___media_files_publications_fund_report_2004_may_a_five_nation_hospital_survey__commonalities__differences__and_discontinuities_blumenthal_5nathospsuvrey_734_pdf.pdf.

Topol, E. (2015). The future of medicine is in your smartphone. *Wall Street Journal*. Retrieved October 20, 2017, from https://www.wsj.com/articles/the-future-of-medicine-is-in-your-smartphone-1420828632.

Tuttle, B. (2016). 21 incredibly disturbing facts about high prescription drug prices. *Money*. Retrieved October 20, 2017, from http://time.com/money/4377304/high-prescription-drug-prices-facts/.

Ungar, L., & O'Donnell, J. (2015). Dilemma over deductibles: Costs crippling middle class. *USA Today*. Retrieved October 20, 2017, from http://www.usatoday.com/story/news/nation/2015/01/01/middle-class-workers-struggle-to-pay-for-care-despite-insurance/19841235/.

United Health Group. (2016). Facts: 2016 Q3. Retrieved October 20, 2017, from https://www.uhc.com/content/dam/uhcdotcom/en/AboutUs/PDF/Q3-2016-Fact-Book.pdf.

Vainieri, M., Ferre, F., Giacomelli, G., et al. (2017). Explaining performance in health care: How and when top management competencies make the difference. *Health Care Management and Review*. (Epub ahead of print).

Vasquez, F. (2016). The sun rises for medical tourism in 2017. *PXCom.* Retrieved October 20, 2017 from https://pxcom.aero/blog/sun-rises-medical-tourism-2017/

Walston, S. (2017). *Strategic health care management: Planning and execution.* Second Edition, Chicago, IL: Health Administration Press.

Walter, B. A., & Priem, R. (1999). Business strategy and CEO intelligence acquisition. *Competitive Intelligence Review, 10,* 15–22.

Watson, T. (1963). *A business and its beliefs.* New York: McGraw-Hill.

Weinstein Organization. (2017). 5 health care marketing assumptions that could cost you. Retrieved October 20, 2017, from http://www.twochicago.com/blog/index.php/2017/03/21/5-health care-marketing-assumptions-cost/.

Wernerfelt, B. (1984). A resource-based view of the firm. *Strategic Management Journal, 5,* 171–180.

Chapter 11

Managing Strategic Alliances: Neither Make Nor Buy but Ally

Edward J. Zajac, Thomas A. D'Aunno, and Lawton R. Burns

CHAPTER OUTLINE

- Make, Buy, or Ally?
- Alliances in Health Care
- Types and Forms of Alliances
- What Are Alliances Meant to Do?
- The Alliance Process: A Multistage Analysis
- Frameworks for Analyzing Alliance Problems
- Alliance Capabilities and Performance Drivers

LEARNING OBJECTIVES

After completing this chapter, the reader should be able to:

1. Distinguish between different vehicles that organizations use to access external resources, that is, outsourcing, mergers and acquisitions, and strategic alliances
2. Explain why strategic alliances have become increasingly important, particularly among health care organizations
3. Identify the relevant dimensions that distinguish different types of strategic alliances
4. Classify an alliance both in terms of its form and its function
5. Discuss the link between alliance motivations and alliance structures and outcomes
6. Explain the extent to which your motivations for a strategic alliance are compatible with those of your alliance partner
7. Discuss how, that as strategic alliances evolve along different stages of development, the critical issues facing the alliance will also evolve, suggesting different implications for managerial intervention
8. Explain why alliances often have both strong advocates and detractors
9. Identify why some alliances in health care succeed and others fail

KEY TERMS

Alliance Objectives	Ownership
Alliance Problems	Partner Orientation
Alliance Process	Pooling Alliances
Alliance Risk	Revenue Enhancement
Alliance Symptoms	Strategic Alliance
Control	Trading Alliances
Cost Reduction	Turbulent Environment
Equity-Based Alliances	Uncertainty Reduction
Joint Venture	

• • • IN PRACTICE: Hospital Purchasing Alliances: Creating Leverage, Reducing Costs—and Stirring Up Controversy

Hospitals set up purchasing alliances (also known as group purchasing organizations or GPOs) starting in 1910. The GPO industry developed throughout the latter half of the twentieth century and consolidated in the 1990s into seven large firms, with lots of regional and smaller players. GPOs exist primarily to pool the purchase of medical-surgical supplies, medical devices, pharmaceuticals, and capital equipment across multiple hospitals to leverage manufacturers, gain lower prices, and thereby reduce hospital costs (Burns and Lee, 2008). Such purchasing alliances are quite common in other industries. Research shows that purchasing alliances reduce input spending anywhere from 10 to 15 percent of costs, consistent with common sense about volume purchasing.

However, in health care, these alliances became incredibly controversial. The GPOs, for example, were the subject of four U.S. Senate hearings during 2002–2006, three Government Accountability Office (GAO) reports, and a panel workshop convened by the Federal Trade Commission in 2002. Why all the attention? The source of the controversy was a small set of small manufacturers, typically makers of medical devices, who claimed in a series of reports published in the *New York Times* that the GPOs have developed contracts with larger manufacturers that were anticompetitive in nature and therefore exclude them from the market. They claimed that hospital efforts to contract for lower prices had the consequence of preventing innovative products from getting to market and thus harming patients.

What is remarkable here is that the anticompetitive practices alleged by the small manufacturers were not attributed to the "usual suspects" in antitrust cases: horizontal combinations of large manufacturers or vertically integrated combinations of manufacturers and downstream distribution channels. Instead, the practices inhered in what were ostensibly arms-length contractual agreements between groups of hospitals, their purchasing alliances, and the manufacturers who sell medical products. The practices at the center of the controversy did not seem that extraordinary—lower prices for a higher percentage of purchases (committed contracts), lower prices for buying from a single vendor (sole-source contracts) or dual vendors (dual-source contracts), and lower prices for buying a range of products (bundled contracts). Such practices are found in other industries (e.g., customer loyalty programs, McDonald's Value Meal). But in health care, these practices came under intense public scrutiny. There were repeated calls by small manufacturers and their trade association to undercut the funding mechanism for hospital purchasing alliances, which might cause them to cease operation. Managing strategic alliances thus became a political hot potato. The GPOs, which used to be faceless and rather unremarkable, found they had a whole new set of constituents that they did not previously serve, including the U.S. Senate, the GAO, the FTC, small manufacturers, and the press.

A recent literature review found that GPOs help hospitals to achieve lower product prices (Burns, 2014). GPO prices may not be the lowest prices observed, given some hospitals' effort to negotiate further discounts using the GPO price and the development of regionally based GPOs below the national level. When aggregated across hospitals, the price discounts obtained through GPO contracting can lower both hospital costs and national spending. With regard to contracting practices, GPOs have diminished their use of sole-source and bundled contracts that rankled the small manufacturers. However, such practices are still popular among their hospital members.

The GPO marketplace is competitive, with substantial rivalry not only among the handful of large national GPOs but also with the growing number of regional and local GPOs. GPOs not only compete with one another but also foster competition in supplier markets for GPO contracts. There is little evidence that GPO contracts have excluded smaller and innovative suppliers from the market. In fact, the evidence suggests that GPOs improve hospital awareness of new products and technology. Overall, hospitals have been consistently satisfied with the services provided by GPOs, as reflected in their historical reliance on and membership in multiple GPOs.

CHAPTER PURPOSE

There is no doubt that the current U.S. health care environment can be characterized as complexly turbulent, a summary term used to capture both the rapid pace and the unpredictability of changes in the environment. This turbulence, we suggest, is rooted in the fact that health care organizations are themselves highly interconnected and also highly interdependent with the broader society in which they find themselves.

This emphasis on connectedness and interdependence is an important basis for viewing a specific organization's environment not as some amorphous external force but rather as the set of other organizations that are interconnected or interdependent with it. This organization, in turn, is part of the environment for the other organizations. In other words, when an organization looks out with concern or anticipation at its **turbulent environment**, what it sees is other organizations looking out at that organization (Shortell and Zajac, 1990).

This conceptualization of organizational environments suggests the need to focus more attention on how specific organizations interact with one another. This chapter emphasizes one such type of interaction—cooperative interorganizational relations. We focus most of our attention on those interorganizational relations that are voluntary and entered into primarily for strategic purposes—that is, that are important to an organization's mission and expected to enhance organizational performance. We term such relationships **strategic alliances**, which are defined as any formal arrangements between two or more organizations for purposes of ongoing cooperation and mutual gain/risk sharing.

MAKE, BUY, OR ALLY?

While attention to strategic alliances among companies is a fairly recent phenomenon, the fundamental question motivating the growth of alliances is centuries old. Specifically, as articulated by Adam Smith in 1776, the concept of comparative advantage was advanced to provide guidance when contemplating whether an individual, a company, or a country should do something him/her/itself versus buy it from another. While providing a good answer to this question of "do it yourself" versus "have others do it" continues to be a foundational issue in the field of economics framed in terms of the "make versus buy" choice (Williamson, 1975), it fails to fully consider the relevance of a third option, namely, to ally, that is, "do it with others" (Zajac and Olsen, 1993). Indeed, in the case of modern organizations, we suggest that firms are increasingly considering all three options when deciding how to devote resources to the many activities needed to produce and sell their goods and services: (1) place the activity within the legal and organizational umbrella of the hierarchical organization and rely on employees to perform the activity, (2) access and pay for the activity in a market transaction with another independent organization, or (3) partner with another organization by making permeable the boundaries of the partnering organizations such that the relevant activities and their performance outcomes are shared between/among the partners. Note also that option 1 (the "make" option) could be achieved organically via internal development of the activity or inorganically through absorbing the activity via merger or acquisition.

So what should we call these options? We prefer the term "vehicles," and we suggest that the choice of

vehicles represents one of senior management's most important strategic decisions when faced with the inevitable challenges to their firm's growth and profitability. One of the distinctive features of health care organizations, whether they be provider, insurer, or supplier organizations, is that they typically engage in all of these vehicles. Pharmaceutical firms, in particular, at any given time are likely to utilize a portfolio of vehicles (i.e., engage in a combination of internal development, acquisitions, alliances, and outsourcing activities) in an effort to optimize the important cost, risk, and speed issues involved in drug development (Lungeanu, Stern, and Zajac, 2016). Consider, for example, the many documented pharmaceutical mergers and acquisitions over the past three decades (Burns, Nicholson, and Wolkowski, 2012), along with the multiple pharmaceutical strategic alliances, often involving biotechnology firms and academic research organizations (Stern, Dukerich, and Zajac, 2014).

Changes in preferred vehicles can also be seen among health care providers and payers. For example, as outlined in Chapter 1 of this volume, the last several decades have witnessed the physical–hospital relationship moving away from the traditional medical staff model, where hospitals served as the "doctor's workshop" for physicians working as independent, community-based practitioners. Instead, we see today hospitals investing heavily in physician employment arrangements and physician alliance models using integrated delivery networks (IDNs) and, more recently, accountable care organizations (ACOs). Again, the choice of vehicle is related to optimizing cost, risk, and speed—in this case, increasing market share, gaining patient referrals, and preparing for risk contracting with payers. Hospitals also sometimes address cost concerns vis-à-vis medical suppliers by banding together in a particular type of strategic alliance known as a group purchasing organization (GPOs), a vehicle that provides an opportunity to balance out what might otherwise be an asymmetric bargaining power situation between a smaller health care buyer and a larger health care supplier.

Given the variety in vehicles used within and across the health care sector, how should health care executives choose among these options? When might one vehicle be preferable to another? Executives can draw on the broader strategy literature for some insights into the "make versus buy versus ally" decision (Borah and Tellis, 2014; Dyer, Kale, and Singh, 2004; Gulati and Nickerson, 2008; Jacobides and Billinger, 2006; Mellewigt et al., 2017; Wang and Zajac, 2007). In terms of empirical evidence regarding the performance implications associated with the choice of vehicle, results are mixed. For example, research on the pharmaceutical sector (cf. Danzon, Nicholson, and Pereira, 2005; Grabowski and Kyle, 2008, 2012) indicates that there are performance advantages to using alliances (relative to M&A), while

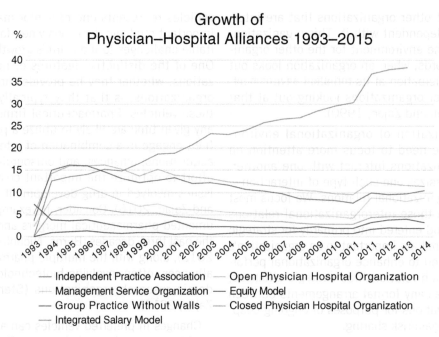

Figure 11.1 Growth of Physician–Hospital Alliances 1993–2015

Legend:
- Independent Practice Association — Open Physician Hospital Organization
- Management Service Organization — Equity Model
- Group Practice Without Walls — Closed Physician Hospital Organization
- Integrated Salary Model

Figure 11.1 Percentage of Total U.S. Community Hospitals in Systems and Networks.

SOURCE: see attached article, Figure 1.

some evidence from the provider sector suggests the opposite (cf. Burns, Goldsmith, and Sen, 2013; Casalino and Robinson, 2003).

Of course, comparative research on organizations opting to use different vehicles over time doesn't fully capture the fact that either choice may be seen as preferable to maintaining the status quo, particularly in turbulent environments. Consider Figure 11.1, which presents data collected by the American Hospital Association regarding hospital participation in hospital networks (ally) and multihospital systems (make) between 2001 and 2015 (data courtesy of Peter Kralovec, Health Forum). It shows that system participation is both more prevalent than network participation (66 percent versus 34 percent in 2015) and also growing more rapidly than network participation. Interestingly, both of these options are at least as popular—if not more so—than standing pat, that is, remaining a freestanding hospital.

ALLIANCES IN HEALTH CARE

Alliances are certainly not without their issues. By their very nature, alliances are risky endeavors: Some claim they face failure rates as high as 50 to 80 percent. The business press has had a penchant for describing, in detail, particular joint ventures or other alliances that failed. The failure of a cooperative alliance between two organizations often involves considerable drama, as interorganizational cooperation turns to conflict and sometimes litigation.

The fragile nature of an alliance between two or more organizations exposes each party to the risk that the other party or parties may not continue to cooperate as expected (Alexander et al., 2016; Hearld et al., 2016).

Although it is very important to recognize the pros and cons of alliances (see Debate Time), we believe that a fixation on the likely failure and inherent riskiness of alliances may be misguided. Specifically, we contend that any assessment of the **alliance risk** should be balanced with an assessment of the expected return or benefit of the alliance in terms of improved financial performance, innovation, and organizational learning, and the opportunity cost of not engaging in a strategic alliance. Regarding the first point, while financial performance is an obvious outcome to consider when analyzing the success or failure of a strategic alliance, it is not clear that it should be considered the most important, direct outcome. For example, innovation may be a driving force behind strategic alliances, and more generally, alliances may be viewed as a desirable way for organizations to learn about new markets, services, and ways of doing business (Zajac, Golden, and Shortell, 1991). These may actually be negatively correlated with financial performance, at least in the short run (Shortell and Zajac, 1988). This issue is discussed in greater detail in the section on how strategic intentions drive alliance activity and specific alliance outcomes.

In terms of opportunity cost, the relevant question is not whether an alliance is risky but, rather, which is riskier: doing nothing and going it alone, merging with another firm, or engaging in an alliance? Riskiness is not necessarily a problem. For example, the virtues of entrepreneurship are often extolled, despite the high risk and high failure rates involved. Strategic alliances may appear risky when the baseline comparison is not made explicit, but when compared with attempting a de novo entry into a new market or ignoring the market altogether, the alliance may actually seem like a relatively low-risk proposition (Shortell and Zajac, 1988). In fact, as discussed below, the creation of a strategic alliance is often motivated by an organization's desire to reduce uncertainty.

The issues just raised are particularly relevant for health care organizations. There has been an increase in hospital alliances in the last few decades, involving roughly one-third of all facilities (Bazzoli et al., 2000), between hospitals and physician groups, between hospitals and managed care organizations (MCOs), and between hospitals, physicians, and agencies of the federal government (Bazzoli et al., 1999; Burns and Pauly, 2002). Beyond health care delivery, alliances are heavily utilized in the life sciences sector (biopharmaceutical firms) to promote research & development (R&D) collaborations, to in-license and out-license promising drugs and molecules, to swap entire clinical franchises (e.g., between Novartis and GlaxoSmithKline), and to develop partnerships with basic research laboratories, either freestanding or housed in universities. Alliances are also utilized by medical technology firms to (a) help commercialize promising inventions developed by physician entrepreneurs and (b) promote R&D efforts with hospital customers and promote cross-selling of products (see below). Alliances known as business coalitions have also emerged among

DEBATE TIME: Positive and Negative Benefits of Alliances

There are a few facts and many more unknowns about strategic alliances. One fact is that we are witnessing a substantial increase in strategic alliances in health care. An unknown, however, is whether this fact reflects a positive or negative development. An interesting example of an ongoing debate is found in Duncan, Ginter, and Swayne (1992). In this section, we consider some of the arguments swirling around the use of strategic alliances. Kaluzny and Zuckerman (1992) argue on the positive side for alliances, while Begun (1992) offers counterarguments on the negative side. The following list of issues summarizes their points of disagreement.

Positive

1. Alliances reflect a fundamental shift in how health service organizations do business; namely, a change from thinking in terms of control to thinking in terms of commitment, trust, shared risk, and common purpose.
2. Alliances provide organizations with a way to manage growing complexity and interdependence while maintaining a fair amount of individual organizational autonomy.
3. Alliances enable organizations to transcend the existing organizational inertia that is often created by complexity and vested interests seeking to maintain the status quo.
4. Alliances have been found to be effective in other sectors of our society, and failure to apply these concepts to health services would be a missed opportunity for meeting the challenges in the future.

Negative

1. Alliances distract organizations from their basic goal, which is to clobber your competitors or at least behave as if you have that need. Managers like the thrill of the competitive chase, and competition creates loyalty and team spirit in an organization.
2. Alliances are essentially a fad whose benefits have been exaggerated, similar to Theory Z, the pursuit of excellence, product-line management, and total quality management.
3. Alliances can lead to collusion between otherwise competing organizations, can lead to legal problems related to antitrust challenges, and are attractive only to lazy organizations that are not interested in competition.
4. The process hassles of initiating and managing alliances are tremendous and costly, and these arrangements are quite fragile.
5. Governing an alliance means governing by committee, which we know to be an ineffective way to run a business. In particular, this problem reduces the speed and flexibility of an organization.
6. Cooperative strategy makes sense for large, multinational firms seeking to enter new and unknown markets or share expensive research and development projects but not for health care organizations that face well-known local markets and do not need to finance much research and development.

Which of the above perspectives do you favor? How would you justify your position?

buyers of care, that is, employers who band together to increase their effectiveness as purchasers of care for their employees. The variety of possible alliance partners is quite high, given the myriad number of players in the different health care sectors (see Figure 1.1 in Chapter 1) and the number of key relationships between adjacent organizations (see Table 11.1).

The causes for this increase in activity are not difficult to identify. Perhaps the most important and obvious factor is that health care organizations have experienced what Meyer (1982) long ago referred to as a series of "environmental jolts." These are relatively abrupt, major, and often qualitative changes in an environment that threaten organizational survival. Such jolts have included the rapid ascent of health maintenance organizations (HMOs) as the dominant form of managed care, as well as the proposed Clinton Health Plan ("Health Security Act")—both in the early 1990s. The latter served as a major spur to the horizontal and vertical integration of providers that began during that decade.

However, the major jolts to the health care system that providers can neither anticipate nor control have included a long string of changes to the Medicare program: the Prospective Payment System (PPS, 1983), the Resource-Based Relative Value Scale (RBRVS, 1992),

the Balanced Budget Act (BBA, 1997), the Medicare Modernization Act (MMA, 2003), the Affordable Care Act (ACA, 2010), and, most recently, the Medicare Access and CHIP Reauthorization Act (MACRA, 2015). The ACA, for example, encouraged hospitals and physicians to voluntarily form alliances to contract with the federal government as ACOs in the Medicare Shared Savings Program (MSSP). Between 2012 and 2016, over 800 ACOs formed to work with public and private payers. The federal government also may impose such changes, often with little period for public comment, understanding, or assessment as to their impact. They have the potential for significant effects on provider reimbursement as well as on provider requirements to respond to mandates to improve quality of care (e.g., pay-for-performance, Hospital Readmissions Reduction Program).

These jolts create great uncertainty for health care managers. Alliances may reflect the reality that it is sometimes better to face life's uncertainties with partners than to go it alone. For example, in response to the proposed Clinton Health Plan, many providers embarked on both hospital and physician alliance strategies and deliberated which partners they should "take to the big dance" (Kaluzny, Zuckerman, and Ricketts, 1995).

Table 11.1 Key Alliance Relationships between Organizations in Various Health Care Sectors

Alliance Relationships within and across Sectors

Suppliers and Suppliers
- Pharmaceutical and biotechnology firms (drug development and commercialization)
- Pharmaceutical and medical device firms (development of drug-eluting stents)
- Medical device and information technology firms (remote monitors)
- Medical products firms and wholesalers (key distribution partners)

Suppliers and Providers
- Medical device firms and physician inventors (device innovation)
- Medical imaging firms and hospital scientists (imaging advances)
- Group purchasing organizations and hospitals (group buying)

Providers and Providers
- Hospitals and physicians (PHOs, MSOs, etc.)
- Pharmacies and retail clinics (MinuteClinic, TakeCare)
- Hospitals and retail clinics (retail medicine feeder for hospitals)

Buyers and Providers
- Employers and retail clinics (on-site primary care for employees)
- Managed care/insurers and hospitals/physicians (pay-for-performance programs)

Buyers and Buyers
- Employers and managed care/insurers (risk-based contracts)
- Employers and pharmacy benefit managers (carve out pharmacy benefits)
- Employers and business groups (pooled purchasing of health insurance)
- Managed care and pharmacy benefit managers (carve out pharmacy benefits)

Of course, alliances are but one response to the environmental changes described above. There has also been a marked increase in other types of multiorganizational arrangements, particularly multihospital systems and other forms of horizontal integration (Burns and Pauly, 2002; Burns et al., 2012; Shortell, 1988), vertical integration (Burns, Goldsmith, and Sen, 2013), and diversification (Goldsmith et al., 2015). In short, as Starr (1982) observed long ago, the landscape of the health care field is itself changing: Where there were once many small and independent organizations, there are now clusters of organizations, including alliances and other types of multiorganizational arrangements.

TYPES AND FORMS OF ALLIANCES

Alliances vary in regard to ownership, control, size, governance, and nature of participation.

Ownership and Control

Researchers have traditionally arrayed multi-institutional systems on a continuum of more autonomy to more **control**. These rankings often reflect the degree of **ownership**, with complete ownership being equated with the highest form of control. While it seems reasonable to view ownership as related to control, we argue that this can sometimes be misleading.

For example, it is well known that McDonald's Corporation is very interested in maintaining control over its raw materials to ensure that quality is highly consistent. In dealing with its exchange partners who supply these raw materials, one might therefore expect that McDonald's would prefer an interorganizational arrangement that would involve substantial ownership interest in suppliers to have greater control. This is not the case, however. Even with no ownership interests, McDonald's simply communicates its quality requirements to the supplier organizations, and the organizations are typically quick to oblige.

How can this be? Two factors seem to be relevant. The first is obvious. McDonald's, by virtue of its size, enjoys substantial relative power in its relationship with suppliers; McDonald's represents a very large portion of a food supplier's business. This obviates, at least in large part, the need for McDonald's to also own some or all of the suppliers' assets. Ownership and control are essentially separated in this case. The second reason has much less to do with the relative power of the organizations involved and more to do with the establishment of a tradition of mutual gain and cooperation. Specifically, McDonald's has made it a policy to be loyal to high-quality suppliers and to use its size to protect the supplier from dramatic swings in sales revenue. In this way, both parties have incentives to ensure a long-term cooperative relationship—with no ownership interests.

This simplified example is not intended to show that ownership and control are usually unrelated, of course. Rather, the example demonstrates that tight control can exist even in cases where there is no ownership interest. In fact, Bazzoli and her colleagues (1999) analyzed all U.S. hospital systems (i.e., two or more hospitals have a common owner) and alliances (i.e., two or more hospitals agree to work together without common ownership) for the years 1994 and 1995 and found that there were alliances that exercised centralized control over a variety of decisions and systems in which control was decentralized.

Furthermore, it is not at all clear that the pursuit of control through higher levels of ownership should be the paramount consideration in designing strategic alliances. As Li, Zhou, and Zajac (2009) show, an overemphasis on one dimension of alliances, such as the degree of control implied by ownership, can lead to negative outcomes on other dimensions of alliances, such as degree of active collaboration between partners. Similarly, one could dimensionalize alliance ownership without direct reference to control by simply considering contractual versus **equity-based alliances** (Salvato, Reuer, and Battigalli, 2017). Contractual alliances, such as preferred buyer–supplier arrangements or licensing agreements, are likely to spell out the terms of partner engagement, including control questions, in legal documents. Equity-based alliances include minority equity investments, which are often observed between large and small firms in the medical device industry, or formal **joint ventures**, in which two organizations give birth to a joint venture "child," with the specific equity percentages agreed upon by the two parent organizations. In these joint ventures, control issues are partly determined by ownership stakes and shareholder vote but also partly determined by the negotiated joint venture operating agreement.

The lesson emerging from our discussion of ownership and control is that there are many dimensions upon which one can categorize strategic alliances, and that one must exercise caution in interpreting what the dimension really represents and how it relates to other relevant dimensions. We now turn to discussing several additional dimensions upon which one can distinguish one type or form of strategic alliance from another.

Number of Members

Alliances vary greatly in size. They can consist of two organizations, but they often consist of many more. For example, some national purchasing alliances of hospitals (known as group purchasing organizations or GPOs) can include thousands of hospitals. Size makes a substantial difference in several ways. Larger alliances are more difficult to govern because it is more difficult to represent all members on a single board of directors. Such alliances may need to develop smaller, more regional versions to facilitate cooperation. Larger size may also entail greater diversity among members, which in turn may make it more difficult to find common ground on important issues ranging from alliance strategy (i.e., what are the alliance objectives—that is, the overall purpose and goals of the alliance) to the management of alliance programs. Further, even when agreements are reached on alliance strategy and operations, larger size makes it difficult to coordinate members' efforts.

On the other hand, size has virtues. It creates power, as noted earlier. Larger alliances typically have more purchasing power because they can buy in larger volume (assuming, of course, that all members can agree on a particular vendor, which is often difficult). Large GPOs can make more than $50 billion worth of purchases per year. Similarly, larger alliances have more clout in lobbying at various levels of government. Further, larger alliances can generate capital easier simply from having a larger number of members' fees to collect.

Nonetheless, the costs and benefits of alliance size are difficult to assess in the abstract. What often matters most in determining an effective size for an alliance is its strategic purpose and particular situation. For example, a local or regional hospital network will have a relatively small number of members compared to other hospital alliances. Yet, it may have exactly the number of members it needs for its purpose, which is to provide the local area with a comprehensive service system.

Governance Structure

While much is known about the antecedents and consequences of organizations' decision to opt for strategic alliances, much less is known about what goes on inside alliances (Albers, Wohlgezogen, and Zajac, 2016). Much of what goes on inside alliances can be discussed in terms of governance structures and processes. Even in the relatively simple situation of an alliance among two entities, there are decisions to be made regarding interface questions (e.g., who will be the boundary spanners? How many? How often will they interact?) and intraface questions (e.g., how will boundary spanners connect back to their own organizations).

When one considers multiparty alliances, governance issues can become even more complex. For example, the governing bodies of many alliances, especially hospital alliances, tend to include at least one member from each participating organization, often the director or CEO of the member organization. This practice stems largely from important distinguishing features of alliances; that is, that they are a form of organization in which the members are equal and have a great deal of autonomy.

Further, the boards of health care organizations traditionally have been based on what Fennell and Alexander (1989) term a philanthropic model, which assumes that "bigger is better." In other words, boards were viewed as a key link to the local community and its resources; having more individuals on a board provided a hospital, for example, with greater community support and access to donors. Similarly, we have observed that alliance boards often are large so as to represent various interest groups.

As just noted, however, this means that larger alliances can have boards with dozens of members that, in turn, can make it difficult to achieve consensus and can slow decision making. Of course, large alliance boards can, and sometimes do, have executive committees that consist of a smaller subset of elected members who have the authority to make key decisions. Thus, an important choice for larger alliances is whether to represent all or some members on the alliance board and to determine what kinds of individuals (CEOs, physicians, trustees) should be alliance board members.

ACOs have perhaps even more diverse and complex structures, which can impact their performance (Shortell et al., 2015). ACOs can include a range of providers (hospitals, physicians, nursing homes, and other post-acute care sites) under a variety of governance models. These can include a local physician-hospital organization (PHO), a more broadly distributed clinically integrated network (CIN), a primary care or multispecialty group practice, a network of hospital providers organized as an IDN, or a large hospital system with an employed medical group. A key challenge for the ACO participants is agreeing to work together to jointly improve performance on a host of quality metrics and reducing costs below historical benchmarks to earn the shared savings. Hospital members may want to increase inpatient utilization (to fill beds) while physician members may focus on outpatient utilization and prescription drug therapy. This may require more centralized rather than decentralized governance and decision making, which may mean that one provider assumes a more superordinate role.

Mandated versus Voluntary Participation

Another important dimension on which alliances vary is whether they are voluntary or mandated by an external group with legal or legitimate authority (Oliver, 1990). Most health care alliances are voluntary. These alliances reflect the efforts of individual organizations to strategically adapt to external changes by choosing to band together. But, it is important to recognize that even voluntary alliances may emerge in large part as a result of external pressure from powerful actors.

A central issue to note in comparing mandated and voluntary alliances is the extent to which the former are characterized more by style than by substance and by instability than by longevity. Scott (1987) argues that mandated forms of organization tend to be adopted only superficially and, as a result, also tend to be short-lived. Many international alliances (including the League of Nations and the United Nations) come to mind in this regard. Superficial compliance with a mandate to form an alliance is especially likely to occur when the participating organizations lack other motives for forming a relationship (Oliver, 1990). In general, managers and other organization members chafe under external constraints and regulation, even when such rules have some merit.

A variation on the mandated versus voluntary alliance question can also be seen as a design choice within a single alliance. GPOs, also described as purchasing co-ops in other industries, can be organized as a mandated or as a voluntary GPO. In a mandated GPO, organizations choosing to join the GPO are required to channel their purchase requirements through the GPO entity. In the voluntary GPO, members maintain their own purchasing capability and can elect to "opt in" or "opt out" when a specific group purchasing opportunity arises.

As one might imagine, there are costs and benefits to both approaches. The major advantage of a mandated GPO is that GPO representatives enter into negotiations with suppliers having greater certainty regarding order sizes, thus maximizing the GPO's leverage vis-à-vis suppliers. A voluntary GPO, on the other hand, has the advantage of providing flexibility to its hospital members, many of whom may value the autonomy to continue purchasing directly from suppliers as they see fit and customize purchasing to suit the needs of the local hospital medical staff. One hybrid approach that seeks to offer the best of both worlds is to institute purchase minimums for each GPO member, enabling the GPO to harness the power of aggregation for the benefit of all members, while also allowing individual members the desired discretion to pick and choose those purchasing opportunities best suited to their specific needs.

Discussion

Existing typologies have been useful in documenting and describing the common and different features of a wide range of interorganizational arrangements in health care. However, it is also important to ask what difference an organization should expect to see if it were to choose one form versus another.

In other words, what is the alliance intended to accomplish? For example, Zajac (1986), in an analysis of contract management arrangements, argues that organizations choosing to engage in a similar type of strategic alliance may have widely varying strategic intentions and that expected performance will vary accordingly. In other words, the form of the alliance is not necessarily a good predictor of what the alliance can achieve.

WHAT ARE ALLIANCES MEANT TO DO?

Pooling versus Trading Alliances

Most broadly, one can distinguish between pooling alliances that bring together organizations seeking to contribute similar resources and trading alliances that bring together organizations seeking to contribute different resources (Doz and Hamel, 1998). This distinction is more precise than the often-made statement that organizations generally seek "complementarities" in alliances. The term "complementarity" suggests differences, but it is important to remember that similarities can often drive alliance activity as well.

An example of a pooling or similarity-driven strategic intent for an alliance is one that seeks to gain purchasing power over a supplier or group of suppliers. As discussed above, such alliances are often seen in health care in the form of (a) business coalitions that contract with payers and hospital networks or (b) hospital GPOs that contract with product manufacturers and distributors. Examples of a trading or difference-driven alliance are (a) a health plan partnership with a pharmacy benefit manager (PBM) to manage drug procurement and utilization, (b) a physician group–hospital joint venture, (c) joint ventures between two biopharmaceutical firms, which combine the development skill of one with the commercialization skill of the other (see end of chapter), and (d) a hospital–supplier joint venture, where the two parties jointly conduct research on new iterations of the supplier's technology (see end of chapter).

These examples highlight how strategic intent can often drive the form of a strategic alliance. Pooling alliances tend to involve more organizations and take the form of federations, consortia, or coalitions; by contrast, trading strategies tend to involve fewer (often only two) organizations and take the form of joint ventures, licensing agreements, and related arrangements. Note also that the reason pooling alliances can accommodate larger numbers of members is that they typically seek to achieve a single common goal, while trading alliances seek to achieve multiple (and hopefully compatible) goals.

Cost Reduction versus Revenue Enhancement

The strategic intent of alliances can also be examined in terms of their expected outcomes. An emphasis on expected alliance outcomes is relevant for several reasons. The success of an alliance will generally be defined by the degree to which the desired outcomes are achieved; some performance outcomes may be largely incompatible with others; and one alliance partner's perception of the expected outcome may not be shared by that of other partners.

The first and most basic expected outcome refers to financial performance and addresses the issue of whether the alliance is primarily conceived for **cost reduction** or **revenue enhancement**. While this is not to say that the two outcomes are mutually exclusive, there are differences in the challenges for success for alliances, in how one gauges success, and in how cost-reducing versus revenue-enhancing alliances might be organized.

For example, consider a local alliance of four hospitals with historically complementary specialties (or distinctive competencies) that seeks to increase the volume of patients to be treated in these specialties. Compare this alliance with a similarly sized and similarly located hospital alliance seeking to share the costs of providing indigent care to the local community. One would not measure success the same way, nor would the interaction between partners be the same in the two alliances. One might expect that the alliance motivated by the desire to increase patient volume would require substantial coordination, given that there is a reciprocal interdependence between the partners. In the case of the cost-sharing alliance, one would likely observe a combining of similar resources requiring relatively less active coordination, given that there is a pooled interdependence among the partners (Thompson, 1967).

Quality, Innovation, and Learning

Another way of classifying the intent of an alliance is the degree to which the alliance seeks to enhance outcomes such as innovation, organizational learning (Inkpen and Tsang, 2007), and quality (Doz and Hamel, 1998; Nembhard, 2012; Zajac, Golden, and Shortell, 1991). These outcomes are distinct from those discussed above in that, while they may lead to revenue enhancement or cost reduction, their relationship to such financial performance measures may be difficult to discern or, in a more extreme case, may be negatively related to financially oriented targets (Shortell and Zajac, 1990).

For example, Zuckerman and D'Aunno (1990) noted that hospitals can increase their reputation for quality by joining a strategic alliance that involves other prestigious organizations. Membership in such an alliance may require only a minor contribution of time, effort, or capital. An interesting feature of such an alliance is that one partner's actions can damage the reputation of another by not delivering the expected level of quality. This suggests the need for appropriate screening of partners in terms of their commitment to quality. There may also be regional differences in the degree to which membership is prestige-enhancing. For example, alliances with a large national, for-profit hospital system may be viewed positively by the local community in some parts of the country as an asset (particularly where investor-owned hospitals are prevalent) but not so in other parts of the country where investor-owned hospitals have less market presence.

Other motives driving alliance activity, such as innovation and learning (Inkpen and Tsang, 2007), are also conceptually distinct from other, more straightforward motives. The payoffs from alliances that are driven by innovation and learning motives are often slow to emerge. This requires a particularly high level of partner commitment and patience. An additional factor to consider is that many organizations underestimate the involvement necessary to realize benefits such as innovation and learning. In these alliances, a more substantial personnel flow between partners can often accelerate the learning and innovation process.

Power Enhancement, Uncertainty Reduction, and Risk Sharing

Power enhancement and **uncertainty reduction** are grouped together because one often has implications for the other. Specifically, alliances can be motivated by an organization's desire to gain influence over, or reduce dependence on, an aspect of the organization's environment. This reduction in dependence may also represent a reduction in uncertainty, although the two are conceptually distinct. An organization might be dependent on another organization, but if the more powerful organization is reliable, then the dependent organization may face little uncertainty.

Uncertainty reduction as an alliance motive can also be compared with a similar, yet distinct, motive: risk sharing. The difference between the two motives is that the former highlights one organization's attempts to reduce its own uncertainty, whereas the latter emphasizes the joint reduction of uncertainty for both (or more) partners. Not surprisingly, the former is equated more with gaining influence of an exchange partner, while the latter is used more in terms of pooling resources to reduce common risk.

CEO Rationales for Alliances

Our discussion of the above-mentioned strategic intentions that can drive alliance activity is intended to be illustrative, rather than exhaustive. Indeed, if one were to ask CEOs the question of "Why ally?" it would not be surprising to hear a myriad of broad and narrow reasons as to why their organizations turn to strategic alliances to further their goals. In fact, one survey of CEOs on this question bears out this expectation. Specifically, in a Coopers and Lybrand CEO survey in 1996, U.S. CEOs highlighted the following top reasons for alliance formation:

- Improve competitive position   77%
- Increase sales of existing products   77%
- Create new products or business lines   76%
- Improve operations or technology   71%
- Improve employee skills   48%
- Decrease cost of existing operations   44%

• • • IN PRACTICE: Strategic Alliances between Buyers and Suppliers of Medical Imaging Equipment

Over the past 20 years, the manufacturers of medical imaging equipment (e.g., General Electric, Siemens, Philips) have developed strategic alliances with their downstream customers, such as academic medical centers, hospital systems, and large integrated physician groups (Mayo Clinic, Cleveland Clinic). These alliances have sought to transform the traditional buyer–seller relationship from selling more product (supplier goal) and lowering unit product cost (buyer goal) to fostering new product development for sellers and developing solutions to buyers' operational problems.

Imaging equipment manufacturers have developed two types of alliances with providers: research alliances and equipment/service alliances. In the former, the manufacturer contributes equipment (e.g., MRIs, scanners, etc.), research scientists and other personnel, and some research funding to the customer site; the hospital's research personnel work with the manufacturer's scientists on mutually agreed-upon research projects, which typically focus on developing the next-generation technology. Intellectual property may be shared between the two partners, including academic research papers. Manufacturers value these alliances because they allow them to tap the insights and product development capabilities of researchers in academic medical centers, invent the next-generation equipment, and leapfrog their competitors. In the latter, multiyear agreements stipulate technology upgrades, the hospital's service as a clinical show site for the manufacturer's latest technology, and the hospital's access to the manufacturer for their consulting expertise (e.g., GE's lean and Six Sigma techniques). Hospitals seek to tap this expertise to redesign their workflows and reengineer core patient processes. In both cases, the alliances serve as platforms for learning and new capability development on behalf of both partners.

Nevertheless, these alliances are not without their problems and frictions. Primary among these are the amount of time consumed in alliance meetings, the conflict in time horizons of the two partners, turnover in key positions overseeing the alliance as well as among researchers, technical problems with the imaging equipment, and difficulties in migrating solutions developed in one site (one hospital of a multihospital system, one clinical area within that hospital) to other clinical sites. Unlike alliances observed in other industries, these alliances typically have underdeveloped coordinative and governance mechanisms to improve alliance functioning, as well as dedicated alliance personnel on the hospital side.

Overall, these supplier–provider alliances are important for an industry where there has historically been much mistrust between the two parties and little successful alliance formation in the past. Moreover, the two parties in these alliances are large, important stakeholders in the entire health care system and involved in arguably the fastest-rising component of health care spending: imaging procedures. Finally, these alliances constitute a growing set of efforts to enable firms in the health care supply chain to access complementary resources, to promote innovation while also improving quality and efficiency, and ultimately to develop true value chains.

What this survey also shows, however, is that the reasons for pursuing strategic alliances are likely not mutually exclusive. Returning to a health care example, a business coalition may be formed because it wants to gain influence over local area hospitals, but it also has as its major objective a reduction in the cost of health care that the coalition members have had to pay. Thus, power and cost-reduction motives are both driving alliance formation. Similarly, a joint venture between a hospital and a multispecialty physician group may have as its objective the creation of new innovative services, yet also have the intent of increasing power over insurers and increasing its reimbursement (Longest, 1990).

Understanding the strategic intent of an alliance can be a critical success factor for the alliance (Kale and Singh, 2009). The understanding has several components, including understanding your own motivation for considering an alliance, expressing this understanding to your alliance partner, eliciting and then listening carefully to your partners' expression of their strategic intentions, and examining the compatibility (which could be compatibly similar or compatibly different) of your intentions and those of your partners. The lack of an articulated mission statement is often cited as the root of many failures in organizational strategy. The same is equally if not more true for strategic alliances, particularly given the potential for incompatible intentions across partners.

Physician–Hospital Trading Alliances

Physician–hospital alliances have exhibited several growth spurts in response to distinct environmental jolts. The Medicare PPS altered the financial incentives of hospitals by using fixed, per-case payments but left physician incentives untouched. Because physicians control (directly or indirectly) up to 80 percent of hospital expenditures, hospitals began to develop relationships with their physicians in order to influence their thinking and practice behavior. The rapid increase in managed care (e.g., penetration by HMOs) in the late 1980s and early 1990s provided an additional spur to alliance formation. As HMOs sought to reduce their inpatient costs (e.g., through lower payments), hospitals looked for ways to cut costs through partnerships with their physicians. Moreover, some HMOs looked to pass on to providers the financial risks for their enrollees. Physicians and hospitals sought to develop alliances to accept and manage this risk. By the mid-1990s, HMO consolidations served to increase managed care's bargaining power over providers in local markets. Providers responded to this threat by forming vertical alliances to pose a countervailing force (Burns et al., 1997). The Clinton Health Plan further stimulated the spread of these alliances by calling for "accountable health plans" comprised of local insurers and providers (not the same as ACOs) to contract with state-level health insurance purchasing cooperatives (Goldsmith et al., 2015).

Finally, the ACA encouraged the formation of ACOs to contract with the Medicare program. Physician–hospital alliances served as one possible chassis for erecting an ACO (Shortell et al., 2015). They also served as platforms for hospitals to work with their physicians to promote quality improvement and clinical integration.

Physician–hospital alliances take many forms, which contribute to the growing list of acronyms managers must now understand. The two most prominent forms are PHOs and independent practitioner associations (IPAs). To return to the beginning of the chapter, PHOs and IPAs reflect an "ally" approach while ISMs reflect a "make" approach. PHOs constitute joint ventures between a hospital and its medical staff and are designed to develop new services (e.g., ambulatory care clinic) or, more commonly, provide a platform to collaborate and thereby attract managed-care contracts. IPAs similarly constitute a mechanism to turn the medical staff and/or other community physicians into a body that can collectively contract with payers. Both PHOs and IPAs are distinct from integrated salary models (ISMs). ISMs constitute vertically integrated arrangements in which the hospital acquires the physician's practice, establishes an employment contract with the physician for a defined period, and negotiates a guaranteed base salary with a variable component based on office productivity, with some expectation (or anticipation) that the physician will refer or admit patients to the hospital.

Besides PHOs, IPAs, and ISMs, there is now a growing, diverse array of alliance relationships developing between these two parties (Burns and Muller, 2008). The relationships fall into three broad categories: noneconomic integration, economic integration, and clinical integration. Noneconomic integration includes marketing of physicians' practices, medical office buildings, physician liaison programs, physician leadership development, and catering to physicians' technology requests. Economic integration includes the PHO and ISM models above as well as physician recruitment, part-time compensation, leases and participating bond transactions, service line development, equity joint ventures, and funds flow models. Clinical integration, finally, encompasses practice profiling, performance feedback, medical/demand/disease management programs, continuous quality improvement programs, linkages via clinical information systems, and development of care management practices (CMPs).

These alliances are pursued by each party for many reasons, only some of which overlap. Hospitals pursue physician alliances to capture their outpatient markets, to increase their revenues and margins, to improve care processes and outcomes, to increase the loyalty of their physicians, to bolster physicians' practices and incomes, and to address pathologies in the traditional hospital medical staff. Physicians likewise enter these alliances to increase their practice incomes and improve the quality of service to patients. But after this, their goals diverge from those of the hospitals. Physicians also want to increase their access to capital and technology, to increase their control in care delivery, and to increase their own lifestyle satisfaction.

Physician–hospital partnerships might be best characterized as a trading alliance. Hospitals contribute capital, legal, managerial, and payer expertise to managed care contracting vehicles such as PHOs, IPAs, and CINs. For their part, physicians contribute their (a) professional control over resource utilization (prescriptions, admissions, referrals) and (b) medical knowledge about and control over quality of care (low-value care)—both of which are necessary to succeed under shared savings models and risk contracting.

How well have these alliances performed? The prevalence of these alliances has waxed, waned, and waxed again. Figure 11.2 shows that alliances such as PHOs and IPAs grew from 1993 to 1996, declined from 1997 to 2011, and started to spread again from 2012 to 2015—due to the ACA and its encouragement of ACOs. Empirical evidence suggests that alliances have yet to demonstrate their promise. Alliances based on economic integration exert few consistent impacts on cost, quality, or clinical integration. Alliances based on noneconomic integration are widespread but have not been subjected to rigorous academic study. Finally, alliances based on clinical integration are developing with positive, but weaker-than-expected impacts on quality of care (Burns and Muller, 2008). There is also recent evidence that physician groups are retreating from some forms of CMPs (Rodriguez et al., 2016).

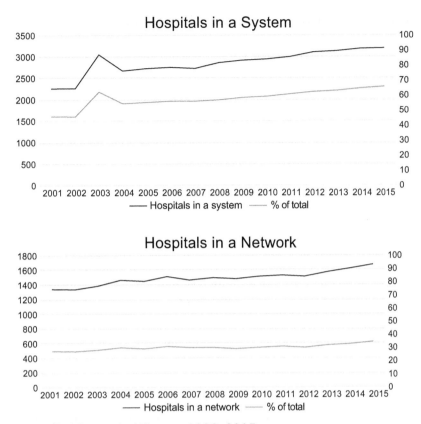

Figure 11.2 Physician–Hospital Strategic Alliances 1993–2015.

SOURCE: American Hospital Association Annual Survey.

Why are the results so disappointing, especially given the prevalence of alliances and the attention received in the literature? One reason is the structural form used to implement the alliance. These alliances are typically organized, financed, and controlled by the hospital, with little physician participation. Not surprisingly, physicians balk at partnerships in which they have not participated. A second, related explanation is the lack of infrastructure found in many alliances. Too often, hospitals will develop the alliances as external contracting vehicles to approach the managed-care market but fail to develop the internal mechanisms that will help the alliance partners to manage risk (Kale and Singh, 2009). Such mechanisms include physician compensation and productivity systems, quality monitoring and measurement, and physician selection (Burns and Thorpe, 1997). Third, the alliances have often served as vehicles to leverage managed care payers and thus run afoul of antitrust actions taken by the Federal Trade Commission (FTC) and Department of Justice (DOJ) (Casalino, 2006). Fourth, alliances often focus on taking advantage of fee-for-service reimbursement systems and seeking to increase patient and procedural volumes, rather than delivering more appropriate care.

These findings suggest that implementation of the alliance and careful attention to developing its infrastructure are critical for the success of any alliance that physicians and hospitals form. In the absence of the mechanisms discussed above, one would expect alliances to exert little impact on hospital quality and cost of care. In fact, two studies addressed this issue directly. Cuellar and Gertler (2005) and Madison (2004) report that PHO alliances do not lower the cost of care. Indeed, they may lead to higher prices paid for care (for either the hospital or its physicians) due to the combined bargaining leverage of the two parties in the IDN model. Moreover, there is no evidence that alliances improve quality of care and, in fact, may damage it.

THE ALLIANCE PROCESS: A MULTISTAGE ANALYSIS

Early studies of alliances focused primarily on why they emerge, how they are structured, and what they do. For example, among the key results from studies on why alliances emerge is that, compared to mergers or acquisitions, they are more likely to form when challenges of integrating two or more organizations are great (e.g., when they have dissimilar cultures), the partner organizations do not understand each other's resources and potential well, and market uncertainty is high (Salvato, Reuer, and Battigalli, 2017).

Table 11.2 A Life Cycle Model of Organizational Alliances in Health Care

Stages			
Emergence	**Transition**	**Maturity**	**Critical Crossroads**
Key Factors in Development at Each Stage			
Environment poses threat to and uncertainty about valued resources	Motivation to achieve purposes of the alliance	Willingness to put alliance interests first	Increased centralization and dependence on alliance motivates members to seek hierarchy or to withdraw from alliance
Organizations share ideologies and similar dependencies	Increased dependence on alliance for valued resources	Members receive benefits from previous investments	
Examples of Tasks at Each Stage			
Define purposes of the alliance	Hire or form a management group	Attain stated objectives	Manage decisions about future of the alliance
Develop membership criteria	Establish mechanisms for coordination and control	Sustain member commitment	

More attention has been given recently to the **alliance process**—how alliances evolve and behave over time (D'Aunno, Alexander, and Jiang, 2017; Hearld et al., 2015; Kale and Singh, 2009; Zajac and Olsen, 1993). Based on this work, we develop a life-cycle model that managers can use to understand how alliances develop as they do and what can be done to improve their chances for success (Table 11.2). This model suggests that organizations often move through predictable stages of development, with one or more factors triggering such movement.

Gulati, Wohlgezogen, and Zhelyazkov (2012) identify two categories of challenges that are common to each stage in the life cycle of alliances. These are challenges of cooperation, specifically, how to align partners' commitment and interests, and challenges of coordination—how to effectively align and adjust partners' actions. Each stage of development also brings distinctive tasks that alliance leaders and members need to address. We turn to these challenges and tasks below.

Emergence: Finding Partners

Research shows that, in the first stage, organizations are likely to select other organizations as partners for alliances based on several factors. These include the potential partner's prior experience in alliances or similar collaborative efforts, indirect ties (e.g., CEOs of two potential partners have a mutual colleague), status, identity and ideology (e.g., shared religious affiliation), and compatibility of resources and routines (Gulati, Wohlgezogen, and Zhelyazkov, 2012). Further, this dance often begins when the potential partners relate to each other symbiotically as well as competitively—that is, when they have complementary relationships such that one organization uses some services or products of the other as opposed to the case when two organizations are vying for the same resources.

A common example of such complementarity or symbiosis is a rural community hospital that refers cases for tertiary care to an urban teaching hospital. A review of 40 studies of alliances concluded that the complementarity of partners not only promotes alliance formation but also contributes to alliance performance (Shah and Swaminathan, 2008).

In this early stage, organizations also engage in the process of projecting exchange into the future and constructing net present valuations of alternative exchange relationships on a continuum ranging from markets (i.e., arm's-length transactions with another independent organization), through strategic alliances (i.e., a formal cooperative arrangement between organizations, preserving the independent identity of each partner), and finally to hierarchies (i.e., the merging of two or more organizations into one organization) (Macneil, 1983). Perceptions of what each exchange partner seeks also emerge more clearly, enabling the more precise identification of similarities and differences that can form the basis for mutually beneficial exchange.

Thus, in the early stage, there is preliminary communication and negotiation concerning mutual and individual organizational interests. As a result, the partners learn not only about each other's interests but also about their compatibility—that is, the fit between their working styles and cultures (Inkpen and Tsang, 2007). An organization's behavior in this stage can set a precedent for future exchange and provide information through which a firm can learn about the expected behavior of its partner. During this phase, initial norms for exchange are forged and commitments tested in small but important ways to determine credibility (Macneil, 1983). To summarize, in this initial stage, the purposes and expectations of the partners are stated and group norms begin to evolve.

Transition

In this stage, the alliance establishes mechanisms for decision making and overall control of its activities or what is generally termed governance (Gulati, Wohlgezogen, and Zhelyazkov, 2012; Salvato, Reuer, and Battigalli, 2017). Governance mechanisms include (1) joint ownership, in which the partners share control of some or all alliance assets; (2) contracts that specify the rights and obligations of alliance partners; (3) informal agreements that rely on trust and goodwill; or (4) some combination of these (Puranam and Vanneste, 2009).

Research to date suggests that, overall, the governance mechanism of joint ownership (equity-based alliances) provides stronger alignment of incentives and better management control of alliance activities (e.g., by representation of partners on the governing board) than other approaches to governance (Salvato, Reuer, and Battigalli, 2017). At the same time, we believe that it is important to match an approach to governance to the particular needs of an alliance. Informal agreements may work effectively, for example, when the partners know each other well and the alliance activities are not complex or do not involve a high degree of risk.

In any case, establishing a governance mechanism may be rocky because, as just noted, organizations are reluctant to grant authority to others or to sacrifice their own autonomy. It is thus critical that alliance managers ensure that their efforts and programs are responsive to members' needs so as to build their commitment to the alliance.

Alliances vary in the extent to which their members are willing to commit resources to initiate and sustain programs and activities. An important weakness of many alliances is their inability to gain adequate commitment of members' resources. For example, there may be free-rider problems in that some members make little commitment but yet can benefit from the investments of others. It is likely that such problems are directly proportional to the value that members perceive in committing resources to the alliance. The more value that members perceive from active participation, the more resources (including autonomy) they are willing to commit to the alliance.

Of course, this leads to a challenging "chicken-and-egg" dilemma. On the one hand, members increase their commitment in proportion to threats from their environment and the alliance's ability to reduce threats and uncertainty. On the other hand, for the alliance to be effective in meeting members' needs, it may require the investment of valued resources from members as well as their willingness to coordinate efforts with each other. At some point, alliances require an investment of resources that are risked by members who have no certainty of return equal to their investment. At this point, trust becomes particularly important.

Maturity

The third stage of an alliance's life cycle is that of maturity and growth. In this stage, it is critical that the alliance begins to achieve its objectives and aid members in coping with external threats (D'Aunno, Alexander, and Jiang, 2017). Such success enables an alliance to continue and to grow. It is also central that members be willing to put the interests of the alliance, at least sometimes, ahead of their own interests. This is necessary because alliances often cannot meet the needs of all of their members, at least not simultaneously. Members must recognize that they will not necessarily benefit equally from alliance activities; it is essential, however, that they benefit as equitably as possible.

Successful alliances seem to share two key characteristics at this stage of development: a dedicated manager or group of managers who focus exclusively on alliance work and processes that enable an alliance to learn from its experience and to build capabilities (Hoang and Rothaermel, 2005; Inkpen and Tsang, 2007; Kale and Singh, 2009). Dedicated alliance managers play several roles. They promote work on important projects, including garnering resources; they signal the legitimacy of the alliance both to its members and to external stakeholders; and they monitor performance and progress toward objectives and provide timely feedback to members.

Finally, alliance managers may develop tools and processes that enable the alliance to learn from its experience. These processes may include, for example, regular meetings to review factors that have contributed to success and failure in alliance projects. Tools that codify this learning include guidelines, checklists, and manuals that specify best practices and make future projects more efficient and effective.

As alliances seek to attain objectives and sustain member commitment, several issues may arise. For example, alliances that add members may find it impossible to avoid having partners with overlapping market areas. If such overlap does occur, what role, if any, should the alliance play in mediating disputes that may arise among members?

Relationships between the members and alliance managers (if there are any) also become more complex. For example, are new programs initiated through the alliance manager's office, through individual members, or both? If through the alliance office, what happens to similar programs already developed by individual members? For instance, suppose that a hospital alliance wishes to develop an alliance-wide insurance plan, but some members already have their own plans. Further, are there or should there be incentives for members to produce innovative programs that can be shared by all alliance members? In the absence of such incentives, how will the alliance develop innovations in management or services?

Zajac and Olsen (1993) note that alliances in this stage of development face some particularly sensitive issues because value is not only created but also claimed and distributed. Surrounding the issue of claiming and distributing value is the question of interorganizational conflict. Explicit or implicit norms for managing the divergence of interests will often arise. To the extent that these norms—defined as shared and reasoned expectations that may arise from agreement or past acts—emphasize the importance of maximizing joint value, alliance partners should search for mutually satisfactory resolutions of conflict.

On the other hand, if norms do not develop in this way, the pursuit of individual firm interests could lead to a destructive escalation of conflict. The use of accepted conflict-resolution systems can limit the potential damage of interorganizational conflict (Salvato, Reuer, and Battigalli, 2017).

The continued development of trust is a key issue in this stage. Trust stems from a growing confidence in an organization's expectations of the future. Schelling (1960) notes that "trust is often achieved simply by the continuity of the relation between parties and the recognition by each that what he might gain by cheating in a given instance is outweighed by the value of the tradition of trust that makes possible a long sequence of future agreement."

Trust and conflict-management systems are subsets of other relational norms underlying the processes of exchange. These norms, including shared expectations of reciprocity between alliance partners and a growing sense of the value of preserving the relationship (Macneil, 1983), set the tone for the continued execution of either contracts or informal agreements.

Critical Crossroads

As they evolve into the fourth stage of development, alliances move to what may be a critical crossroads. To this point, members became increasingly dependent on each other for needed resources, and there was growing pressure for greater member commitment to the alliance and more centralized decision making. In many ways, however, these developments run counter to the reasons why many organizations join an alliance. That is, alliances are attractive because they provide a relatively low-cost vehicle to gain a variety of benefits while maintaining organizational autonomy. Thus, this stage may be a critical crossroads at which some members conclude that the price of belonging to an alliance is too high and withdraw. In contrast, others may decide that it is necessary to move toward more hierarchical arrangements to gain the full benefits of collective action.

The underlying issue is whether there is sufficient commitment or "glue" to hold alliances together over time. Though there may be common goals, ideologies, values, and inducements that keep members together, alliances typically remain loose arrangements. Can the degree of commitment required of members be secured in the long run? Will members be willing to sacrifice autonomy to allow for greater discipline in decision making? What coordination mechanisms are most appropriate and under what circumstances (Gulati, Wohlgezogen, and Zhelyazkov, 2012; Salvato, Reuer, and Battigalli, 2017)? To survive, alliances must balance the need for and benefits of collective action with the need for individual members to retain adequate autonomy.

This critical crossroads represents a reconfiguring stage in the development of a strategic alliance (Zajac and Olsen, 1993). It is usually triggered by reaching the end of the expected duration of the relationship or by changes in the partners' perceived level of the relationship's value. Reconfiguring may imply that an exchange partner will choose to leave, or it may mean that partners will join more tightly together by widening the scope of exchange processes. For example, a group of hospitals may move from a shared purchasing arrangement to developing a joint preferred provider network to contract with payers.

With respect to perceived changes in the value of the strategic alliance, such changes may emerge from a new and changing environment or a historical comparison of actual to expected value creation (Alexander et al., 2016). While this performance gap can lead to a reevaluation (positive or negative) of the interorganizational relationship itself, it may simply lead to a reassessment of the developmental processes. In other words, the reconfiguring stage may not involve a change in the type of strategic alliance per se but only a change in the process of interaction within the existing strategic alliance. These change options suggest that this stage may loop back to either the emergence stage, where value forecasts are respecified and strategic motivations are clarified for a new forecast period, or the transition stage, where the forms of exchange are revised and updated based on the continued experiences of the partners.

Thus, the model of strategic alliance development outlined here does not propose a one-way, deterministic path for alliances. Indeed, we agree with de Rond (2003), who argued on the basis of several careful case studies of alliances, that their development is often complex and nonlinear. Nonetheless, the model presented here highlights a sequence of likely phases that many alliances may experience and emphasizes a set of critical issues that health care organizations may face at the various stages of alliance development.

FRAMEWORKS FOR ANALYZING ALLIANCE PROBLEMS

A major difficulty that organizations face in addressing alliance problems is actually their inability to identify the problem correctly. By that we mean that individuals within an organization often do not know, or disagree strongly on, what the problem is, and this is compounded by differences of opinion between partners in alliance problem identification and diagnosis. These disagreements, we contend, can often lead to false diagnoses and the treatment of alliance symptoms rather than the root alliance problems facing the alliance. These incorrect interventions subsequently lead to greater friction, gridlock, and, ultimately, an increased likelihood of alliance failure (see Case at the end of the chapter). The three simple frameworks offered below are intended to lessen the likelihood of such failure.

Locating the Problem

If one were to ask several involved individuals why a particular alliance was in trouble, it is possible that one would get a uniform response. In such cases, locating the problem is simple. We argue, however, that such agreement is the exception rather than the norm. Typically, there are a host of possible reasons why an alliance might be facing difficulties. Without some way of organizing these reasons, there may be little hope of remedying the situation. We propose that alliance problems can be usefully categorized as follows:

- Environmental problems: that is, "the market changed"
- Strategy problems: that is, "it was a bad idea from the beginning"
- Structure problems: that is, "it was not organized correctly"
- Behavior problems: that is, "we had the wrong person at the top"

These categories follow a macro-to-micro continuum, but more important for purposes of this chapter, they also tend to follow an uncontrollable-to-controllable continuum.

The categories themselves are useful in assessing the degree to which intervention can be effective. For example, after analyzing the categorized reasons, a manager may believe that the primary problem is environmental—that is, the market conditions no longer support the alliance. This is largely an uncontrollable factor and, therefore, suggests that the alliance is not likely to succeed. On the other hand, the manager may believe the primary problem is structural—that the number or composition of the alliance is not right or that the incentives for participation are inadequate. This is more of a controllable factor and suggests that the alliance can be modified and thus face improved odds for success.

• • • IN PRACTICE: Problems in Physician–Hospital Alliances

Consider the problems in health care alliances that require collaboration among professional groups with different training, time horizons, and economic incentives. For example, trading alliances between physicians and hospitals are particularly vulnerable to these difficulties. An analysis of six integrated systems in Illinois suggests that physician–hospital alliances have polarities to be resolved rather than problems to be solved (Burns, 1999). These polarities consist of nine areas in which the integrated system must seek to manage in two directions simultaneously (i.e., pursue the physicians' interests simultaneously with the hospital's interests). For example, the hospital system seeks to expose its physicians to practicing in a risk-based environment; at the same time, it is purchasing primary care physicians who are then given guaranteed salaries for several years—in effect, exempting them from all risk. As another example, the hospital system wishes to become "an organization of physicians," and yet the system is developed and controlled almost exclusively by hospital executives and serves primarily hospital purposes in the short term. For such alliances to be credible to physicians and work effectively, they need to satisfy the interests of both parties simultaneously. In terms of our framework, the problems lie not in uncontrollable environmental issues, or in the basic strategy of deepening physician–hospital relationships, but in the fundamental structural decisions made and the behavioral problems created or exacerbated by those structural decisions. The framework can be particularly valuable in highlighting disagreement as to what fundamental problems are facing a strategic alliance.

In this way, the Environment → Strategy → Structure → Behavior framework can be a useful tool in identifying and diagnosing alliance problems.

Separating the Root Cause from the Symptom

If you had a rash and were to go to a physician, what would be the first thing the physician would do? Would the physician treat the rash or first ask a set of questions to discern why you have the rash? Hopefully, the latter approach is the more common. Unfortunately, many organizations involved in strategic alliances take the former approach. There is a problem; let us fix it. This "can do" attitude is laudable in one sense but potentially reckless (possibly even rash) in another sense. Specifically, when one observes friction in strategic alliances, we argue that the most important response is to first delve more deeply to understand the source of that friction before attempting to treat the problem.

This advice regarding diagnosis before treatment may seem obvious, but it often is not done in alliances. The reason it is often not done stems from alliance partners' unwillingness or inability to put themselves in their partners' shoes. By this we mean that signs of noncooperative behavior from a partner are often viewed with hostility on the part of other partners. The other partners then devise their own response strategy before an analysis or diagnosis is done as to why the partner may appear to be acting noncooperatively. Quite simply, we are stating that the noncooperative behavior is only a symptom of a deeper problem.

The obvious questions then become, "What could the deeper problems be, and how do we treat them?" We propose that there are several classes of problems:

1. Parochial self-interest or cheating behavior
2. Misunderstanding, culture clashes, and a lack of trust
3. Different assessments, asymmetric investments, and temporary alliance arrangements without a long-term plan
4. Alliance performance ambiguity and low tolerance for such ambiguity
5. Overly optimistic expectations of alliance performance
6. Weak infrastructure and strategic management of the alliance or lack of alliance experience

These categories, interestingly, match discussions of problems that exist in managing change (Kotter and Schlesinger, 1979). While the categories are not mutually exclusive, they are quite distinct from one another. For example, the first category represents rational, calculative, noncooperative behavior in which one partner knowingly acts in his own interest to the detriment of the other partner. The second type of problem is based less on selfishness than on the absence of accepted and well-developed norms; that is, a trusting relationship between partners has yet to emerge, and cultural clashes dominate. The third category differs from the first in that, while the first category (i.e., selfish, noncooperative behavior) reflects disagreement on ends and means, the third category reflects agreement on ends but not means. In other words, partners may share the same goal but diverge in their views on how to achieve that goal. They consequently make different investments in the alliance relationship. Fourth, some alliance partners simply feel uncomfortable with the ambiguity and fluidity of alliances. The absence of full control, as is typical in strategic alliances, may not agree with some reluctant partners. The fifth category reflects the partners' initial euphoria with alliance formation without anticipating its subsequent problems, while the sixth category reflects the failure of the partners to sufficiently invest in alliance management and development.

Identifying different categories of problems is in and of itself useful as a way to move beyond the symptom and toward the problem. Treating the problem is the next step, and we propose a simple principle: the treatment should match the problem. Again, while this seems obvious, we find that all too often in alliances the treatment is either insufficient or too harsh. Both of these situations are unfavorable. There are at least 10 ways of dealing with alliance problems:

- Partner selection and due diligence
- Education
- Participation and sharing of alliance management
- Facilitated negotiation
- Swapping capabilities
- Exchange of personnel and information
- Co-optation
- Coercion
- Strategic implementation of the alliance
- Knowledge accumulation

Matching this set of treatments with the set of problems identified earlier represents a step toward effective alliance management. Consider the case where a partner faces a particularly calculative, self-interested partner. That partner is not lacking information; he knows what the situation is but does not want what his partner wants. In this case, an approach that emphasizes negotiation or co-optation is likely to be more effective than one that emphasizes participation or education. Contrast such a case with a partner whose actions are based on a misunderstanding. Here, negotiation as a response does not address the root problem; education and participation are more appropriate. We invite the reader to draw further matches between problem and treatment.

Know Thy Partner

A third framework that can be useful in addressing potential and ongoing alliance problems focuses more directly at understanding your partner's "type." Specifically, we suggest that it is a mistake to assume that your partner thinks about your alliance the same way that you do. Ideally, you will know what type of alliance partner you are dealing with at the earliest stages of the alliance. Unfortunately, it is our experience that many times a partner fails to take into adequate account the variety of partner types or **partner orientations** that exist. In our experience, there are five types of partners, ranging from the most desirable to the least desirable; each is discussed briefly below.

The Cooperative Partner

This partner is primarily interested in maximizing the joint gains in the alliance relationship and recognizes that such maximization requires attention to what you need to achieve in the alliance. Thus, this partner will work with you in helping you achieve your goals as well as her own. This is what you hope you have in an alliance partner, but it may be rarer than one thinks. This partner sees the alliance as win-win and is interested in seeing that both sides win. A major pharmaceutical firm embodies this philosophy with the goal of being "the partner of choice" for biotech firms. This company employs numerous alliance managers who see their role as "ombudspersons" for the alliance.

The Quasi-Cooperative Partner

This partner is interested in making sure that you receive just enough value from the alliance so that you will not exit. By providing you with the minimally acceptable amount of value, you still prefer the alliance above other alternatives, but not by much. This relationship is unbalanced in terms of power and dependence but can be stable, albeit not as rewarding for the weaker party. This partner sees the alliance in terms of keeping you interested, but barely.

The Indifferent Partner

This partner—for better or worse—is not particularly interested in your strategic aspirations at all. The partner sees the alliance primarily as a vehicle for the achievement of that partner's strategic goals, and you are simply along for the ride. The partner has no objections to your expending effort for your purposes, as long as (1) he does not need to help you do this and (2) the attainment of his objectives is not impeded as a result. This partner sees the alliance in terms of "I'll get mine, you find yours."

The Competitive Partner

This partner is worse than indifferent, insofar as he perceives your gains as implying a loss for him, even when really there is no such tradeoff. This person is oblivious to the positive-sum possibilities of the alliance and very sensitive to the zero-sum aspects. This partner cannot abide any asymmetry in alliance success that might favor you, even if such variation is a natural or short-term occurrence. This partner is so fixated on the relative comparison aspects of the relationship that he sees the alliance in terms of "your gain must mean my loss." Another major pharmaceutical firm had this philosophy, in that managers in this firm viewed a win-win alliance situation as one in which they felt they had "left money on the table." They would often seek to renegotiate win-win alliances.

The Vengeful Partner

This partner is even worse than a competitive partner, because he is primarily focused on ensuring that you lose, even if he loses, as well. You might not think that such partners exist, and it is unlikely that you would knowingly ally with such a partner; but a partner can develop this orientation when problems in the alliance become personalized and negative emotion plays a larger role. Note that we readily accept the notion of positive emotion in alliances when we claim that trust between partners is a beneficial aspect of an alliance relationship. However, we suggest that when one partner feels that the other has somehow violated that trust, a sense of betrayal emerges that can lead a partner to act irrationally. This partner sees the alliance in terms of "I may lose, but you'll lose more." While this is admittedly rare, several alliances have had protracted legal battles when one party feels that the other party did not act "in good faith."

Partner Assessment

As you can see, there are multiple partner types, and most of them are not particularly attractive. So, how can you "know thy partner" in advance? First and foremost, you must pay careful attention during the alliance emergence process for cues from your alliance partner that suggest one type versus another. For example, we have observed in working with health care organizations that some alliance partners have little idea what their partners' strategic goals are. A cooperative partner would know this, and a lack of interest in the partner's goals is an early indication that your partner is indifferent, or worse. Similarly, explore with your partner alternative scenarios for the alliance, including some in which you do better initially, and gauge your partner's reaction.

If your partner objects to the slightest asymmetries in alliance outcomes, this suggests a problem that will likely emerge again and again.

Finally, assuming you are comfortable with your partner's orientation at the inception of the alliance, you must still be vigilant to changes in that orientation that may arise due to changes in the context of the alliance, whether it be changes in environmental conditions or in personnel. Ideally, this type of "early warning system" will serve you well as the alliance relationship evolves. However, we also encourage you to utilize another valuable feature of strategic alliances: Be sure to have a clear written statement of exit provisions, by which you and your partner can extricate yourselves from an alliance that may no longer be serving its intended valued purpose.

ALLIANCE CAPABILITIES AND PERFORMANCE DRIVERS

Hundreds of studies over the past decades have examined factors that can promote and inhibit the success of alliances (Gulati, Wohlgezogen, and Zhelyazkov, 2012; Kale and Singh, 2009; Salvato, Reuer, and Battigalli, 2017). We discussed several of these factors above, but it is useful to summarize them here and to consider some key capabilities that alliances need to be successful. Factors that affect alliance success can be grouped into the first three stages of the life-cycle model depicted in Table 11.2: emergence, transition, and maturity.

In the stage of emergence, or alliance formation, three characteristics of partners are critical. Specifically, alliance success depends, as noted above, on the extent to which partners are complementary such that one organization uses some services or products of the other, as opposed to the case when two or more organizations are vying for the same resources. Similarly, alliances will be more successful to the extent that partners are compatible, sharing similar cultures, expectations, and capabilities. A third partner characteristic that seems critical to success is commitment, the extent to which each partner wants to make the relationship work well.

In the next stage of alliance development, or what Kale and Singh (2009) term the phase of governance and design, results from many studies show that alliance success depends on the extent to which partners can find effective and efficient ways to coordinate and control their joint efforts (Gulati, Wohlgezogen, and Zhelyazkov, 2012; Salvato, Reuer, and Battigalli, 2017). Three approaches

are particularly useful: shared ownership of some or all of alliance projects, contracts that specify the rights and obligations of partners, and goodwill and trust among the partners. As noted above, research to date suggests that shared ownership is particularly important for alliance success; yet, it is important to match an approach to governance to the particular needs of an alliance.

Finally, in the stage that we term maturity, research results show that alliance success depends on the extent to which mechanisms for coordinating alliance projects (that were established in the transition or design stage) work well and, perhaps more importantly, trust develops among partners. In turn, trust is important because it is more or less inevitable that conflicts or disagreements among partners will occur, and they are more likely to be resolved effectively to the extent that the partners trust each other. Nonetheless, even without high levels of trust, or perhaps especially when trust levels are low, it is important to have mechanisms in place to deal with conflicts or disagreements (e.g., regular meetings that are dedicated specifically to reviewing and resolving potential and actual disagreements). Of course, in the absence of trust, it will be difficult to establish even straightforward mechanisms to deal with disagreements among alliance partners.

Underlying many of the factors noted above are two fundamental capabilities that seem to drive alliances' success. The first is a dedicated manager or group of managers who focus exclusively on alliance work and processes (Hoang and Rothaermel, 2005; Kale and Singh, 2009). For example, one important task for these managers is to monitor performance and progress toward objectives on projects and provide timely feedback to members (D'Aunno, Alexander, and Jiang, 2017).

Second, alliances and their members need to be able to learn from their experience and to build additional capabilities as needed (Inkpen and Tsang, 2007). Learning processes may include, for example, regular meetings to review factors that have contributed to success and failure in alliance projects. Further, tools are needed to codify this learning and may include guidelines, checklists, and manuals that specify best practices and make future projects more efficient and effective.

In sum, research on alliances has produced useful results that can guide managerial action (see the Summary and Managerial Guidelines). Together with the frameworks for analyzing alliance problems introduced above, understanding factors and capabilities that often drive alliance success provides a strong foundation for effective managerial action.

SUMMARY AND MANAGERIAL GUIDELINES

1. In assessing the risk of forming or entering an alliance, managers should compare the potential costs and benefits of alliances to doing nothing or to alternative strategies that involve going it alone or merging with another firm; alliances may well be less risky than other strategies.

2. The form or structure of alliance should follow from its function—that is, what it is intended to do.

3. Managers should consider their options with respect to several important aspects of alliance structure, including ownership and control, number of members, governance structure, and mandated versus voluntary participation.

4. Many of the benefits of control in interorganizational relationships can be achieved without ownership; trust, commitment, and even power may be important substitutes for control based on ownership.

5. Increased size brings greater complexity and often more difficulty in coordinating efforts, but larger alliances tend to be more powerful for certain purposes (e.g., lobbying, purchasing in volume).

6. Large alliances often need more complex governance structures, and a key issue is who will be represented on an alliance board. It may be a mistake to have only CEOs or executive directors on alliance boards because the interests of other groups may be neglected; further, turnover among top managers is common and may disrupt the alliance if the board has no other types of members.

7. Mandated participation in an alliance is often less preferable to voluntary participation. Alliances are not likely to succeed if members' only or most important motive for participation is to comply with external demands.

8. Recognize that alliances can be created to achieve one or more of the following objectives: to pool similar resources (e.g., as in joint purchasing arrangements); to trade dissimilar resources (e.g., as in a symbiotic relationship between a hospital and physician group); to reduce costs; to enhance revenues; to promote innovation, learning, or quality of services; or to enhance power, reduce uncertainty, or share risks among members.

9. From the above list, it is important to understand your own motives for seeking an alliance and to express these motives to potential or current partners.

10. Similarly, managers need to listen carefully to the intentions of potential or current partners in order to assess compatibility; failure to articulate a shared mission is an important reason for alliance failure.

11. Two kinds of problems are typical when it comes to alliance objectives. First, even though alliance objectives may be shared by members, the objectives may conflict with each other, especially over time. Second, there may be a lack of consensus among members concerning alliance objectives. Both problems highlight the need for effective communication.

12. Recognize that alliances often develop in several stages, each of which brings distinctive threats and opportunities.

13. In the first stage (emergence), it is important to define the purposes of the alliance and select partners accordingly. Clear communication and acknowledgment of interests are critical.

14. After forming an alliance, managers must find ways to coordinate and control activities; this may entail hiring or forming a management group to focus specifically on alliance concerns.

15. As alliances mature, managers are likely to face complex issues about how much individual members must conform to and, indeed, place alliance interests ahead of their own. Further, there may be conflict about how to distribute the benefits (resources) that alliances have generated. Thus, managers need to focus on ways to sustain member commitment through trust, goal attainment, and the use of appropriate mechanisms to resolve conflict.

16. Mature alliances face the task of measuring up to members' original and changing expectations. Such alliances need to rethink their structure and objectives to make sure that they keep pace with members' needs.

17. More specifically, managers can diagnose alliance problems according to whether they are primarily environmental (i.e., stemming from external sources such as shift in market demands), strategic (i.e., concerning the overall purpose and direction of the alliance), structural (i.e., alliance form fits poorly with its purposes), or behavioral (i.e., skills are not adequate for carrying out alliance activities).

18. It is important to match alliance problems with appropriate means to deal with them, ranging from educating members, to negotiating with them, to coercing them.

19. Alliances can be just a management fad—be careful that you are forming one for the right reasons.

20. Recognize that alliances have their costs for managers in terms of time spent in understanding and negotiating with potential and current partners. In fact, alliances can slow decision making and make organizations less flexible—precisely what they are designed to avoid.

21. Select partners and develop ways of relating to them so as to avoid charges of collusion and antitrust problems.

22. Do not let alliance arrangements make your organization lazy and lose its interest in continuous improvement.

DISCUSSION QUESTIONS

1. Under what circumstances would you agree with someone who said that alliances are very risky?

2. What dimensions would you use to classify the various types of strategic alliances? Why those dimensions?

3. Which alliance motivations do you think are the most compatible with each other?

4. What do you consider to be the likely stages of strategic alliance development? Does every alliance have to go through each stage?

5. What is the difference between an alliance problem and an alliance symptom, and what does this difference mean in terms of managerial intervention?

6. When can you tell if your partner is not likely to have a cooperative orientation?

CASE

Strategic Alliances in the Pharmaceutical and Biotechnology Industry

In the past two decades, alliances between pharmaceutical and biotechnology firms have become an increasingly important and popular strategy (Gottinger and Umali, 2008; Haeussler and Higgins, 2014; Schweizer, 2014). What has prompted these two different sectors of the life sciences to enter such strategic interactions? For their part, *pharmaceutical firms* have felt pressure from the patent expiry of their blockbuster drugs, which drove firm success in the 1990s and early 2000s and, thus, slowing sales and eroding profit margins. They have also faced increased public scrutiny of their pricing practices, increased regulatory oversight of manufacturing processes, and more conservative drug reviews by the U.S. Food and Drug Administration (USFDA). Finally, they are now confronting greater difficulties discovering new products, due to the growing complexity and uncertainty of the science. Alliances have also become important for *biotechnology firms* that also face huge risks of failure in their drug projects (and thus firm failure) as well as enormous capital needs to sustain their research operations until they develop a commercial product with sufficient sales. Biotechnology firms also lack the scale and vertical integration of pharmaceutical firms to conduct their own clinical trials and field their own sales and marketing forces.

Alliances allow these two sets of firms to contribute unique capabilities to try to achieve greater success in new drug development. Pharmaceutical firms contribute capital, sales, and marketing expertise; biotechnology firms contribute knowledge stocks in biology and genomics that more chemistry-based pharmaceutical firms historically lacked. In essence, the former are adept at commercialization while the latter are more adept at research and development (R&D)—the twin pillars of innovation (Burns, Nicholson, and Wolkowski, 2012). More generally, these alliances can serve a range of R&D objectives, such as risk diversification, cost reduction, shortening of product development cycles, broadening the breadth and depth of knowledge stocks, and risk diversification. They can also serve a range of commercialization objectives such as increased access to marketing assets, market access, and market share.

This division of labor is evident from an analysis of the origin of USFDA new drug approvals (NDAs) between 2011 and 2016. The top 25 pharmaceutical firms are the marketer in nearly 70 percent of NDAs, while small/mid-sized biopharma firms are the originator in over 60 percent of NDAs (Rhodes, 2016). Overall, biological products represented 22 percent of NDAs in 2013 and then 39 percent in 2014. A sizeable percentage (30 percent) of the new products developed by biotechnology firms was acquired by their pharmaceutical counterparts. By contrast, a much smaller percentage (12 percent) of innovative products originating in pharmaceutical firms was acquired by biotechnology companies.

A historical review of "priority reviews" and "fast track designations" by FDA paints an even sharper picture (Drakeman, 2014). Products that undergo priority reviews treat serious or life-threatening conditions and represent significant improvements in safety or effectiveness; products designated for fast track address serious conditions with unmet clinical need. Both sets reflect more innovative therapies. Between 1998 and 2012, the FDA granted priority review to 162 products; 70 of these products received fast track status. Among the 162 priority review products, 89 (55 percent) originated in a handful ($n = 53$) of biotechnology firms; among the 70 fast track products, 49 (70 percent) originated in biotechnology firms. Not surprisingly, biotechnology firms dominated pharmaceutical firms in the priority review of new biological entities (NBEs) (24 of 26); more surprisingly, biotechnology firms nearly equaled pharmaceutical firms in the priority review of new chemical entities (NCEs) (65 versus 71).

There are at least four explanations for the development success of biotechnology companies (Sammut and Burns, 2017). First, biologics have greater specificity: They bind to the target and wrap themselves around the target using their larger mass. This means they have lower potential for off-target toxicity and side effects as well as greater success in clinical trials in terms of product safety. Second, biotech firms have targeted "orphan diseases" where there is huge unmet clinical need (which leads to rapid adoption by clinicians and patients). Orphan diseases also require clinical trials with smaller patient sizes and may not need to undertake expensive Phase III trials, thereby reducing the amount of capital needed to develop them. Orphan products also have no competitors, which allows companies to charge a higher price for their products, and due to their complexity face fewer threats by generics, which makes them more immune to patent cliffs. Third, biotech firms are perpetually raising funds to stay in operation, need to move their products forward as quickly and inexpensively as possible at every stage of development, and always have to operate more efficiently than their pharmaceutical counterparts. Fourth, biotech firms begin as small start-up operations focused on discovery and then development of one or a small number of drugs. They thus did not suffer from the diseconomies of scale and scope often found in large pharmaceutical firms (Sammut and Burns, 2017).

There is empirical evidence that products developed in strategic alliances have a higher probability of success in Phase II and Phase III clinical trials than products developed independently by either the pharmaceutical or biotechnology firm (Danzon, Nicholson, and Pereira, 2005). Historical evidence shows that in-licensed drugs have a greater likelihood of moving from Phase I to commercial launch compared to a firm's internal R&D projects. The success rate for the former is nearly double that of the latter. This suggests that biopharmaceutical firms may want to de-emphasize the number of internal R&D programs and spend more time monitoring R&D programs conducted externally at smaller firms and academia (Rhodes, 2016).

Co-development of new drugs via an alliance adds value that outweighs any potential moral hazard problems arising from the two partners sharing development responsibilities (Nicholson, Danzon, and McCullough, 2005). In 2001–2002 alone, there were 923 new (publicly announced) strategic alliances in this industry. This figure includes biotech–biotech, biotech–pharma, and pharma–pharma alliances, and each type offers different benefits to its partners.

For example, in the realm of biotech–pharma alliances, a recent report focusing on licensing alliances between biotech and pharma firms suggests that "the number of biopharmaceutical licensing alliances has remained fairly constant over the past several years, but their value trebled from $30 billion USD to $90 billion USD between 2004 and 2007" (Business Insights, 2009).

Of the 923 alliances mentioned above, a large number of new alliances (217) occurred between pharmaceutical and biotechnology firms, probably reflecting pharmaceutical firms' needs for access to new products that the smaller, but more research-intensive, biotechnology firms have been generating. These are typically trading alliances that allow pharmaceutical firms to gain access to innovations, while enabling biotechnology firms to gain access to capital, clinical trial expertise, and the marketing capabilities that pharmaceutical firms possess (Danzon, Nicholson, and Pereira, 2005). Some support for the view that pharmaceutical firms are using alliances to gain access to technical innovations is found in the fact that almost one-third of the new alliances involved genomics, the path-breaking science that can be used to develop treatments tailored to individuals' genetic types, making them highly effective.

Indeed, a high proportion of new alliances (404 of the 923 mentioned above) were between partners who already had an ongoing relationship. New agreements among established partners may signal that the relationship has matured, as indicated in the life-cycle model of alliances presented in Table 11.2.

Interestingly, of the 923 alliances mentioned above, the highest percentage (one-third) occurred between biotechnology firms. This suggests that these relatively small firms found alliances to be an especially important strategy to build the scale (and perhaps scope) needed to compete and perform well. Biotechnology firms may be creating pooling alliances that can allow them to reduce uncertainty and enhance market power.

Finally, it appears that firms are using alliances to enhance their capabilities in key therapeutic areas. Most new alliances that focused on a specific therapeutic area were focused in the area of oncology, where there is both high demand for new, more effective treatments and the willingness to pay high prices for them (Reuters Business Insight, 2004).

Alliance dynamics between the two types of biopharmaceutical firms have become more interesting due to the growing success of biotechnology firms relative to their larger pharmaceutical counterparts. Certainly in the past five years, and perhaps going back as far as the last 15 years, biotechnology stocks have outperformed pharmaceutical companies. Data from Cowen shows that, between 2011 and 2015, the "Biotech Index" rose 258 percent compared to the "Pharma Index" (+84 percent) and the S&P 500 (+73 percent) (Schmidt, 2015). The R&D and cost advantages of biotech firms may suggest that alliances now represent "a second best option" for biotechnology firms (Veilleux, 2014). Going forward, they may increasingly favor in-house R&D programs supported by venture capital and capital markets over licensing deals with large pharmaceutical firms.

Questions

1. What do you think are the possible major tensions that exist when a pharmaceutical firm forms an alliance with a biotechnology firm?

2. How would you try to address those tensions?

3. Identify different challenges that exist for maintaining or strengthening an ongoing alliance versus beginning a new relationship.

REFERENCES

Albers, S., Wohlgezogen, F., & Zajac, E. J. (2016). Strategic alliance structures: An organization design perspective. *Journal of Management, 42*, 582–614.

Alexander, J. A., Hearld, L. R., Wolf, L. J., et al. (2016). Aligning forces for quality & multi-stakeholder healthcare alliances: Do they have a sustainable future? *The American Journal of Managed Care, 22*(12 Suppl.), s423–s436.

Bazzoli, G. J., Chan, B., Shortell, S. M., et al. (2000). The financial performance of hospitals belonging to health networks and systems. *Inquiry, 37*, 234–252.

Bazzoli, G. J., Shortell, S. M., Dubbs, N., et al. (1999). A taxonomy of health networks and systems: Bringing order out of chaos. *Health Services Research, 33*(6), 1683–1717.

Begun, J. W. (1992). Cooperative strategies weaken the competitive capabilities of health care organizations. In W. J. Duncan, P. M. Ginter, & L. E. Swayne (Eds.), *Strategic issues in health care management: Point and counterpoint* (pp. 44–50). Boston, MA: PWS-KENT.

Borah, A., & Tellis, G. (2014). Make, buy, or ally: Choice of and payoff from announcements of alternative strategies for innovations. *Marketing Science, 33*(1), 114–133.

Burns, L. R. (1999). Polarity management: The key challenge for integrated delivery systems. *Journal of Healthcare Management, 44*(1), 14–33.

Burns, L. R. (2014). *The performance of group purchasing organizations (GPOs) in the health care value chain: A literature review.* Philadelphia, PA: The Wharton School. Retrieved June 12, 2017, from http://c.ymcdn.com/sites/www .supplychainassociation.org/resource/resmgr/Rescarch/AHA_ AHRMM_Wharton_2014_LitRe.pdf.

Burns, L. R., & Lee, J. A. (2008). Hospital purchasing alliances: Utilization, services, and performance. *Health Care Management Review, 33*(3), 203–215.

Burns, L. R., & Muller, R. W. (2008). Hospital-physician collaboration: Landscape of economic integration and impact on clinical integration. *Milbank Quarterly, 86*(3), 375–434.

Burns, L. R., & Pauly, M. V. (2002). Integrated delivery networks: A detour on the road to integrated health care? *Health Affairs, 21*(4), 128–143.

Burns, L. R., & Thorpe, D. P. (1997). Physician-hospital organizations: Strategy, structure, and conduct. In R. Conners (Ed.), *Integrating the practice of medicine* (pp. 351–371). Chicago, IL: American Hospital Association Publishing.

Burns, L. R., Bazzoli, G. J., Dynan, L., et al. (1997). Managed care, market stages, and integrated delivery systems: Is there a relationship? *Health Affairs, 16*, 204–218.

Burns, L. R., Goldsmith, J. C, & Sen, A. (2013). Horizontal and vertical integration of physicians: A tale of two tails. *Advances in Health Care Management, 15*, 39–117.

Burns, L. R., Nicholson, S., & Wolkowski, J. (2012). Pharmaceutical strategy and the evolving role of mergers and acquisitions (M&A). In L. R. Burns (Ed.), *The business of healthcare innovation* (Chap. 3). Cambridge, UK: Cambridge University Press.

Burns, L. R., Wholey, D., McCullough, J., et al. (2012). The changing configuration of hospital systems: Centralization, federalization, or fragmentation? In L. Friedman, G. Savage, & J. Goes (Eds.), *Annual review of health care management: Strategy and policy perspectives on reforming health systems* (Vol. 13, pp. 189–232). Bingley, UK: Emerald Group Publishing.

Business Insights. (2009, March). *Evolving trends in biopharmaceutical licensing: Deal assessments, drivers, and resistors.* Retrieved August 15, 2010, from http://www .globalbusinessinsights.com.

Casalino, L. P. (2006). The Federal Trade Commission, clinical integration, and the organization of physician practice. *Journal of Health Politics, Policy and Law, 31*, 569–585.

Casalino, L. P., & Robinson, J. C. (2003). Alternative models of hospital-physician affiliation as the United States moves away from tight managed care. *Milbank Quarterly, 81*(2), 331–351.

Cuellar, A., & Gertler, P. (2005, January). How the expansion of hospital systems has affected consumers. *Health Affairs, 24*(1), 213–219.

Danzon, P. M., Nicholson, S., & Pereira, N. S. (2005). Productivity in pharmaceutical-biotechnology R&D: The role of experience and alliances. *Journal of Health Economics, 24*, 317–339.

D'Aunno, T. A. , Alexander, J. A., & Jiang, L. (2017). Creating value for participants in multistakeholder alliances: The shifting importance of leadership and collaborative decision-making over time. *Health Care Management Review, 42*(2), 100–111. https://10.1097/HMR.0000000000000098.

De Rond, M. (2003). *Strategic alliances as social facts: Business, biotechnology and intellectual history.* Cambridge: Cambridge University Press.

Doz, Y. L., & Hamel, G. (1998). *Alliance advantage: The art of creating value through partnering.* Boston, MA: Harvard Business School Press.

Drakeman, D. (2014). Benchmarking biotech and pharmaceutical product development. *Nature Biotechnology, 32*(7), 621–625.

Duncan, W. J., Ginter, P. M., & Swayne, L. E. (1992). *Strategic issues in health care management: Point and counterpoint.* Boston, MA: PWS-KENT.

Dyer, J. H., Kale, P., & Singh, H. (2004). When to ally & when to acquire. *Harvard Business Review, 82*(7–8), 108–115.

Fennell, M. L., & Alexander, T. A. (1989). Hospital governance and profound organizational change. *Medical Care Review, 46*(2), 157–187.

Goldsmith, J., Burns, L. R., Sen, A., et al. (2015). *Integrated delivery networks: In search of benefits and market effects.* Washington, DC: National Academy of Social Insurance.

Gottinger, H-W., & Umali, C. (2008). Strategic alliances in global biotech pharma industries. *Open Business Journal, 1*, 10–24.

Grabowski, H., & Kyle, M. (2008). Mergers and alliances in pharmaceuticals: Effects on innovation and R&D productivity. In K. P. Gugler & B. B. Yurtoglu (Eds.), *The economics of corporate governance and mergers* (Chap. 11, pp. 262–287). Cheltenham, UK: Edward Elgar Publishing.

Grabowski, H., & Kyle, M. (2012). Mergers, acquisitions, and alliances. In P. Danzon & S. Nicholson (Eds.), *The Oxford handbook of the economics of the biopharmaceutical industry* (Chap. 18, pp. 552–577). Oxford, UK: Oxford University Press.

Gulati, R., & Nickerson, J. (2008). Interorganizational trust, governance choice, and exchange performance. *Organization Science, 19*(5), 688–708.

Gulati, R., Wohlgezogen, F., & Zhelyazkov, P. (2012). The two facets of collaboration: Cooperation and coordination in strategic alliances. *Academy of Management Annals, 6*(1), 531–583. doi:10.1080/19416520.2012.691646.

Haeussler, C., & Higgins, M. (2014). Strategic alliances: Trading ownership for capabilities. *Journal of Economics and Management Strategy, 23*(1), 178–203.

Hearld, L. R., Bleser, W. K., Alexander, J. A., et al. (2016). A systematic review of the literature on the sustainability of community health collaboratives. *Medical Care Research and Review, 73*(2), 127–181. https://doi.org/10.1177/1077558715607162

Hoang, H., & Rothaermel, F. (2005). The effects of general and partner-specific experience on joint R&D project performance. *Academy of Management Journal, 48*(2), 332–345.

Inkpen, A. C., & Tsang. E. W. K. (2007). Learning and strategic alliances. *Academy of Management Annals, 1*(1), 479–511. https://doi.org/10.1080/078559815.

Jacobides, M. G., & Billinger, S. (2006). Designing the boundaries of the firm: From "make, buy, or ally" to the dynamic benefits of vertical architecture. *Organization Science, 17*(2), 249–261.

Kale, P., & Singh, H. (2009). Managing strategic alliances: What do we know now, and where do we go from here? *Academy of Management Perspectives, 23*(3), 45–62.

Kaluzny, A., & Zuckerman, H. (1992, Winter). Strategic alliances: Two perspectives for understanding their effects on health services. *Hospital and Health Services Administration, 37*, 477–490.

Kaluzny, A. D., Zuckerman, H. S., & Ricketts, T. C. (1995). *Partners for the dance: forming strategic alliances in health care.* Ann Arbor, MI: Health Administration Press.

Kotter, J. P., & Schlesinger, L. A. (1979). Choosing strategies for change. *Harvard Business Review, 57*, 106–114.

Li, J., Zhou, C., & Zajac, E. J. (2009). Control, collaboration, and productivity in international joint ventures: Theory and evidence. *Strategic Management Journal, 30*, 865–884.

Longest, B. B. (1990). Interorganizational linkages in the health sector. *Health Care Management Review, 15*, 17–28.

Lungeanu, R., Stern, I., & Zajac, E. J. (2016). When do firms change technology-sourcing vehicles: The role of poor innovative performance and financial slack. *Strategic Management Journal, 37*, 855–869.

Macneil, I. R. (1983). Values in contract: Internal and external. *Northwestern University Law Review, 78*, 340–418.

Madison, K. (2004). Hospital-physician affiliations and patient treatments, expenditures, and outcomes. *Health Services Research, 39*(2), 257–278.

Mellewigt, T. A., Thomas, A., Weller, I., et al. (2017). Alliance or acquisition? A mechanisms-based, policy-capturing analysis. *Strategic Management Journal, 38*(12), 2353–2369. https://doi.org/10.1002/smj.2664.

Meyer, A. (1982). Adapting to environmental jolts. *Administrative Science Quarterly, 27*, 515–537.

Nembhard, I. M. (2012). All teach, all learn, all improve? The effect of interorganizational learning on performance improvement. *Health Care Management Review, 37*(2), 154–164.

Nicholson, S., Danzon, P. M., & McCullough, J. (2005). Biotech-pharmaceutical alliances as a signal of asset and firm quality. *Journal of Business, 78*, 1433–1464.

Oliver, C. (1990). Determinants of interorganizational relationships: Integration and future directions. *Academy of Management Review, 15*(2), 241–265.

Puranam, P., & Vanneste, B. (2009). Trust and governance: Untangling a tangled web. *Academy of Management Review, 34*(1), 11–28.

Reuters Business Insight. (2004). Pharmaceutical strategic alliances: Benchmarking 21st century deal-making. Retrieved August 16, 2004, from http://www.the-infoshop.com.

Rhodes, J. (2016, Fall). Life sciences investment. Presentation to the Wharton School.

Rodriguez, H., Henke, R., Bibi, S., et al. (2016). The exnovation of chronic care management processes by physician organizations. *Milbank Quarterly, 94*(3), 626–653.

Salvato, C., Reuer, J. J., & Battigalli, P. (2017). Cooperation across disciplines: A multilevel perspective on cooperative behavior in governing interfirm relations. *Academy of Management Annals, 11*(2), 960–1004. https://doi.org/10.5465/annals.2014.0001.

Sammut, S., & Burns, L. R. (2017). Life sciences investment and biotechnology in China. In L. R. Burns & G. Liu (Eds.), *China's healthcare system and reform* (Chap. 16, pp. 428–450). Cambridge, UK: Cambridge University Press.

Schelling, T. C. (1960). *The strategy of conflict*. Cambridge, MA: Harvard University.

Schmidt, E. (2015, November). Biotechnology. Presentation to the Wharton School.

Schweizer, L. (2014). Strategic alliances or M&A as the road to innovation for pharmaceutical companies? *Entrepreneurship & Organization Management, 3*(2), 1–2.

Scott, W. R. (1987). The adolescence of institutional theory. *Administrative Science Quarterly, 32*, 493–511.

Shah, R., & Swaminathan, V. (2008). Factors influencing partner selection in strategic alliances: The moderating role of alliance context. *Strategic Management Journal, 29*(5), 471–494.

Shortell, S. M. (1988). The evolution of hospital systems: Unfulfilled promises and self-fulfilling prophecies. *Medical Care Review, 45*(2), 177–214.

Shortell, S. M., & Zajac, E. J. (1988). Internal corporate joint ventures: Development processes and performance outcomes. *Strategic Management Journal, 9*, 527–542.

Shortell, S. M., & Zajac, E. J. (1990). Health care organizations and the development of the strategic

management perspective. In S. Mick & associates (Eds.), *Innovations in health care delivery: New insights into organization theory* (pp. 141–180). San Francisco, CA: Jossey-Bass.

Shortell, S. M., Colla, C. H., Lewis, V. A., et al. (2015). Accountable care organizations: The national landscape. *Journal of Health Politics, Policy and Law, 40*(4), 647–668.

Starr, P. (1982). *The social transformation of American medicine*. New York: Basic Books.

Stern, I., Dukerich, J. M., & Zajac, E. J. (2014). Unmixed signals: How reputation and status affect alliance formation. *Strategic Management Journal, 35*, 512–531.

Thompson, J. T. (1967). *Organizations in action*. New York: McGraw-Hill.

Veilleux, S. (2014). International strategic alliances of small biotechnology firms: A second-best option? *International Journal of Biotechnology, 13*(1/2/3), 53–65.

Wang, L., & Zajac, E. J. (2007). Alliance or acquisition? A dyadic perspective on interfirm resource combinations. *Strategic Management Journal, 28*(13), 1291–1317.

Williamson, O. E. (1975). *Markets and hierarchies: Analysis and antitrust implications*. New York: Free Press.

Zajac, E. J. (1986). Organizations, environments, and performance: A study of contract management in hospitals. Unpublished doctoral dissertation, University of Pennsylvania, Philadelphia.

Zajac, E. J., & Olsen, C. P. (1993). From transaction costs to transactional value analysis: Implications for the study of interorganizational strategies. *Journal of Management Studies, 30*, 131–146.

Zajac, E. J., Golden, B. R., & Shortell, S. M. (1991). New organizational forms for enhancing innovation: The case of internal corporate joint ventures. *Management Science, 37*, 70–84.

Zuckerman, H. S., & D'Aunno, T. A. (1990). Hospital alliances: Cooperative strategy in a competitive environment. *Health Care Management Review, 15*(2), 21–30.

Chapter 12

Health Policy and Regulation

Kristin Madison, Gary Young, Aditi Sen, and Peter D. Jacobson

CHAPTER OUTLINE

- Federal Policy and Regulation
- State Policy and Regulation
- Organizational Strategies for Regulatory Compliance
- Recent Policy and Regulatory Initiatives

LEARNING OBJECTIVES

After completing this chapter, the reader should be able to:

1. Explain why regulations matter
2. Describe the policy and operational context of health care regulations
3. Identify the most important state and federal regulations that affect health care organizations
4. Identify the key regulatory agencies and summarize their current policies
5. Explain how regulatory compliance will affect health care organizations' strategic decision making
6. Formulate strategies for regulatory compliance
7. Discuss recent policy initiatives that have regulatory implications
8. Evaluate strengths and weaknesses in current regulatory efforts to achieve policy goals

KEY TERMS

ACA (Patient Protection and Affordable Care Act)	EMTALA
Accountable Care Organization	ERISA
Accreditation	False Claims Act
Anti-Kickback Statute	Federal Trade Commission
Antitrust Law	HCQIA
Centers for Medicare and Medicaid Services	HIPAA
Certificate of Need	Licensure
Clayton Act	Medicare Payment Advisory Commission
Community Benefit Standard	National Practitioner Data Bank
Compliance	Notice of Proposed Rulemaking
Corporate Integrity Agreement	Office of the Inspector General
Deeming Authority	Preemption
Department of Health and Human Services	Recovery Audit Contractor
Department of Justice	Regulation

Safety Zones

Sherman Act

Stark Physician Self-Referral Law

Tax Exemption

Transparency

Value-Based Payment

CHAPTER PURPOSE

The purpose of this chapter is to introduce regulatory challenges that managers of health care organizations (HCOs) are likely to encounter. With the increasing intersection between health care delivery and the law, health care executives must confront a wide range of regulatory **compliance** issues that affect how health care institutions operate. Recent changes in health insurance regulation, publicly financed coverage programs, health care payment models, and health information technology have increased the complexity of the health care regulatory and policy environment. This chapter helps health care managers navigate this environment by describing major laws and programs, explaining the regulatory process, and highlighting organizational compliance issues.

FEDERAL POLICY AND REGULATION

The health care industry is heavily regulated at both the federal and state levels. By **regulation**, we mean governmental oversight of the private marketplace. This oversight is often intended to increase access, control costs, or improve quality in a world in which market competition may fail to achieve these goals. Regulation can be economic, such as when governments create reimbursement mechanisms or monitor financial arrangements between physicians and health systems; it can also serve a social function, such as when governments require the provision of emergency care regardless of a patient's ability to pay (Shortell and Walshe, 2004). Because federal health care regulations affect so many facets of HCOs' operations, it is important for managers to understand the nature of these regulations and the agencies that implement them.

Federal Agencies and Their Oversight

The federal government plays three key health roles: payer, regulator, and promoter of public health. As a payer for health care services, the government makes decisions about which benefits to cover and how to pay providers and suppliers for their efforts. The implications of these decisions extend beyond government insurance programs such as Medicare and Medicaid, since commercial insurers tend to follow Medicare coverage decisions. As a regulator, the government monitors how federal dollars are spent and takes steps to protect the health and safety of the public. As a promoter of public health, the government finances research, collects and disseminates data, undertakes educational initiatives, and supports efforts to improve health. These functions are performed through a number of agencies, each with its own distinct responsibilities.

• • • IN PRACTICE: Antitrust Policy and Limits of Licensing Bodies to Regulate Healthcare Delivery

In North Carolina, the State Board of Dental Examiners (Board), the licensure body for dentists in the state, took several actions to deter nondentists from providing teeth whitening services to the public. These actions included issuing cease-and-desist letters threatening criminal liability. North Carolina legislation authorized the Board to regulate dentistry and required that six of the eight board members be licensed, practicing dentists.

The Federal Trade Commission filed an administrative complaint noting that a majority of the Board's decision makers comprised individuals who themselves were practicing dentists and thus market participants and alleging that the Board's actions were anticompetitive and in violation of federal antitrust law. The Board took the position that its activities were immunized from federal antitrust review because they constituted state action. The case eventually reached the U.S. Supreme Court. In 2015, the Court handed down its decision holding that the Board's actions in this case were not covered by state action (*North Carolina State Board of Dental Examiners v. Federal Trade Commission*, 135 S.Ct. 1101).

The Court determined that the supervision requirement for state action immunity was not met because "there is no evidence of any decision by the State to initiate or concur with the Board's actions against the nondentists." According to the Court, the Board acted without state action even in deciding whether or not teeth whitening constituted a form of dentistry, a question that the North Carolina authorizing statute did not address.

• • • IN PRACTICE: Antitrust Policy and Limits of Licensing Bodies to Regulate Healthcare Delivery (Continued)

Given that state licensure boards often consist of practitioners who are market participants, the Court's decision has important implications for state licensing boards and other entities that make decisions affecting entry into an occupation or industry. State licensure has often figured into turf disputes for competing health care professionals. For example, in many states physicians and nurse practitioners have been wrestling over the efforts of nurse practitioners to modify licensure restrictions so that they have greater autonomy for patient care. While, as noted elsewhere in this chapter, state licensing bodies play an important role in regulating the delivery of health care services, the Court's decision makes clear that federal antitrust law may impose substantial limits on these boards' involvement in such disputes.

The magnitude of federal antitrust law's implications for state licensing actions will depend in part on states' responses to the Supreme Court's decision. States may attempt to shield boards from federal antitrust law by putting in place supervisory mechanisms that will enable boards to avail themselves of state action protections. It is not clear, however, what forms of supervision will satisfy the requirements of the state action doctrine. Future litigation may focus on just how closely a state must supervise a licensing body for state action immunity to apply. In a dissenting opinion in the North Carolina case, three of the nine members of the Court asserted that state action immunity exists under much broader circumstances than those recognized by the Court's majority. Given the continued lack of clarity with respect to the doctrine's reach, we are likely to see more antitrust litigation in the licensure area in the future.

The principal federal government agency for health care is the **Department of Health and Human Services** (HHS), which aims "to enhance and protect the health and well-being of all Americans" by "providing for effective health and human services and fostering advances in medicine, public health, and social services." With programs addressing health care, public health, health information technology, and civil rights in health care, among many other areas, and hundreds of billions of dollars of spending each year, HHS exerts significant influence over the American health system (HHS, 2017).

Some of the largest programs in HHS include the **Centers for Medicare and Medicaid Services** (CMS), which manages the Medicare and Medicaid programs; the Food and Drug Administration (FDA), which ensures the safety and efficacy of medical devices, food, drugs, and other biological products; and the National Institutes of Health (NIH), which conducts and supports biomedical research in order to prevent, treat, and cure diseases. Other areas of HHS support specific vulnerable populations within the United States, such as children and older Americans, along with marginalized groups, such as Native Americans. Table 12.1 briefly describes the HHS agencies.

Congressional Committees

Regulatory agencies derive their authority from the legislative branch. Congress and state legislatures often enact broad policy statements, delegating the details to the appropriate regulatory agency. Regulatory agencies must act within the bounds of any specific legislation. For instance, Congress enacted broad language to protect

patient privacy and confidentiality under the Health Insurance Portability and Accountability Act (HIPAA) but did not specify how the goals of the act should be accomplished. Congress delegated the details of developing regulatory guidance to the Department of Health and Human Services. Similarly, Congress imposed obligations on tax-exempt hospitals in the Patient Protection and Affordable Care Act (ACA) but left the details of these requirements to be determined by the Internal Revenue Service (IRS).

Because Congress delegates authority to federal regulatory agencies, congressional committees play important roles in health care regulation. First, these committees develop and introduce legislation that provides executive branch agencies with the authority to issue regulations. Second, the committees have oversight responsibility for ensuring that the regulatory process is consistent with legislative intent.

In the Senate, the Health, Education, Labor and Pensions (HELP) Committee has jurisdiction over matters involving health policy. The Senate's Finance Committee contains a health care subcommittee that has jurisdiction over taxation and revenue measures as well as oversight powers to evaluate existing laws and the agencies that implement them.

In the House of Representatives, the Ways and Means Committee is responsible for taxation, tariffs, and other revenue-generating activities. Its jurisdiction is similar to that of the Senate Finance Committee but differs in one important way: It deals only with matters related to Medicare, not Medicaid, while the Senate Finance Committee

Table 12.1 Operating Divisions within the Department of Health and Human Services

The Centers for Medicare and Medicaid Services (CMS)

The Centers for Medicare and Medicaid Services is responsible for managing the provision of government health insurance through the Medicare and Medicaid programs. It works in conjunction with state governments to administer Medicaid and the Children's Health Insurance Program (CHIP).

Food and Drug Administration (FDA)

The Food and Drug Administration is responsible for ensuring the safety and efficacy of medical devices, food, drugs, biological products, cosmetics, radiation-emitting products, and veterinary products. It also provides education to the public regarding proper nutrition and use of medication.

The National Institutes of Health (NIH)

The National Institutes of Health conducts and supports research into methods of preventing, treating, or curing both common and rare diseases. In addition to engaging in its own internal research efforts, it provides financial support for scientific research to universities and other institutions.

The Centers for Disease Control and Prevention (CDC)

The Centers for Disease Control and Prevention tracks health indicators, monitors and responds to emerging health threats, and works to prevent disease and foster healthy communities. It partners with both state and international health agencies to promote public health.

Agency for Healthcare Research and Quality (AHRQ)

The Agency for Healthcare Research and Quality works to improve the quality, safety, efficiency, and effectiveness of health care in the United States. AHRQ seeks new ways to increase access to care, promote evidence-based medicine, and reduce costs without compromising quality. By conducting, sponsoring, and disseminating research, it enables more Americans to become informed health care decision makers.

Administration for Children and Families (ACF)

The Administration for Children and Families administers more than 60 programs that promote the economic and social well-being of families, children, individuals and communities. ACF's programs address child care, child support, and early childhood development, among other areas.

Administration for Community Living (ACL)

The Administration for Community Living has a mission to "maximize the independence, well-being, and health of older adults, people with disabilities across the lifespan, and their families and caregivers" (ACL, 2017). It funds services and supports provided by state and community organizations, invests in research, and manages programs that prevent abuse, facilitate employment, and promote health and wellness, among other goals.

Agency for Toxic Substances and Disease Registry (ATSDR)

The Agency for Toxic Substances and Disease Registry was created in 1980 through the Comprehensive Environmental Response, Compensation, and Liability Act, also known as the Superfund Act. Its purpose is to conduct public health assessments of waste sites, respond to emergency hazardous substance outbreaks, and support research and dissemination of information related to hazardous substances.

Health Resources and Services Administration (HRSA)

The Health Resources and Services Administration is responsible for ensuring that uninsured, isolated, or medically vulnerable populations receive adequate care. It serves tens of millions of Americans through more than 90 programs and thousands of grantees (HRSA, 2017).

Table 12.1 Operating Divisions within the Department of Health and Human Services *(Continued)*

Indian Health Service (IHS)

The Indian Health Service is focused on ensuring that culturally acceptable and comprehensive care is provided for American Indians and Alaska Natives. It operates a comprehensive health service delivery system for over 2.2 million people in 567 recognized tribes in 36 states (IHS, 2017).

Substance Abuse and Mental Health Services Administration (SAMHSA)

The Substance Abuse and Mental Health Services Administration promotes behavioral health and provides treatment and services for individuals with mental or substance use disorders.

---

has jurisdiction over both programs. The House Committee on Energy and Commerce contains a subcommittee on health that has legislative oversight over Medicaid, hospital construction, and public health measures.

The House and Senate both have appropriations committees, which determine funding for HHS and other health services. The appropriations committees must approve all federal treasury expenditures.

The Regulatory Process

Agencies carry out their core functions by issuing and enforcing regulations. At the federal level, the Administrative Procedures Act determines the process of promulgating regulations. The process begins when the agency publishes a **Notice of Proposed Rulemaking** in the *Federal Register*. Stakeholders and interested citizens then have a certain time period to submit comments; after reviewing these comments, the agency may choose to revise the regulation. It then publishes the final regulation in the *Federal Register*, along with its responses to the comments. The final regulation is then incorporated into the Code of Federal Regulations.

An alternative approach, negotiated regulation, has become increasingly popular. In the negotiated regulation process, the regulatory agency meets with the affected industry to develop a regulatory approach that is acceptable to each side to avoid contentious and time-consuming litigation (Jacobson, Hoffman, and Lopez, 2006).

Largely because of the expanding federal investment in health care, the scope and number of regulations have expanded exponentially. At best, the current health care regulatory structure is a fragmented, ad hoc arrangement with overlapping and sometimes inconsistent requirements that can be difficult for health care managers to interpret and implement.

Medicare and Medicaid Law and Policy

If an agency's importance is measured by its budget, then CMS is among the most important federal agencies;

in 2015, spending on the Medicare program was $646 billion (20 percent of total national health expenditures), and spending on Medicaid was $545 billion (17 percent of total national health expenditures). These expenditures contribute to both the physical health of many millions of individuals and the financial health of many thousands of HCOs. To understand the importance of Medicare and Medicaid to health care operations, health care managers must understand the programs' coverage policies, their payment mechanisms, and their oversight and administration.

Medicare

Medicare, created by a 1965 statute, is a federal health insurance program for individuals 65 or older and certain individuals with disabilities. Today, Medicare has become a major federal financial commitment: In 2015, 15 percent of total federal spending was devoted to Medicare. The program covers 48.2 million Americans 65 or older. Most individuals who have been legal residents of the United States for at least five years are automatically eligible to receive benefits when they reach age 65; there is no means-testing for eligibility. The program also covers individuals who have end-stage renal disease and 8.8 million individuals with specific disabilities.

Medicare is composed of four distinct parts (A, B, C, and D) that cover different services. Medicare Part A provides hospital insurance. It covers inpatient care and also skilled nursing facility, hospice, and home health care. Medicare Part A is financed through a payroll tax on employers and their employees. For individuals who have paid Social Security taxes for at least 10 years (or who have a spouse who has paid them), no monthly premium is required for coverage. Those who have not been paying Social Security taxes for at least 10 years may purchase Part A coverage for a premium that depends on work history.

Medicare Part B covers some medically necessary services, including outpatient care, doctors' services, some home health services, mental health services, and durable medical equipment, as well as some preventive care, such as wellness visits and a range of cancer and chronic disease screenings. Automatic enrollment occurs at age 65 for those who are eligible for Social Security benefits or Railroad Retirement Board benefits; it also occurs for those who are under 65 and receive Social Security or Railroad Retirement Board disability benefits. Individuals who have Lou Gehrig's disease are also eligible to receive Part B benefits. Unlike Part A, Part B requires premium payments from all enrollees; however, individuals may choose to opt out of Part B enrollment. Enrollees receiving Social Security will have Part B premiums automatically deducted from Social Security payments; others will pay a standard premium which, as of 2007, is income-adjusted for those making above a certain amount.

Medicare Part C provides coverage through Medicare Advantage Plans, an alternative to the standard Medicare coverage under Parts A and B. Operated by private insurers, these plans take on a number of forms, including preferred provider organizations and health maintenance organizations. Those who choose to enroll in a Medicare Advantage Plan will have both Part A and Part B coverage through their selected provider. All services covered by Medicare, except for hospice care (which will continue to be available through the traditional Medicare program), must be included in Medicare Advantage Plans. The distinguishing feature of these plans is that they may also offer additional coverage, including hearing, dental, vision, and drug coverage and/or health and wellness programs. Medicare Advantage Plan enrollees pay the Part B premium and may also pay an additional fee to the plan for the extra services provided. Enrollment in Medicare Advantage plans has been growing over time, rising from 17 percent of all Medicare beneficiaries in 2000 to 31 percent in 2016.

Medicare Part D provides prescription drug coverage through Medicare-approved insurance companies to people with Medicare. Individuals enrolled in Medicare Part A and/or Part B are eligible to enroll in Part D as well. Individuals enrolled in Medicare Advantage Plans that do not already include drug coverage can also choose to enroll in a Medicare prescription drug plan. Different Part D plans may cover different drugs.

While Medicare covers many services, enrollees are still financially responsible for coinsurance, co-payments, deductibles, and products and services that Medicare does not cover. Enrollees in traditional Medicare (not Medicare Advantage) who want supplemental insurance to cover these "gaps" may purchase Medigap policies, which are sold by private insurance companies. An enrollee must pay all Medigap premiums.

Medicare enrollee premiums finance only some of the costs of the Medicare program. Medicare Part A is financed through a federal payroll tax, while Part B and Part D are financed in part through general tax revenues. It has been projected that given the current structure of the Medicare program and the taxes that support it, there will be insufficient funds to pay full Medicare Part A benefits by 2028 (Boards of Trustees, 2016). The worker-to-beneficiary ratio is declining; the number of beneficiaries will grow rapidly as the baby boom generation enters Medicare. In addition, the volume and intensity of services provided is expected to increase. It is likely that Congress will need to alter the benefits package, increase taxes, or both in order to maintain the financial viability of the Medicare program.

Medicaid

Medicaid is a combined federal and state program that provides medical assistance to low-income individuals and families. Largely operated at the state level, it provides care to 76 million people, including 34 million children, 27 million adults, and 15 million elderly and disabled people, at an estimated cost to the federal and state governments of $574 billion in 2016. Unlike Medicare, Medicaid requires that individuals and families meet certain financial and other eligibility criteria to enroll in the program. Under the current program, the federal government matches state expenditures based on a formula that compares each state's per capita income to the national average. Ongoing policy debates are considering the potential for alternative financing mechanisms, such as block grants, for Medicaid.

Medicaid has long served three broad purposes. First, it finances health care for families receiving cash assistance through welfare or the Supplemental Security Income (SSI) program. Those who have minimal income and assets and are aged, blind, disabled, or members of families with dependent children fall into this category. Second, it covers low-income children and pregnant women, regardless of their eligibility for cash assistance programs. Table 12.2 provides more details about both of these "categorically needy" groups. Third, Medicaid provides catastrophic insurance for people whose otherwise-adequate income is consumed by medical bills. Individuals who need nursing home care or other long-term care often fall into this category. Medically needy individuals are those who have too much money to be considered categorically needy, such as qualified working disabled individuals.

The ACA greatly expanded Medicaid eligibility, extending the program to all individuals with incomes below 133 percent of the federal poverty level, including non-disabled adults without children. The Supreme Court ruled that the ACA's mandated Medicaid expansion was unconstitutional, however; as a result, states could choose whether to adopt the expansion. Under the ACA, the federal government covered all costs associated with this expansion for the first three years and 90 percent or more of costs thereafter. As of January 1, 2017, 31 states and Washington, DC, had chosen to expand Medicaid.

Table 12.2 Categorically Needy Groups

- Families who meet states' Aid to Families with Dependent Children (AFDC) eligibility requirements in effect on July 16, 1996.

- Pregnant women and children under age 6 whose family income is at or below 133% of the federal poverty level.

- Children ages 6 to 19 with family income up to 100% of the federal poverty level.

- Caretakers (relatives or legal guardians who take care of children under age 18 [or 19 if still in high school]).

- Supplemental Security Income (SSI) recipients (or, in certain states, aged, blind, and disabled people who meet requirements that are more restrictive than those of the SSI program).

- Individuals and couples who are living in medical institutions and who have monthly income up to 300% of the SSI income standard (federal benefit rate).

SOURCE: Retrieved March 2010 from CMS website: http://www.cms.hhs.gov/MedicaidGenInfo/Downloads/MedicaidAtAGlance2005.pdf.

In addition, increased coverage has been provided for children through initiatives such as the Children's Health Insurance Program and for disabled individuals through the Ticket to Work and Work Incentives Improvement Act of 1999.

Although Medicaid programs vary from state to state, federal statutes and regulations set forth minimum requirements in terms of benefits provided. Beyond federally required services, states may offer certain optional services, for which they receive matching federal dollars. Of the optional services, the most commonly offered include prescription drugs (which are offered in all states), dental care, prosthetic devices, hearing aids, and intermediate care facilities for individuals with intellectual disability. States may also seek waivers to offer services in innovative ways.

Payment

Medicare's payment mechanisms have changed over time. Historically, hospitals that sought to maximize their profits or net revenues from Medicare patients could do so by maximizing the number of services they provided, because Medicare reimbursed hospitals based on their costs. This system contributed to Medicare program cost excesses, however, and Congress ultimately decided to take a different approach.

To maximize their net revenues today, hospitals must consider both Medicare's fixed payment rates and their own costs of providing services. In 1983, Medicare implemented the Prospective Payment System (PPS), a fixed-payment system for inpatient services based on a patient's specific diagnosis. Under PPS, the government pays hospitals for admitted patients according to a formula based on the admitted patient's diagnosis and certain other criteria that are not tied directly to the hospital's actual costs. If the cost of care is less than the payment, the hospital keeps the difference, but if the

cost of care is higher, the facility loses money. With PPS, hospitals have an incentive to provide cost-effective care and curtail excessive institutional spending.

In the 1990s, Medicare changed its mechanism for physician reimbursement. Instead of paying usual and customary fees, a practice modeled after commercial insurance reimbursement policies, Medicare adopted a Resource Based Relative Value System (RBRVS) to compensate physicians. In this system, physicians are reimbursed on a fee-for-service basis under a formula based on expected resource use. Three separate relative value units (RVUs) are calculated to determine physician payment. The "Work RVU" captures the relative time and intensity associated with a service; the "Practice Expense RVU" reflects the cost of maintaining a physician practice; and the "Malpractice RVU" captures the costs of malpractice insurance. After adjustment for geographic costs, the three RVUs are summed and then multiplied by a dollar conversion factor to determine the payment rate. Today, Medicare is increasingly moving away from fee-for-service payment and toward payment tied to performance on quality and efficiency metrics. We discuss the trend toward value-based payment further below.

Medicare's payment systems for inpatient and outpatient services allow payment for covered technologies. For those technologies that do not fit into a bundled payment category, the Social Security Act requires Medicare to ensure that they are "reasonable and necessary" for diagnosis and treatment. Determining whether to cover the latest technology is an important and highly contested Medicare function.

Oversight and Administration

Because most health care providers serve Medicare and/or Medicaid patients, and accept reimbursement from these programs, they become subject to the rules associated with these programs. These rules relate not just to the reimbursement process but also to the nature of health care operations. Medicare and Medicaid programs will only reimburse HCOs that have met specific eligibility requirements, including federal conditions of participation, which impose minimum health and safety standards. Fulfillment of these conditions is determined by a state agency that conducts random and unannounced surveys on behalf of CMS. If a national accreditation organization, such as the Joint Commission has more stringent requirements, CMS may grant it "deeming" authority, which allows it to deem a HCO as meeting CMS certification requirements.

Thus, while the Medicare and Medicaid programs' primary functions are to increase health care access, they may also significantly influence providers' structures and operations. As described previously, the programs' payment mechanisms affect providers' incentives to control costs. In addition, as described later in the chapter, these programs have recently taken a more proactive approach to encouraging quality improvement through value-based purchasing initiatives. Toward this end, the ACA created the CMS Innovation Center, which develops, tests, and lays the groundwork for more widespread adoption of new care and payment models that have the potential to lower costs and improve quality.

An independent congressional agency, the Medicare Payment Advisory Commission (MedPAC), has played a significant role in shaping a variety of Medicare reform initiatives. MedPAC advises Congress on a broad range of issues: "In addition to advising the Congress on payments to private health plans participating in Medicare and providers in Medicare's traditional fee-for-service program, MedPAC is also tasked with analyzing access to care, quality of care, and other issues affecting Medicare" (MedPAC, 2017). To the extent that MedPAC's recommendations are translated into legal and program reforms, they may substantially alter the financial and regulatory environments in which health care providers function.

The Patient Protection and Affordable Care Act

While much of the federal government's influence on health care financing and delivery stems from its operation of the Medicare and Medicaid programs, the 2010 enactment of the ACA significantly increased federal responsibilities. In addition to expanding Medicaid, the ACA sought to enhance Americans' access to care through federal regulation of insurance markets. It mandated that all individuals obtain "minimum essential coverage" or pay a fee and penalizes certain (large) employers if they do not offer affordable coverage of "minimal value" to their employees. The ACA also called for the creation of state-based marketplaces where individuals without

access to affordable employer-based insurance could purchase insurance on their own. Some states have opted out of creating their own marketplace; residents of these states can access a federally facilitated marketplace to shop for and purchase health insurance. The ACA provides for subsidies designed to make marketplace insurance affordable for low-income individuals; the subsidies are tied to both the level of individuals' income and the cost of the policies.

The ACA also introduced a series of federal requirements intended to ensure that coverage was available, affordable, and effective in protecting consumers against major financial losses. It prohibited insurers from turning down customers or placing limits on coverage based on preexisting conditions. It limited the factors that insurers could use to set individual insurance premiums; premiums could be tied to enrollee age, geography, tobacco use, and family size but not health status or other factors. It required plans in the individual and small group markets to cover "essential health benefits" which include a range of ambulatory, hospital, and emergency services as well as maternity and newborn care, behavioral health services, and preventive services. Further, the Act prohibited the application of annual and lifetime dollar limits to essential health benefits. It allowed young adults to remain on their parents' insurance up to age 26. The ACA also required that insurers spend at least 80 to 85 percent of premium dollars on medical care. In addition, it introduced the first federal provider network adequacy standards for insurance plans offered through the marketplaces. There has been some concern that limited or "narrow" networks in ACA plans may restrict enrollee choice and access; federal and state standards for network adequacy are currently being developed and tested. CMS has engaged in oversight and enforcement of the insurance components of the ACA through its Center for Consumer Information and Insurance Oversight (CCIIO).

Food and Drug Law

The FDA, like CMS, is a federal agency responsible for decisions that have a profound effect on both patients and HCOs. While CMS exercises its influence primarily through its coverage and payment policies and related rules, the FDA exercises its influence through its regulatory efforts to ensure the safety and efficacy of drugs and medical devices.

The first step in developing a new drug is generally to perform laboratory and animal testing to determine whether it has promise for human use. If so, the developers submit an Investigational New Drug Application to the FDA to obtain approval to conduct clinical trials. After receiving approval, researchers can begin Phase I trials, in which they give the drug to a small number of people to test its safety and identify its side effects.

If a drug's performance in Phase I is sufficiently successful, the drug will then be tested in a Phase II trial, in which researchers study its effectiveness as well as its safety in a larger group of people. In Phase III, the drug is tested on still more people; results are used to assess the drug's benefits and risks and to provide the necessary information for the drug's label.

Drug development may be halted at any stage of clinical trials. If Phase III trials are successfully completed, however, the drug's sponsor can submit a New Drug Application to obtain the necessary FDA approval before marketing the drug. Based on the information supplied in the application, the FDA will weigh the drug's benefits and risks in determining whether the drug is safe and effective for the specified indication. It will also review the drug's proposed label and assess the adequacy of the drug's manufacturing process.

The FDA also regulates medical devices. Depending on the characteristics and uses of the devices, they are classified as Class I, Class II, or Class III devices, with Class III devices being subject to the most intensive regulatory scrutiny. Many Class I devices are exempt from premarket notification requirements, for example, while those seeking to market Class III devices must generally obtain premarket approval, just as developers of new drugs must obtain approval.

Regulatory Challenges

The FDA faces many regulatory challenges; this chapter highlights three. The first challenge is to balance the public demand for speedy access to newly developed drugs against the risk that an accelerated approval process might fail to identify the dangers that new drugs present. More generally, if regulators impose requirements that are too stringent, they will deprive people of access to beneficial drugs; if they impose requirements that are too lax, they will expose people to significant risks of harm.

A second challenge is to ensure continued monitoring of drugs once they reach the marketplace (Institute of Medicine, 2012). Because some drug risks may emerge only after a drug is used by a large number of patients, it is important to track adverse events that occur after a drug has been approved. In some cases, the FDA asks drug sponsors to conduct Phase IV, or postmarketing, clinical trials designed to permit further assessment of drugs. The FDA also relies on individual reports of adverse events submitted by drug sponsors, physicians, and consumers. The FDA also engages in more systematic surveillance of adverse effects through its Sentinel Initiative, which brings together data on hundreds of millions of patients from multiple sources, such as medical records and insurance claims databases (Kuehn, 2016).

A third challenge is to ensure that information is appropriately disseminated to physicians and patients. With respect to physicians, debate has long surrounded the FDA's policies with respect to a practice known as off-label promotion. The FDA approves drugs for specific indications, but physicians are free to prescribe drugs for other uses. Drug manufacturers, however, are not permitted to promote these off-label uses; federal authorities have pursued legal action against a number of manufacturers for illegal marketing practices. The prohibition of off-label promotion may encourage drug sponsors to systematically study off-label uses and seek formal FDA approval for additional indications. At the same time, it may impede the dissemination of data that physicians would find useful in making prescribing decisions. The First Amendment's free speech protections may apply to some forms of information sharing; in the aftermath of successful First Amendment-based arguments in suits involving off-label promotion, the FDA has sought to reformulate its policies (Richardson, 2016).

With respect to patients, the challenge is finding a way to appropriately regulate direct-to-consumer advertising. Regulations require that advertisements for prescription drugs "present a fair balance between information relating to side effects and contraindications and information relating to effectiveness of the drug"; they cannot be "false or misleading with respect to side effects, contraindications, and effectiveness" (21 CFR § 202.1[e][5]). Office of Prescription Drug Promotion reviews broadcast advertising but has taken a limited number of regulatory actions against advertisers, eliciting criticism from those who believe that the FDA should engage in more extensive oversight.

Antitrust Law

Because Medicare and Medicaid law and food and drug law are directed specifically at the provision of health care products and services, it is not surprising that they can be important factors in health care managers' decision-making processes. Other areas of federal law may have a less obvious connection with the health care industry but nonetheless often play a key role in shaping managerial strategies. **Antitrust law** is one example.

The purpose of the antitrust laws is to promote competition based on the conviction that competitive markets bring benefits of relatively lower consumer prices, higher output, and greater innovation. Antitrust laws exist at both the federal and state levels. However, because much of the enforcement activity in the health care industry is at the federal level, we focus here on federal antitrust law. Additionally, most state antitrust provisions parallel what exists at the federal level.

There are three primary federal antitrust provisions that apply to the health care industry. Section 1 of the

Sherman Act prohibits contracts and other agreements that unreasonably restrain trade. This provision applies to situations where individuals or organizations that are in a competitive situation with one another also collaborate to achieve common business objectives. Section 2 of the Sherman Act prohibits activities that are undertaken to obtain or achieve a monopoly. This section is aimed at the conduct of a single entity that undertakes anticompetitive activities to strengthen its competitive position. The third provision, Section 7 of the **Clayton Act**, prohibits mergers, acquisitions, and joint ventures that threaten to substantially lessen competition or are likely to create a monopoly. Because these provisions are broad in scope, over time the courts and antitrust enforcement officials have developed analytic frameworks for deciding when business arrangements and activities constitute violations of the antitrust laws.

Federal enforcement of the antitrust laws is the responsibility of both the U.S. **Department of Justice** (DOJ) and the **Federal Trade Commission** (FTC). These federal agencies coordinate their efforts in investigating and prosecuting antitrust cases. The Sherman Act permits both civil and criminal sanctions, including imprisonment, whereas the Clayton Act carries civil sanctions only. Also, the FTC can pursue antitrust cases under a provision within its own authorizing statute, Section 5 of the Federal Trade Commission Act, which prohibits unfair methods of competition and unfair or deceptive acts affecting commerce. Although Section 5 is technically even broader in scope than the previously noted antitrust provisions, the FTC typically invokes Section 5 to prosecute arrangements or activities that would otherwise violate the Sherman or Clayton acts.

Of the previously noted antitrust provisions, Section 1 of the Sherman Act has perhaps the greatest relevance to the health care industry. The health care industry is highly diverse, with numerous types of health care providers and other entities who often are in a position to compete as well as collaborate with one another. Some of the earliest antitrust cases in the health care industry involved physicians who were competitors but also agreed to boycott prepaid health plans as a means to protect their fees. Many Section 1 Sherman Act cases have involved physician networks that have been formed principally to facilitate joint price negotiations on behalf of network members with insurance plans and other payers of health care services. These networks often comprise physicians who are otherwise competitors but have formed a joint venture to strengthen their negotiating position with payers.

However, Section 1 is not a blanket prohibition on all collaborations among competitors. The courts have long recognized that collaborative arrangements can often have beneficial as well as harmful consequences for competition. Although collaborations involving competitors

necessarily impose some limits on competition that can result in harms such as higher consumer prices, they may also generate efficiencies in the participating entities' legitimate business activities or foster innovations that could not possibly be achieved by any one of the entities alone. Accordingly, to decide whether an arrangement is a violation of Section 1, enforcement officials and courts assess whether the benefits outweigh the harms for a given arrangement. Two primary legal standards are applied: per se and rule of reason.

The per se standard is applied to types of arrangements for which it is well established that the arrangement only harms competition. Price fixing is perhaps the best example of such an arrangement. In the case of price fixing, competitors collaborate for the sole purpose of agreeing on certain prices for their services or products so that they no longer are effectively competing on price. For example, consider eight dermatologists who in the past have competed for patients and collectively comprise 80 percent of the dermatologists in a market area. These dermatologists get together to agree on certain prices that they will charge for office visits and other services they provide. As a result, the dermatologists now gain what would likely be considerable negotiating leverage with local health plans for dermatology services. Because such an arrangement entails some degree of harm to competition (because the health plans have to pay higher prices for dermatology services that get passed down to consumers in the form of higher insurance premiums) but would not produce any efficiencies or innovations, it is treated as per se illegal under the antitrust laws.

The rule of reason standard is applicable when the arrangement has potential for both harm and benefit to competition. Consider the case of physician networks. If joint price negotiation was all that a particular network, one comprised of physicians or physician practices who were otherwise competitors, was designed to accomplish, the arrangement would raise concerns from an antitrust perspective. However, in addition to facilitating joint price negotiations, these networks are often designed to allow physicians to share clinical resources and administrative services that promote the efficiency of their separate practices. The arrangement may also be used to enhance quality of care through shared personnel and clinical resources, such as electronic medical records. The resolution of such cases under the rule of reason standard therefore calls for very fact-based examinations as to their net effects on competition. This examination entails a delineation of the affected market in terms of geographic boundaries, number and types of competing physicians within the market, and the degree to which a network is designed to promote efficiencies or quality in patient care.

Although antitrust enforcement officials are most concerned about collaborative arrangements that bring together competitors ("horizontal" arrangements), they also may scrutinize arrangements that involve entities that do not compete directly but rather have ongoing business relationships with each other as suppliers and purchasers ("vertical" arrangements). For example, physician-hospital organizations, which have been organized to enable a hospital and members of its medical staff to jointly negotiate prices with payers, have sometimes fallen under antitrust scrutiny on the ground that they are being used to boycott a health plan or competitively disadvantage certain physicians.

In the health care industry, Section 2 cases are less common but do arise from time to time amid concerns about an entity's ability to thwart competition. One Section 2 case involved an insurance plan that sought to strengthen its competitive position by refusing to contract with a hospital that was owned by a competing insurance plan. In such cases, antitrust enforcement officials look closely at an entity's market power or its ability to influence prices based on market share. The higher the entity's market share, the more enforcement officials will be inclined to scrutinize any possible anticompetitive actions undertaken by that entity.

Section 7 of the Clayton Act has been most frequently invoked in health care cases for proposed mergers between hospitals or between physician practices. For Section 7 of the Clayton Act, the basic analytic framework applied is similar to that already discussed for Section 1 of the Sherman Act. That is, there is a balancing of potential harms and benefits that may be associated with the merger or other combination of entities. For example, a merger between two hospitals in a six-hospital market may raise concerns about the combined entity's ability to raise prices. At the same time, the combined entity may be able to operate more efficiently than either of the two entities separately due to economies of scale.

Organizations that are planning mergers or acquisitions and meet certain financial criteria are required under the Hart-Scott-Rodino Act to report their plans to the federal government. Once a report is submitted, the federal government has a specified window of time to request additional information and to decide whether it believes the merger or acquisition would be an antitrust violation.

In addition, the DOJ and FTC have jointly issued enforcement guidelines for the health care industry. These guidelines include so-called **safety zones** that outline the factual elements of certain business arrangements the agencies view as acceptable and thus will not prosecute, barring extraordinary circumstances. Two such safety zones relate to physician networks, which, as noted, have been a major source of concern for enforcement officials because of their potential to reduce competition for physician services. These safety zones specify the percentage of physicians from the relevant clinical specialty and geographic market that is acceptable to

include in a network without raising antitrust concerns. One safety zone permits physician participation up to 20 percent whereas the other one permits participation up to 30 percent, but to qualify for the 30 percent safety zone the network must be nonexclusive (i.e., participating physicians must be allowed to join other networks). Additionally, for a network to qualify for safety zone status, its participating physicians must share some degree of financial risk through the contracts that it has with health plans and other purchasers of physician services. This can entail contracts that link revenue to selected network-wide performance metrics for the quality or efficiency of patient care.

For additional guidance, there is also the option of submitting a letter to the DOJ or FTC that outlines a proposed arrangement. An agency's response to such letters is purely advisory but does constitute an important source of additional guidance for industry participants.

States may choose to insulate or immunize certain activities that are potentially anticompetitive from federal antitrust review. However, for state action immunity to apply, state officials must meet two requirements. Specifically, they must (1) declare explicitly a policy decision to substitute state regulation for competition regarding the activity in question and (2) establish a regulatory arrangement through which the activity is in fact closely supervised. If these requirements are not met, those engaged in the activity may be found in violation of federal antitrust laws (see In Practice: "Antitrust Policy and Limits of Licensing Bodies to Regulate Healthcare Delivery").

Tax Exemption Law

Like antitrust law, **tax exemption** law is not necessarily directly targeted at HCOs but nonetheless has significant implications for managers' strategic decision making. The U.S. health care industry comprises a relatively large number of organizations that are exempt from paying most if not all taxes, including income, property, and sales taxes. Most of these tax-exempt organizations are nonprofit hospitals. Indeed, almost all nonprofit hospitals are exempt from at least federal income tax. However, some physician organizations, nursing homes, and other types of provider organizations have tax exemptions as well.

Organizations qualify for federal income tax exemption under Section 501(c)(3) of the Internal Revenue Code, which applies to corporations organized and operated exclusively for religious, charitable, scientific, or educational purposes. Although this provision does not refer to health care specifically as an exempt purpose, most 501(c)(3)-exempt HCOs have qualified on the basis of having a charitable purpose. Organizations that qualify for a federal tax exemption also are able to issue tax-exempt bonds, which enables them to issue bonds at relatively lower interest rates (and thus reduce their financing costs) because bondholders do not pay federal tax on the interest.

The IRS is responsible for determinations as to whether an organization qualifies for a Section 501(c)(3) exemption. In making 501(c)(3) determinations, the IRS applies two tests, one focusing on organizational criteria and the other focusing on operational criteria. For the organizational test, the IRS examines the applicant's formative documents (e.g., articles of incorporation) as to whether they limit the organization to pursue one or more exempt purposes (e.g., charitable, scientific). All organizations seeking to qualify as a charitable organization must be organized on a nonprofit basis.

For the operational test, the IRS examines the applicant's actual activities relative to three requirements. One is that the organization is operated to achieve an exempt purpose. The IRS has established a **community benefit standard** for assessing whether hospitals are operated to serve a charitable purpose. A second requirement prohibits so-called private benefit and private inurement, which are somewhat complex concepts but essentially mean that the earnings of an exempt organization cannot be distributed to any individual or organization as a form of dividend. The earnings of an exempt organization must be directed to further the organization's exempt purpose. Of course, this requirement does not prevent exempt organizations from paying salaries, even very high ones, to employees needed to carry out the organization's activities. However, the salaries must be in line with what is required to secure individuals with the necessary skills in a given market area. In this vein, all of an exempt organization's business transactions need to be conducted in an arm's-length manner and in accordance with fair market value, or else they jeopardize its exempt status.

The third requirement pertains to political activity by exempt organizations. Specifically, exempt organizations are prohibited from lobbying or otherwise campaigning on behalf of any political candidate. Exempt organizations may engage in lobbying activities to influence legislation or other policy action, but these activities must be limited to less than a "substantial" part of the organization's total activities. The IRS does not apply a quantitative threshold for defining a substantial part but rather looks at the facts and circumstances of each situation.

The IRS established the community benefit standard in 1969, thereby effectively replacing a standard that had required exempt hospitals to provide services to the poor to the extent of their financial ability. The agency's decision to replace this charity care standard was a response to the recently adopted Medicare and Medicaid programs, which at that time many health policy experts believed would greatly reduce the number of uninsured citizens and thus greatly reduce the need for hospitals to provide charity care. The community benefit standard reflected on the part of the IRS an expanded concept of charitable purpose for hospitals—one encompassing the promotion of health itself rather than strictly the provision of care to the poor.

The community benefit standard consists of several factors: providing charity care to the extent of the hospital's financial ability, operating a 24-hour emergency room, accepting payment from the Medicare and Medicaid programs on a nondiscriminatory basis, extending medical privileges to all qualified physicians in the area, and maintaining a governing board drawn largely from representatives of the community. Although the IRS does not require that an applicant meet all or even any specific combination of these factors, based on past IRS determinations, the presence of a 24-hour emergency room appears to carry considerable weight.

Despite the IRS' expanded concept of charitable purpose as formalized in the community benefit standard, in practice it has treated hospitals differently than it does other types of HCOs. For most other types of HCOs, the IRS appears to require evidence that the applicant provides care to the poor as part of its activities.

At the same time, however, in recent years hospitals have been subject to several new requirements for maintaining federal tax exemption. Since 2009, tax-exempt hospitals have been required to report annually to the IRS how much they spend for each of seven defined community benefits (e.g., charity care, unreimbursed costs for Medicaid enrollees, community health improvement). Hospitals report this information on Schedule H of the IRS Form 990. The ACA also added four new requirements for tax-exempt hospitals as codified in 501(r) of the Internal Revenue Code. Under one of the new requirements, federally tax-exempt hospitals must conduct a community health needs assessment (CHNA) at least once every three years, and develop an implementation plan to address community needs as identified in the CHNA. This is the first federal requirement for hospitals to engage in community health activities. The other three requirements relate to hospitals' own financial assistance policies and bill collection practices. Specifically, hospitals must establish a written financial assistance policy and a written policy governing emergency medical care. Also, in the case of emergency or medically necessary care, hospitals are prohibited from charging patients eligible for financial assistance more than amounts generally billed to insured patients. One additional requirement is that hospitals must make reasonable efforts to determine whether patients are eligible for financial assistance before initiating extraordinary collection efforts for unpaid bills (Internal Revenue Service, 2018).

A 501(c)(3) exemption does not necessarily apply to all of the income earned by an exempt organization. Income earned from activities that are unrelated to an entity's charitable purpose may trigger what is known as unrelated business income tax (UBIT). Under UBIT rules, exempt organizations must pay taxes at federal corporate rates on income earned from any activity meeting three criteria: the activity constitutes a trade or business, the activity is regularly carried on, and the activity is not substantially related to the organization's exempt purpose. For example, many hospitals have investment interests in for-profit businesses through either a parent–subsidiary relationship or a partnership arrangement. The income that hospitals earn from these businesses will often qualify for UBIT treatment as their underlying activities are not related to the hospital's exempt purpose—providing hospital services to the local community.

Exemptions for most other taxes are granted at the state and local level. With respect to state income, sales, and property tax exemptions, the overriding issue is whether the applicant has a charitable purpose. Whereas some states and local taxing authorities grant exemption based on an entity's 501(c)(3) status, others have their own criteria that may require or attach considerable weight to the actual provision of charity care, regardless of whether the applicant is a hospital or another type of provider. A number of high-profile court cases have involved a state's revocation of a hospital's property tax exemption. Indeed, most challenges of a hospital's tax-exempt status have come from state and local government rather than the IRS, which at least in part can be explained by the fact that an exempt hospital can constitute a potentially important source of revenue for a municipality that is facing budgetary pressures (Rubin, Singh, and Young, 2015). As such, hospitals must be attentive to the requirements associated with their tax-exempt status.

Other Federal Laws and Regulations Affecting Hospital and Health System Operations

While Medicare and Medicaid law, insurance regulations, food and drug law, antitrust law, and tax exemption law are all important areas of federal law, many other areas of federal law affect health care providers. Many federal statutes and regulations are relevant for day-to-day operations; executives must develop a culture of regulatory compliance and implement measures to identify and remediate noncompliance. Federal regulations also shape and constrain strategic decision making. Executives must work closely with their attorneys to identify potential regulatory barriers to business arrangements with physicians.

Consider the following questions as you read this section: What organizational strategies would you adopt to ensure compliance with these complex regulations? What disciplinary measures would you recommend for individuals within your organization who fail to comply with applicable regulations?

Federal Fraud and Abuse Laws

The federal fraud and abuse laws prohibit three principal types of conduct. First, the **Anti-Kickback Statute** (AKS) prohibits the knowing and willful solicitation or receipt of remuneration by any person in connection with items or services for which payment could be made by Medicare or Medicaid. While the most obvious violation of the AKS would be a bribe for a referral of a Medicare patient, providers engaged in other kinds of arrangements, such as payments of financial incentives in connection with physician recruitment, may also run afoul of the AKS. Second, the **Stark Physician Self-Referral Law** (Stark) prohibits physicians from referring patients to certain health services providers with which the physicians have a financial relationship. Third, the **False Claims Act** (FCA) prohibits knowingly submitting or causing to be submitted a false claim to the government, such as a Medicare claim for a service that was not provided or a service different from the one that was actually provided.

The secretary of HHS retains discretion to promulgate regulations to define the scope of these prohibitions and establish specific exceptions. These regulations run for hundreds of pages, with numerous safe harbors (which are defined as arrangements that the regulatory agencies believe are not abusive and hence are acceptable) and exceptions that are difficult to interpret and apply. There are safe harbors or exceptions for personal services and management contracts, payments to employees, practitioner recruitment activities, space rentals, equipment rentals, referral services, warranties, discounts, coinsurance waivers, obstetrical malpractice insurance subsidies, group practice investments, and ambulatory surgery centers, among other areas, but these safe harbors or exceptions may be limited in important ways or require satisfaction of a long list of criteria.

The activities prohibited by the fraud and abuse laws concern policy makers because they provide incentives to deliver more health care than is necessary, increasing the costs of Medicare and Medicaid, and they also expose patients to health risks attributable to too much treatment or poor-quality treatment. As much as 10 percent of the annual federal health care budget may be lost to fraud and abuse, while federal fraud recoveries total several billion dollars each year. Because there is a great deal of money involved, the federal government has made fraud and abuse enforcement a primary focus of its regulatory efforts. As a result, the issue is one of ongoing importance to health care executives. Virtually every issue of trade publications, such as *Modern Healthcare*, will have an article discussing various aspects of compliance with the fraud and abuse laws, along with complaints about the government's enforcement policies and the resulting burden.

The HHS **Office of the Inspector General (OIG)**, with the cooperation of the Department of Justice, dedicates considerable resources to enforcing federal fraud and abuse laws. State authorities may also bring enforcement actions; many states have their own fraud and abuse statutes. Government authorities are not the only entities involved in fraud and abuse enforcement, however. Many FCA suits are initiated not by government entities but instead by individual employee whistle-blowers pursuant to the *qui tam* provisions of the FCA. Individuals who bring *qui tam* actions inform the government of a potential violation and then share in any proceeds the government acquires from a judgment or settlement. Thus, the FCA's *qui tam* provision significantly increases the probability of detection of false claims.

The sanctions associated with statutory violations are significant. They include civil monetary penalties and possible exclusion from participation in Medicare and Medicaid under the Stark Law, AKS, and the FCA, as well as criminal penalties under AKS. Failure to comply with fraud and abuse regulations may also lead the government to impose a **corporate integrity agreement**, whereby the organization essentially loses control of the compliance process and must adhere to strict governmental oversight.

That all of this imposes substantial compliance requirements on health care providers is clear. Providers must remain vigilant about their practices; their organizations must be structured to identify and respond to potential issues, particularly given current enforcement efforts and the ACA's introduction of a requirement for prompt return of overpayments, which includes payments submitted in violation of fraud laws. What remains uncertain is the degree to which this extensive regulatory framework adversely affects efficient organizational arrangements. In particular, critics of the current regulations complain that the regulations impede legitimate market arrangements that can advance public policy goals of reducing costs and improving patients' quality of care. Other commentators question whether the fraud and abuse laws "fit" the medical marketplace (Healthcare Leadership Council, 2017).

As an example, take the issue of gainsharing, which occurs when physicians and health systems enter into agreements to share cost savings based on certain efficiency and quality-of-care metrics. Initially, OIG stated in an advisory bulletin that gainsharing violated the fraud and abuse regulations. This interpretation was in tension with the policies of the IRS (with respect to tax exemption criteria) and the Department of Justice and Federal Trade Commission (with respect to antitrust enforcement), which encouraged integration and risk-sharing in arrangements between physicians and health systems. Over time, OIG has relaxed its categorical opposition to gainsharing, allowing some arrangements to proceed, as long as they incorporate clear protections against abuse, such as quality-of-care metrics. In 2015, Congress removed a legal barrier to gainsharing by amending a statutory provision penalizing hospitals that make payments to physicians as inducements to limit patient services.

Health care executives and physicians have also raised concerns about the impact of fraud and abuse laws on physician payment arrangements and joint ventures between physicians and health systems. To fall within the relevant AKS safe harbor, for example, payment to physicians under personal services contracts must reflect fair market value and cannot be tied to the volume of referrals. Joint ventures must be carefully structured to avoid both the AKS and self-referral laws. The complexity of the regulations governing these and other arrangements may hinder efforts to engage in efficiency-enhancing practices.

Undoubtedly, the government's concern for fraud and abuse is legitimate. Whether it is systematic fraud and abuse that results in the filing of false claims, upcoding for insurance reimbursement, or kickbacks for prescribing pharmaceuticals or ordering durable medical equipment, a regulatory presence to restrain bad behavior is necessary. At the same time, the fraud and abuse regulatory structure suffers from excessive complexity, an undetermined compliance burden, and a lack of empirical evidence to support the current approach.

• • • IN PRACTICE: Physician Recruitment and the Fraud and Abuse Regulations

Health care managers often find themselves in the difficult position of having to navigate through complex and voluminous fraud and abuse laws and regulations. These provisions prohibit many practices, while at the same time creating exceptions and "safe harbors" for others. The safe harbors outline various payment and business practices that, although potentially capable of inducing referrals of business reimbursable under the federal health care programs, will not be treated as offenses under the anti-kickback statute.

Imagine that you are a hospital manager who seeks to expand hospital service offerings by bringing a new physician to your area. Physician recruitment potentially implicates the fraud and abuse regulations, including both the anti-kickback statute and the Stark statute. If you are contemplating offering some form of remuneration to the physician, you would first want to consider the requirements of 42 C.F.R. § 411.357. By providing that certain compensation arrangements do not constitute a financial relationship, this federal regulation removes them

• • • IN PRACTICE: Physician Recruitment and the Fraud and Abuse Regulations

(Continued)

from the reach of the Stark statute, which applies when a financial relationship exists. The regulation's complex provisions read in part as follows:

. . . the following compensation arrangements do not constitute a financial relationship:

(e) Physician recruitment. (1) Remuneration provided by a hospital to recruit a physician that is paid directly to the physician and that is intended to induce the physician to relocate his or her medical practice to the geographic area served by the hospital in order to become a member of the hospital's medical staff, if all of the following conditions are met:

(i) The arrangement is set out in writing and signed by both parties;...

(iii) The amount of remuneration under the arrangement is not determined in a manner that takes into account (directly or indirectly) the volume or value of any actual or anticipated referrals by the physician or other business generated between the parties; and

(iv) The physician is allowed to establish staff privileges at any other hospital(s) and to refer business to any other entities (except as referrals may be restricted under an employment or services contract that complies with § 411.354[d][4]).

(2)(i) The "geographic area served by the hospital" is the area composed of the lowest number of contiguous zip codes from which the hospital draws at least 75 percent of its inpatients. The geographic area served by the hospital may include one or more zip codes from which the hospital draws no inpatients, provided that such zip codes are entirely surrounded by zip codes in the geographic area described above from which the hospital draws at least 75 percent of its inpatients....

(iv) A physician will be considered to have relocated his or her medical practice if the medical practice was located outside the geographic area served by the hospital and...

(B) The physician moves his medical practice into the geographic area served by the hospital, and the physician's new medical practice derives at least 75 percent of its revenues from professional services furnished to patients (including hospital inpatients) not seen or treated by the physician at his or her prior medical practice site during the preceding 3 years, measured on an annual basis (fiscal or calendar year). For the initial "start up" year of the recruited physician's practice, the 75 percent test in the preceding sentence will be satisfied if there is a reasonable expectation that the recruited physician's medical practice for the year will derive at least 75 percent of its revenues from professional services furnished to patients not seen or treated by the physician at his or her prior medical practice site during the preceding 3 years....

(4) In the case of remuneration provided by a hospital to a physician either indirectly through payments made to another physician practice, or directly to a physician who joins a physician practice, the following additional conditions must be met:...

(iii) In the case of an income guarantee of any type made by the hospital to a recruited physician who joins a physician practice, the costs allocated by the physician practice to the recruited physician do not exceed the actual additional incremental costs attributable to the recruited physician...

Before undertaking a transaction that might implicate the fraud and abuse regulations, managers need to discuss the transaction with an attorney to ensure that the business arrangement complies with the relevant regulations. Keep in mind, too, that physician recruitment may also involve other regulatory issues, such as IRS regulations on private inurement and private benefit.

This example is adapted from Gostin and Jacobson (2006).

HIPAA Privacy and Security

Fraud and abuse regulations have affected HCOs' daily operations for many years and will likely continue to do so for many more. There is another, newer set of regulations, however, that has emerged over the last few years and promises to become increasingly important in the future: privacy and security-related regulations.

In 1996, Congress passed HIPAA. As the act's title suggests, many of its provisions are aimed at health insurance plans. For example, HIPAA prohibits group health plans from discriminating against employees or dependent family members based on health factors in determining eligibility or premiums; it also offers opportunities to enroll in new plans due to life-changing events.

HIPAA's protections extend beyond its regulation of insurance coverage, however, to include privacy and security of health information. Specifically, these regulations, which apply to both health providers and health plans, are intended to safeguard the privacy and security of protected health information (PHI), which includes anything that could identify an individual patient. The use of medical records, billing information, and other personally identifiable health data must follow stringent guidelines. Absent specific authorization from patients, PHI may only be shared for certain purposes, such as provider payment, treatment, and health care operations. Institutions are required to have security measures in place to protect the data from unnecessary dissemination to parties who are not involved in a patient's care and to ensure that contracted entities protect the information as well. Employees must be trained to follow appropriate procedures for protecting health information. HIPAA also requires providers to grant patients access to their own medical records.

From an operational perspective, HIPAA regulations do not require major changes in how providers and staff communicate but, outside of treatment and other specified contexts, permit only the minimum necessary PHI to be exchanged. The regulations do not define what would constitute the minimum necessary information but leave it to providers to determine.

HIPAA also mandates that providers and health plans notify patients, HHS, and in some cases, the media, when breaches of unsecured PHI occur. Many millions of Americans have been impacted by such breaches, which may result from the loss of physical records or storage devices, theft, hacking, or other forms of unauthorized access or disclosure (Office for Civil Rights, 2017).

HIPAA requires providers to devote significant attention to regulatory compliance. HHS' Office for Civil Rights conducts audits and investigates compliance issues, including impermissible uses and disclosures of PHI, lack of patient access to their information, violations of the minimum necessary rule, and lack of appropriate safeguards. Recent enforcement actions have generated million dollars of fines for violating HIPAA's privacy and security provisions.

In addition, state laws may impose more stringent privacy protections. In that sense, HIPAA sets a floor of privacy protection rather than a ceiling.

EMTALA

A third statute that affects the daily operations of health care providers is the Emergency Medical Treatment and Labor Act (EMTALA) of 1986, which is designed to prevent institutions from denying care to anyone seeking emergency medical treatment, regardless of citizenship, insurance status, or ability to pay. EMTALA's broad purpose is to prevent private hospitals from dumping uninsured patients on hospitals of last resort without first screening and stabilizing them. Hospitals that accept Medicare reimbursement and have emergency departments are subject to EMTALA's two primary requirements.

First, hospitals must perform an initial patient evaluation. Specifically, the statute states that "if any individual . . . comes to the emergency department and a request is made on the individual's behalf for examination or treatment for a medical condition, the hospital must provide for an appropriate medical screening examination within the capability of the hospital's emergency department . . . to determine whether or not an emergency medical condition . . . exists." Individuals who arrive at the hospital in a location other than the dedicated emergency department must specifically state that they are seeking treatment for an emergency medical condition for EMTALA to apply.

The statute's second requirement is that hospitals stabilize individuals who are determined to have an emergency condition before discharge or transfer to a more appropriate facility. If a hospital elects to transfer, it still has an obligation to mitigate risks to the health of the individual, and in the case of a woman in labor, to the health of the unborn child.

Health Care Quality Improvement Act

A fourth example of a statute that affects providers' operations is the Health Care Quality Improvement Act (HCQIA) of 1986. At the time of its enactment, HCQIA reflected two primary concerns: one relating to weaknesses in existing peer review processes and the other to the ease with which incompetent physicians were able to move between states without a record of their malpractice experience or professional disciplinary action. HCQIA is designed to address these issues by encouraging physicians to identify and discipline fellow physicians who are incompetent or who engage in unprofessional behavior, so as to improve the quality of care.

HCQIA provides limited immunity to physicians and dentists who engage in the peer review process, mitigating the risk associated with lawsuits from physicians who face sanctions or the loss of staff privileges after formal peer review. HCQIA provides immunity only if the peer review decision was taken (1) in the reasonable belief that the action was in the furtherance of quality health care, (2) after a reasonable effort to obtain the facts of the matter, (3) after adequate notice and hearing procedures were afforded to the physician involved or after such other procedures as were fair to the physician under

DEBATE TIME: Health Care Provider Integration

U.S. health policy reflects a deeply conflicted attitude toward the clinical integration of hospitals and physicians. During much of the twentieth century, there was little or no integration between these two types of providers. Most hospitals maintained a so-called dual structure whereby their medical staff, those physicians who have authority to admit patients to the hospital and use its clinical resources, was organized as a largely separate and self-governed entity. Hospitals and the members of their medical staff rarely collaborated in pursuit of common patient care goals. Indeed, the hospital–physician relationship was predicated largely on the mutual but distinct financial interests of the two types of providers; hospitals relied on physicians for admissions, and physicians relied on hospitals for the equipment and technology that they needed to provide services. This relationship was supported, even promoted, by fee-for-service reimbursement under which the incomes of hospitals and physicians were tied to the volume of services they provided to patients.

Although in more recent years, several industry forces have motivated hospitals and physicians to collaborate in some areas of patient care, many health care leaders believe that hospitals and physicians continue to function far too independently from each other. The lack of integration between hospitals and physicians may translate into a fragmented delivery system that is prone to error, inefficiency, and poor quality of care. Health care leaders have called for hospitals and physicians to collaborate in developing policies and procedures for ensuring continuity of care for patients across clinical settings, sharing expertise and experience for identifying cost-effective medical technologies and devices, and assuming joint financial accountability for managing the care of patients. Toward this end, various policy initiatives have been put forth to create incentives, financial and otherwise, to encourage hospitals and physicians to work more collaboratively to improve patient care. One example is Medicare's shared savings program, which allows health care providers to come together to form **accountable care organizations** (ACOs), which can receive bonuses if they are able to reduce costs while meeting quality targets.

However, such initiatives are impeded by various U.S. laws and regulations, some of which have been enacted for the very purpose of keeping hospitals and physicians from integrating too closely. In particular, federal fraud and abuse laws impose many restrictions on the ability of hospitals and physicians to form partnerships for sharing financial risks and rewards in the delivery of patient care services, such as through gainsharing arrangements. Hospitals with a federal income tax exemption may jeopardize their exemption when they invest in health care organizations that are controlled by physicians who are members of their medical staff. The antitrust laws also present legal risks for hospitals and physicians that engage in collaborative arrangements as these arrangements can be seen as anticompetitive tactics to strengthen the participants' negotiating leverage with health plans. Although both the Federal Trade Commission and Department of Justice, the two government agencies that are responsible for antitrust enforcement, have encouraged health care providers to integrate clinically to reduce their risk of antitrust violations, the regulatory guidance has not been entirely consistent and, in some instances, has been contradictory to the policies of other government agencies with oversight responsibility for the health care industry. Further, some states have corporate practice of medicine laws that prohibit or otherwise restrict hospitals from employing physicians directly.

In light of these legal barriers to collaboration, some health care leaders believe that significant legal reforms are a necessary first step for promoting meaningful hospital–physician integration. When the rules governing the ACO program were issued, government regulators also issued waivers that shielded certain ACO activities from the reach of fraud and abuse laws. The FTC and DOJ issued a statement of enforcement policy applicable to ACOs, while the IRS issued a notice regarding tax-exempt organizations' participation in ACOs. But ACOs still face regulatory challenges, and Medicare ACOs are not the only vehicle through which hospitals and physicians could seek to work together.

So what do you think? An argument in favor of more comprehensive legal reforms is that many of the previously noted laws are overly broad as they relate to the health care industry and deter hospitals and physicians from engaging in collaborative arrangements that are good for patient care. A counterargument is that wide-scale legal reforms may usher in an era of highly undesirable conduct in the health care industry as some providers exploit legal exemptions and loopholes for their own financial gain rather than to improve patient care.

the circumstances, and (4) in the reasonable belief that the action was warranted by the facts known after such reasonable effort to obtain facts and after meeting the requirements of (3) above. Most courts have held that bias or malice in the peer review process is irrelevant, as long as those involved in the peer review process made a good-faith effort to ascertain the facts.

HCQIA also established the **National Practitioner Data Bank** (NPDB) to store information regarding physicians' and dentists' professional competence and conduct, increasing the accessibility of information about medical liability awards and settlements and peer review sanctions. Hospitals, state licensing bodies, entities making malpractice payments, and other organizations are required to report certain actions to the NPDB. Health care managers must also consult the NPDB when considering offering staff privileges, and every two years for all health care practitioners with current staff privileges. Today, the NPDB contains over a million reports related to adverse licensure, certification, and clinical privileges actions; medical malpractice payments; and civil judgment and criminal convictions. NPDB records are confidential and not available to the public but may be accessed by hospitals, health plans, licensing agencies, and professional societies, among other entities.

While the NPDB has helped to ensure wider access to information about physicians, it has also been subject to criticism, particularly with respect to its inclusion of malpractice payment data. It does not include all payments made in connection with an allegation of substandard care; for example, payments made solely for the benefit of a corporation, such as a group practice or hospital, are not reported to the NPDB. Furthermore, the NPDB may have unintended consequences. Physicians concerned about the long-term impact of an NPDB report may be less willing to settle disputes, preferring instead to go to trial in the hope of successfully defending against claims. The NPDB may also increase physicians' reluctance to disclose errors, undermining recent efforts to promote transparency when errors arise.

STATE POLICY AND REGULATION

While the scope of the federal government's involvement in health care has increased significantly over time, state and local governments have traditionally played a far more central health-related role. State and local governments provide care through public hospitals and clinics, finance care through Medicaid and other programs, and create and enforce health care-related laws and regulations. Whether acting as providers, payers, or regulators, state and local governments can have a dramatic impact on health care delivery and, ultimately, public health.

As providers, state and local governments have a direct impact on the availability of care. For example, a local government hospital can provide much-needed services to communities that might otherwise be significantly underserved. As payers, governments affect access and quality through the incentives created by the reimbursement policies they adopt.

State and local governments also affect access and quality through the regulations they implement. States' regulations of health insurance, for example, affect both the scope and cost of private insurance policies. Even before the enactment of the ACA, some states limited insurers' ability to turn away applicants, prohibited refusals to renew policies, or regulated premium setting. States may mandate that insurance policies sold within the state include certain benefits, increasing access to the covered providers or services, but also increasing the costs of policies. They may also attempt to ensure access to care through mechanisms such as requirements for external reviews of claims denials.

State regulation also affects public health more generally. In addition to engaging in general health promotion activities, public health departments enforce laws intended to prevent the spread of contagious disease through quarantines or immunization requirements. State laws support public health departments' surveillance efforts through requirements that health care providers report certain injuries and diseases. State agencies regularly become involved in a wide range of public health issues, including foodborne illnesses and environmental health hazards, such as lead. State agencies also have responsibility for oversight of the quality and safety of health care facilities. It is in this role that state agencies have the most direct interaction with health care providers.

Licensure

Licensure serves as a primary mechanism by which states regulate the quality of care provided by health care professionals and HCOs. As licensure is a strictly state-level activity, it constitutes an important form of local control over the delivery of health care services. State licensure of health care professionals, such as physicians, nurses, and dentists, is carried out through licensure bodies that a state has authorized for this activity. Some states have had such occupational licensure arrangements in place for health care and other types of professionals for well over 100 years. These entities are composed of individuals from the relevant profession, though they may also include one or more individuals who are selected to represent consumers. Within legislative parameters, these entities decide the requirements necessary for securing a license, including educational background, clinical training, and any examinations that a candidate must take.

Among the states, relatively uniform licensure requirements exist for the most common types of health care professionals, including physicians and nurses. However, state licensure requirements often vary quite substantially for relatively new types of health care professionals that are less established within the health care delivery system. For example, many states require individuals seeking to practice acupuncture to complete formal educational training and pass a written examination. However, some states recognize apprenticeship as an acceptable route to licensure and a few states have no licensure requirements at all.

Many types of HCOs must also secure a license before they can begin to operate. The major impetus for statelevel licensure of HCOs was the 1946 Hill-Burton Act. Through this legislation, the federal government made hospital funding available to states but tied the funds to a state's adoption of a hospital licensure statute. Since then, states have expanded their licensure programs to cover more types of HCOs.

The types of HCOs required to obtain a license vary somewhat across states. Although all states require licensure for certain types of organizations, namely hospitals and nursing homes, they differ in their treatment of other organizations, such as home health agencies, freestanding clinics, and ambulatory surgical centers (ASCs). States uniformly do not require licensure for physician offices as these entities are not treated as distinct HCOs but rather as an extension of the physician practice itself and thus exempt from licensure. In most states, the department of health or a comparable government agency is responsible for the licensure of HCOs. This is in contrast to the licensure of health care professionals where, as noted, responsibility is vested in occupational licensure boards that are largely composed of individuals with the same professional background as the applicants. The state agencies that are responsible for licensure of HCOs typically subdivide regulatory responsibilities by type of organization, such as hospitals or nursing homes, and these regulatory responsibilities are carried out by state employees who develop expertise as to the relevant licensure requirements and procedures.

For any type of HCO, the specific licensure requirements and procedures will differ somewhat from state to state. Typically, not all licensure requirements are located in the state authorizing statute itself; the state licensing agency will have responsibilities for issuing additional licensure requirements. In general, licensure requirements tend to focus on structural features of organizations, such as resources and policies, rather than the actual quality provided. For example, state licensing requirements for hospitals typically focus on such characteristics as physical layout, equipment, governance policies, and staffing. Because of this focus on structural features, licensure is often considered to be a minimal form of quality oversight.

All states require as a condition of licensure that an organization undergo a site inspection. In an on-site inspection, state agency personnel visit the organization to observe its campus and review documents and other materials pertaining to licensure requirements. The inspectors will conduct interviews with the administrative and clinical staff regarding the implementation of relevant policies and procedures. At least one inspection will be conducted prior to the time the organization first opens its doors. Subsequent inspections may be announced or unannounced. Also, in some states, certain types of organizations are deemed to be in compliance with licensure requirements if they are accredited by a state-approved accrediting body. For example, in some states, a hospital that is accredited by the Joint Commission is deemed to be in compliance with the state's hospital licensure requirements and does not need to undergo a separate state inspection.

Certificate of Need Regulation

In many states, a health care facility cannot be constructed, renovated, or expanded without obtaining a **certificate of need** (CON). Existing HCOs may also need to secure a CON before purchasing major equipment or offering new services. A CON is a form of approval from a state agency, usually the department of public health or a comparable agency, that is responsible for determining whether a need exists for the requested organization, service, or equipment. Thus, like licensure, CON is a regulatory hurdle that must be overcome before a provider can begin to offer services. Numerous empirical studies have examined the effect of CON on health care costs (Conover and Sloan, 1998; Hellinger, 2009; Polsky et al., 2014). While the results are by no means entirely consistent, the weight of the evidence has not been highly supportive of CON as a form of cost control. CON has also been criticized for being highly politicized in many states and insufficiently transparent.

During the 1970s, almost every state had a CON law because federal policy, specifically the 1974 National Health Planning and Resources Development Act, promoted this type of regulatory mechanism as a form of cost control for health care services. The basic idea was to establish within each state a central planning and regulatory structure for overseeing the use and allocation of health care resources to prevent excess capacity from driving up costs. However, since the 1970s, a number of states have eliminated their CON programs, preferring to approach cost control from the standpoint of market competition rather than relying on a regulatory and central planning structure. Still, as of 2018, 38 states had some form of CON or CON-like programs in place (NCSL, 2018).

Among states that have retained their CON programs, there is considerable variation among key program elements, namely the organizations that are covered; the types of projects, equipment, or services for which a CON must be secured; and the expenditure thresholds under which a CON is not required. For example, a state CON program may exempt all projects with an expenditure target of under $200,000.

States also differ in the way they review CON applications. All states require applicants to put forward evidence of need in support of their request that speaks to issues of access, cost, and quality. However, some states require applicants to support their request with a high level of quantitative data and analytic models, whereas other states accept applications that are less formal in their presentation.

Relationships between State and Federal Law

States' involvement in health-related regulation extends well beyond the insurance, public health, licensure, and CON areas. State law relating to medical negligence is an important consideration for health care providers, for example. Other state laws, such as those related to antitrust, fraud, or privacy, may exist alongside similar federal laws.

State and federal laws interact in varied ways. For example, as previously noted, states have antitrust statutes that generally parallel federal antitrust statutes. Under the state action doctrine, however, certain activities that might otherwise be found to violate federal antitrust law are exempted because a state has taken an active role in supervising those activities. State action arguments may be relevant in situations involving seemingly anticompetitive actions of state licensing boards or medical staffs of public hospitals. In addition, providers who turn to state governments for approvals of various forms of collaboration may hope to invoke the state action doctrine (Havighurst, 2006).

Preemption principles also affect the interaction between federal and state laws. At the core of preemption analysis is a simple idea: If federal and state laws directly conflict, the federal law applies. (State law may also preempt local laws.) Preemption may mean that someone who seeks a remedy for an injury under state law, such as the law relating to negligence, may not be able to pursue the claim.

But the forms of preemption are numerous, and the analysis involved is not always straightforward. Litigation involving the federal Employee Retirement Income Security Act (**ERISA**), which imposes minimum requirements on retirement and health benefit plans, illustrates the complexity of preemption issues. The statute itself

states that it supersedes all state laws that "relate to" employee benefit plans. Arguably, such laws may include certain statutes intended to encourage employers to expand employee access to health care benefits. Federal appeals court cases have come to differing conclusions about whether ERISA preempts state and local efforts to expand access through various forms of employer mandates, such as a mandate that employers spend a minimum amount on health insurance or pay an equivalent amount to the state. One court found a Maryland law preempted, while another rejected a similar challenge to a San Francisco ordinance.

Other ERISA preemption cases have found their way to the Supreme Court. The Supreme Court has ruled, for example, that ERISA does not preempt a state statute requiring health maintenance organizations to permit review of denied claims by independent reviewers. It has also ruled, however, that ERISA preempts certain claims based on a state law permitting managed care enrollees to sue their plans for injuries resulting from benefit denials. ERISA was also found to preempt a state requirement that employer health benefit plans provide data to an all-payer claims database that could be used to support state health policy initiatives.

As these examples make clear, both state law and federal law can have a significant influence over health care entities' activities.

ORGANIZATIONAL STRATEGIES FOR REGULATORY COMPLIANCE

In view of the numerous regulatory requirements and challenges that hospitals and other HCOs face, they need to develop strategies for complying with regulatory demands. Noncompliance could result in costly lawsuits and regulatory sanctions that disrupt daily operations. As noted earlier, the imposition of a corporate integrity agreement is very disruptive to the regulatory compliance process. In rare instances, systematic regulatory failures could result in the loss of eligibility for Medicare and Medicaid reimbursement. To avoid such results, it is advisable for health care executives to adopt regulatory compliance practices that are thorough, systematic, and capable of adapting to the continuously changing environment in which HCOs operate.

Patient Safety

One important strategy for maintaining regulatory compliance involves mitigating risk of harm to patients. The 1999 report by the Institute of Medicine, *To Err Is Human: Building a Safer Health System*, stated that between 44,000 and 98,000 deaths could be attributed to preventable medical errors (IOM, 1999). To promote patient safety, HCOs have a responsibility to create and enforce policies that ensure recruitment and retention of competent physicians and other care providers, prevent the spread of infectious disease through safe practices (such as appropriate handwashing), and maintain facilities and equipment properly. Evidence-based practices for safeguarding patients are constantly evolving, and organizations must have a system in place to demonstrate due diligence toward protecting patient safety.

In the event that a patient's safety is compromised as a result of an error or negligence, there are a number of steps an organization could take to protect the institution. First, while care providers and institutions have historically attempted to cover up their mistakes, research has shown that patients may be less likely to pursue litigation if they are provided with information about what happened during their care process (Boothman et al., 2009). Although this approach remains controversial because it may increase risk exposure, acknowledging that an error has occurred and demonstrating that the HCO is taking reasonable steps to both mitigate harm to the patient and prevent harm to future patients may deter litigation.

Second, HCOs are often subject to reporting requirements. They may be required to report errors to an appropriate state agency, and the Joint Commission strongly encourages accredited organizations to report to the Joint Commission as well. In 1996, the Joint Commission introduced a sentinel event reporting policy to help HCOs identify errors and take steps toward preventing future occurrences. Patient safety events, defined as "events not primarily related to the natural course of the patient's illness or underlying condition," become sentinel events if they result in death, permanent harm, or "severe temporary harm and intervention [is] required to sustain life" (The Joint Commission, 2017). HCOs can conduct root cause analyses to determine and address the underlying systemic or procedural issues that resulted in the error.

The Role of the Regulatory Compliance Officer

To successfully navigate through the complex regulatory environment, HCOs often appoint a regulatory compliance officer. This individual is responsible for conducting all activities related to regulatory compliance, including educating staff on regulatory compliance protocols through training programs, monitoring compliance, and implementing consistent enforcement policies. Officers also actively respond to compliance violations and seek out opportunities to prevent future violations. In addition to serving as internal monitors, they act as liaisons between HCOs and appropriate regulatory agencies to ensure proper reporting occurs. Collaboration with other departments in the HCO, such as Risk Management, Internal Audit, Employee Services, and Human Resources, is essential to addressing compliance issues as well as fostering the development of a compliance culture.

Regulatory compliance officers must pay special attention to certain areas as a result of their potentially serious consequences for HCOs. Officers often conduct internal audits of practices that might constitute fraud or abuse. For example, Medicare payments to HCOs are based on codes that reflect patients' severity of illness. When upcoding occurs, patients are misrepresented as sicker, thereby allowing an organization to obtain greater compensation for services provided and placing it at risk for fraud and abuse sanctions. A proper internal auditing system will allow for appropriate code assignments and reimbursement commensurate with a patient's disease category. Organizations should prepare for audits under Medicare's Recovery Audit Program; **Recovery Audit Contractors** identify improper Medicare payments to correct errors involving both overpayment and underpayment. Due diligence in preparation for such audits is essential for preventing FCA whistle-blower claims concerning an organization's improper conduct. Organizations must have proper policies and procedures to respond to employees who raise compliance concerns.

RECENT POLICY AND REGULATORY INITIATIVES

Federal, state, and local governments; public and private payers; professional and trade organizations; providers; and others continually search for new ways to improve health care's quality and reduce its cost. This section illustrates a few of the many approaches, both legal and nonlegal, that have been taken in recent efforts to reform the health care system.

For health care managers, familiarity with health reform efforts is important because of their power to transform the regulatory and market environments in which HCOs operate. Imagine, for example, a proposed law that required the disclosure of a hospital's prices, or mandated reporting of surgery outcomes, or tied Medicare reimbursement to specific quality measures. If you were a health care executive, would you support or oppose such a law? What actions would you take in support of or in opposition to the law? Would you seek to modify the content of the law, and if so, how? If the proposed law were enacted, how might you alter your organization's operations? Consider these questions as you review each of the following examples of recent policy and regulatory reform initiatives.

Transparency

In most marketplaces, consumers consider the price and quality of available goods and services before making purchasing decisions. This is not the case, however, when it comes to health care. Most patients know little about the price or quality of medical services. This lack of information creates significant hurdles for patient efforts to obtain low-cost, high-quality care. It also undermines the competitive process that might otherwise drive prices lower and quality higher. A number of recent initiatives attempt to address these problems by increasing price and quality **transparency**.

Prices

Insured patients who are responsible for only fixed co-payments or limited coinsurance have little reason to care about medical prices. For the increasing number of patients who are enrolled in high-deductible health plans or who are uninsured, however, health care prices have become critically important. Without price information, these patients will not be able to take financial considerations into account when deciding on a course of treatment. Nor will they be able to choose providers on the basis of price. As a result, providers will have little reason to compete over price.

A number of state governments have responded to the paucity of pricing data (de Brantes and Delbanco, 2016; NCSL, 2017). In 2003, for example, the California legislature passed a "Payers' Bill of Rights" that mandated that hospitals publicly disclose their charges. Subsequently, it added a requirement that hospitals provide price estimates to uninsured patients upon request. Maine uses an all-payer claims database to create a public website that allows consumers to compare average costs for health services and procedures across many different facilities (CompareMaine, 2017). New Hampshire also maintains a website that reports the median amounts paid by insurers and patients for a variety of medical services (CSHSC, 2009).

These initiatives may partially remedy patients' pricing information deficit, but unless accompanied by other reforms, they are unlikely to achieve effective competition in health care markets. Patients are not likely to know the precise nature of the hospital services they will require, and even if they do, they will not be able to easily wade through the thousands of items on hospital price lists. In addition, a study shows that patients may not always succeed in obtaining hospital cost estimates, despite California's mandate (Farrell et al., 2010). New Hampshire's program may assist patients in learning more about health care costs, but price variation among providers has persisted, suggesting that it may not generate significant patient shopping on the basis of price (CSHSC, 2009). Insurers may provide information about

costs or fees, but many enrollees—particularly enrollees in traditional, as opposed to high-deductible, health plans—never take advantage of it (Fronstin, 2017). There is also a worry that detailed price disclosure might sometimes raise prices, because it could lead lower-paid providers to seek higher rates or facilitate price coordination among otherwise-competing providers. While price transparency has potential as a tool to encourage more efficient provision of care, the barriers to achieving this potential are considerable.

Quality and Safety

Most patients lack information about health care quality, just as they lack information about price. Patients have traditionally turned to friends, family members, and their own physicians for recommendations for health care providers but have had little access to more systematic assessments of clinical quality. This lack of information hinders patients' abilities to select providers and payers' abilities to compensate providers on the basis of quality. As a result, providers might seek to deliver high-quality care for reasons of professional ethics or regulatory compliance but might not feel significant reputational or financial pressure to increase quality. In addition, limited availability of quality measures may undermine providers' efforts to assess and improve their own quality.

Governments and other organizations have sought to fill this information void through public quality and safety reporting. Many states, including California, Colorado, Illinois, New York, and Pennsylvania, have established reporting systems for hospital health care quality information, while other states require public reporting of errors or hospital infection rates (Hanlon et al., 2015; Madison, 2009). Patients in some states can obtain hospital-specific quality and safety information, such as cardiac bypass surgery mortality rates or infection rates, through state-operated websites. These legal reporting mandates complement efforts by public and private payers and other organizations to increase public quality information. HHS, for example, provides structure, process, and outcome-based hospital quality measures, as well as measures based on hospital patient surveys, on its Hospital Compare website. For-profit companies also provide quality ratings.

Measures of quality of other providers are available, but less common. Medicare, for example, publishes quality ratings for nursing homes, dialysis facilities, and home health agencies. A few states publish physician-specific mortality rates for bypass surgery. California publishes quality ratings for medical groups, as does a Massachusetts-based broad coalition of providers, payers, and others. Medicare's Physician Compare website provides quality measures for some physicians.

Efforts to improve the quality of care through reporting face considerable challenges. Quality measures must be appropriately selected; ideally, they would reflect important dimensions of care without leading providers to neglect unmeasured aspects of care. They must be appropriately designed so that they accurately capture quality and are not biased by underlying patient illness. Poorly designed measures could encourage providers to try to improve ratings by avoiding sicker patients, while at the same time misleading users about where to obtain high-quality care. Measures must be appropriately presented so that users understand them; confusing measures could lead to poor choices of providers. They must not be overly burdensome; particularly given the numerous and varied organizations involved in quality reporting efforts, providers may face considerable administrative costs in collecting quality data. Finally, people must use them. Report cards can improve quality only if patients respond by selecting higher-quality providers, or providers respond by increasing their own quality of care.

Some patients are aware of report cards, and some of these patients use them (Harris and Buntin, 2008; Scanlon et al., 2015); anecdotal evidence suggests that some providers respond to them (Chassin, 2002). But many patients do not use them. Lack of awareness, lack of interest, and illness itself can all serve as barriers to use. In addition, studies have suggested that report cards may have unintended consequences, as providers attempt to improve their ratings by changing the mix of patients they treat, rather than by improving the care they deliver (Dranove et al., 2003; Werner and Asch, 2005). The technical challenges involved in creating measures are formidable, particularly for physicians, who may not treat enough patients to create meaningful measures. Moreover, studies evaluating the early effects of report cards on quality have had mixed results (Fung et al., 2008). Nevertheless, quality reporting has become ubiquitous and researchers continue to investigate ways to make quality reporting more effective (Bardach et al., 2015; Pronovost et al., 2016; Sinaiko, Eastman, and Rosenthal, 2012). Public reporting may become an even more important tool for quality improvement in the future, as reporting technologies improve and familiarity with report cards grows.

The Move toward Value-Based Payment Models

In recent years, the trend away from fee-for-service payment models has increased. Some early innovators in this area embraced "pay-for-performance" models in which they would pay providers quality-based incentives in addition to fee-for-service payments. Today, payers are adopting more diverse forms of **value-based payment** (VBP) as a strategy for improving the performance of HCOs. In concept, VBP entails linking financial incentives to the accomplishment of assigned performance goals related to efficiency, productivity, or quality.

Most existing VBP programs follow a similar structure. A typical program focuses on individual physicians, physician groups, or hospitals as the entities accountable for achieving assigned quality and, potentially, cost goals. For example, a health plan may assign a set of quality targets for diabetes care to the physician organizations with which it contracts. One of these quality targets may specify that a certain percentage of the group's diabetic patients will receive an annual blood test to monitor for glucose control. The group's score on this and other measures will then be used to compute an incentive payment. The financial incentives can be structured in various ways, including bonuses, penalties, or fee adjustments. Beyond incentives that may layer on top of fee-for-service payments, VBP also refers to emerging alternative payment models where providers take on financial risks for costs of care. In these global or bundled payment models, providers are paid a set amount for any services associated with an episode of care or condition, such as all services associated with a coronary artery bypass graft surgery, even if these services are provided by multiple providers in a range of settings. The VBP label may also be applied to contracts between suppliers and purchasers in which a price for a drug or device is tied to the outcomes experienced by patients using the drug or device.

At present, both the private and public sectors have embraced VBP. Many private payers have now adopted VBP arrangements that hold providers accountable for costs and quality of patient care, including global budgets, shared savings, and bundled payments (Health Care Transformation Task Force, 2016). In the public sector, the use of VBP in both Medicaid and Medicare has increased rapidly.

By the end of 2014, 20 percent of Medicare fee-for-service payments were linked to value. This figure was due largely to the growth of accountable care organizations and bundled payments. In January 2015, CMS announced the goal of making 85 percent of payments through VBP or P4P by 2016 and 90 percent by 2018 (CMS, 2015). The Medicare Access and CHIP Reauthorization Act (MACRA) of 2015 accelerated the adoption of "alternative payment models" (APMs) that focus on performance. MACRA introduced the Quality Payment Program, a new infrastructure for physician payment, which includes two payment options for physicians: the Merit-Based Incentive Payment System, a traditional fee-for-service payment model with quality-based incentives, and an APM in which payment will be tied to value and providers will assume a certain level of risk. The details of the Quality Payment Program remain uncertain even as MACRA's payment formulas are set to determine payment beginning in 2019.

Over one-third of state Medicaid programs have also adopted some type of VBP. For example, Medicaid programs have used bundled payments, monthly per-patient payments to physicians to coordinate care, and population-based payments, where providers are given a set fee for meeting the health care needs of a predetermined population. Under Section 1115 of the Social Security Act, state Medicaid programs can introduce pilot or demonstration projects focused on innovative delivery and payment reforms, including Delivery System Reform Incentive Payment (DSRIP) initiatives. Under DSRIP initiatives, provider payment is tied to meeting performance metrics; the specific metrics and program designs vary across states. DSRIP initiatives were in place in 10 states as of 2017. Overall, 40 states in 2017 had delivery system or payment reform initiatives in place in their Medicaid program, including patient-centered medical homes, ACA health homes, accountable care organizations, bundled payments, and DSRIP initiatives (Kaiser Family Foundation/National Association of Medicaid Directors, 2017).

This interest in VBP is in large part a response to a growing body of evidence indicating that the quality of care in the United States is suboptimal. Some health policy experts attribute at least part of the quality problem to a lack of provider reimbursement for high quality of care. The promise of VBP is that by linking financial incentives to important quality and value goals, providers will be motivated to improve quality. Whether this promise is being realized is not entirely clear based on a growing body of studies that addresses the impact of early pay-for-performance efforts and VBP on quality and generally finds mixed results (RAND, 2014; Rosenthal et al., 2005; Young et al., 2007). Critics of VBP suggest that successes have been limited to date for a range of reasons, including that current models do not ensure that patients receive appropriate, high-quality care or that payments are sufficient to cover the costs of care. Further, providers have been reluctant to join VBP efforts in some cases because payments under VBP are often less transparent than under fee-for-service and because they may be held financially accountable for patient characteristics that are outside their control but impact outcomes and, therefore, payment (Miller, 2017). As the use of VBP in the private and public sectors becomes more mainstream, it will be increasingly important to evaluate this type of payment reform as a strategy for improving quality.

Specialty Hospitals and Other Nontraditional Health Care Organizations

A number of new HCOs and settings have emerged over the past two decades, including specialty hospitals, retail clinics, and ASCs. Proponents of these new care settings suggest that they can provide quality health care at lower costs and improve consumer access to care, such as by reducing wait times. In contrast to general hospitals, these organizations are generally characterized by a narrow scope of practice, provider or retail ownership, and a higher likelihood of being for-profit. Due to these and other characteristics, new forms of policy and regulation are likely needed to monitor these organizations.

Whether or not they achieve their intended effects, laws and regulations often have unintended consequences. The recent growth in specialty hospitals illustrates this point. The federal Stark statute, which is intended to prevent physician self-referrals, contains an exception for physician referrals to hospitals they own when "the ownership or investment interest is in the hospital itself (and not merely in a subdivision of the hospital)" (42 U.S.C. § 1395nn[d][3][C]). This exception permits physician financial support for general hospitals while at the same time blunting the financial impact of a physician-investor's own referrals on his or her investment return. But what if the only services available within the whole hospital were cardiac services? The Stark statute exception would seem to apply, permitting providers to refer despite their ownership interests. The whole hospital exception, along with the profitability of the services involved, contributed to the growth of specialty hospitals in areas such as cardiac care (Iglehart, 2005). Under the ACA, additional requirements were placed on physician-owned hospitals to qualify for the whole hospital exception, effectively blocking the expansion of existing or creation of new physician-owned hospitals (Plummer and Wempe, 2016).

Specialty hospitals are controversial. In theory, their narrow focus may help them deliver more efficient and higher-quality care than traditional general hospitals. In addition, their existence may spur competing hospitals to improve their own quality. At the same time, however, physician-owned specialty hospitals are subject to the general concerns underlying the fraud and abuse laws, such as the concern that physician-investors may overrefer patients, increasing costs and perhaps worsening outcomes. Evidence to date suggests that single-specialty hospitals are no more efficient than other hospitals and, in some cases, may be less efficient (Carey, Burgess, and Young, 2008). In terms of quality, physician-owned and non-physician-owned hospitals appear be comparable on measures of patient satisfaction, process, and outcomes such as readmissions and mortality (Blumenthal et al., 2015). ASCs, which provide outpatient surgeries in freestanding clinics or hospital outpatient departments, and are largely provider-owned, face similar concerns, and there is evidence that physician-ownership of ASCs has resulted in higher surgical volumes (Hollingsworth et al., 2010).

There is some fear that if physician-investors refer patients with generous payers to the specialty hospitals and ASCs they own, local general hospitals will be left with patients they perceive as money-losers due to either the severity of their illnesses or the identity of their payers. A recent study, however, suggests that while patients at physician-owned hospitals were slightly younger and less likely to be admitted through the emergency room, they were equally likely to be from a racial or ethnic minority or enrolled in Medicaid and had similar rates of chronic conditions compared to patients in non-physician-owned hospitals (Blumenthal et al., 2015).

More broadly, while general hospitals may be concerned about competition from specialty hospitals and ASCs, the ACA effectively blocked the growth of physician-owned specialty hospitals, considerably mitigating this threat (Plummer and Wempe, 2016). In the future, other new health care delivery settings such as ASCs and retail clinics are likely to emerge. Given the uncertainties about both the beneficial and detrimental effects of specialty hospitals and other alternative health care settings, debate continues about how best to respond to their growth. It will be important to understand how these new organizations affect existing providers and, ultimately, access to and quality of care.

DEBATE TIME: Regulation of Pharmaceutical Promotion

Pharmaceutical companies spend billions of dollars each year to promote products to physicians (Kornfield et al., 2013). Pharmaceutical companies advertise in professional journals; make regular visits to physician offices for conversations about their products, a practice called "detailing"; and provide free samples of their products. Pharmaceutical companies may also influence physicians' prescribing efforts through the financial relationships they establish. Pharmaceutical companies have funded catered lunches at physicians' offices; offered payments for advising, consulting, or speaking; and contributed toward the costs associated with continuing medical education and other meetings. In 2016, more than 600,000 physicians received more than $2 billion from drug and device companies in general payments for things like food and beverages, consulting fees, and speaking fees (OpenPaymentsData.CMS.gov, 2017).

Studies suggest that pharmaceutical companies' financial ties to physicians may affect prescribing patterns (Rothman and Chimonas, 2008; Wazana, 2000). The changes in prescribing patterns could potentially increase health costs or worsen health outcomes, relative to a world in which prescriptions were written by fully independent physicians. The proliferation of financial ties could in the long run reduce patient trust in physicians, potentially undermining treatment relationships.

Concerned about the effects of pharmaceutical company promotional efforts, many academic medical centers and health systems now limit drug company interactions with their physicians. Pharmaceutical manufacturers have also altered their practices. The Pharmaceutical Research and Manufacturers of America's 2009 Code on Interactions with Healthcare Professionals, for example, bans distribution of promotional pens and mugs to physicians and restricts the circumstances under which restaurant meals can be provided. Policy makers have also taken actions to limit pharmaceutical marketing. Vermont, for example, bans most gifts to physicians, while Massachusetts has restricted the provision of meals and prohibited the provision of entertainment or recreational items, such as sports tickets. The ACA mandated the creation of the federal Open Payments database, which increases transparency by providing data about payments that pharmaceutical and device companies make to individual physicians.

Despite these steps, pharmaceutical company promotional efforts continue and so does the debate. Do you think the Open Payments database will have a significant impact on pharmaceutical company practices? Would you argue for more widespread adoption of legal restrictions on these practices? Would you advise health system executives to limit interactions between their physicians and pharmaceutical and device companies? Or would you argue that current policies are problematic, and that the public would be better served by different or more limited forms of regulation?

SUMMARY AND MANAGERIAL GUIDELINES

1. State and federal governments have a significant impact on health care delivery through the statutes they enact, the regulations they impose, and the policies they adopt.

2. Governments use varied tools to achieve varied goals. Many governmental initiatives, including FDA regulations, licensure statutes, HCQIA, pay-for-performance programs, and quality reporting programs, are intended to ensure health care quality. Others, including antitrust law, fraud and abuse laws, and CON laws, may in theory help lower health care costs. EMTALA and the tax code may increase health care access, as do programs such as Medicare and Medicaid. Government initiatives may sometimes achieve several of these goals simultaneously, may achieve one goal but sacrifice progress on another, or, if poorly designed or poorly executed, may achieve no goals at all.

3. Given the large number of applicable laws and regulations, as well as their potential consequences for providers, health care managers must treat regulatory compliance with the importance given to other areas of health care operations. Due diligence is essential, both for internal compliance and responses to governmental inquiries. To ensure that the appropriate attention is devoted to regulatory issues, appoint a regulatory compliance officer who reports directly to the CEO.

4. To ensure ongoing compliance, identify regulatory requirements and develop monitoring procedures for activities that implicate these requirements. Identify troublesome areas that could result in bad publicity or substantial sanctions, and conduct routine audits in these areas.

5. Identify potential violations and establish mechanisms for reporting and correcting them. Determine appropriate internal sanctions for compliance failures and apply enforcement procedures consistently throughout the organization. To increase the likelihood of compliance and reduce the likelihood of legal sanctions, create opportunities for building relationships and resolving conflicts within your organization.

6. Governmental entities continuously experiment with new approaches to achieve policy goals. Health care managers must remain aware of the evolving content of laws, regulations, and policies, because it will necessarily affect day-to-day operations. To ensure continued compliance in a dynamic regulatory environment, maintain lines of communication throughout your organization and create and regularly update training and educational programs.

DISCUSSION QUESTIONS

1. Identify the major laws and regulations affecting HCOs. Why is the health care industry so heavily regulated? What are the central goals of these laws and regulations? Who benefits from them?

2. What problems do these regulations present? If you could eliminate one of these laws or regulations, which one would you eliminate, and why? Are there alternative regulatory approaches that would achieve regulatory objectives in a less burdensome way?

3. Critics of formal governmental health care regulation suggest that mechanisms such as self-regulation or accreditation would provide more effective oversight. Do you agree?

4. Nonprofit organizations must meet a community benefit test to take advantage of the federal income tax exemption. Should a facility be allowed to use population health interventions to meet the test instead of the measures noted in this chapter? If so, what measures of population health should the IRS accept?

5. Do you think government entities should devote more resources to developing health care quality report cards? Why or why not?

6. How should we regulate emerging market arrangements, such as pay-for-performance initiatives, and emerging health care providers, such as specialty hospitals?

CASE

An Ambulatory Surgical Center Joint Venture

David Donaldson is the special assistant to the CEO of Tri-County Hospital, a 350-bed community hospital. Last week, he attended a meeting at which four of the hospital's orthopedic surgeons proposed a joint venture between them and the hospital to establish a freestanding ambulatory surgical center. The proposal they outlined had the following features:

- Tri-County will contribute 70 percent of the capital needed for construction of the facility and purchase of equipment and initial supplies. The other 30 percent will be financed by the surgeons with a bank loan.

- All business issues and questions related to the ambulatory surgical center will be decided by a majority vote of the center's managing directors. Three of the six positions will be occupied by representatives of the surgeons; the other positions will be occupied by representatives of the hospital. The partnership agreement will contain a binding arbitration clause in the event that a decision before the managing directors receives a tie vote.

- The surgeons will receive 65 percent of the profits from the ambulatory surgical center. The hospital will receive the remaining 35 percent.

- The hospital and surgeons will jointly develop a protocol addressing the types of surgical cases that should be handled on an inpatient basis at the hospital versus those that will be referred to the ambulatory surgical center. The hospital will be expected to promote the ambulatory surgical center and encourage medical staff members to make appropriate referrals. Also, profit margin thresholds will be established in advance for the ambulatory surgical center, and as these thresholds are reached, the division of profits between the hospital and the surgeons will be adjusted in favor of the hospital.

- As a next step, David plans to prepare a memorandum for the hospital's CEO regarding the proposed joint venture. David generally believes that the CEO should seriously consider the joint venture. Although the surgeons did not say so explicitly, he suspects that if the CEO declines the deal, the surgeons may very well leave the hospital completely and form the ambulatory surgical center on their own. The four surgeons who have proposed the deal account for a substantial percentage of the income the hospital earns from its surgical department. At the same time, David knows that the formation of such joint ventures is a complicated matter and requires careful planning to comply with legal and regulatory issues. His initial take on the proposal outlined by the surgeons is that some legal problems in fact may arise.

Questions

1. Consider what David should say in his memorandum to the CEO about the joint venture. Which laws or regulations might this joint venture violate?

2. What changes, if any, in the proposed arrangement might be needed to keep the ambulatory surgical center in compliance with legal and regulatory requirements?

3. What course of action should David recommend?

REFERENCES

Administration for Community Living (ACL). (2017). About ACL. Retrieved August 4, 2017, from https://www.acl.gov/about-acl.

Bardach, N. S., Hibbard, J. H., Greaves, F., Dudley, R. A. (2015). Sources of traffic and visitors' preferences regarding online public reports of quality: Web analytics and online survey results. *Journal of Internet Medical Research, 17*(5), e102.

Blumenthal, D. M., Orav, E. J., Jena, A. B., Dudzinski, D. M., Le, S. T., & Jhu, A.K. (2015). Access, quality, and costs of care at physician owned hospitals in the United States: Observational study. *BMJ, 351,* h4466.

Boards of Trustees of the Federal Hospital Insurance and Federal Supplementary Medical Insurance Trust Funds.

(2016). *2016 Annual Report.* Retrieved October 8, 2018, from https://www.cms.gov/Research-Statistics-Data-and-Systems/Statistics-Trends-and-Reports/ReportsTrustFunds/Downloads/TR2016.pdf.

Boothman, R. C., Blackwell, A. C., Campbell, D. A., Jr., et al. (2009). A better approach to medical malpractice claims? A University of Michigan experience. *Journal of Health and Life Sciences Law, 2*(2), 125–159.

Carey, K., Burgess, J. F., & Young, G. J. (2008). Specialty and full-service hospitals: A comparative cost analysis. *Health Services Research, 43*(5), 1869–1887.

Center for Studying Health System Change (CSHSC). (2009). Impact of health care price transparency on price variation: The New Hampshire experience. Issue Brief No. 128.

Retrieved October 8, 2018, from https://www.apcdcouncil .org/publication/impact-health-care-price-transparency-price-variation-new-hampshire-experience.

Centers for Medicare and Medicaid Services (CMS). (2015). Better care. Smarter spending. Healthier people: Paying providers for value, not volume. Retrieved August 23, 2017, from https://www.cms.gov/Newsroom/MediaReleaseDatabase/ Fact-sheets/2015-Fact-sheets-items/2015-01-26-3.html.

Chassin, M. R. (2002). Achieving and sustaining improved quality: Lessons from New York State and cardiac surgery. *Health Affairs, 21*(4), 40–51.

CompareMaine. (2017). About CompareMaine. Retrieved August 4, 2017, from http://www.comparemaine.org/?page=about.

Conover, C. J., & Sloan, F. A. (1998). Does removing certificate-of-need regulations lead to a surge in health care spending? *Journal of Health Politics, Policy and Law, 23*(3), 455–481.

De Brantes, F., & Delbanco, S. (2016). Report card on state price transparency laws. Retrieved October 8, 2018, from https://www.catalyze.org/product/2016-report-card/.

Dranove, D., Kessler, D., McClellan, M., et al. (2003). Is more information better? The effects of "report cards" on health care providers. *Journal of Political Economy, 111*(3), 555–588.

Farrell, K. S., Finocchio, L. J., Trivedi, A. N., et al. (2010). Does price transparency legislation allow the uninsured to shop for care? *Journal of General Internal Medicine, 25*(2), 110–114.

Fronstin, P. (2017). Consumer engagement in health care: Findings from the 2016 EBRI/Greenwald & Associates consumer engagement in health care survey. Employee Benefit Research Institute Issue Brief No. 433. Retrieved October 8, 2018, from https://www.ebri.org/pdf/briefspdf/EBRI_IB_433_ CEHCS.25May17.pdf.

Fung, C. H., Lim, Y. W., Mattke, S., et al. (2008). Systematic review: The evidence that publishing patient care performance data improves quality of care. *Annals of Internal Medicine, 148*(2), 111–123.

Gostin, L. O., & Jacobson, P. D. (2006). *Law and the health system.* New York: Foundation Press.

Hanlon, C., Sheedy, K., Kniffin, T., et al. (2015). 2014 guide to state adverse event reporting systems. Retrieved October 8, 2018, from https://nashp.org/wp-content/ uploads/2015/02/2014_Guide_to_State_Adverse_Event_ Reporting_Systems.pdf.

Harris, K. M., & Buntin, M. B. (2008). Choosing a health care provider: The role of quality information. Robert Wood Johnson Foundation Research Synthesis Report No. 14. Retrieved October 8, 2018, from http://citeseerx.ist.psu.edu/viewdoc/ download?doi=10.1.1.670.6295&rep=rep1&type=pdf.

Havighurst, C. C. (2006). Contesting anticompetitive actions taken in the name of the state: State action immunity and health are markets. *Journal of Health Politics, Policy & Law, 31*(3), 587–607.

Health Care Transformation Task Force. (2016). Health care transformation task force reports increase in value-based payments. Retrieved October 8, 2018, from http://hcttf.org/ releases/2016/4/12/healthcare-transformation-task-force-reports-increase-in-value-based-payments.

Health Resources and Services Administration (HRSA). (2017). About HRSA. Retrieved August 4, 2017, from https:// www.hrsa.gov/about/index.html.

Healthcare Leadership Council. (2017). Health system transformation: Revisiting the federal anti-kickback statute and physician self-referral (Stark) law to foster integrated care delivery and payment models. Retrieved October 8, 2018, from https://www.hlc.org/app/uploads/2017/02/HLC_ StarkAntiKickback-White-Paper.pdf.

Hellinger, F. J. (2009). The effect of certificate-of-need laws on hospital beds and healthcare expenditures: An empirical analysis. *American Journal of Managed Care, 15*(10), 737–744.

Hollingsworth, J. M., Ye, Z., Strope, S. A., et al. (2010). Physicianownership of ambulatory surgery centers linked to higher volume of surgeries. *Health Affairs, 29*(4), 683–689.

Iglehart, J. K. (2005). The emergence of physician-owned specialty hospitals. *New England Journal of Medicine, 352*(1), 78–84.

Indian Health Service (IHS). (2017). About IHS. Retrieved August 4, 2017, from https://www.ihs.gov/aboutihs/.

Internal Revenue Service. (2018). New requirements for 501(c)(3) hospitals under the Affordable Care Act. Retrieved October 8, 2018, from https://www.irs.gov/charities-non-profits/charitable-organizations/new-requirements-for-501c3-hospitals-under-the-affordable-care-act.

Institute of Medicine (IOM). (1999). *To err is human: Building a safer health system.* Washington, DC: National Academies Press.

Institute of Medicine (IOM). (2012). *Ethical and scientific issues in studying the safety of approved drugs.* Washington, DC: National Academies Press.

Jacobson, P. D., Hoffman, R. E., & Lopez, W. (2006). Regulating public health: Principles and application of administrative law. In R. A. Goodman, R. E. Hoffman, W. Lopez, G. W. Matthews, M. A. Rothstein, & K. L. Foster (Eds.), *Law in public health practice* (2nd ed.). New York: Oxford University Press.

Kaiser Family Foundation/National Association of Medicaid Directors (2017). Medicaid moving ahead in uncertain times. Retrieved October 25, 2017, from http://files.kff.org/ attachment/Report-Results-from-a-50-State-Medicaid-Budget-Survey-for-State-Fiscal-Years-2017-and-2018.

Kornfield, R., Donohue, J., Berndt, E. R., et al. (2013). Promotion of prescription drugs to consumers and providers, 2001–2010. *PLoS One, 8*(3), e55504. Retrieved from https:// doi.org/10.1371/journal.pone.0055504.

Kuehn, B. M. (2016). FDA's foray into big data still maturing. *JAMA, 315*(17), 1934–1936.

Madison, K. (2009). The law and policy of health care quality reporting. *Campbell Law Review, 31*(2), 215–255.

Medicare Payment Advisory Commission (MedPAC). (2017). About MedPac. Retrieved August 1, 2017, from http://www .medpac.gov/-about-medpac-.

Miller, H. D. (2017). Why value-based payment isn't working, and how to fix it. Center for Healthcare Quality and Payment Reform. Retrieved October 8, 2018, from http://www.chqpr .org/downloads/WhyVBPIsNotWorking.pdf.

National Conference of State Legislatures (NCSL). (2018). CON-certificate of need state laws. Retrieved October 8, 2018, from http://www.ncsl.org/research/health/con-certificate-of-need-state-laws.aspx.

National Conference of State Legislatures (NCSL). (2017). Transparency and disclosure of health costs and provider payments: State actions. Retrieved August 4, 2017, from http://www.ncsl.org/research/health/transparency-and-disclosure-health-costs.aspx.

Office for Civil Rights, Department of Health and Human Services. (2017). Breach portal. Retrieved August 4, 2017, from https://ocrportal.hhs.gov/ocr/breach/breach_report.jsf.

OpenPaymentsData.CMS.gov. (2017). The facts about open payments data (2016 totals). Retrieved August 5, 2017, from https://openpaymentsdata.cms.gov/summary.

Plummer, E., & Wempe, E. (2016). The Affordable Care Act's effects on the formation, expansion, and operation of physician-owned hospitals. *Health Affairs, 35*(8), 1452–1460.

Polsky, D., David, G., Yang, J., et al. (2014). The effect of entry regulation in the health care sector: The case of home health. *Journal of Public Economics, 110,* 1–14.

Pronovost, P. J., Austin, J. M., Cassel, C. K., et al. (2016). Fostering transparency in outcomes, quality, safety, and costs. Vital directions for health and health care series, Discussion paper, National Academy of Medicine, Washington, DC. Retrieved October 8, 2018, from https://nam .edu/wp-content/uploads/2016/09/Fostering-Transparency-in-Outcomes-Quality-Safety-and-Costs.pdf.

RAND. (2014). Measuring success in health care value-based purchasing programs: Findings from an environmental scan, literature review, and expert panel discussions. Retrieved October 8, 2018, from http://www.rand.org/content/dam/rand/pubs/research_reports/RR300/RR306/RAND_RR306.pdf.

Richardson, E. (2016, June 30). Health policy brief: Off-label drug promotion. *Health Affairs.* Retrieved from http://www .healthaffairs.org/healthpolicybriefs/brief.php?brief_id=159.

Rosenthal, M. B., Frank, R. G., Li, Z., et al. (2005). Early experience with pay-for-performance: From concept to practice. *Journal of the American Medical Association, 294*(14), 1788–1793.

Rothman, D. J., & Chimonas, S. (2008). New developments in managing physician relationships. *Journal of the American Medical Association, 300*(9), 1067–1069.

Rubin, D. B., Singh, S. R., & Young, G. J. (2015). Tax-exempt hospitals and community benefit: New directions in policy and practice. *Annual Review of Public Health, 36,* 545–558.

Scanlon D. P., Shi, Y., Bhandari, P., et al. (2015). Are healthcare quality "report cards" reaching consumers? Awareness in the chronically ill population. *American Journal of Managed Care, 21*(3), 236–244.

Shortell, S. M., & Walshe, K. (2004). Social regulation of healthcare organizations in the United States: Developing a framework for evaluation. *Health Services Management Research, 17*(2), 79–99.

Sinaiko, A. D., Eastman, D., & Rosenthal, M. B. (2012). How report cards on physicians, physician groups, and hospitals can have greater impact on consumer choices. *Health Affairs, 31*(3), 602–611.

The Joint Commission. (2017, August 4). Sentinel event policy and procedures. Retrieved October 8, 2018, from https://www .jointcommission.org/sentinel_event_policy_and_procedures/.

United States Department of Health and Human Services (HHS). (2017). About HHS. Retrieved August 4, 2017, from https://www.hhs.gov/about/index.html.

Wazana, A. (2000). Physicians and the pharmaceutical industry: Is a gift ever just a gift? *Journal of the American Medical Association, 283*(3), 373–380.

Werner, R. M., & Asch, D. A. (2005). The unintended consequences of publicly reporting quality information. *Journal of the American Medical Association, 293*(10), 1239–1244.

Young, G. J., Meterko, M., Beckman, H., et al. (2007). Effects of paying physicians based on their relative performance for quality. *Journal of General Internal Medicine, 22*(6), 872–876.

Chapter 13

Health Information Technology and Strategy

Karen A. Wager and Mark L. Diana

CHAPTER OUTLINE

- Terms and Definitions
- Historical Overview and Today's Health Information Technology Landscape: A National Perspective
- Changing Health Environment Relies on Effective Use of Health IT
- Health IT Ramifications of Payment Reform and New Models of Care
- Strategic Alignment
- Assessing Health IT Performance and Value to the Health Care Organization

LEARNING OBJECTIVES

After completing this chapter, the reader should be able to:

1. Define key terms including health information technology (health IT), electronic health records (EHRs), and interoperability

2. Describe the history, evolution, and current state of health IT adoption and use and current issues

3. Discuss the health IT implications of recent legislation, payment reform, and new models of care (such as accountable care organizations and patient-centered medical homes) and the IT capabilities needed to effectively lead in this new environment

4. Discuss the importance of aligning health IT plans and capabilities with the overall strategic plans of a health care organization

5. Describe the process that health care organizations generally use to manage and enhance value of health IT

KEY TERMS

Care Management

Data Analytics

Electronic Health Record (EHR)

Health Information Exchange (HIE)

Health Information Technology (Health IT)

HITECH Act of 2009

Interoperability

Patient Engagement Tools

Population and Patient Registries

Revenue Cycle and Contracts Management

Telehealth and Telemedicine

CHAPTER PURPOSE

In today's health care environment, no health care management book would be complete without a chapter on health information technology (health IT) and strategy. The terms "health IT" and "health care information system" are often used interchangeably to describe the technology, data, people, and processes that are needed to provide timely, accurate, and relevant health information where and when it is needed. Advances in technology, consumer engagement, payment reform, and the massive infusion of federal resources have led to widespread adoption and use of health IT including electronic health record (EHR) systems in U.S. hospitals and office-based physician practices. Leadership and management of health care organizations are now grappling with how to optimize the use of such systems in practice, ensure that the systems can "talk to each other," and share relevant health information securely within and across the continuum of care. They are also investing in the use of data analytics, care management IT capabilities, telehealth, and patient engagement strategies to effectively manage care and resources under value-based payment models. Such investments require substantial resources and should be well aligned and integrated with the strategic plans of the organization.

This chapter provides the reader with a broad historical overview of the health IT landscape including current adoption and use of EHR systems as well as the external factors that are impacting the use of health IT to manage population health under new payment models. Included is a brief description of the EHR incentive programs and major payment reform initiatives. The health IT ramifications of payment reform and new models of care are discussed. The chapter emphasizes the importance of aligning health IT investments and plans with the overall strategic plans of the organization. It concludes with a discussion of how to assess the value of health IT investments and a real-world case study of an organization struggling to share health information effectively across a care delivery network.

TERMS AND DEFINITIONS

Health IT is a general term that describes a broad range of technologies and applications that are used to store, transmit, and manage health information electronically. For our purposes, we focus on technologies and systems (data, people, and processes) that are used to support the strategic and operational needs of health care provider organizations and the patients and/or communities in which they serve. Health IT includes both administrative/financial systems as well as clinical information systems that are commonly used to diagnose, treat, and manage the patient's care across a continuum. An *EHR* is a computer-based patient health record that is maintained by the provider over time and may include demographics, progress notes, problems, medications, vital signs, past medical history, immunizations, laboratory data, and radiology reports. EHR systems have core capabilities and functions including provider order entry, clinical decision support (CDS), alerts and reminders, and access to evidence-based knowledge aids. EHR systems should be able to share information electronically with others in a secure manner.

EHRs have eight main functions as defined by the Institute of Medicine (IOM) (see Table 13.1). The first four core functions enable the EHR to electronically collect and store data about patients, supply that information to providers on request, permit providers to directly enter orders into the computer, and provide health care professionals with advice in making decision about a patient's care (e.g., alerts, reminders, CDS) (Blumenthal and Glaser, 2007). The other four functions of an EHR are designed to enable health information exchange (HIE) across organizational boundaries and more fully engage the patient in his or her own care through home monitoring, telehealth, and other means. To achieve HIE, the systems must be interoperable. **Interoperability** is the ability of a system to exchange electronic health information with and use electronic health information from other systems without special effort on the part of the user (ONC, 2015). It is often referred to as systems being able to "talk to each other."

Table 13.1 Functions of an EHR System as Defined by the Institute of Medicine

Core Functionalities	Other Functionalities
Health information and data: Includes medical and nursing diagnoses, a medication list, allergies, demographics, clinical narratives, and laboratory test results	*Electronic communication and connectivity*: Enables those involved in patient care to communicate effectively with each other and with the patient; technologies to facilitate communication and connectivity may include e-mail, Web messaging, and telemedicine
Results management: Manages all types of results (e.g., laboratory test results, radiology procedure results) electronically	*Patient support*: Includes everything from patient education materials to home monitoring to telehealth

Table 13.1 Functions of an EHR System as Defined by the Institute of Medicine *(Continued)*

Core Functionalities	Other Functionalities
Order entry and support: Incorporates use of computerized provider order entry, particularly in ordering medications	*Administrative processes*: Facilitates and simplifies such processes as scheduling, prior authorizations, insurance verification; may also employ decision-support tools to identify eligible patients for clinical trials or chronic disease management programs
Decision support: Employs computerized clinical decision-support capabilities such as reminders, alerts, and computer-assisted diagnosing	*Reporting and population health management*: Establishes standardized terminology and data formats for public and private sector reporting requirements

SOURCE: IOM Committee on Data Standards for Patient Safety (2003).

HISTORICAL OVERVIEW AND TODAY'S HEALTH INFORMATION TECHNOLOGY LANDSCAPE: A NATIONAL PERSPECTIVE

More than 25 years ago, the IOM published a landmark report that outlined numerous problems inherent with paper-based record systems and called for the widespread adoption of EHRs (Institute of Medicine, 1991). Studies had shown that paper-based medical record systems can lead to medical errors and duplication of services; in addition, they are often incomplete, illegible, and frequently unavailable when and where the information is needed (Burnum, 1989; Hershey, McAloon, and Bertram, 1989). Computer-based record systems could provide an electronic record of the patient's care and therefore make an abundance of information instantly available to multiple care providers, providing them with alerts and reminders and giving them access to knowledge aids and the latest research findings. The computer-based record could essentially "follow" a patient throughout his or her lifetime and instantly track all relevant health, mental, and social well-being information electronically (Institute of Medicine, 1991). However, EHR adoption rates remained limited in the two decades following the 1991 IOM report, despite the many potential benefits to be gained from using them.

In the intervening years, the IOM issued other seminal reports that detailed critical quality problems in the U.S. health care systems and recommended the increased use of health IT as a significant opportunity to address those quality issues (Institute of Medicine, 1999, 2001). There were significant technological advances in the broader society during this time, including Web-based technologies, smartphones, and other personal digital devices, such as the Fitbit and Apple Watch. Consumers are far more active in the management of their own care, with the Internet and their personal devices serving as their personal library of health information. The ubiquity of personal digital devices that track and collect individual's health information has led to a new category of data, often referred to as patient-generated data (as opposed to the data generated by health care providers). Social networks have created new ways for patients with similar conditions to connect and share information with one another. Health care organizations and providers have invested in a host of clinical applications designed to ensure patient safety, improve quality, and increase efficiency. Such systems included laboratory, radiology, and pharmacy information systems; medication administration systems with bar-coding technology; computerized provider order entry (CPOE); and other ancillary clinical systems. Despite the advances and the implementation of these applications, however, U.S. health care organizations continued to lag in the adoption and use of EHR systems (Wager, Lee, and Glaser, 2017).

Three U.S. presidents have called for the widespread adoption of EHR systems since the IOM report was first published. Most recently, President Obama included in the American Recovery and Reinvestment Act of 2009 (also known as ARRA or the stimulus act) a section known as the Health Information Technology for Economic and Clinical Health Act, otherwise known as the HITECH Act. The HITECH Act set forth a plan for advancing the adoption and appropriate use of health IT to improve quality of care and establish a foundation for the electronic exchange and use of information (Blumenthal, 2009). The main method of stimulating EHR adoption and use was through incentives payments from Medicare and Medicaid to eligible hospitals and providers that implemented certified EHRs in a way that fully integrated these tools into the care delivery process and led to "meaningful use." The term "meaningful use" had a specific meaning that provided detail on how eligible providers had to use these systems to receive incentive payments (Blumenthal and Tavenner, 2010). In general, eligible providers included nonfederal acute care hospitals and office-based physician practices.

The Office of the National Coordinator for Health Information Technology (ONC) was established by George W. Bush in 2004 but substantial funding for HIT adoption and use did not appear before the HITECH Act. The HITECH Act allocated more than $30 billion in stimulus funding to achieve the widespread adoption and meaningful use of health IT (Blumenthal and Tavenner, 2010). This was the largest investment in federal funds ever made to help spearhead the widespread adoption and meaningful use of health IT in the United States, including funding for workforce development and health IT training. Whether this was enough funding to achieve an interoperable and secure nationwide health information system is as yet an unanswered question.

Since 2009, EHR adoption and meaningful use among eligible providers has increased dramatically. Initially, eligible hospitals that had already adopted some level of EHRs were the main beneficiaries of incentive payments, but eventually eligible hospitals that did not have EHRs at the start of the program also adopted them.

Currently, according to the ONC, nearly 84 percent of eligible nonfederal hospitals have adopted at least a basic EHR system by 2015 (EHR systems can be classified in several ways, most commonly by the degree of functionality. See Table 13.2 for a classification of basic and fully functional EHRs), a ninefold increase from 2008, before the HITECH Act was passed (The Office of the National Coordinator for Health Information Technology, 2015) (see Figure 13.1). While there was some concern when the HITECH Act was first passed that the amount of money allocated was not sufficient to spur significant advances in health IT adoption, the ensuing increase was unprecedented in the United States compared to the incredibly slow progress during the two preceding decades following the first IOM report.

Even with this significant increase, evidence suggests that small and rural hospitals continue to lag in EHR adoption and meaningful use, and that up-front and ongoing costs, physician cooperation, and the complexity of meeting meaningful use requirements continue to be barriers (Adler-Milstein et al., 2015). Further, noneligible hospitals, including psychiatric, long-term care, and rehabilitation hospitals continue to have low EHR adoption rates of approximately 10 percent compared to

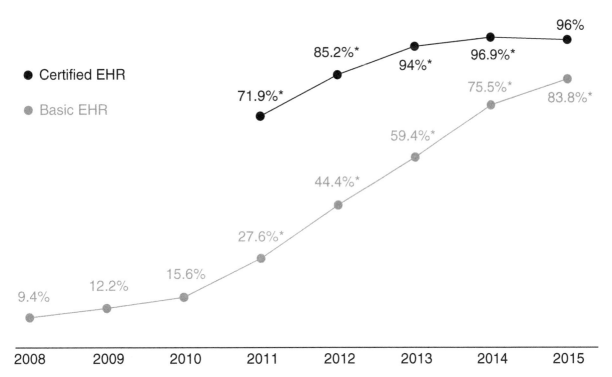

Figure 13.1 Percentage of Nonfederal Acute Care Hospitals with Adoption of at Least a Basic EHR with Notes System and Possession of a Certified EHR, 2008–2015.

NOTE: Basic EHR adoption requires the EHR system to have a set of EHR functions defined in Table 13.1. A certified EHR is EHR technology that meets the technology capability, functionality, and security requirements adopted by the Department of Health and Human Services. Possession means that the hospital has a legal agreement with the EHR vendor but is not equivalent to adoption. *Significantly different from previous year (p < .05).

SOURCE: ONC (2015).

the 84 percent among eligible hospitals. There also continue to be low levels of interoperability, including low participation in HIEs, that facilitate sharing information across care settings, and the number of HIEs in general is declining (Adler-Milstein, Lin, and Jha, 2016; Walker et al., 2016). On the other hand, the ability of eligible hospitals to report public health data, including electronically reporting to immunization registries, laboratory results, and syndromic surveillance, has significantly increased (Walker and Diana, 2015). Federal government hospitals were not eligible for incentive payments, but the Veteran's Administration had already established its own system-wide interoperable EHR system.

In addition to acute care hospitals, the growth in the adoption and use of EHRs in office-based physician practice settings has also increased considerably. As of 2014, 79 percent of primary care physicians and 70 percent of medical and surgical specialties had adopted a certified EHR system (Heisey-Grove and Patel, 2015). Considering that the main goal of adopting health

IT is to improve the quality, effectiveness, and efficiency of health care delivery, there is some evidence that hospitals adopting EHRs have improved their adherence to process measures and patient satisfaction (Adler-Milstein, Everson, and Lee, 2015; Kazley, Diana, and Menachemi, 2012).

The dramatic increase in EHR adoption since the passage of the HITECH Act, at least among eligible providers, has led to a shift in emphasis away from adopting health IT to how the data and information derived from it can be used to improve quality, effectiveness, and efficiency. Adoption alone is not sufficient to achieve these goals. Optimization and integration of the systems is vital to providing key stakeholders (patients, providers, payers, etc.) with the information needed to effectively manage population health. Therefore, we will focus our discussion in this chapter on the external environment that health care providers face and on how health IT capabilities can help support strategic initiatives to respond to the rapidly changing environment.

Table 13.2 Functions Defining Use of EHRs

	Basic System	Fully Functional System
Health Information Data		
Patient demographics	X	X
Patient problem lists	X	X
Electronic lists of medications taken by patients	X	X
Clinical notes	X	X
Notes including medical history and follow-up		X
Order Entry Management		
Orders for prescriptions	X	X
Orders for laboratory tests		X
Orders for radiology tests		X
Prescriptions sent electronically		X
Orders sent electronically		X
Results Management		
Viewing laboratory results	X	X
Viewing imaging results	X	X
Electronic images returned		X
Clinical Decision Support		
Warnings of drug interactions or contraindications provided		X
Out-of-range test levels highlighted		X
Reminders regarding guidelines-based interventions or screening		X

SOURCE: DesRoches et al. (2008).

CHANGING HEALTH ENVIRONMENT RELIES ON EFFECTIVE USE OF HEALTH IT

The Affordable Care Act

President Obama signed the Affordable Care Act (ACA) in 2010. The goals of the ACA are to improve access; reduce the cost of services and bend the overall cost curve; and improve the quality of health care service delivery, health outcomes, and public health. These goals are consistent with the Triple Aim of improving the patient experience, including quality and satisfaction; improving population health; and reducing cost (Whittington et al., 2015). The components of the ACA that address these goals include coverage expansion and insurance market reforms to expand access, payment reforms to reduce costs, and delivery system reforms to improve quality. Many of these reforms have implications for health care providers and health IT. Furthermore, other delivery system models have implications for using health IT including, for example, patient-centered medical homes.

One of the key components of the ACA that affects health IT is coverage expansion. The ACA included provisions to expand Medicaid eligibility and to offer a variety of health insurance plans for people who do not qualify for Medicare or Medicaid and who do not have employer-based insurance. Coverage expansion means that health care providers are likely to have more patients, and many of these may be sicker and have more complicated heath care needs, although this is still somewhat uncertain.

Among the most important reforms under the ACA that influence health IT are the various payment reforms. Most of these programs represent a shift in emphasis from paying for service delivery to paying for value. Value refers to the level of quality given the level of cost. The major initiatives that focus on paying for value include the EHR Incentive Program, originated in the ARRA legislation and now replaced in the Medicare Access and Chip Reauthorization Act (MACRA) of 2015; the value-based purchasing (VBP) program; the Medicare Shared Savings Program; and various other initiatives.

Hospital Value-Based Purchasing

The hospital VBP program uses previously reported quality measures to compare hospital performance. Quality measures include performance in the areas of acute myocardial infarction (MI), heart failure, pneumonia, certain surgeries, hospital-acquired conditions, and patient experience of care. In general, hospitals with higher-quality performance are paid more than hospitals with lower performance, all else equal. Quality performance scores are based on achievement, that is, hospitals are compared to a threshold and benchmark for all other hospitals and on improvement over time by an individual hospital.

For hospitals to determine the amount of potential VBP incentive payments they could receive in any given year, they must determine how well they are performing on the various quality measures and be able to calculate the quality performance scores they will receive based on a comparison of their own quality scores to the benchmarks for all hospitals and on their own improvement. For example, if a hospital has an acute MI mortality rate below the benchmark for all hospitals, and it is then able to improve its acute MI mortality rate in the following year, that hospital would earn 10 achievement points. Similarly, because this hospital improved its acute MI mortality rate above its own prior rate, it would earn 9 improvement points. In subsequent years, if our imaginary hospital's acute MI mortality rate stayed above the benchmark of all hospitals, it would still earn the 10 achievement points, but it would not earn improvement points if its own acute MI mortality rate did not improve. These points accumulated through the various quality measures result in incentive payments to the hospital.

Most, if not all the quality measures can be captured by various health IT applications, including EHRs. If these measures are captured in health IT applications, and if they can be shared with other parts of the organization, for example, the financing function, then the hospital can set quality improvement targets and determine the potential impact on its financial performance. In this way, the hospital can determine strategic priorities for its quality improvement efforts under the VBP program.

Accountable Care Organizations

The Medicare Shared Savings Program is an option for providers to participate in that offers the potential to share savings with the Centers for Medicare and Medicaid Services (CMS) if certain benchmarks are met. Participating organizations are known as accountable care organizations (ACOs). Providers organized as ACOs can share in cost savings to the Medicare program for meeting cost and quality benchmarks. This model attempts to promote accountability, care coordination, and process redesign. Providers are eligible for ACO participation under a formal legal structure and shared governance mechanism. ACOs represent a cooperative effort of providers that come together to provide care to a defined population, but that are not necessarily organized as a single integrated organization. Participating providers can include physicians and other health care providers in group practice arrangements, networks of individual practices of ACO professionals, partnerships or joint ventures between hospitals and ACO professionals, and others as determined by HHS. An ACO must be accountable for cost, quality, and overall care of Medicare beneficiaries assigned to it. Private insurers are also operating ACOs with the same essential goals but with varying details of participation and risk sharing.

Providers that choose to participate in ACOs must be able to track the cost and quality of care they provide to ACO beneficiaries, much like the description in the section on VBP above. However, ACOs face the additional challenge of sharing information on cost and quality performance across organizational settings. Further, they need to share information on care coordination for patients who receive care across the various ACO participants. This means that organizations participating in ACOs need to not only have adequate health IT internally, such as EHRs, but the health IT must also be interoperable across organizations to be successful in generating savings.

Bundled Payments

Another payment reform introduced in the ACA is bundled payment (Kaiser Family Foundation, 2016). This is a five-year pilot program to develop Medicare bundled payment for "episodes of care," which includes an acute inpatient episode and physician, outpatient, and post-acute services. This program focuses on coordination, quality, and efficiency of services around hospitalization for one or more selected conditions (Kaiser Family Foundation, 2016). Like the ACO program, CMS will calculate a target price for an episode of care, such as a knee replacement. If the provider can deliver the care for less cost than the target price, they can share in the savings, and if they deliver the care for higher cost than the target price, then the provider may lose money on that episode. Once again, in this scenario, providers must have access to timely and accurate information about the cost of all the components of the episode of care and use that information to determine if and how they can deliver the care below the target price.

There are a variety of other payment reduction programs, many of them focused on inpatient settings, that also have implications for the use of health IT. These programs include efforts to reduce hospital 30-day readmissions, reduce health care–associated infections, and the VBP program. Hospitals are at risk of having Medicare reimbursement reduced if the 30-day readmission rate is too high, the rate of health care–associated infections is too high, or they do not meet quality benchmarks set by the VBP program. The strategic application of health IT can support efforts to be successful under these various programs. An example would be using predictive analytics to identify patients at high risk of readmission within 30 days to allow for targeted interventions to reduce such a readmission.

Medicare Access and Chip Reauthorization Act of 2015

The EHR Incentive Program originated in the HITECH Act has been replaced by MACRA, which means changing requirements for health IT. MACRA consolidates various quality-based payment initiatives (e.g., the EHR Incentive Program and the Physician Quality Reporting System) into one program called the Quality Payment Program (QPP). The QPP has two paths—the Merit-Based Incentive Payment System (MIPS) and Alternative Payment Models (APMs). MIPS is a program that combines various quality reporting programs into a single incentive payment program that measures eligible professionals (EPs) on quality, resource use, clinical practice improvement, and meaningful use of certified EHR technology (also called advancing care information). Advancing care information represents changes to the previous EHR Incentive Program. The CMS has six objectives with associated measures that participating providers are required to report: protecting patient information, electronic prescribing, patient electronic access (patient portals), coordination of care through patient engagement, HIE, and public health and clinical data registry reporting. Providers have some choice in selecting the measures in each of these objectives. This approach differs from the EHR Incentive Program by removing the all or nothing measurement threshold, removing redundant measures, and dropping the CPOE and CDS objectives.

Providers can also receive incentive payments for participating in APMs. Examples of APMs include ACOs, patient-centered medical homes (PCMHs), and bundled payment models. MACRA does not change how any APM functions or rewards value but creates extra incentives for APM participation. To be considered an APM, entities must require participants to use certified EHR technology, payments must be based on quality measures comparable to those in the MIPS quality performance category, and entities must either (1) bear more than nominal financial risk for monetary losses (as defined by CMS) or (2) be a Medical Home Model expanded under the Center for Medicare & Medicaid Innovation (CMMI). To illustrate the importance of health IT in these kinds of care delivery models, consider that a Medical Home Model that qualifies as an APM has the following features:

- Participants include primary care practices and offer primary care services (they may also offer specialty services).
- Each patient is empaneled to a primary care clinician.
- It at least displays four of the following characteristics:
  - Planned coordination of chronic and preventive care
  - Patient access and continuity of care

- Risk-stratified care management
- Coordination of care across the medical neighborhood
- Patient and caregiver engagement
- Shared decision making
- Payment arrangements in addition to, or substituting for, fee-for-service payments

Many of these features require sophisticated and integrated health IT systems to support such activities as care coordination, continuity of care, and risk stratification. Health IT can also be valuable in patient and caregiver engagement activities. Since many of the payment models that emphasize value include a variety of quality performance metrics, the ability to apply health IT to improve the quality of care is critical to successfully functioning in this new environment.

HEALTH IT RAMIFICATIONS OF PAYMENT REFORM AND NEW MODELS OF CARE

The Context and Shift in Perspective

The shift to APMs and new care delivery models requires integration and coordination of care among providers and strategies for engaging patients in managing their health. Consequently, health care leaders and provider organizations are considering a wide range of integration options including everything from direct ownership through vertical and horizontal integration to looser forms of integration exemplified by accountable care. Many are starting small by participating in demonstration projects that test Medicare payment models, such as ones designed to improve care management of high-risk patients (PwC Health Research Institute, 2015). Regardless of the APM or model of care employed, to be successful in achieving the Triple Aim, data integration is critical. The industry must come together with a common purpose and focus on care coordination, quality improvement, and cost reduction (Glaser, 2012). Those assuming financial risk must have an effective population health management strategy in to keep their "cohort" of patients healthy, minimizing the need for expensive interventions, such as emergency department visits, hospitalizations, diagnostic and imaging tests, and procedures (Felt-Lisk and Higgins, 2011). And, although PHM often focuses largely on high-risk patients who generate the majority of health costs, it also systematically addresses the preventive and chronic care needs of every patient (Population Health Management, 2012). This requires a fundamental shift in industry perspectives and health care delivery practice and a greater reliance on data and health IT as illustrated in Figure 13.2.

- From care providers working independently of each other to collaborative teams of providers
- From treating individuals when they get sick to keeping groups of people healthy
- From emphasizing volumes to emphasizing outcomes
- From maximizing the use of resources and assets to applying appropriate levels of care at the right place
- From offering care at centralized facilities to offering care at sites convenient to patients
- From treating all patients the same way to customizing health care for each patient
- From avoiding the sickest chronically ill patients to creating venues to provide special chronic care services
- From being responsible for those who seek services to being responsible for the needs of the community
- From putting forth best efforts to becoming high-reliability organizations

Figure 13.2 Changes in Health Industry Perspectives and Care Delivery.

SOURCE: Glaser (2016).

The shift in perspective and practice has profound implications on data management and the issue of how health IT is used to support clinical and financial accountability. Health systems and providers will need to ensure that patients have access to the right resources and services, at the right time, and in the right setting based on the patients' needs and preferences. Care coordination is critical. Equally important, health systems and providers must be able to provide the patient-centered, coordinated quality care in a cost-effective manner.

To this end, health systems and providers need ready access to accurate, timely, and complete patient information across the continuum of care. The need for aggregated data across the continuum of care has been understood as an essential element to reforming the U.S. health care delivery system for decades. It was not until this past decade, however, that it truly seemed within reach. Much of the change can be attributed to the dramatic growth in the adoption and use of EHR systems, largely attributed to the HITECH Act and the CMS EHR incentive programs.

The widespread adoption and use of EHR systems alone, however, is not enough to facilitate care coordination and population health management. Effective data exchange and the translation of data into meaningful improvements in health outcomes remain largely unrealized (Phillips et al., 2015). Lack of interoperability remains a significant barrier. In short, interoperability is "the ability of systems to exchange and use electronic health information from other systems without special effort on the part of the user" (Institute for Electrical and Electronics Engineering [IEEE], n.d.). The ONC issued a report *Connecting Health and Care for the Nation: A Shared Nationwide Interoperability Roadmap* (ONC, 2015) that outlines three critical pathways to achieving health IT interoperability: (1) requiring standards; (2) motivating the use of those standards through appropriate incentives; and (3) creating a trusted environment for the collecting, sharing, and using of electronic health information. The roadmap requires collaboration and partnership. Providers must be willing to share the information they have generated, different health care information systems must be able to communicate with each other securely, and health IT vendors must have incentives to play together (Glaser, 2015). A recent qualitative study among clinicians and IT leaders from six regions of the United States found that significant care coordination gaps exist due to the lack of interoperability (Samal et al., 2016). The researchers found that the largest gaps were in information transfer, systems to monitor patients, tools to support patients' self-management goals, and tools to link patients and their caregivers with community resources (Samal et al., 2016). Similarly, another study found that among physicians who used EHRs, at least one-third, and sometimes more than half, of them did not routinely receive patient information needed to coordinate care (Hsiao et al., 2015). Additionally, many of the health care organizations that invested early and heavily in PHM and risk-based contracts found that they were confused by an unclear vision of IT capability requirements, lack of internal expertise, and build versus buy considerations for what is emerging as a new business model (Hunt et al. 2015). Core IT capabilities and functions including the use of data analytics, however, should be considered in any population health management strategy and in preparing for value-based reimbursement.

Core Health IT Features and Functions

Although EHRs are useful patient documentation tools and can aid in adherence to evidence-based practice guidelines and reducing errors, they alone are not sufficient in assisting health care organizations and providers with the tools needed to grow their ability to manage population health effectively. Again, in an era of increased clinical and financial accountability, other core health IT functionality and capabilities are needed including the following:

- *Revenue cycle and contracts management application*: Beyond performing the routine tasks of registering patients, scheduling appointments, and administering bills, systems that support the revenue cycle must be able to support payments based on quality and performance, requiring capabilities, such as the following:
  - Aggregating charges to form bundled payments, with aggregation logic that supports different groupings for different payers
  - Managing the distribution of payment(s) among a team of health care providers and organizations
  - Facilitating retrospective and prospective analysis of clinical and administrative data to identify opportunities to improve quality and reduce costs (Glaser, 2012)

- *Population and patient registries*: The ability to compile and use population and patient registries from different sources in order to monitor patients, provide outreach, engage in care management, stratify population/patients based on risk, identify care gaps, and report on quality metrics. Registries can be useful tools in tracking when patient was last seen, treatment received, and current health status. They can also be used for patient monitoring, point-of-care reminders, and public health reporting (Handmaker and Hart, 2015).

- *Health information exchange*: The ability to share health information with patients and among different care providers and settings in a standardized electronic format in safe/secure environment. Having relevant and timely information available in the format needed is critical to the success of accountable care. For example, through HIE primary care providers may be notified when their patients visit the emergency department or are hospitalized. They can also access recent test results leading to reduction in duplicate tests. The goal is to enable health care providers to share information seamlessly when and where it is needed.

- *Care management*: Care management is a set of systems and capabilities that support proactive, preventative, and cost-effective care for individuals and populations. Specific capabilities include managing transitions of care, care coordination, disease management, and population management (Glaser, 2012). Many care management functions can be automated to facilitate the appropriate level of care and intervention needed.

- *Patient engagement tools*: A wide range of health IT tools and applications are available that may be useful in engaging patients in managing their health and care and in communicating with care givers. Examples include personal health records (PHRs), patient portals (which are typically Web portals that enable patients to access their health record, schedule appointments, refill prescriptions, send a nonurgent message to their provider, and pay bills online), remote monitoring at home or through mobile devices, automated reminders and messages, and online health assessments, to name a few. Patients are also using social media platforms, such as *Patients Like Me* to find patients with similar conditions or as a means of support, sensor devices, and apps, such as MyFitness Pal and Fitbit to monitor blood sugar, exercise, and diet.

- ***Data analytic tools including predictive analytics***: The massive increase in the collection of patient and financial data in electronic form has led to the rise of "Big Data" and health systems leveraging its use of analytics to make better clinical and financial decisions. Advanced population analytics can be used to assess how different segments of patient populations are doing as well as assess the clinical and financial performance of individual care providers, team care, and the organization.

- ***Performance and quality reporting measures***: Measuring performance including quality and financial outcomes requires business intelligence and advanced workflow and rules engines. These tools can be used to monitor process performance; integrate disparate types of data with evidence-based guidelines; and assist clinical decision making by presenting care givers with alerts, reminders, and changes in patient conditions. Dashboards can also be used to analyze data over time to identify trends and gaps in care.

- ***Ability to migrate to precision medicine***: Health care has been designed historically for the average or typical patient; however, much is changing with the emergence of precision medicine. Precision medicine is an innovative approach to disease prevention and treatment that takes into account individual differences, genetics, environments, and lifestyles. It provides care givers with tools to better understand the complex mechanisms underlying a patient's health, disease, or condition, and to better predict which treatments will be most effective (Fact Sheet: President Obama's Precision Medicine Initiative, 2015). In the future, a health system or organization's ability to support precision medicine may have profound implications for providing the "right" care to each patient.

- ***Telemedicine and telehealth***: Hospitals, physician practices, and other organizations are using telemedicine and telehealth technologies to provide patients with greater convenience and access to health care services. Examples include two-way interactive video, equipping patients with devices that can be used to collect and monitor vital health information, e-visits, remote monitoring of e-ICUs, and patient access to health education and self-management through the Internet (Kvedar, Coye, and Everett, 2014).

Many health systems and providers are still in the early stages of dabbling in designing and implementing alternative models of care for managing a defined population under value-based payment. In fact, some are focusing efforts on optimizing the use of EHRs into practice and exploring how best to use the systems to transform care processes, patient experiences, and outcomes (Creswell, Bates, and Sheikh, 2016). There are examples of leaders in the field, such as the 17 Beacon Communities located across the nation, that received grant funding under the HITECH Act to use health IT in innovative ways and measure its impact on achieving care coordination, quality, and cost reduction (Singer et al., 2015). Experiences and outcomes of the Beacon Community projects and initiatives may be found on the ONC's website (Health IT.gov., n.d.).

STRATEGIC ALIGNMENT

Within the ever-changing health care environment and the shift to value-based reimbursement, it is increasingly critical that the health IT plans align with the overall strategic plan of the organization or health system. Health IT investments are not one-time activities. They are significant and ongoing. Health IT resources include not only the specific data, applications, security, and infrastructure described above but also the human resources or staff needed to maintain, support, train, and ensure systems are available all day every day.

The ability to align the health IT strategy with the organizational strategy is a key factor for the successful adoption of health IT. There are many ways an organization can make strategic decisions about what kind of health IT capabilities it needs to achieve its goals and objectives. Among these are the standard strategic planning tools, including analysis of the internal and external environments and the identification of strategic opportunities and threats. Such activities should result in a set of long- and short-term goals and objectives for the organization. The development of goals and objectives may be impacted by the availability of new technology that enables new ways of doing things, which requires a thorough and thoughtful assessment of the potential of emerging technologies.

Organizational strategies can drive the development of health IT strategies and result in a set of IS goals and objectives that are explicitly linked to higher-level goals and objectives. This is an explicit approach to strategic alignment that would require, for example, any health IT proposal to demonstrate a clear link to the organization's goals and objectives. This approach may be used regardless of how alignment is achieved, but it is sometimes problematic, particularly for infrastructure types of projects. For example, it may be difficult to link an enterprise-wide network upgrade to specific goals and objectives, but such an upgrade could have a significant impact on the success of other health IT projects.

Other approaches can also link directly to an organization's strategic outlook. For example, an organization may be committed to continuous improvement, which could be reflected in a health IT strategy of continuous improvement in processes and management. The development of a health IT strategy may be driven by fundamental views about the nature of competition and the role of health IT in facilitating competitive advantage (Wager, Lee, and Glaser, 2017).

Successful strategic alignment should result in a set of health IT projects that the organization has identified as important to its strategic direction or for sustaining existing capabilities. This portfolio of projects typically includes pending requests, projects approved but not begun, and projects that are in progress. This portfolio of health IT projects should be managed by an executive-level team that includes both senior business and health IT executives. This team prioritizes projects in the portfolio and determines which project to fund in the current period, which to fund later, and which will have to wait. In this way, the strategic direction of the organization is linked directly to the ongoing health IT projects.

To be successful in health IT adoption, the strategic-level questions must eventually give way to questions of execution. In other words, an organization must move from the "what and why" to the "how" of adopting and using health IT. One advantage of achieving strategic alignment is that it tends to lead to another critical factor in the success of health IT projects, which is executive level and clinical leadership support. High-level support for health IT projects not only communicates to the rest of the organization that they are serious about adopting the system in question, but it also increases the chances of having the necessary resources dedicated to the project. Executive leadership can allocate the financial and human resources needed to increase the chances of project success. These resources should be directed toward such critical activities as user involvement and training, change management, and incentive programs.

It is crucial to understand that health IT includes the data, processes, people, information technology, and the way these components interact to collect, process, store, and present information that supports the organization (Whitten and Bentley, 2005). Health IT is not simply a collection of computers and software. They are generally complex systems, and therefore it is critical to approach their acquisition, implementation, and management with proven methodologies. The obvious analogy is architecture. Architects have perfected a methodology for successfully completing highly complex projects. Anyone who has worked with an architect to build a house or a hospital have been exposed to at least parts of this methodology (see Zachman [1987] for an early description of this analogy). One should no sooner attempt to build a complex information system without a methodological approach than they should try to build a hospital without one.

Even though many providers have adopted EHRs and other health IT, they are continually faced with several fundamental challenges to its ongoing use. First, health care organizations must integrate the technology into their systems of care delivery. This means moving beyond the period of adoption to one of appropriate and effective use of the technology. For example, assume that hospital leadership has decided that reducing 30-day readmissions is a strategic priority. One way to do this might be to establish the ability to share information with primary care physicians in the community, perhaps as a part of an ACO the hospital belongs to, or a patient-centered medical home. The proposal for a health IT project to enable this kind of information sharing—perhaps to implement an HIE—rests on the assumption that implementing the health IT solution would both enable information sharing across the involved organizations, and that the number of 30-day readmissions would decline as a result. Thus, the health IT implementation is appropriate in that it has been implemented in response to a strategic priority and it is effective if it has enabled the hospital to reduce 30-day readmissions.

Second, adopting any technology is only the beginning, as that technology must be maintained and managed as any organizational asset. A health IT application does not function by itself. People must be trained to use it in specific ways for it to perform its intended function. Much like any tool, the ability to achieve the desired results depends on choosing the right tool and on being able to use the tool effectively. Effective training also required evaluating the use of the technology to identify weaknesses and opportunities for improvement. Further, there must be plans for upgrading and replacing the technology, and the systems they support, as advances in technology and our understanding of the best methods of care delivery increase. This means that the organization must maintain a certain level of human resource capability with managing its technology and system to continue benefiting from the technology, and all of this must be done in alignment with the overall strategy of the organization.

ASSESSING HEALTH IT PERFORMANCE AND VALUE TO THE HEALTH CARE ORGANIZATION

If we accept the notion that health IT can support the strategic goals of the organization, and if we go about managing it with the expectation that it will support those goals, it makes sense that we should evaluate how well our health IT has achieved its intended goals. This is a more difficult proposition than it may seem at first, however. This is partly because the nature of health IT varies, as discussed previously, from enterprise-wide infrastructure technologies to department-specific clinical information systems. How does one assess the value of laying fiber optic cable, an enterprise-wide technology, as it relates to the strategic goals of the organization? It is unlikely that the organization strategy would include investing in fiber optic cable or even increasing the bandwidth of its network. Further, the performance of these systems in terms of achieving strategic value may hinge more on their collective performance than their individual performance. For example, analyzing the ability to integrate and share data across a single institution may be a different assessment than the ability to integrate and share data across a continuum of care.

To try to make this clearer, go back to the example we gave above of a hospital with the strategic goal of reducing 30-day readmissions that decides to implement an HIE to be able to share information with primary care providers that are participating in an ACO with the hospital. The hospital and primary care providers must all have functioning EHR systems in place that can provide the information to be shared through the HIE before the HIE itself can be useful. Each health care organization would need to assess the value it has achieved from its EHR implementations. All the health care organizations participating in the ACO would need to assess the value achieved through implementing the HIE. These are likely to be quite different assessments, and the value of the HIE hinges on the collective performance of all of these systems.

One key to a meaningful assessment of health IT performance is to choose the correct metric or metrics for assessment. For example, not all health IT projects will yield a positive return on investment (ROI), but if the system is designed to enable achievement of a strategic goal of the organization, the ROI of that system is not the appropriate metric, even if it were positive. This is complicated by the fact that many information systems have diverse value propositions within and across proposals. A single system can potentially improve service and productivity, reduce cost, and generate revenue, while other proposals under consideration may cost significantly

more or less, and have widely differing risks and benefits. This is not to say that formal financial analysis of proposals and implemented systems is not warranted, but that such an analysis may not be the only or the best measure of the outcome of a health IT investment.

For the organization to assess the impact of health IT on the ability of the organization to achieve its strategic goals, the organization must link its health IT investments to its organizational strategy. Without this linkage, the IS function may be performing at a high level but doing the wrong things, or it may be that the IS function is supporting the overall strategy, but that strategy may be the wrong one. The Agency for Healthcare Research and Quality (AHRQ) has developed a useful toolkit for evaluating IT projects (Cusack et al., 2009). The evaluation process begins with defining the goals of the project and the goals of the evaluation itself, which should include a discussion of who the intended audiences are for the evaluation.

The next step in the evaluation process is to link the health IT project goals to outcome measures. This linking should be explicit and a range of outcome measures should be considered, both quantitative and qualitative. The key is to choose valid measures that will allow you to determine how well the project is meeting its stated goals. Once measures are chosen, they should be assessed for validity, importance, and feasibility. Linking the potential impact of the project on the measure can assess validity; the greater the potential impact on the measure, the more suitable the measure is for evaluating the project. Similarly, rate each measure on its importance to the stakeholders or to those who will receive the evaluation report. Then, determine the feasibility of obtaining the data necessary for the measure. Those measures that are both high in importance and highly feasible are sure candidates for inclusion on the evaluation. Last, choose the study design, including an assessment of the cost of the study. The study design should include both a timing approach and data collection strategies. Once these activities have been concluded, an overall evaluation plan should be developed. The plan should include all the components discussed.

Health IT projects are largely costly investments, with often widely varying impacts. They are difficult to implement in any industry setting but perhaps more so in health care—and particularly across a spectrum of care. Such costly investments are difficult to justify without a clear understanding of the impact throughout the organization. A solid evaluation plan that is an integral part of the project from the beginning provides a means of assessing such impacts and of the overall value of the project. This information can be invaluable when considering whether to engage in future projects and in an organization's ability to successfully conduct such projects.

SUMMARY AND MANAGERIAL GUIDELINES

1. In recent years, EHR systems have been widely adopted in U.S. acute care hospitals and physician practice settings, largely due to financial incentives made available through the HITECH Act of 2009. The EHR incentive program has been replaced by MACRA, which has health IT implications and reporting requirements for health care providers.

2. Changes in the health environment, such the movement to value-based payment and new models of care delivery (such as accountable care organizations and PCMH), have implications for data management and the use of health IT to support clinical and financial accountability.

3. Core health IT features and functions needed in the era of increased clinical and financial accountability include the following:

    a. Revenue cycle and contracts management application

    b. Population and patient registries

    c. Health information exchange

    d. Care management

    e. Patient engagement tools

    f. Data analytic tools including predictive analytics

    g. Performance and quality reporting measures

    h. Ability to migrate to precision medicine

    i. Telehealth and telemedicine

4. Investing in EHR and other types of health IT is not something that should be taken lightly. It is critical that information systems plans are well aligned with the overall strategic plans of the health care organization and their value to the organization should be managed and assessed.

DISCUSSION QUESTIONS

1. What are the primary features and functions of an EHR system? How does an EHR differ from merely automating the patient's record?

2. The IOM called for the CPR or EHR to become the standard in 1991, yet it wasn't until 2015 that it became a reality. Why was that? What were barriers to EHR adoption and use, and how were the primary barriers overcome? To what extent have the goals of the HITECH Act been achieved?

3. Discuss the health IT implications of today's health care environment, which is focused on increased clinical and financial accountability and value-based payment and new models of care.

4. Review the literature or interview health leaders in your community to find examples of how health IT tools are being employed to facilitate the organization's ability to manage patient care and population health more effectively.

5. Interview a senior leader in a local organization in your community. To what extent do the organization's health IT plans align with the overall strategic plans of the organization. How are health IT priorities established? How does the organization assess the value of its health IT investments?

CASE: THE COLLABORATIVE CARE NETWORK

The following case was written by Dayle Benson, a doctoral student in the executive health administration and leadership program at the Medical University of South Carolina. The case has been edited for educational purposes. It is used with permission.

The Setting

Six months ago, leaders from the Mason Clinic, Franklin Medical Clinic, Landmark Clinic, Optimum Medical Group, Banner Clinic, and the University Medical Group came together with the intent to form a physician-led delivery network or independent physician association (IPA) capable of improving the health status of the community by fostering exceptional outcomes and patient experience at an appropriate cost. The new entity is called the Collaborative Care Network.

Across the country, patients, employers, and payers are demanding greater accountability from the health care system. Multiple initiatives, some sponsored by employers and others by the federal government, are designed to incent providers to pursue the "Triple Aim"—a better patient experience, improved health for the population, and reduced cost (Berwick, Nolan, and Wittingham, 2008). Traditional fee-for-service models that reward providing more care are being replaced by so-called "value-based reimbursement," which places a greater onus on providers to better manage both quality and cost.

Providers recognize the need to adapt and are pursuing a variety of approaches with the intent to achieve and document improved outcomes, better control utilization and costs, and improve access and patient satisfaction. Physicians and health systems recognize that broader access, more effective alignment, and significant capital resources will be required to achieve these ends. As a result, hospitals are employing more physicians, physician groups are consolidating, and there is an increase in participation in clinically integrated networks.

The Collaborative Care Network is to be built upon the strong and trusted patient–physician relationship to develop a care philosophy and model capable of providing differentiated outcomes. Through clinical integration, the independent groups will work collectively to improve the clinical care processes and serve the population more effectively. One of the design components critical to the success of the network's market position is that information will be shared freely across the network, emphasizing a data-driven approach for protocol development, intervention design, and patient management.

A core competency of the Collaborative Care's success is the ability to share information with patients and health care providers that allows for better care management, improved clinical outcomes, and effective use of clinical resources. The network will provide data aggregation, analytics, and reporting to support care management, while the practices may utilize their own population health management tools. Data will be used to stratify population and manage performance. Network physicians and leadership will use that data to analyze performance for continuous improvement and to be able to meaningfully document that same performance for patients, payers, and employers. Those metrics will include quality metrics (e.g., patient-reported outcomes, specialty society outcomes, HEDIS), utilization measures (e.g., hospital admissions and readmissions, ED admits, high-cost imaging studies), and cost profiles (e.g., per member per month by physician).

The Network's Information Systems (IS) Challenge

The IS challenge is that each of these groups has their own governance structure and a different EHR system. Payers in market do not currently share patient-level data across different organizations. Although a HIE exists, it is uncertain as to how much information is being submitted and whether or not those data are retrievable in a manner that allows for coordinated population health management and monitoring. In order to be successful, the Collaborative Care Network will need to develop an analytical platform that can be used across the groups. At a minimum, the network will need data sharing to stratify patient populations and measure quality and utilization performance. Based on the data, care management interventions can be developed and implemented at the practice level. Developing the information systems to do this effectively will require significant investment. Capabilities must include the following:

- Ability to collect information from multiple systems and organizations
- Systems to analyze and report on aggregated data to identify opportunities to improve quality and reduce cost and unnecessary utilization
- Actionable data, analytics, and reporting that will be pushed out to the medical groups and providers in a secure environment

Questions

1. Assume you were an integral part of the executive leadership team involved in developing a strategic IS plan that is well aligned with the goals of the new Collaborative Care Network. Who would you recommend serve on the planning team? How would you assess the IS capabilities and functions needed to support the goals of the Collaborative Care Network? What challenges might you face? How might you overcome these challenges?

2. To what extent is interoperability a critical success factor in sharing data among the physician practices? And among different EHR systems? Conduct a review of the literature to examine the current state of interoperability and HIE within your community.

3. Describe the process you would employ to identify and evaluate IS internal capabilities, IS needs/capabilities, present alternatives, and gain buy in and support from key stakeholders.

4. How will you assess success of the plan? Give examples of processes and metrics you might use.

REFERENCES

Adler-Milstein, J., DesRoches, C. M., Kralovec, P., et al. (2015). Electronic health record adoption in US hospitals: Progress continues, but challenges persist. *Health Affairs (Millwood)*, *34*(12), 2174–2180. doi:10.1377/hlthaff.2015.0992.

Adler-Milstein, J., Everson, J., & Lee, S. Y. (2015). EHR adoption and hospital performance: Time-related effects. *Health Services Research, 50*(6), 1751–1771. doi:10.1111/1475-6773.12406.

Adler-Milstein, J., Lin, S. C., & Jha, A. K. (2016). The number of health information exchange efforts is declining, leaving the viability of broad clinical data exchange uncertain. *Health Affairs (Millwood), 35*(7), 1278–1285. doi:10.1377/hlthaff.2015.1439.

Berwick, D., Nolan, T., & Wittingham, J. (2008). The triple aim: care, health, and cost. *Health Affairs, 27*(3), 759–769. doi:10.1377/hlthaff.27.3.759.

Blumenthal, D. (2009). Stimulating the adoption of health information technology. *New England Journal of Medicine, 360*(15), 1477–1479.

Blumenthal, D., & Glaser, J. P. (2007). Information technology comes to medicine. *New England Journal of Medicine, 356*(24), 2527–2534.

Blumenthal, D., & Tavenner, M. (2010). The "Meaningful Use" regulation for electronic health records. *New England Journal of Medicine, 363*(6), 501–504.

Burnum, J. F. (1989). The misinformation era: The fall of the medical record. *Annals of Internal Medicine, 110*, 482–484.

Cresswell, K. M., Bates, D. W., & Sheikh, A. (2016). Ten key considerations for the successful optimization of large-scale health information technology. *Journal of the American Medical Informatics Association, 0*, 1–5.

Cusack, C. M., Byrne, C. M., Hook, J. M., et al. (2009). *Health information technology evaluation toolkit.* Rockville, MD: Agency for Healthcare Research and Quality. Retrieved from https://healthit.ahrq.gov/sites/default/files/docs/page/health-information-technology-evaluation-toolkit-2009-update.pdf.

DesRoches, C. M., Campbell, E. G., Rao, S. R., et al. (2008). Electronic health records in ambulatory care: A national survey of physicians. *New England Journal of Medicine, 359*(1), 50–60.

Fact Sheet: President Obama's Precision Medicine Initiative. (2015). Retrieved May 1, 2017, from https:// www.whitehouse.gov/the-press-office/2015/01/30/fact-sheet-president-obama-s-precision-medicine-initiative.

Felt-Lisk, S., & Higgins, T. (2011). Exploring the promise of population health management programs to improve health. Mathematic Policy Research—Issue Brief. Retrieved from https://pdfs.semanticscholar.org/7606/d9d0ed45173b91e014c9fac8ef3b601c6f36.pdf

Glaser, J. P. (2012, April 10) Six technologies to support accountable care. *Hospitals and Health Networks Weekly.* Retrieved from https://www.hhnmag.com/articles/5529-six-key-technologies-to-support-accountable-care.

Glaser, J. P. (2015, April 14). Interoperability: A promised unfulfilled. *Hospitals and Health Networks.* Retrieved from https://www.hhnmag.com/articles/3554-interoperability-a-promise-unfulfilled.

Glaser, J. P. (2016, June 13). All roads lead to population health management. *HHN Daily.* Retrieved from https://www.hhnmag.com/articles/7332-all-roads-lead-to-population-health-management.

Health IT.gov. (n.d.). Beacon community programs. Retrieved May 5, 2017, from https://www.healthit.gov/policy-researchers-implementers/beacon-community-program.

Handmaker, K., & Hart, J. (2015). 9 steps to effective population health management. *Healthcare Financial Management, 69*, 70–76.

Heisey-Grove, D., & Patel, V. (2015, September). *Any, certified or basic: Quantifying physician EHR adoption.* No. 28. Washington, DC: Office of the National Coordinator for Health Information Technology.

Hershey, C. O., McAloon, M. H., & Bertram, D. A. (1989). The new medical practice environment: Internists' view of the future. *Archives of Internal Medicine, 149*, 1745–1749.

Hsiao, C., King, J., Hing, E., et al. (2015). The role of health information technology in care coordination in the United States. *Medical Care, 53*(2), 184–190.

Hunt, J. S., Gibson, R. F., Whittington, J., et al. (2015). Guide for developing an information technology investment road map for population health management. *Population Health Management, 18*(3), 159–171.

Institute for Electrical and Electronics Engineering (IEEE). (n.d.). Standards glossary. Retrieved January 5, 2017, from https://www.ieee.org/education_careers/education/standards/standards_glossary.html.

Institute of Medicine. (1991). *The computer-based patient record. An essential technology for health care.* Washington, DC: National Academy Press.

Institute of Medicine. (1999). *To err is human: Building a safer health system.* Washington, DC: National Academy Press.

Institute of Medicine. (2001). *Crossing the quality chasm: A new health system for the 21st century.* Retrieved from Washington, DC: Institute of Medicine.

IOM Committee on Data Standards for Patient Safety. (2003). *Key capabilities of an electronic health record system.* Washington, DC: Institute of Medicine.

Kaiser Family Foundation. (2016). Payment and delivery system reform in Medicare. A primer on medical homes, accountable care organizations, and bundled payments (#8837-03). Retrieved from http://kff.org/medicare/report/payment-and-delivery-system-reform-in-medicare/.

Kazley, A. S., Diana, M. L., & Menachemi, N. (2012). Is EHR use associated with patient satisfaction in hospitals? *Health Care Management Review, 37*(1), 23–30. doi:10.1097/HMR.0b013e3182307bd3.

Kvedar, J., Coye, M. J., & Everett, W. (2014). Connected health: A review of technologies and strategies to improve patient care with telemedicine and telehealth. *Health Affairs, 33*(2), 194–199.

Office of the National Coordinator for Health Information Technology (ONC). (2015). Connecting health and care for the nation: A shared nationwide interoperability roadmap. Retrieved January 5, 2017, from https://www.healthit.gov/sites/default/files/hie-interoperability/nationwide-interoperability-roadmap-final-version-1.0.pdf.

Phillips, R. L., Bazemore, A. W., DeVoe, J. E., et al. (2015). A family medicine health technology strategy for achieving the triple aim for US health care. *Family Medicine, 47*(5), 628–635.

Population Health Management: A roadmap for provider-based automation in a new era of health care (2012). *Institute for Health Technology Transformation.* Retrieved April 28, 2016, from http://ihealthtran.com/whitepapers.

PwC Health Research Institute. (2015). Healthcare's alternative payment landscape. Retrieved from https://www.pwc.com/us/en/health-industries/health-research-institute/publications/alternatives-payments-2015.html.

Samal, L., Dykes, P. C., Greenberg, J. O., et al. (2016). Care coordination gaps due to lack of interoperability in the United States: A qualitative study and literature review. *BMC Health Services Research, 16*(143), 1–8.

Singer, R. H., Torres, G., Liffman, D., et al. (2015). Evaluation of the Beacon Community Cooperative Agreement Program. NORC at the University of Chicago. Report prepared for the Office of the National Coordinator for Health IT.

The Office of the National Coordinator for Health Information Technology. (2015). *Adoption of electronic health record systems among US non-federal acute care hospitals: 2008–2014.* Washington, DC.

Wager, K. A., Lee, F. W., & Glaser, J. P. (2017). *Managing health care information systems: A practical approach for health care management* (4th ed.). San Francisco, CA: Jossey-Bass.

Walker, D. M., & Diana, M. L. (2015). Hospital use of health information technology to support public health infrastructure. *Journal of Public Health Practice and Management. 22*(2), 175–181. doi:10.1097/PHH.0000000000000198.

Walker, D. M., Mora, A., Demosthenidy, M. M., et al. (2016). Meaningful use of EHRs among hospitals ineligible for incentives lags behind that of other hospitals, 2009–13. *Health Affairs (Millwood), 35*(3), 495–501. doi:10.1377/hlthaff.2015.0924.

Whitten, J., & Bentley, L. (2005). *Systems analysis and design methods* (7th ed.). New York: McGraw-Hill/Irwin.

Whittington, J. W., Nolan, K., Lewis, N., et al. (2015). Pursuing the Triple Aim: The first 7 years. *Millbank Quarterly, 93*(2), 263–300.

Zachman, J. A. (1987). A framework for information systems architecture. *IBM Systems Journal, 26*(3), 276–292.

Chapter 14

Consumerism and Ethics

Ann Leslie Claesson-Vert and Gregory L. Vert

CHAPTER OUTLINE

- Consumerism: Key Concepts and Challenges
- Health Care Reimbursement and Consumerism
- The Role of Consumers in Health Management
- Retail Medicine
- Ethical Considerations in Health Care

LEARNING OBJECTIVES

After completing this chapter, the reader should be able to:

1. Identify key concepts of consumerism and how they impact health care
2. Define the impact of consumer-driven health care trends and associated electronic risks on the health care environment
3. Identify different types of health care reimbursement that are a result of the consumer-driven health market
4. Describe the interrelationship between retail medicine, consumer's choice, and health marketing
5. Explain the role of social networking and health literacy in consumer-driven health care
6. Explain the influence of Microsoft and Google's investment in PHRs on the health care environment
7. Differentiate different ethical principles and how they are demonstrated in health care

KEY TERMS

Autonomy

Belmont Report

Beneficence

Bioethics

Confidentiality

Consumer-Driven Health Care

Consumer-Directed Health Plan (CDHP)

Consumerism

Consumers

Convenient Care Association (CCA)

Convenient Care Clinic

Electronic Health Record (EHR)

Ethics

Fidelity

Flexible Spending Accounts or Arrangement (FSAs)

Health Insurance Portability and Accountability Act (HIPAA)

Health Literacy

Health Reimbursement Account (HRA)

Health Savings Account (HSA)

High-Deductible Health Plan (HDHP)

Human Subjects

Institutional Review Boards (IRBs)

Justice

Medical Savings Accounts (MSAs)

Nonmaleficence

Office for Human Research Protections (OHRP)

Personal Health Record (PHR)

Privacy

Research

Retail Medicine

• • • IN PRACTICE: Consumer-Driven Markets

Richard pauses from his morning run to upload cardio data to his iPod from the sensor in his Nike running shoe. He then sends today's fitness data directly to his online Nike+ account where it will be stored for future use and possible integration into his personal health record at Microsoft's HealthVault.

Across town, Patti, a health care manager for an integrated health care system, checks her lab results online and receives an e-mail reminder for an upcoming doctor's appointment. Her employer offers a high-deductible health plan (HDHP) that includes options for health care reimbursement arrangements (for health services not covered by the plan) and a wellness option. Jennifer has chosen to utilize the wellness option and is tracking her exercise and weight loss on a "tethered PHR" based out of her hospital system. She then checks the PatientsLikeMe website for new information in the ALS and fibromyalgia blogs before she goes to lunch.

The above situations are examples of applications targeting the consumer-driven health care movement. Consumers are choosing to take more responsibility for their own health and wellness and expect increased access to health information from a variety of sources. Advances in technology and telecommunications have contributed to enhanced expectations and needs by consumers for rapid access to health information and services, instant communications, and customer satisfaction. Health care environments need to remain current in the latest health information technology, treatment advances, and consumer needs in order to remain competitive. Consideration of health-related advances and applications, such as personal health records (PHRs), health network sites (e.g., PatientsLikeMe), and changes in health care reimbursement structures (e.g., HDHP) contribute to an increased awareness of health and wellness by consumers. Consumers have changed the face of health care in today's marketplace and will continue to do so in the near future.

CHAPTER PURPOSE

The purpose of this chapter is to provide information and resources concerning the role of consumerism and ethics in our health care environment. In the past few decades, our society has seen a shift toward a greater emphasis on consumerism and how consumer decision making can impact health care service delivery. Consumers increasingly play a more active role in negotiating and maintaining their own health care. This includes specific services required to fulfill their needs and the associated health-based trends.

Ethical scenarios and choices are de rigueur in many health care environments, with issues, such as end-of-life decisions, health care disparities (who gets the care?), birth control and right-to-life, and religious/cultural preferences in health care treatments. Hence, ethical decision making and health care could easily take up an entire chapter on its own. For the purposes of this chapter, the focus is on the interrelationships between consumerism and ethics and how these relationships influence effective health care delivery.

The chapter begins with an exploration of consumerism, key concepts, and challenges, such as shared decision making, transparency, the Health Insurance Portability and Accountability Act (HIPAA) of 1996, and consumer-driven marketing. Next follows an examination of how the health care reimbursement market has changed due to an increased emphasis on the role of consumer-driven health care with potential revisions

due to political environments and the expanded role of the consumer in health care management and personal wellness. The concept of retail medicine and its influence on the current and future health care market is the third area of discussion. Finally, ethical considerations in health care, key concepts, challenges, and guidelines for health care managers and consumers provide a baseline for ethical decision making.

CONSUMERISM: KEY CONCEPTS AND CHALLENGES

Health care has traditionally been considered a provider or medical-driven environment with an emphasis on medical services provided by physicians based on clinical judgment and research. Recent trends and advances in health care treatment, increased use of technology, higher demands and expectations by consumers, and a change from the acute-care model to the chronic-care model as the population ages have contributed to a shift toward a more consumer-oriented or **consumer-driven health care** system.

As the population ages and the baby boomer generation retires, increased pressure is placed on generations X, Y, and millennials to fill the expectations and roles set by the previous generations. Due to recent advances in health care treatment and technology, people are living longer with more chronic diseases as a daily part of their lives (Cahin and Lancashire, 2008, March 27; Federal Interagency Forum on Aging-Related Statistics, 2008, March; Hajat and Kishore, 2018, para 1). In 2018, the Agency for Healthcare Research and Quality (2018, para 1) noted that over one-quarter of all Americans, with two out of three older Americans, have a minimum of two chronic behavioral or physical health problems. This increase in multiple chronic conditions has contributed to a shift from the acute-care to the chronic-care model (Saver, 2006; Agency for Healthcare Research and Quality, 2018, para 1). The change in demographics and socioeconomics, shortages of health care professionals, a shift toward more chronic-care needs for health care service delivery, and increased consumer expectations have provided impetus for alternative forms of health care. These include a more consumer-driven health care system that caters to the specialized needs and well-being of individuals, groups, populations, and payers.

With increased access to the Internet and health care–related education, **consumers** expect care to be delivered in different settings. For instance, care once delivered in a hospital setting has moved into the home under the name of wellness (Agency for Healthcare Research and Quality, 2018, paras 1–7; Saver, 2006). Health care recipients are no longer merely "clients" or "patients" who accept the health care provider's decisions as their treatment; instead, they are active participants in their own health care decision making.

Traditional approaches to health care service delivery in the United States have been paternalistic in nature. As such, services given to patients were decided upon without significant input from the patients concerning their own needs or expectations. With the advent of the consumer-driven health movement, more health care consumers are rejecting this paternalistic approach and demanding greater choice and control over health care decisions and treatment choices. If their needs are not met, they do not hesitate to complain to elected officials or use litigation to express their dissatisfaction (Jarousse, 2015, para 1; Ransom et al., 2008). A report by the Kellogg Foundation noted that 65 percent of health care consumers felt they should have control over health care decision making (Ransom et al., 2008).

Customer satisfaction has been a recognized marker for quality in many industries, and particularly in health care. Consumers have grown accustomed to e-commerce, service guarantees/warranties, 1-800-number information call centers, and higher standards for quality for many products and services. Health care is expected to be no different with the same level of high quality, instant service, and customer satisfaction (Jarousse, 2015, paras 28, 53, 56; Ransom et al., 2008). The U.S. health care system has not kept pace with other industries in its provision of support to maintain customer satisfaction and loyalty. The consumer-driven health movement has provided the momentum for a fundamental change in our health care environment, and health organizations and providers are moving toward a more customer-friendly, consumer-driven product: consumer-driven health care (Cordina, Kumar, and Moss, 2015).

Consumers, Consumerism, and Economics

The *Oxford English Dictionary* (OED, 1989h) defines a consumer as "a person who uses up a commodity; a purchaser of goods or services, a customer," as opposed to one who produces goods or services (producer or provider). Consumer expectations are what drive a market. Consumers' expectations and perceptions of what should be available, accessible, convenient, and safe are primary indicators of who and what is successful in an economy.

Consumerism is defined as "doctrine advocating a continual increase in the consumption of goods as a basis for a sound economy" or "advocacy of the rights of consumers" (OED, 1989h). Consumer-driven health care is health care that is directly motivated and impacted by what its consumers expect and demand. Today's health care consumer expects and demands high-quality, safe, and accessible health care services. They research health problems, and they seek information and second opinions on diagnosis and treatment options through available media and personal networking, such as online support groups (e.g., PatientsLikeMe), social networking sites (e.g., Facebook, Twitter), disease-specific associations, public service and government websites, alternative/complementary medicine, and other health care professionals.

Key Principles of Health Care Consumerism

Many key concepts have previously been identified regarding health care consumerism. Havlin, McAllister, and Slavney (2003) referred to consumerism in health care as a strategy that encourages and enables people to take charge of their personal health through (1) knowledge of their health status and needs, (2) informed decision making, (3) wise use of health care dollars, and (4) confident and active participation in their own health care decisions and treatment choices. Potter (1988) recognized five basic principles needed for a consumer-driven market structure that can also be applied to health care: access, choice, information, redress, and representation. Consumers need to have access to services and products, accurate information to assist them in making informed choices, a method for communicating dissatisfaction with service or product choices, and some process to ensure that their interests are represented to decision makers impacting their well-being and welfare (Cordina, Kumar, and Moss, 2015; Potter, 1988).

Bachman (2006) noted in his report *Healthcare Consumerism: The Basis of a 21st Century Intelligent Health System* that our health care environment was moving toward a more demand-control model influenced by specified economic forces. This concept aligns health care more closely with consumer purchasing behaviors seen in other industries. He identified six "mega trends" that impact the demand-control model, one of which is consumerism:

1. Personal responsibility
2. Self-help, self-care
3. Individual ownership
4. Portability
5. Transparency (right to know)
6. Consumerism (empowerment) (Bachman, 2006)

In addition to these six mega trends, Bachman also noted five key "building blocks" of health care consumerism that are important for health care managers to consider:

1. Personal accounts (FSAs, HRAs, HSAs)
2. Wellness/prevention and early intervention programs
3. Disease management and case management programs
4. Information and decision support programs
5. Incentive and compliance reward programs (Bachman, 2006)

Cordina, Kumar, and Moss (2015) noted that individuals, as consumers, were taking a more active role in decision making expecting greater control and transparency in the products they choose. These findings support prior studies by Havlin, McAllister, and Slavney (2003); Bachman (2006); and Potter (1988) on this shift toward a stronger consumer presence and personal responsibility.

Shared Decision Making, Transparency, and Health Literacy

Consumer awareness of service/product quality and cost are key drivers of transparency in health care. Many people are more aware of the price of a new cell phone or automobile than health care services that they depend upon for their own well-being and health status (Goodman, 2006). As health care insurance reimbursement options now include **consumer-driven health plans (CDHPs)**, such as **high-deductible health plans (HDHPs)**, flexible spending accounts (FSAs), and **health reimbursement accounts (HRAs)**, employees are being asked to take more responsibility for their own health care needs. As more employees are being asked to make choices in their health care coverage, the question remains: do they have the information to effectively make these decisions?

To make informed choices, certain health care information needs to be readily available and *visible* to the public. Therefore, our health care environment needs to become more *transparent* in its approach to information utilization and access. Though this does suggest the need for several reforms, a move toward increased transparency does not mean that all health information should be made publicly available. Extensive regulations and legislation exist to protect individual health information, such as the Health Insurance Portability and Accountability Act (HIPAA) and the Patient Safety and Quality Act.

Access to and *an understanding of* available health care information is a requirement for consumers to make informed health care decisions (Berkman et al., 2011, p. 97; Potter, 1988; The Joint Commission, 2015, para 2).

Health Information Privacy

Consumers versus Providers: Users of Published Information

Increased transparency in health care has made visible a plethora of information on health, wellness, treatment options, and disease management. Conventional and nonconventional forms of medicine are often frequented daily by health consumers. Increased access to information and communication through a variety of formats (e.g., the Internet, social networking, media advertisements, and personal contacts) has brought about questions, such as "What information should be made available?" and "To whom?"

HIPAA and the "Need to Know"

As advances in technology and telecommunications began to change the face of our health care environment in the late twentieth century, the privacy of health information, portability of insurance and utilization, and exchange of electronic data became primary focuses of concern. In 1996, the **Health Insurance Portability and Accountability Act (HIPAA)**, Public Law 104-191, was enacted by Congress to combat waste, fraud, and abuse in health care (Maryland Department of Mental Health and Hygiene, 2007; U.S. Department of Health and Human Services, n.d. a). It became effective in 1997 with a Privacy Rule finalized in 2002.

The HIPAA legislation specifies regulations for the privacy of personal health information, portability of health insurance, and the organization of the interchange of electronic data for certain financial and administrative operations (Maryland Department of Mental Health and Hygiene, 2007). HIPAA rules limit the use and disclosure of personal health information by "covered entities" who qualified on a "need-to-know" basis according to HIPAA criteria. These "covered entities" include health plans (e.g., individual, group, and government insurance plans), health care providers (e.g., physicians, dentists, and other providers, hospitals, health care organizations, and "any other person or organization that furnishes, bills, or is paid for health care"), as well as health care clearinghouses (e.g., health care billing services, health information management systems) who conduct standard health care transactions electronically (U.S. Department of Health and Human Services, n.d. a).

HIPAA also included Administrative Simplification (Title II, Subtitle f of HIPAA), which required the U.S. Department of Health and Human Services (HHS) to adopt national standards for the use of electronic health information, such as unique health identifiers, code sets, and health care transactions (U.S. Department of Health and Human Services, 2009). The HIPAA Privacy Rule and Security Rule are enforced by the HHS Office for Civil Rights. Additional information pertaining to the HIPPA Administrative Simplification can be found at 45 CFR Parts 160, 162, and 164. (U.S. Department of Health and Human Services, 2009).

Another federal regulation that protects the privacy and disclosure of personal health information is the Patient Safety and Quality Improvement Act (PSQIA). Passed in 2005, the PSQIA created a voluntary reporting system pertaining to data utilized in patient safety and health care quality concerns (U.S. Department of Health and Human Services, n.d. a). The PSQIA ensures federal protection for patient safety data and enforces civil monetary penalties for violations of patient safety confidentiality.

Health care consumers and managers should be aware that while HIPAA does provide protection and privacy for personal health information, it pertains only to those entities listed in its criteria (health care providers, health plans, and health clearinghouses). Many online health-related services and locations are not included under the HIPAA regulations, including personal health information uploaded to websites, support groups, social health networks (e.g., PatientsLikeMe), or **personal health records (PHRs)** (e.g., Google Health or Microsoft's Health-Vault). While these online vendors do have compliance agreements which consumers sign prior to participation, they are not considered covered entities; hence, there is no recourse via HIPAA protection for consumers or users of these online services (Stewart, 2009).

When health care professionals and providers consider patient health literacy status, it is generally assumed to mean the individual capacity to acquire, process, and comprehend basic health information and associated services required to make appropriate decisions about health (NNLM, 2017). Yet how many consumers actually understand what is being said or marketed to them through social media or the Internet pertaining to their health? **Health literacy** is described as the ability of individuals to acquire, understand, process, and ultimately apply basic health information to make fully informed and appropriate health decisions (Healthy People 2020, 2014, para 1; NNLM, 2017, para 1). The National Network of Libraries of Medicine recognizes that health literacy involves a plethora of complex processes, such as reading, listening, comprehending, as well as specific analytical and decision-making skills (NNLM, 2017, para 2). These skills encompass the ability to comprehend health provider instructions and to read the labels on medications, appointment reminder slips, education brochures, or consent forms (para 3). The Joint Commission stated that effective communication was a crucial factor to the effective delivery of health care services (2017, para 1). In its 2017 publication on patient-centered communication, it identified that over 90 million Americans have low health literacy status resulting in a limited capacity to understand and apply health information. The Joint Commission also noted more than 300 different languages are spoken in the U.S., which can contribute to this decrease in health literacy and comprehension (2015, para 2). Low health literacy was also identified as a barrier to receiving high-quality health care especially for those living with chronic diseases (The Joint Commission, 2015, para 2; U.S. Department of Health and Human Services, 2012). The Joint Commission recommends an approach for clearer communication of health information that incorporates individual language needs, literacy levels, cultural expectations, and methods to determine individual understanding (2015, paras 1–3). Part of this recommendation is the inclusion of the assessment of individual health literacy status with application of these results to effective communication techniques for patient education and treatment regimes.

Older adults and other population groups may have may lower health literacy levels that could contribute to additional barriers to learning, health compliance, or poor patient outcomes (Berkman et al., 2011; Blais and Bolinger, 2014, p. 133; Guzys et al., 2015; Health and Human Services, 2012). These potentially lower levels of understanding should be taken into consideration by health professionals and others, in addition to the marketing efforts aimed at these consumers, in order to provide appropriate information for the consumer to make fully informed decisions.

HEALTH CARE REIMBURSEMENT AND CONSUMERISM

Consumers now demand a more active voice into choices regarding their health and wellness, and the consumer-driven health movement is in full swing. The movement is propelled by consumers' revolt against organized methods for cost-containment and the limitations on health services and treatment options that have been commonplace in the era of managed care. Although managed care proposed to control health costs by managing resource allocation and access to care, many have rebelled against these constraints, resenting HMO organizations and the health providers who participate in them (Robinson and Ginsburg, 2009). HMOs offered a comprehensive benefit design, a limited provider network, and a means of capping health expenditure with an emphasis on medical management but also imposed limits on care due to precertification, restricted second opinions, and exclusion of treatment for specified populations (Robinson and Ginsburg, 2009).

The consumer-driven health care movement has spurred changes to health plans and approaches to health care reimbursement. Health care expenditures have increased due to advances in technologies, treatments, pharmaceuticals, and the public's expectations for rapid, quality health care that is cost-effective, accessible, and understandable. Additional drivers of health care cost are the aging workforce, the move from a chronic disease model to an acute care model, increased consumer demand for life-enhancing or life-sustaining therapies, increased drug company direct-to-consumer advertising, and elevated health risks in the population due to stress, obesity, smoking, high blood pressure, diabetes, heart disease, a lack of perceived personal responsibility in self-care and wellness, or a lack of understanding of the impact of not taking responsibility for one's health or health options (Frakt, 2015, paras 1–5; Havlin, McAllister, and Slavney, 2003). People make daily choices impacting their own health and well-being, but how much time do they spend choosing a health plan?

Choosing a Health Insurance Plan

"Evaluating health insurance plans can be daunting and confusing, and most people don't get much guidance, research shows" (Frakt, 2015, para 1). Whether the choice is a Medicare plan, an employer-based plan, one of the marketplace health exchanges from the Affordable Care Act, or another option based on health care reform, research shows that little guidance is often provided to consumers, can be confusing, or presented at a literacy level incompatible with the average consumer (Frakt, 2015, para 1; Olen, 2017, para 2). Research by George Loewenstein, economics and psychology professor at Carnegie Mellon (Frakt, 2015, para 5), revealed that consumers in the study not only misunderstood plan cost and features but also could not correctly define what a co-pay was (28 percent) or what "maximum out of pocket" meant (41 percent).

While some individuals may consider choosing their health insurance plan as type of shopping activity,

Senator Shaheen of New Hampshire notes that it should be taken seriously, as the type of coverage and size of premiums can make a significant difference in the ability to really afford what is chosen. "I encourage you to shop around," stated Senator Jeanne Shaheen, Democrat of New Hampshire, to followers on Facebook considering how to choose a health plan from the Affordable Care Act marketplaces (Olen, 2017, para 2). Author Helaine Olen noted in her New York Times op-ed that marketing efforts linking health plan choice with the consumer shopping experience were used by organizations such as the American Diabetes Association, American Institute of Architects, Aetna, the Robert Wood Johnson Foundation, and Mercer (Olen, 2017, para 2). A Harris poll conducted for Jellyvision, Inc., software company from April 1 to 8, 2016, noted that approximately one half of employees found choosing a health plan to be stressful (The Jellyvision Lab, Inc., 2016, pp. 2–3), which correlates with an Aflac poll that they would rather "talk to an ex or walk across hot coals than enroll in a health plan" (para 5).

What can consumers do to help ensure they choose the best and most affordable plan for themselves? HealthCare.gov (https://www.healthcare.gov/choose-a-plan/comparing-plans/) provides a resource listing tips for consumers to aid them in choosing a health insurance plan. The website presents materials on the levels of health plans (Bronze, Silver, Gold, and Platinum), potential total cost, and plan types (HMO, PPO, POS, EPO) (HealthCare.gov, 2017a). A YouTube video is also linked to aid in a better understanding of the process and targeted at a different literacy level (https://www.youtube.com/embed/XOkPAANg3R8).

Consumer-Directed Health Plans

CDHPs are designed to allow the employee greater choice in their health care, thus enabling them to be wise consumers (Patterson, 2004). These plans contribute to collective decision making in health care with more responsibility on the employee. CDHPs are designed specifically to enable consumers greater input into their plan and wellness choices. These plans (1) provide more information to aid in the selection of providers, treatment options, and facilities; (2) offer greater choices in services; and (3) may allow the employee to design their own health plan, including benefits covered, deductible, co-pay, and providers. It is common for CDPHs to offer service quality evaluations of health care providers as well as to provide health coaches or designated specialist coaches for specified health conditions (Patterson, 2004). Additional features of CDHPs appealing to the modern consumer are 100 percent coverage of preventative care and saving accounts that may be carried over to traditional PPO health plans (Havlin, McAllister, and Slavney, 2003).

Some characteristics of enrollees in CDHPs were identified in the 2016 Employee Benefit Research Institute/Greenwald & Associates Consumer Engagement in Health Care Survey. This annual survey reports nationally representative data concerning CDHPs and HDHPs (Fronstin and Emlinger, 2017). Information on consumer behavior, attitudes, and impact of the health plan are identified, which is important to health care managers who are considered redesigning existing services and programs.

The 2016 survey was conducted with a consumer panel of 3,295 adults with private insurance through their employer, government-based market exchange, or purchased directly from the insurance provider. Fourteen percent of the population participated in CDHPs that were associated with a health savings account (HSA) or health reimbursement arrangement (HRA), 14 percent also had HDHP not linked to a HSA or HDP, and 73 percent had more traditional coverage (Fronstin and Emlinger, 2017, p. 1). Over half of those enrolled in CDHPs took advantage of employer contributions by opening a HSA with 20 percent noting a 10 percent increase in employer contributions of at least $2,000 in 2014. In addition, 42 percent stated an increase of employer HSA contributions of $1,000 to $1,999 which is a 36 percent increase since 2104 (Fronstin and Emlinger, 2017, p. 1).

When compared with individuals enrolled in traditional health plans, individuals enrolled in CDHPs were:

1. More likely to demonstrate cost-conscious behaviors
2. More likely to engage in wellness programs
3. More likely to realize financial incentives for healthy behaviors
4. Less likely to have a health problem
5. Less likely to smoke
6. More likely to exercise
7. Less likely to be obese
8. More likely to have a higher household income and be highly educated (Fronstin and Emlinger, 2017).

CDHPs members are more likely to be proactive in determining the coverage available in their health plan, ask for a generic drug as opposed to a brand name, talk with their physician regarding treatment options and choices, develop a budget to manage health care costs, and use online cost-tracking tools (Fronstin and Emlinger, 2017).

High-Deductible Health Plans

One form of CDHPs is the HDHP. These health plans offer a broad provider network, limited involvement with medical management, higher deductibles, and lower premiums (Internal Revenue Service, 2017;

Robinson and Ginsburg, 2009). Minimum annual deductibles for HDHPs as noted by the IRS for the year 2018 are as follows:

- Self-coverage minimum annual deductible: $1,350 ($50 increase since 2017); $6,650 (maximum deductible and other out-of-pocket expenses)
- Family coverage minimum annual deductible: $2,700 ($100 increase since 2017); $13,300 (maximum deductible and other out-of-pocket expenses) (Thompson Reuters, 2017).

Typical deductibles for HDPHs range from $500 to tens of thousands of dollars. This is critical because health care is paid for by the enrollee until the deductible has been met. Additional benefits include optional participation in HSAs or HRAs. For basically healthy individuals who expect limited health care expenses per year, HDHPs may be a viable option.

HDHPs focus on the premise that health insurance should function similarly to other forms of insurance, covering high-cost, unpredicted, and catastrophic health needs but not necessarily providing coverage for everything. They have also been referred to as "catastrophic" health insurance (Treasury, U.S., 2008) and have a higher annual deductible than typical plans and a maximum limit on the total of annual deductible and out-of-pocket expenses, such as co-payments (Internal Revenue Service, 2017). Predictable and low-cost health needs are the responsibility of the individual to finance. The structure of HDHPs generally includes an account where pretax monies can be set aside for these predictable low-cost health expenses through a HSA or HRA (Robinson and Ginsburg, 2009). In order to be eligible for HSAs, individuals must be enrolled in an HDHP (Treasury, U.S., 2008).

Generally, HDHPs provide exceptions for preventive care, such as well-baby/well-child services, certain health evaluations, immunizations, weight loss and smoking cessation programs, routine prenatal care, and specified screenings (Treasury, U.S., 2004). Under these guidelines, preventive care generally does not include treatment of existing conditions but rather stresses the early identification of new conditions that may require treatment (Treasury, U.S., 2004).

Survey results published by the America's Health Insurance Plans (AHIPs) noted a modest increase of 3.4 percent in HSA/HDHP plan enrollment from 19.7 million to 20.2 million as of January 2016 (AHIP, 2017, p. 2). Still, these numbers remain relatively small when compared to total enrollment of individuals in private health insurance (AHIP, 2017, p. 2). The most popular HSA/HDHP product identified was that offered by preferred provider organizations (PPOs) with over 54 percent of enrollment (AHIP, 2017, p. 2). This accounts for more than three-quarters of all enrollment as found in the

2015 study. For additional information on HSA/HDHPs, review the report at https://www.ahip.org/wp-content/uploads/2017/02/2016_HSASurvey_Draft_2.14.17.pdf.

As noted earlier by Fronstin and Emlinger (2017, pp. 1–2) in their consumer survey of insurance type with a consumer panel of adults with private insurance through their employer, government-based market exchange, or purchased directly from the insurance provider, 14 percent participated in CDHPs that were associated with a HSA or HRA, 14 percent also had HDHP not linked to a HSA or HDP, and 73 percent had more traditional coverage (Fronstin and Emlinger 2017, p. 1). AHIP (2017) also recognized that the most popular HSA/HDHP product identified was PPOs with over 54 percent of enrollment (AHIP, 2017, p. 2). This accounts for more than three-quarters of all enrollment as found in the 2015 study.

Reimbursement Accounts for Noncovered Health Expenses: HSAs, MSAs, FSAs, and HRAs

Historically, health care plans have not included coverage for all health services. Optional savings accounts were established so that qualified individuals could deposit pretax monies to use on specified health-related expenses. These accounts may be linked directly to other health plans, such as an HDHPs. Examples of these types of health-related savings accounts include **flexible spending accounts or arrangements (FSAs)**, HSAs, medical savings accounts (MSAs), and HRAs. These types of accounts offer tax advantages to assist in offsetting health care expenses (Department of the Treasury, Internal Revenue Service, 2008, 2016; Fronstin and Emlinger, 2017).

Before 2004, these financial health accounts were the creation of the IRS regulatory processes, employer-funded only, and called HRAs or other similar names due to the labeling of each individual vendor (Internal Revenue Service, 2018; Patterson, 2004). Sometimes, these accounts were referred to as a personal care account and were funded by the employer only. The balance in the account was carried over, or "rolled over," annually (Internal Revenue Service, 2018; Patterson, 2004). Starting in 2004, a new type of medical carryover account, the **health savings account (HSA)** or health FSA was established by the Medicare Prescription Drug, Improvement, and Modernization Act (Fronstin and Emlinger, 2017; Patterson, 2004). These accounts were funded by the individual, the employer (with employee pretax monies or through an employer-provided cafeteria plan), or another individual on the behalf of the account owner (IRC section 125; TASC, 2008b). Participation in an HDHP was required, and the account was able to be carried from employer to employer. HSAs also received

rollovers from Archer MSAs (Department of the Treasury, Internal Revenue Service, 2008, 2016; Fronstin and Emlinger, 2017; Patterson, 2004). This change in IRS restrictions on spending in these types of accounts was a key factor in the consumer-driven health movement. The IRS Code (IRC) Section 125 now allowed employees to carryover unused monies from year to year for noncovered health expenses as opposed to FSAs, where all monies were spent annually (Patterson, 2004).

Health Savings Accounts

HSAs are tax-exempt financial accounts used to reimburse medical expenses not covered under existing health plans. These noncovered medical expenses include periodical health evaluations (annual visits), routine prenatal and well-child care, smoking cessation programs, obesity/weight-loss programs, and health screenings (e.g., cancer, heart disease, infectious diseases, substance abuse, mental health conditions, pediatric conditions, etc.) (Department of the Treasury, Internal Revenue Service, 2008, 2017; TASC, 2008b).

Requirements for participation in a HSA are as follows: participation in a HDHP and no other health coverage except for certain specified areas (such as long-term care, accidents, vision care, dental care, liabilities under workman's compensation, tort or other liabilities incurred via property requirements, etc.), not enrolled in Medicare, and not being claimed as a dependent on another individual's tax return (Department of the Treasury, Internal Revenue Service, 2008). Two main benefits of HSAs are that contributions are tax-exempt, and contributions can be made by the individual, another individual on the owner's behalf, or the employer. Additionally, funds accrued in the HSA do not need to be spent during a single year, and can be rolled over on an annual basis, and the HSA is "portable"—you are able to take it with you when changing employers or leaving the workforce (Department of the Treasury, Internal Revenue Service, 2008).

Medical Savings Accounts

Created in 1997, **medical savings accounts (MSAs)**, also known as Archer MSAs, are another type of tax-exempt financial account and were created to offset uncovered medical expenses for self-employed individuals or employees in small businesses (those with fewer than 50 workers). MSA participation requires employment by a small business that maintains an HDHP (or being a spouse of employee) or self-employment (or being a spouse of self-employed person) (Department of the Treasury, Internal Revenue Service, 2008, 2017).

Benefits for MSAs are similar to those for HSAs (see Table 14.1), but there are some differences. Contributions are tax-exempt and can be made by the individual owner (or an individual on the owner's behalf) or by the employer

Table 14.1 Financial Reimbursement Accounts for Noncovered Health Expenses

Account Type	Participation in HDHP	Tax Considerations	Monies Can Be Rolled Over Annually	Contribution Type	Who Establishes Account	Portable?
HSA	Yes	Tax-deductible contributions; employer contributions are pretax and excluded from gross income	Yes	Individual or employer; both in same year allowed	Self or employer	Yes
MSA	No	Tax-deductible contributions; employer contributions are pretax and excluded from gross income	Yes	Employer or self, but not both	Employer	Yes
FSA	Optional	Tax-deductible contributions; employer contributions are pretax and excluded from gross income	No	Employer-funded through voluntary salary reduction agreement	Employer	No
HRA	Yes	100 percent tax deductible for employer; tax-free for employee	Discretion of employer	Employer-funded	Employer	No

but not by both during the same year (Department of the Treasury, Internal Revenue Service, 2017, 2018). Like in the HSA, funds accrued in the MSA do not need to be spent during a single year and can be rolled over on an annual basis. Also like an HSA, the owner is allowed to move their MSA when changing employers or leaving the workforce (Department of the Treasury, Internal Revenue Service, 2017). Contributions to Archer MSAs are limited by the employee's income and annual deductible limits (Department of the Treasury, Internal Revenue Service, 2017, 2018). In IRS Publication Number 969, a tax map is provided to aid the public in better understanding this unique form of tax-deferred savings for future health expenses with link to required forms and detailed instructions (Internal Revenue Service, 2018).

Another type of Archer-designated MSA is the Medicare Advantage MSA. Medicare Advantage MSAs are a tax-exempt trust arranged through financial institutions such as insurance companies or banks. They can only be funded by Medicare and the monies used to pay for medical expenses accrued by the account holder who is a Medicare enrollee (Department of the Treasury, Internal Revenue Service, 2008, 2017, 2018). Participants must be enrolled in an HDHP that meets Medicare guidelines and must be enrolled in Medicare.

Flexible Spending Arrangements

Flexible spending arrangement (FSA) is a blanket term for financial accounts where pretax funds are accumulated in order to be used for reimbursement of uncovered medical expenses. Contributions to FSAs are generally made by the employer through a voluntary salary reduction arrangement with the employee (Department of the Treasury, Internal Revenue Service, 2008, 2017, 2018). Employers can offer FSAs in addition to other benefits or as a part of a cafeteria plan. Employees do not have to participate in other health plans, and they can decide to participate only in an FSA if they so choose (Department of the Treasury, Internal Revenue Service, 2008, 2017, 2018). The Internal Revenue Service (2017) identified a cap on salary reduction contributions to FSAs at $2,550 annually (adjusted for inflation). More information on FSAs can be found at www.irs.gov/irb/2015-44_IRB/ar10.html.

FSAs require that all funds held in the account must be spent annually. Unlike HSAs and MSAs, the balance of an FSA cannot be carried over from year to year (Department of the Treasury, Internal Revenue Service, 2008, 2017, 2018; Patterson, 2004). Additionally, self-employed individuals do not qualify for FSAs. Reimbursement for medical expenses through FSAs may occur through employer-sponsored debit cards, credit cards, and stored-value cards (Department of the Treasury, Internal Revenue Service, 2008, 2017, 2018).

Health Reimbursement Arrangements

HRAs are financial arrangements that are used for reimbursement of substantiated medical expenses. These substantiated or qualified medical expenses are determined by the employer and may include deductibles, co-payments, coinsurance, prescription medications, dental and vision expenses, or other uncovered medical expenses (TASC, 2008a).

HRAs are employer-funded with pretax monies only, but they cannot be funded through an employer–employee salary reduction agreement as with FSAs (Department of the Treasury, Internal Revenue Service, 2017, 2018; TASC, 2008a). They are generally offered in combination with HDHPs. All contributions to the HRA are 100 percent tax deductible for the employer and tax-free for the employee, which makes them an attractive consideration for many individuals and families with identified uncovered annual medical expenses.

Unused funds in the HRA can be carried over in full annually, partially carried over, or required to be spent annually. This determination is made at the discretion of the employer (Department of the Treasury, Internal Revenue Service, 2008, 2017, 2018; TASC, 2008a) and is subject to the Consolidated Omnibus Budget Reconciliation Act (COBRA) laws. COBRA was passed in 1986 to provide a continuation of employer-based health coverage for a temporary time that may otherwise be ended (U.S. Department of Labor, n.d., paras 1–3). For additional information on COBRA benefits, review the information provided at the website https://www.dol.gov/agencies/ebsa/about-ebsa/our-activities/resource-center/faqs/cobra-continuation-health-coverage-compliance.

Reimbursement for uncovered medical expenses may be accomplished using employer-distributed debit cards, credit cards, or stored-value cards (Department of the Treasury, Internal Revenue Service, 2008, 2017, 2018; TASC, 2008a).

For additional information on HSAs and other health plans (Publication 969: Health Savings Accounts and Other Tax-Favored Health Plans), visit http://www.irs.gov/pub/irs-pdf/p969.pdf.

The Patient Protection and Affordable Care Act

The Patient Protection and Affordable Care Act (PPACA) of 2010 (Public Law 111–148) is a type of health insurance reform with the goal of revising the health insurance market and accessibility to health insurance for individuals and small business employers (Burke, 2014, p. 94; Leonard and Rosenbaum, 2011, p. 597; Roland, 2015). Full implementation of the PPACA took place in 2014 (Rosenbaum, 2011, p. 130). The law consists of two parts: (1) the Patient Protection and Affordable Care Act (https://www.gpo.gov/fdsys/pkg/PLAW-111publ148/pdf/PLAW-111publ148.pdf) and (2) the Health Care and Education Reconciliation Act (https://www.gpo.gov/fdsys/pkg/PLAW-111publ152/pdf/PLAW-111publ152.pdf). The first part of the law, outlines reforms targeting Medicare, Medicaid, revenues, and health insurance coverage. The second part, stresses education and health, such as higher education, student loans grant options, removing exclusions for pre-existing medical conditions and expansion of community health centers (Congress.gov, 2018).

This reform included the incorporation of approved health insurance exchanges or health insurance marketplaces to be managed by each state. States established their own exchange or opted for a federal government-managed exchange to assist in making insurance more accessible for qualified individuals and small business owners (Burke, 2014, p. 94). These insurance products are also called qualified health plans (QHPs). The three main objectives of the PPACA are (1) to make health insurance affordable to more people, (2) to expand the Medicaid program, and (3) to support innovative health care services and delivery designed to decrease general health care cost (HealthCare.gov, 2017b). While political debate continues regarding the advantages and disadvantages of the PPACA, consumer benefits include removal of limitations on coverage for preexisting conditions, preventive care and health screening coverage, while disadvantages include increased cost for some consumers and difficulty maneuvering in the government websites when signing up for health plans.

THE ROLE OF CONSUMERS IN HEALTH MANAGEMENT

A major demographic change will occur in the year 2030 as the baby boomer generation will be age 65 to age 84, which will significantly impact the economic and workplace structure of this nation (United States Census Bureau, 2018, para 1–2). This increases the size of the older population to one in every five residents being of retirement age. Jonathan Vespa, a U.S. Census Bureau demographer stated that by the year 2035, 78.0 million people will be aged 65 and older as compared to 76.7 million (previously 76.4 million) under the age of 18 years (U.S. Census Bureau, 2018, para 1–2). By 2012, the global population increased to seven billions with 8 percent (or 562 million) being aged 65 years or older (He, Goodkind, and Kowal, 2016, p. 1). Three years later in 2015, this aging population increased another 55 million (or 0.5 percent) with a projection to increase approximately 236 million throughout the world over the next eight years and almost doubling to 1.6 billion between 2025 and 2050 globally (p. 1). How will the face of health care change as the baby boomer generation retires and other generations assume the responsibilities for our fast-paced, demanding health care market? What is the impact of the aging baby boomer generation, increasing diversity in our patient and health care populations, and increased responsibilities on Generations X and Y?

Personal Health Management: Key Concepts and Responsibility

Societal changes have influenced how Americans perceive their health and wellness status. Technology, instant messaging, and instant communications have contributed to the public's expectations of instant service, customer satisfaction, and a more prominent role in their own health care. The public is more aware of health concerns and the personal responsibility required in maintaining health and well-being.

Reports by the Institute of Medicine (IOM), the U.S. Census Bureau, and Health People 2010 have escalated the public's awareness of the health status of the American people and identified issues of concern, including prevalence of overweight and obesity, type 2 diabetes, cardiac disease, cancer, health care disparities, as well as lack of access to health service and treatment options. New technologies and advancements in medicine and pharmaceuticals have contributed to increased longevity. However, as longevity increases, so does the propensity for chronic disease and the need for self-help and self-care in order to achieve a higher quality of life. Key areas for improvement for the American population include obesity and weight loss, increased exercise, health eating and nutrition, regular health screenings for diseases, such as heart disease, diabetes, high blood pressure, and certain types of cancer and genetic diseases.

Ten leading health indicators were identified by Healthy People 2010 as key areas of concern in the U.S. population at the beginning of the twenty-first century (Healthy People 2010, n.d.) (Table 14.2). Each indicator is directly linked to Healthy People 2010 objectives. Each indicator and objective was chosen for its ability to be measured (available data to measure progress), its importance as a public health issue, and its ability to motivate the public to action (Healthy People 2010, n.d.).

Why are these leading health indicators important for health care managers? Since many of these areas have been targeted by media and specific private and publicly funded health care initiatives, gaining awareness of what the U.S. public as consumers is looking for can assist health care managers in tailoring their organizational and departmental goals to fit those needs.

Wellness and the Consumer

While the public is taking more responsibility for its own health and wellness, not everyone has embraced or can embrace the need for self-improvement or personal responsibility. Technology has increased access to information for many people (Ryan, 2018, p. 1), but what does the public do with that information once received? According to the Current Population Survey in 2016, 89 percent of all U.S. households had a computer and/or smartphone with 81 percent with a broadband Internet subscription (Ryan, 2018, p. 1, Milani & Franklin, 2017, p. 487). Differences in socioeconomic status and language barriers have contributed to lack of understanding and often lack of access to health care services for certain population groups. Health care managers who work with these populations should be aware that differences in culture or socioeconomic status do not mean that health and wellness are not areas of concern. Strategies for health and wellness promotion that may work in one population or culture may not work in another. Health information disseminated via social networking sites (e.g., Twitter, Cyworld, Facebook), by the Internet, or the use of PHRs (e.g., Microsoft's HealthVault, Google Health) may be effective for certain populations or age groups, whereas television advertisements, telephone calls, and personal interaction may be better techniques for reaching other populations and age groups. Consumer-driven health care seeks to tailor offerings to fit the population served including health and wellness choices with respect for culture and traditional viewpoints and methods.

Health information technology (HIT) has changed the way in which medicine and health care is delivered. HIT can be defined as the computer-based storage, usage, retrieval, and sharing of health care information, data, and knowledge for communication and decision-making purposes (Cohen and Stussman, 2010). Examples of HIT include electronic medical or health records (EMRs/EHRs), PHRs, health networks (e.g., PatientsLikeMe), social network sites (e.g., Facebook, Twitter), telecommunications applications (e.g., iPhone, Android), and personal data storage devices (e.g., PDAs, eBook, iPad).

Table 14.2 Healthy People 2010 Leading Heath Indicators

Physical Activity	Mental Health
Overweight and obesity	Injury and violence
Tobacco use	Environmental quality
Substance abuse	Immunization
Responsible sexual behavior	Access to health care

SOURCE: For additional information on the Healthy People 2010, see http://www.healthypeople.gov/LHI/lhiwhat.htm.

In a report on HIT use among U.S. men and women by the Pew Internet & American Life Project in 2013, researchers noted over 93 million Americans (80 percent of Internet users) reported searching for a health-related topic online. This was an increase from the 62 percent reporting health-related Web searching in 2001. What were these 93 million people looking for? When asked this question and focusing on 16 specified topics ranging from mental health to immunizations, the most common online searches pertained to a specific disease or medical issue (63 percent) or a specific health care treatment or procedure (47 percent) (Weaver, 2013, paras 2–3).

Additional major topics for online searches were diet, nutrition, and vitamins (44 percent); fitness and exercise information (36 percent); over-the-counter drugs (34 percent); health insurance (25 percent); and specific health care providers or hospitals (21 percent).

What does this mean for health care professionals and health care managers? HIT is being used by more adults to access health information and to communicate with health providers. Health care managers who choose to embrace HIT and telecommunications in their practice and health care service delivery will enhance their appeal to consumers, particularly younger generations and those who are technologically savvy, but how safe are they (Agency for Healthcare Research and Quality, 2018, para 1; Moscovitch, 2018; Musgrave, 2018, para 1)?

Social Network Sites and Health Management

Social networking has become a household word and a common method of communication for many people. Social networking is defined as the creation and maintenance of business and personal relationships accomplished digitally or online (Merriam-Webster, 2017). Social networking is done through social network sites (SNS), which are defined as "web-based services that allow individuals to (1) construct a public or semi-public profile within a bounded system, (2) articulate a list of other users with whom they share a connection, and (3) view and traverse their list of connections and those made by others within the system" (Boyd and Ellison, 2007). While social networking (implying the initiation of a relationship or place to meet) may occur on these sites, it is generally not the primary focus of many of these sites; rather, they provide a medium for their users to verbalize and make their social networks visible and expressive to others (Agrawal, 2016; Boyd and Ellison, 2007). Many users of large SNSs already have an extended in-person social network, and their use of SNSs is simply a means of extending communication within their existing network (NCSBNInteract, 2011; NCSBN, 2011). Agrawal (2016)

identified five advantages of social networking for the good of society: (1) increased teen awareness of events, news, and to feel like they are part of something; (2) sending safety messages regarding the distractions caused by social media use while driving (pictures of crashes or statistics of accidents); (3) increased marketing exposure to larger numbers of potential consumers; (4) increased ability for cross-global communication; and (5) rapid dissemination of global news events and disasters reporting.

SNSs are used by individuals to connect with others based on common interests, language, political or religious views, and racial, sexual, ethnic, or nationality-based identities (Boyd and Ellison, 2007; Cordina, Kumar, and Moss, 2015; Stewart, 2009) or to "stay in touch" with those we do not see very often sharing details about lives and thoughts (Piscotty, Martindell, and Karim, 2016). SNSs may vary in the extent to which they cater to diverse audiences or how they incorporate new information and communication tools (e.g., blogging, mobile connectivity ability, or photo sharing).

What does this mean for consumer-driven health care and health care managers? Social network sites have contributed to increased public awareness of health and wellness issues and have been used to disseminate information to larger numbers of people at one time. For example, when an emergency department nurse in Salt Lake City refused to allow police to draw blood on an unconscious patient and was subsequently arrested, this event was shared quickly around the globe via social media.

Social marketing has been utilized by the public sector to elicit the interest of the public in policy and governmental issues by aligning key issues and initiatives with the needs of the people and to disseminate research and news events (Balasubramani, 2014; Stewart, 2009). Applying social marketing techniques to health care, with its emphasis on understanding people and their needs, and using this understanding to design interventions, may be a good strategy for appealing to the consumer-driven health care market (Piscotty, Martindell, and Karim, 2016; Stewart, 2009).

One example of the power of social marketing can be seen in the popularity of health SNSs and PHRs. Health social network sites are a type of online social network that links users to common health or medical themes or areas of interest (e.g. PatientsLikeMe) or genetics (e.g., 23andMe) (Stewart, 2009). Users of health social network sites may be linked together through common personal experience, shared health information, or shared camaraderie.

Health networks and personal health tracking were made popular by Nike with the introduction of its Nike+ website in April 2008 and the use of running shoes with sensors implanted in them to gather and transmit fitness data through its website to monitor performance. Other technologies targeting health and wellness monitoring include smartphone applications and wearable monitors, such as FitBit or the iPhone health applications. A workshop conducted by the National Institutes of Health in 2018 focused on the use of artificial intelligence (AI) and application of machine learning and other technologies to improve health and wellness in clinical settings (Garnett, 2018, paras 1, 16, 30, 31). With such ventures into health and wellness management such as Nike's HealthVault and fitness monitors (Fitbit), Dr. Dina Katabi of MIT's Center for Wellness Networks and Mobile Computing previewed a "health-aware home" that monitors heart rate, breathing, falls, sleep, and other behaviors without physical sensors being attached to the body (paras 31–32). The data can be uploaded via an iPod to the Nike+ website (Stewart, 2009). A number of websites and smartphone or smartwatch applications offer to track and monitor cardio, fitness, and health data as well as providing jogging routes, sharing information, and establishing support groups centered around specific health activities or situations (Colon, 2018, Milani & Franklin, 2017, p. 488). Examples for 2018 include Fitbit charge, Garmin Vivoactive 3, Motiv Ring, and Apple Watch Series. PatientsLikeMe was formed as a network centered on amyotrophic lateral sclerosis (ALS, otherwise known as Lou Gehrig's disease) and has since expanded to include 19 disease states and behavioral conditions (Patientslikeme.com, 2018). PatientsLikeMe is one example of a support network where users can manually enter health data and treatment details (e.g., dosage and side effects of treatments) to share with others on the site. In this way, users can see what has and has not worked for others in similar situations and disease stages (Patientslikeme.com, 2018).

Electronic Health Care Records

Electronic Medical Health Records versus Personal Health Records

One of the most common forms of HIT is the EHR (Agency for Healthcare research and Quality, 2018, para 1; Robert Wood Johnson Foundation, 2008). The terms **electronic health record (EHR)** and EMR have been used to describe health or medical information that is stored, utilized, retrieved, or shared electronically. The Health Information Management System Society (HIMSS) defines EHRs as:

> [A] longitudinal electronic record of patient health information generated by one or more encounters in any care delivery setting. Included in this information are patient demographics, progress notes, problems, medications, vital signs, past medical history, immunizations, laboratory data, and radiology reports. (Health Information Management System Society, 2018, para 1)

It is important to remember that EHRs are developed and maintained by health care organizations (e.g., clinic, hospital, physician's office) as a record of care rendered at that facility at that point in time. They are not a complete record of all care provided to an individual over all venues of time (Agency for Healthcare Research and Quality, 2018, paras 1–2: Health Information Management System Society, 2018, para 1; Musgrave, 2018, para 1).

Medical records were initially designed by physicians as a means of documenting and storing information regarding patient encounters. They were designed around the premise of meeting the needs of the physician and contained information that physicians deemed important, though not necessarily everything the patient considered important (Robert Wood Johnson Foundation, 2010). The first EHRs appeared in the 1960s, based on initial research using clinical care projects, such as COSTAR (Computer Stored Ambulatory Record, developed by Harvard), HELP (Health Evaluation through Logical Processing, developed by the Latter Day Saints Hospital at the University of Utah), CHCS (Composite Health Care System—Department of Defense), and DHCP (De-Centralized Hospital Computer System—Veteran's Administration) (Allan and Englebright, 2000). Current versions are more robust and technologically savvy enabling multiple users, sharing of personal health records utilizing HIPAA criteria, and types of technology applications by smartphone applications, doctors office records, hospitals, and other health organizations (Agency for Healthcare Research and Quality, 2018, paras 1, 5, 7–9).

As HIT became more prevalent, medical records began to be digitized and information transferred to electronic files for use by physicians, nurses, and hospital staff. Benefits of the EMR included larger storage capacity (electronic versus paper files), easier access for patients to view their records (through intranet and online portals), and easier transferability of records and data sharing (per HIPAA criteria) (Agency for Healthcare Research and Quality, 2018, paras 1–3, 7: Robert Wood Johnson Foundation, 2010). EMR online portals could be internally accessed through the organization's intranet or externally accessed online portals using predetermined authorization codes and access protocols. As access to personal health information via EMRs and EHRs and organizationally based online portals increased, individuals began to recognize the value in having accessible personal health information.

Personal Health Records

As utilization of HIT and Internet access became commonplace for consumers and health care professionals in the United States, it became evident that access to such health information might assist consumers in their personal wellness efforts and contribute to increased personal responsibility for health care decision making (Robert Wood Johnson Foundation, 2010). Consumers began questioning why they could not see their medical information alongside other information they considered valuable when making health choices. The option of using their own medical or health information in areas they considered important, such as weight or exercise tracking, monitoring of chronic conditions, or personal wellness initiatives, led to the development of the PHR.

PHRs are electronic Web-based repositories for personal health information, whereas EHRs reside in a hospital or health care organization's database. With PHRs, consumers decide what health information will be provided, where it comes from, and who has access to it (Stewart, 2009). PHRs can be freestanding or tied to institutions (tethered) (Robert Wood Johnson Foundation, 2010).

Some larger health care systems have moved toward further integration of tethered PHRs that include basic features of EHRs plus wellness and personal health management options (HealthIT.gov, 2016). Two basic kinds of PHRs are tethered or connected PHRs and stand-alone PHRs (HealthIT.gov, 2016). The tethered or connected PHR is aligned directly to a specified health care organization's EHR. Individuals use a secure portal to access their records, such as health summaries or lab and radiology reports. Conversely, stand-alone PHRs require the individuals to fill in and maintain their own health records (e.g., adding lab results, exercise information, etc.) and use their own computers to store the information as a hard-copy record or in a personal cloud format located in a secured area in the Internet. Examples of freestanding PHRs include Dossia, WebMD, Revolution Health, Google Health, and Microsoft's HealthVault. Freestanding PHRs require consumers to enter health information manually; however for users of Dossia, there is the option to choose to automatically pool information from insurance claims, laboratory tests, or physician medical records into their PHR through the utilization of Indivo, an open infrastructure (Stewart, 2009).

Some differences between PHRs and EMRs or EHRs include privacy concerns, record design and maintenance responsibilities, reason for record development, and ability to move through the PHR or EMR system and accomplish tasks. While some tethered PHRs may provide access to health information and even some limited messaging within the system, they are still constrained by what and where information can be accessed and communication exchanged (Robert Wood Johnson Foundation, 2010).

Some barriers exist regarding the full implementation of HIT, hence the expansion and full capabilities of PHRs. Systemic barriers identified by the Robert Wood Johnson Foundation in their *Project HealthDesign* and research on PHRs (2010) included (1) a fragmented

state of the current health care system, (2) diversity of health care data, (3) interoperability and technical difficulties related to the sharing of health data, and (4) the current reimbursement system (Robert Wood Johnson Foundation, 2010).

Lack of coordinated use of HIT, with EHRs, throughout the U.S. health care system is one area that impedes acceptance and utilization of PHR. Just how prevalent is the use of electronic health (medical) records by health providers in the United States? A report by the Robert Wood Johnson Foundation on "Health Information Technology in the United States: Where We Stand, 2015" (DesRoches, Painter, and Jha, 2015) made some interesting findings:

- A minimum of a basic HER was in place for 75.5 percent of hospitals in 2014, which is a significant increase of 58.9 percent since the year 2013.
- The exchange of health data between hospitals and external health professionals was identified at 62 to 76 percent increase since 2013 and a 41 percent increase since the beginning of this survey in 2008 (DesRoches, Painter, and Jha, 2015).

One of the primary constraints in the full utilization of EHR by physicians was still cost. While the HITECH Act of 2009 encouraged adoption and implementation of EHR, use of technology, and digital sharing of health data, DesRoches, Painter, and Jha (2015) from the Robert Wood Johnson Foundation noted that hospitals continued to face barriers in fully adopting these standards. These barriers were primarily in the form of financial viability and sustainability. Privacy can also be a concern with the use of personal health information in PHR platforms. Web-based applications that are not under the jurisdiction of health care providers raised some privacy concerns by consumers, policy makers, and consumer advocates. HIPAA regulates and provides protection for health information used by "covered entities" (health care providers who transmit health information electronically, health plans, and health care clearinghouses) (Office of Civil Rights, 2018, p. 2). Not all PHRs are not covered under HIPAA privacy regulations. Those offered by a health care provider or health plan are covered by the HIPAA Privacy rule whereas PHRs available by a non-HIPAA-covered vendor or third party such as Google Health or certain applications available for smartphones are not covered (Office of Civil Rights, 2018, p. 2).

For users of current platforms of PHRs and health network sites, consumers should use discretion of who has access to their private health information. "Private" may no longer be equal to confidential under these circumstances including information shared on smartphone applications of Internet sites (Office of Civil Rights, 2018, p. 2–3). Consumers who are familiar with online banking or social network sites, such as Twitter or Facebook are aware of the level of privacy that is currently available. However, discretion over personal health information use, who has access to this data, and what they can do with it may entail stronger information management systems and privacy that are currently available. Advice for consumers and health care managers who supervise employees who use these types of platforms is to caution users to reconsider what they share and what remains private.

Ciampa (2015) identified that the top concern for computer professionals globally is information security with greater than 666 million electronic data record breaches from 2005 to early 2014 (p. xiii). These attacks exposed personal identifying information, such as Social Security numbers addresses, health records, and credit card numbers. Ciampa (2015, p. 607) stated that the question was not how vulnerable we are or if an attack will occur, but when.

How does the average consumer protect him- or herself from inadvertent cyberattack while using the Internet or accessing his or her personal health information? An interview with Dr. Gregory Vert, SAMS/SANS-trained malware expert and a top cybersecurity researcher currently at the Cybersecurity and Intelligence Department in the College of Security & Intelligence at Embry Riddle Aeronautical University, cautioned consumers to "be cautious in what you are doing, don't do anything free, and be prepared for the unexpected" (2017). Consumers should understand how to back up their systems and that the Internet is not safe. The increased potential for cybercrime, such as advance persistent threats (APTs), increases daily for industries, such as health care, financial institutions, military defense, technologies, public utilities, and political entities (Vert et al., 2017).

> When I started into this business about 1982, we thought we would be on top of it and be safe (NSA) as the Internet was just starting to come around. People that were recruited into the program including military officers, but the curve (security of internet and threatscape) has only gotten worse. Nobody can control it anymore. As more people have come into the internet of things, the threatscape increased exponentially due to addition of more electronic access points, such as cell phones, tablets, resulting in the need for cybersecurity and protection of personal information. (Vert et al., 2017)

Vert listed the following four top dangers of the Internet and EHR access for consumers to be aware of:

1. **Free stuff.** Always pay for whatever service you are requesting/purchasing. You always pay for it. Paying for services thus creates a contractual relation that you can litigate if product does not materialize. Free is never anything you want to do. Never click on an e-mail that comes in to you that masquerades as your medical records, a message your father has died, etc.

2. **Spearfishing.** Spearfishing an e-mail from somebody you don't really know asking you to click on a link (or open the message). It gives a short time frame to click on the message due to a perceived risk asking, which in turn downloads malware onto the computer system, cell phone, or tablet.

3. **Questionable websites or companies.** Do not do business with companies that have repeatedly been hacked or that are questionable in their business behaviors (ethics). This includes Facebook's recent exposure of Russian advertising to hack into personal accounts (Shane, 2017; Shane and Goel, 2017). Other questionable sites are WikiLeaks, LinkedIn, and Twitter.

4. **Shared USB drives.** Never swap or share USB drives with anybody. They are self-bootable and can activate even when the device is turned off (Vert et al., 2017).

RETAIL MEDICINE

Key Concepts

Retail medicine has been described as health care services that are provided in "retail settings" or nonhospital, nontraditional medical environments (Nash, Jacoby, and Murtha, 2008). Examples of retail medicine include minor emergency health care clinics, **convenient care clinics**, LASIC centers, dental clinics, and cosmetic services (Cordina, Kumar, and Moss, 2015; Hilgers, 2005). Emphasis on the customer as the consumer of services has changed the health care environment toward a more market-based, sales-oriented approach to health care service delivery.

People's lives have become more complicated. Many find themselves immersed in multiple roles, such as parent, child, spouse, employer, employee, caretaker, student, friend, colleague, or expert that come with increased expectations and requirements. Increased access to information, knowledge, and communication via the media, the Internet, social networking, and personal interaction has caused people to become more aware of and sophisticated in their perceptions of what health services are available and what *they* expect. The use of instant messaging, PDAs, cell phones, and e-mail has become a way of life for many Americans.

Health care consumers expect health services to be readily available when needed, in easily accessible

• • • IN PRACTICE: Microsoft and Google Investments in PHRs

The consumer-driven health care movement has caused consumers to be more aware of health needs and expectations. Consumers are taking more responsibility for their own health and wellness and are turning to health network sites (e.g., CureTogether) and personal health records (PHRs) (e.g., Google Health, Microsoft's HealthVault) to assist them in this venture (Froomkin, 2008; Robert Wood Johnson Foundation, 2010; Stewart, 2009).

Microsoft and Google are two leading vendors in PHRs. PHRs are individual health records that are owned and controlled by the patient, not a health care facility or health provider (Stewart, 2009). The patient decides what is included and who has access to the information. PHRs are usually Web-based and stored on health-related websites that provide PHR platforms, such as Google Health and Microsoft's HealthVault.

Google Health uses a continuity of care (CCR) record, which is a type of standardized health record developed by a collaboration of health care advocacy groups, health providers, and regulators (Stewart, 2009). By choosing this type of health record, Google Health expects that the information contained will be of value to its users and what health care providers hope their patients will track themselves. Information can be either manually entered or imported from a number of partnered sources, such as An Vita Health, Inc., or Medi Connect (Stewart, 2009). One major advantage of PHRs is that your record stays with you even if you change doctors, employers, or health plans.

While Google began its ventures into PHRs in 2006, announcing the advent of Google Health in February 2008, Microsoft released its HealthVault PHR application in October 2007, partnering with 40 health care organizations, such as Johnson & Johnson and the American Heart Association (Anonymous, 2008; McBride, 2008; Stewart, 2009). HealthVault's PHR platform is based on a need to house large amounts of information and health-related transactions. HealthVault is accessed through a Windows LiveID and has additional search capabilities through "Live Health Search." Another interesting feature of HealthVault is its capability to upload information from personal and medical devices, such as blood-glucose monitors, heart rate monitors, bathroom scales, and over 50 Wi-Fi- and Bluetooth-enabled devices (Stewart, 2009).

Both Google Health and Microsoft HealthVault have partnered with additional health clinics, pharmacies, and other health-related groups (e.g., Cleveland Clinic, CVS Pharmacy, Quest Diagnostics) (McBride, 2008; Robert Wood Johnson Foundation, 2010). While Google Health and Microsoft HealthVault have volunteered to comply with current health information privacy standards, HIPAA regulations do not cover health data stored in these PHR sites; hence, consumers should use discretion when considering what to upload and who really has access to their personal health information.

locations, staffed by health care professionals trained in the latest treatments and diagnostic procedures, and to be cost-effective. Many consumers have a basic understanding and recognition of many non-life-threatening health conditions, such as ear infections, urinary tract infections, and influenza. As the pace and stress of their lives increase, rapid accessibility to care and treatment for these routine health concerns has become a market need. Hilgers (2005) noted that retail medicine and health services usually contain at least one of the following characteristics: (1) price competition and marketing emphasis on cost-effectiveness, (2) mass marketing techniques through multiple media formats, (3) corporation of health services via larger multistate organizations, and (4) the targeting of health needs that are not considered to be life-threatening or serious. As customer expectations continue to rise, service providers—especially those who provide health care–related services—must adapt to the needs of their customer base. Retail medicine is one answer to the expanding consumer need for health services as a niche solution (Cordina, Kumar, and Moss, 2015).

Choices and Challenges in Retail Medicine

Convenient Care Clinics

One form of retail medicine that caters to the diagnosis and treatment of non-life-threatening conditions are retail health care clinics often referred to as minor emergency clinics, urgent care clinics, convenient care clinics, or colloquially as "doc-in-a-box" clinics. These clinics tend to be in high-volume areas, such as retail outlets or shopping malls. They may be associated with pharmacies or with large chain department or consumer stores, such as Wal-Mart, Target, CVS, or Walgreens. This type of medical clinic has also been referred to as "Wal-Mart medicine" due to the proximity of the health clinic inside a Walmart, Target, or other large consumer store. Convenient care clinics, minor medical or minor emergency clinics, and their parent organizations do display some of the characteristics noted by Nash, Jacoby, and Murtha (2008), such as incorporation of health services via larger multistate organizations, targeting needs that are not considered to be life-threatening, use of mass-marketing techniques targeting consumers who frequent the stores they are in, and generally not accepting insurance. Cordina, Kumar, and Moss (2015, para 29) noted an increase in the number of retail clinics in the United States from 1,183 in 2010 to 1,866 by 2015 with CVS operating over half of the clinics with plans for expansion to 1,500 CVS clinics by the year 2017.

These retail clinics or convenient care clinics offer walk-in services for a limited scope of medical conditions from minor sore throats and ear infections to preventive services such as flu shots, vaccinations, and health screenings (Nash, Jacoby, and Murtha, 2008). They are usually staffed by advanced practice health professionals, such as nurse practitioners (NPs) or physician's assistants (PAs). Research in 2015 by McKinsey & Company (Cordina, Kumar, and Moss, 2015, para 29) found that greater than 80 percent of participants were aware of these retail services but were not exactly sure what was offered. Of those using these clinics, 51 percent stated they used health services at pharmacies or retail clinics for immunizations and 26 percent for treatment of a minor illness.

Many of the convenient care clinics are members of the **Convenient Care Association (CCA)**. The CCA is an organization of health care systems and companies that offer accessible, cost-effective, quality health services located in retail-based environments (Convenient Care Association, 2018). Executive management for the CCA is provided by a nonprofit public health institute, the Public Health Management Corporation (PHMC).

The first convenient care clinic opened its doors in 2000 in Minneapolis—St. Paul, Minnesota, operated by QuickMedX, and its services were limited to a very small number of illnesses operating on a cash-only basis (Convenient Care Association, 2018). By 2018, CCA member clinics had increased to approximately 2,400 clinics operating in 44 states. Ninety-seven percent of the convenient care retail clinics were noted to be CCA members in 2018 (Convenient Care Association, 2018) with more than 35 million patients treated (Convenient Care Association, 2018).

Despite their rise in popularity, many consumers are left wondering: Is convenient care quality care? How do I know whether the care I receive is up to quality industry standards? Some health care professionals and organizations have questioned the quality of care delivered at retail and convenient care clinics and consider it to be controversial in regard to clinical care (Convenient Care Association, 2018, paras 3–4). Other traditional-based practitioners and health organizations view the impetus of retail medicine as a threat to health care quality and safety by removal of patients from traditional medical practices and services (e.g., hospital- and physician office–based). The Convenient Care Clinic Association requires its member clinics to implement national

guidelines and standards for health care quality and safety in assisting clinical providers with their health care decision making (Convenient Care Association, 2018; Nash, Jacoby, and Murtha, 2008).

Complementary, Integrative, and Alternative Medicine Considerations

Complementary and alternative medicine (CAM) refers to health and medical practices that are not considered to be part of conventional Western medicine or standard care. Conventional medicine or "standard care" is defined as medicine that is practiced by a medical doctor (MD) or doctor of osteopathy (DO) or by allied health professionals, such as registered nurses or physical therapists (MD Anderson Cancer Center, 2009; Medline Plus, 2009). Other terms for conventional medicine are Western medicine, mainstream medicine, or allopathy (MD Anderson Cancer Center, 2009). Alternative medicine pertains to "therapeutic choices taken in place of traditional medicine used to treat or ameliorate disease" (MD Anderson Cancer Center, 2009). Complementary medicine consists of therapies and practices used to "complement" or be used in addition to Western or allopathic medical choices or treatments (MD Anderson Cancer Center, 2009). CAM therapies may include mind–body interventions (e.g., meditation, prayer, music therapy), biologically based and herbal treatments (e.g., herbal medicine or plant therapies), manipulative and body-based therapies (e.g. massage, reflexology), or energy therapies (e.g. Reiki, qi gong, Therapeutic Touch) (MD Anderson Cancer Center, 2009).

The consumerism movement in health care, compounded by changes in socioeconomic status and insurance coverage, has increased the demand for the availability of retail and CAM choices (Hilgers, 2005; Wolsko et al., 2000). Reasons why consumers may choose to utilize CAM include poor results from conventional medical treatments, negative experiences with traditional Western medical practitioners, unpleasant side effects for pharmaceutical therapies, limited available personal capital, or personal views and perceptions of health that are not in alignment with traditional Western medical choices (Barnett, 2007).

Concierge Medicine and Global Competition

Concierge care is an additional form of medical care delivery that caters to the wealthy and upper middle classes. Consumers who can afford to pay for special health services with personalized benefits may choose concierge care over other forms of traditional, alternative, or retail medicine. Second opinions, precertification, and long waiting lists are some of the reasons why the wealthy may choose to select the convenience and instant access of concierge care, even if it means going outside the United States to get it.

Concierge care is not dependent upon insurance reimbursement, and consumers may pay an additional fee of $1,500 per individual or up to $20,000 per couple for personalized health care services. Services provided may include same-day appointments, home visits, provider accompaniment to emergency rooms, and after-hours accessibility via pagers or cell phones. This extra fee is in addition to co-payments or deductibles designated by insurance companies (Nash, Jacoby, and Murtha, 2008). Outside of the United States, surgical procedures, radical oncology treatments, cosmetic reconstruction, and fertility clinics are a few of the services provided by concierge health clinicians. Conventional Western, non-Western, and alternative medical therapies can all be found in various locations across the United States, or in several countries worldwide for those who are able and willing to afford them. There has always been some sort of a concierge care trade for upscale medical services, but the recent trend for a more consumer-based approach to health care increased the potential for this particular market in meeting the real or perceived needs for a knowledgeable, informed, and fiscally sound public.

ETHICAL CONSIDERATIONS IN HEALTH CARE

Key Concepts

The very nature of health care and health care systems evokes certain ethical concerns and considerations for the health care manager. Consumerism and the increasing demands of consumers as active participants in their health care decisions may cause controversies between ethical decision making and treatment options. Does everyone have the right to all treatment options? Should the truth always be told even if it jeopardizes a patient's health or well-being? What key ethical principles are frequently seen in health care decision making, and are they the same for all organizations and industries? These questions reflect some of the ethical concerns raised in health care environments.

In this section, we explore the ethical considerations inherent in health care, particularly those impacted by the expanded consumer role. We consider how consumers have impacted ethical decision making and how choices can impact quality patient care in health care environments. How will these change the interrelationship between ethics and consumerism in the next decade or two? What will be changed and what will remain the same?

Ethics has been a topic of examination, critique, and discussion throughout history. Greek philosophers Socrates and Hippocrates each debated merits and controversies inherent in the study of ethics, logic, and human behavior. As science and medicine have continued to evolve and expand over the centuries, new

perspectives on societal obligation, behavior, and moral considerations began to emerge. Professional standards of quality care and codes of conduct were developed as guides for professional morality and ethical behavior. Professional standards of care and laws regulating behaviors were assumed throughout history with the work by Ignaz Semmelweis in the nineteenth century on handwashing and Florence Nightingale with hygiene and cleanliness standards for disease prevention (Marjoua and Bozic, 2015, p. 265). These became more formalized in the 1960s with the advent of specific bioethical legal decisions (Nuremburg trails, Tuskegee Syphilis studies scandal, etc.) and civil rights issues (Ethics & Compliance Initiative, 2018, para 2), surrounding human subjects protections and bioethics (Marjoua and Bozic, 2015, p. 265, Moffett and Moore, 2011, p. 109, Office of History and Stetten Museum, 2018, paras 1–6). Standards of care refer to usual and customary behaviors and practices ("standards") comprising quality competent care and sound medical judgment (Moffett and Moore, 2011, para 10). Whereas medical malpractice, or the absence of the application of a standard of care, was defined by Chief Justice C. J. Roberson as "the failure of a physician to provide quality of care required by law. When a physician undertakes to treat a patient, he takes an obligation enforceable by law to use minimally sound medical judgment and render minimally competent care in the course of the service he provides . . . A competent physician is not liable per se for a mere error of judgment, mistaken diagnosis or the occurrence of an undesirable result" Moffett and Moore, 2011, p. 110).

The medical and health care fields are unique in respect to certain moral and ethical expectations. Health care professionals are expected to comply with general moral/ethical principles to "do good" (beneficence) and "do no harm" (nonmaleficence) to patients. The Hippocratic Oath (OED, 1989f; AAPS, n.d.; History of Medicine Division, 2012, paras 1-3.), still taken by physicians, is an embodiment of the principle of nonmaleficence and requires physicians to "do no harm" to their patients and others in their professional practice but does not recommend the principle of veracity (truth telling) in professional dealings (Beauchamp and Childress, 2009). Omissions such as this have led to the revision of many of the initial codes of conduct for medicine and health care as societal views and have expectations changed over time. Key moral and ethical principles that pertain directly to health care relationships discussed in this section are respect for autonomy, privacy, confidentiality, fidelity, veracity, nonmaleficence, beneficence, and justice.

Autonomy

Autonomy relates to the freedom to follow or act according to one's own will (OED, 1989a). Personal autonomy pertains to self-rule or self-governance where the individual, organization, institution, or entity is free from limitations or control by others. This includes the capacity to understand and have access to information needed to make meaningful decisions (Beauchamp and Childress, 2009). The majority of ethical theories pertaining to autonomy and respect for autonomy encompass two primary elements: liberty (freedom from controlling factors or influences) and agency (the capacity for intentional choices and actions) (Beauchamp and Childress, 2009). Therefore when a physician, individual, or institution is respectful of autonomy, they display a respect for the rights of others to hold personal views and to make choices based on their own system of values, beliefs, and mores. Respect for others, with particular emphasis on personal autonomy, is evidenced in the Patient's Bill of Rights of 1973 and the patient's ability to obtain, understand, and make informed decisions (consent) for procedures and other health-related choices (American Hospital Association, 2018). In the early 1970s, the American Hospital Association (2018) outlined a set of expectations and rights for patients undergoing health care and hospitalization. Approved in 1973 by the AHA House of Delegates and revised in 1992 and 2010, this document serves to specify standard expectations for health care practice and services (American Hospital Association, 2018, para 1).

Conflicts in autonomy can be seen in ethical dilemmas concerning competence, informed consent, or assumptions of control over others (certain family and organizational situations). Beauchamp and Childress (2009) note that respect for autonomy includes acknowledgment of the value and decision-making rights/capacity of others; hence, disrespect for autonomy may be seen as disrespectful actions, attitudes, or behaviors that demean, insult, or do not include attention to autonomous rights of others.

Privacy

The principle of **privacy** relates to the right or choice of being alone, undisturbed, or free from public attention or intrusion (OED, 1989i). Privacy in health care and medicine also pertains to freedom from intrusion of others, especially concerning personal choice, protection from outside interference or observation, and a reasonable expectation of isolation or seclusion without access of the self by others (Beauchamp and Childress, 2009). Privacy issues have been a cause of concern in health care for a number of years, such as public controversy over abortion or family planning, child rearing, relationships, and other areas of personal choice. An example of the expectation of privacy can be seen in *Griswold v. Connecticut* (1965), where the right to protection of information and privacy from the government and others concerning contraception was upheld (Beauchamp and Childress, 2009).

Five types of privacy have been identified that have relevance to health care: (1) informational privacy, (2) physical privacy, (3) decisional privacy, (4) proprietary privacy, and (5) relational or associational privacy. Informational privacy is emphasized in bioethics and rights to access of certain information. Physical privacy pertains to physical and personal space. Decisional privacy relates to personal choices and decision making. Proprietary privacy is concerned with "property interests in the human person" (Beauchamp and Childress, 2009), and relational or associational privacy pertains to expectations of intimate relationships and family where decisions are made in relation to others (Beauchamp and Childress, 2009). Examples of conflicts concerning privacy and privacy issues seen in health care include invasion of privacy and physical space without the consent of the individual, unauthorized access to personal information, or a lack of respect and privacy concerning personal decisions in intimate or close relationships, such as friends, spouses, or physicians.

Confidentiality

Confidentiality is closely related to the principle of privacy. The term "confidential" has been defined as an expectation of a certain privacy and nondisclosure regarding information relayed to another person (OED, 1989d). **Confidentiality**, therefore, pertains to the nature of a confidence or confiding of secrets or private information from one to another. Inherent in the concept of confidentiality is the expectation that any information confided will remain between the confider and confidant, whether this understanding is implicit or explicit. Agreeing to confidentiality means that the person to whom the information was entrusted agrees to not disclose it to anyone without the permission of the confider (Beauchamp and Childress, 2009).

Breaches of confidentiality and privacy are closely related. The primary differences between the two are that a breach of confidentiality occurs when an individual (organization or institution) who received confidential information discloses (or fails to protect) the information without the permission of the confider (Beauchamp and Childress, 2009). It is important to note, as stated earlier, that HIPAA requirements do not pertain to privacy and confidentiality in the use of PHRs. As mentioned earlier, EHRs are protected under the HIPAA regulations, whereas personal health information that is provided to websites, social networking groups, or PHRs such as Microsoft's HealthVault or Google Health is not.

Information housed in EHRs can generally be considered private and confidential due to its protection under HIPAA. Although this may not always be the case as with Farrah Fawcett and Brittany Spears, whose private medical information was leaked to the press by a health care employee at the UCLA Health System (Dissent, 2008 in phiprivacy.net; Silverman, 2009; UCLA Media Relations, 2008). Privacy and confidentiality of health care information (real or presumed) should be considered by consumers (e.g., individuals and groups) who may choose to use one form of health record maintenance over another.

Fidelity

The principle of **fidelity** refers to the concept of being faithful, loyal, or honest (OED, 1989e). Fidelity also pertains to the obligation to honor commitments. In health care, fidelity pertains to relationships between individuals, such as between a health care professional or physician and a patient. Conflicts can occur when there are cross obligations or instances of divided loyalties (Beauchamp and Childress, 2009). Conventional physician–patient relationships tend to place the patient's interests first; therefore, behaviors that are in contrast to what can be conceived as the patient's best interest may be construed as conflicts of fidelity. Health care providers or managers may encounter conflicts of fidelity regarding multiple allegiances to other colleagues, institutions, religious beliefs, funding agencies for research studies, or patients (Beauchamp and Childress, 2009).

Veracity

Veracity concerns truth-telling or the quality of truthfulness (OED, 1989j). It is a basic assumption in health care that information and relationships will be truthful and honest. Beauchamp and Childress (2009) identified three components that are inherent in the concept of veracity that pertain directly to health care: (1) respect for others; (2) fidelity, promise-keeping, and contract; and (3) health professional–patient relationships based on trust. Relationships between health care provider and patient are based on trust and the assumption that the provider will act in the best interest of the patient. When this does not occur, violations of fidelity in the patient–provider relationship can occur, which can escalate to larger ethical situations that may come to the attention of the health care manager or director.

An example of conflict of veracity in health care is nondisclosure of pertinent health information to patients, such as a potentially terminal disease or impending death. Numerous health-related standards and guidelines, including the Hippocratic Oath (Becker's Hospital Review, 2016, paras 1–2) and Declaration of Geneva of the World Medical Association (Association of American Physicians and Surgeons, Inc., n.d.), do not recommend veracity in professional relationships (Beauchamp and Childress, 2009). The American Medical Association's medical ethics principles did not support the principle of veracity or truth-telling to patients until 1980, when physicians were explicitly encouraged to "deal honesty with patients and colleagues" (Association of American Physicians and Surgeons, Inc., n.d.; Beauchamp and Childress, 2009).

Nonmaleficence

Nonmaleficence relates to the duty to "not inflict harm on others" (Beauchamp and Childress, 2009). Obligations of nonmaleficence pertain to intentionally reframing from doing (or nonparticipation in) actions or behaviors that would hurt others. This includes potential for causing harm as well as placing another into a risk for harm. An example seen in health care would be to not cause pain and suffering or demean others (Beauchamp and Childress, 2009). Negligence is an additional example of nonmaleficence that can be seen in health care. Negligence is the absence of care or treatment that is given or that which is below the expected standards of care in the profession or specialty area (Beauchamp and Childress, 2009). Conflicts related to the principle of nonmaleficence frequently seen in health care can be related to religious beliefs and traditions; withholding (withdrawing) life support, treatments, and technologies used to sustain life; extraordinary (and ordinary) medical treatments; and euthanasia/death (Beauchamp and Childress, 2009).

Beneficence

Beneficence is closely related to the principle of nonmaleficence in that beneficence pertains to the obligation to do good, prevent or remove harm, and to act in a kind or benevolent manner (Beauchamp and Childress, 2009; OED, 1989b). Obligations of beneficence, as opposed to nonmaleficence, contain positive requirements for action, may not provide reasons for legal punishment for noncompliance, and are not required to be followed impartially (Beauchamp and Childress, 2009).

Three key aspects of the principle of beneficence that are expected in professional relationships and health care interactions are as follows: (1) prevent harm or evil, (2) remove harm or evil, and (3) promote and do good. Health care is by definition a "helping" profession in which individuals choose to try to make a difference in a caring manner to others. Many health care organizations are based on an altruistic approach to health and wellness with a love and compassion for the human condition. Other terms for beneficence that have been used in relation to health care professionals are mercy, kindness, and charity (Beauchamp and Childress, 2009).

Justice

The Oxford English Dictionary Online (1989g) defines **justice** as "the quality of being (morally) just or righteous," including just conduct, integrity, and conformity to a moral right or reason. Other words associated with justice are rightfulness, fairness, correctness, and propriety. Justice can take many forms. Distributive justice relates to fair and equal distribution as defined by society. Criminal justice is concerned with the fair (just) infliction of punishment for criminal acts, and rectificatory justice deals with breaches of contracts or malpractice issues (Beauchamp and Childress, 2009). Some beliefs pertaining to distributive justice that can be seen in health care interactions are the concept of equal shares—distribution according to need, effort, contribution, merit, or free-market exchange (Beauchamp and Childress, 2009). Health care disparities, treatment accessibility, and equal employment opportunities are examples of some of these conflicts that can be seen in health care and that the health care manager may encounter.

Clinical Bioethics: Rights and Responsibilities

Bioethics is the discipline concerned with ethical questions and actions in medicine and biology (OED, 1989c). It differs from other forms of ethics in that bioethics concentrates on issues found in medicine, such as clinical treatment, end of life decisions, and research concerns and situations. Clinical bioethics departments can be found at a number of universities and government entities both in the United States and internationally. The Department of Bioethics at the National Institutes of Health was established in 1996 and is divided into three key areas of interest: health policy, human subjects' research, and genetics (National Institutes of Health, n.d.).

Research Considerations and Human Subject Protection

Ethical considerations also pertain to clinical research in health care. Research standards, guidelines, and regulations have been established that delineate criteria for research study design and participation by human subjects. Biomedical and behavioral clinical research, especially pertaining to human subject participation in health care facilities, is overseen by Institutional Review Boards (IRBs) and certain governmental agencies, such as the Office for Human Research Protections (OHRP).

Institutional Review Boards (IRBs) are administrative entities established by institutions to protect the ethical rights of human subjects who participate in research conducted under their supervision (OHRP, Jurisdiction of the Institutional Review Board, n.d. a). IRBs have the capacity to review research protocols, require modifications, or disapprove of and require changes to research activities as specified under federal and local institutional policy. IRBs determine whether the clinical situation presented is considered to be research and if it involves

human subjects. The regulatory definition of research is "a systematic investigation, including research development, testing and evaluation, designed to develop or contribute to generalizable knowledge" [Federal Policy §___.102(d)], and human subjects, as they pertain to research, are defined as "living individual(s) about whom an investigator (whether professional or student) conducting research obtains (1) data through intervention or interaction with the individual, or (2) identifiable private information" [Federal Policy §___.102(f)] (OHRP, Jurisdiction of the Institutional Review Board, n.d. b).

The Office for Human Research Protections (OHRP) is a branch of the U.S. Department of Health and Human Services that provides leadership regarding protection of human subjects involved in research activities. The OHRP oversees and safeguards the rights, welfare, and well-being of human research subjects through regulatory oversight, education, advice on bioethical and regulatory issues, and clarification of existing ethical requirements and standards of conduct (OHRP, 2005, September). The Office for Human Subjects Protections also offers a guidebook for IRBs, which contains valuable resources for IRB formation, new review committee members, basic considerations for IRB review, and institutional administration.

One publication that has been instrumental in the establishment of federal regulations for human subject protection is the Belmont Report. The Belmont Report is the result of work by the National Commission for the Protection of Human Subjects of Biomedical and Behavioral Research in the 1970s, with revisions by the Department of Health and Human Services (HHS) in the late 1970s and early 1980s for the protection of human subjects (OHRP, 2008, November 13). The report by the National Commission was originally entitled "Ethical Principles and Guidelines for the Protection of Human Subjects Research" but was renamed the Belmont Report in 1978 after the Belmont Conference Center where the commission initially met when working on the report (OHRP, 2008, November 13). Three interrelated ethical principles are outlined in the Belmont Report that pertains to biomedical and behavioral research: respect for human persons, beneficence, and justice (Figure 14.1). These three principles are the foundation for HHS human subject protection regulations.

The information contained in the Belmont Report and subpart A of 45 CFR part 46 led to the creation of a code of conduct for the protection of human subjects called the "Common Rule." This was created in 1991 by HHS and 14 other federal agencies and departments (OHRP, 2008, November 13). The Belmont Report remains an integral resource for human subject protection education for researchers and IRBs that involve human subjects. Additional information on 45 CFR part 46 can be obtained at http://www.hhs.gov/ohrp/humansubjects/guidance/45cfr46.htm, and the Belmont Report can

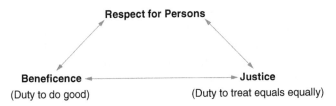

Figure 14.1 Key Principles for Human Subjects Protection from the Belmont Report.

be found at http://www.hhs.gov/ ohrp/humansubjects/guidance/belmont.htm.

Training in human subjects protection is a requirement for researchers in biomedical, behavioral, and other health care–related fields. The Collaborative Institutional Training Initiative (CITI) (n.d.) provides Web-based education and training in human subjects protections including biomedical modules and education. CITI is a joint venture between the University of Miami and the Fred Hutchinson Cancer Research Center and was made available to subscribing institutions in 2000. Additional information on the CITI training initiative may be obtained at https://www.citiprogram.org/aboutus.asp?language=english.

Patient Rights

The existence of the rights of patients in health care has been implied for many years, but it was not until 1973 when the American Hospital Association (AHA) approved the use of the Patient's Bill of Rights that health care providers and organizations began to formally define and agree on what these rights were. The original version of the Patient's Bill of Rights (American Hospital Association, 1992/1998) contained 12 conditions that were expected on the behalf of the patient, many of which echo many of the ethical principles noted in this section:

1. Right to considerate and respectful care.
2. Right to obtain current, relevant, and understandable information concerning diagnosis, treatment, and prognosis.
3. Right to make decisions regarding the plan of care and to refuse treatment to the extent permitted by the law and organizational policy.
4. Right to have an advance directive or designate a surrogate decision maker.
5. Right to every consideration of privacy.
6. Right to expect confidentiality of information and communication.
7. Right to review records pertaining to his or her medical care with explanation (or interpretation) of said records and information.
8. Right to expect reasonable response to the patient's request for appropriate and medically indicated care and treatment according to the organization's capacity and policies.
9. Right to ask and be informed of business relationships among the organization and other internal or external stakeholders that may influence the patient's care and treatment.
10. Right to consent or refuse to participate in research studies that affect care and treatment and to have those research studies or activities fully explained.
11. Right to expect reasonable continuity of care when appropriate and to be informed of available and realistic patient care options when hospital care is no longer appropriate.
12. Right to be informed of organizational policies and practices that pertains to the patient's care, treatment, and responsibilities.

Although the AHA Patient's Bill of Rights was revised in 1992, it was still considered to be difficult to read and understand by most Americans (Gardner, 2010). In an effort toward increased communication and comprehension between provider and patient, the AHA again revised the Patient's Bill of Rights and shortened it to a more consumer-friendly brochure entitled "The Patient Care Partnership: Understanding Expectations, Rights, and Responsibilities," as it is currently provided in 2018 by the AHA website (American Hospital Association, 2018). This brochure includes six rights written in plain language, which include "high quality hospital care, a clean and safe environment, involvement in your care, protection of your privacy, help when leaving the hospital," and "help with your billing claims" (American Hospital Association, 2003; 2018).

Other health and medical organizations and advisory groups have developed their own versions of the Patient's Bill of Rights. The President's Advisory Commission on Consumer Protection and Quality on the Health Care Industry under President Clinton issued a 1997 interim report defining a Patient's Bill of Rights in Medicare and Medicaid emphasizing three goals, seven sets of rights, and one set of responsibilities (U.S. Department of Health and Human Services, n.d. b). Additional information on this version of patient rights can be found at http://www.hhs.gov/news/press/1999pres/990412.html. These revised patient rights expanded existing expectations to include access to emergency services, care without discrimination, right to speedy complaint resolution, and additional patient responsibility and involvement in their own health and welfare (U.S. Department of Health and Human Services, n.d. b).

Ethics and the Health Care Manager

The role of health care managers and directors can vary according to job description and level of responsibility over others. However, all health care managers and directors, regardless of their level, type of facility, or geographic location should function in an ethical and competent manner.

A number of issues impact ethical management in health environment, such as reimbursement issues, organizational change and behavior, situations related to clinical and behavioral research studies, fiscal needs, and public or consumer pressure. Managed care and the move toward pay-for-performance can contribute to questionable behaviors on the part of health care providers, third-party reimbursement organizations, and expectations (versus reality) of patients regarding service delivery and payment.

Temptation to not always act in an ethical manner can become prevalent if an organization does not require high standards for quality and ethics. While societal examples of unethical behavior, such as that seen by leaders in Enron, WorldCom, and Tenet Health Care may not be enough to dissuade leaders or health professionals to avoid unethical temptation, it is important that high-quality professional standards for ethical and professional conduct be set and followed in order to establish and maintain an ethically competent organization. Just as high-quality standards in compliance with industry standards is important from a regulatory and public-perception standpoint, the method by which a facility or organization regulates its ethical standards can be equally important, especially in this age of consumer-driven health care.

Some ways in which health care managers and directors can work to ensure ethical practices at the organizational level have been identified by Hofmann and Nelson (2001):

1. Refuse temptation to incorporate or excuse inefficient business practices through rationalization (e.g., not-for-profit agencies do not need to fully comply with progressive or aggressive policies and procedures).

2. Ensure that your organization's mission, vision, and values statements are fully understood by all staff, and that decisions and actions made are consistent with these statements.

3. Involve physician, board, and management in significant change efforts that may impact the organization's role in the community.

4. Assess all possible potential effects (positive and negative) on the community before starting competitive strategies.

5. Assess and evaluate all potential ramifications (economic, noneconomic, internal, and external) of eliminating programs or services beforehand.

A number of useful tools and resources are available for managers and leaders concerning ethical behavior and practice. Specific health-related organizations, such as the American College of Surgeons, the American Medical Association, the American Organization of Nurse Executives, the National Center for Healthcare Leadership, and the American College of Healthcare Executives provide specific guidelines and resources for ethical practice. For example, the National Center for Healthcare Leadership (NCHL) has a Leadership Competency Model that can be used to guide the design and development of health care management academic programs. This model (version 2.1) contains 26 competency areas (with five or six levels of attainment), such as accountability, professionalism, change leadership, community orientation, and human resource management (NCHL, 2010). Ethics and ethical behavior are emphasized in *L18.4—Understanding the Basics of Organization Governance* ("Understands governance practices, including board relations, committee structure, and fiduciary, *ethics*, and clinical review responsibilities") and *L19—Professionalism* ("The demonstration of *ethics*, sound professional practices, social accountability, and community stewardship. The desire to act in a way that is consistent with one's values and what one says is important.") (NCHL, 2012). Another tool provided by NCHL is a leadership self-assessment test, which leaders can take to determine their current status in the leadership development schemata. Information regarding NCHL and the leadership self-assessment may be obtained at http://www.nchl.org and http://nchl.org/static.asp?path=2852,3241.

The American College of Healthcare Executives has an ethics self-assessment instrument (http://www.ache.org/newclub/career/ethself.cfm) as well as an ethics toolkit (http://www.ache.org/ABT_ACHE/EthicsToolkit/ethicsTOC.cfm) and other useful resources for health care managers and leaders. For additional information on ethical behavior in business and practice for health care environments including biomedical and behavioral research, review the following links:

American College of Healthcare Executives: http://www.ache.org

America College of Surgeons: http://www.facs.org/

American Medical Association—The Council on Ethical and Judicial Affairs: http://www.ama-assn.org/ama/pub/category/4325.html

American Organization of Nurse Executives: http://www.aone.org/

Center for Practical Bioethics: http://www.practicalbioethics.org/

Institute for Global Ethics: http://www.globalethics.org/

IRB Forum: The Institutional Review Board—Discussion and News Forum: http://www.irbforum.org

Office for Human Research Protections (OHRP): http://www.hhs.gov/ohrp

The Petrie-Flom Center for Health Law Policy, Biotechnology, and Bioethics: http://www.law.harvard.edu/programs/petrie-flom

DEBATE TIME: Ethical Dilemmas for Health Care Managers

An ethical or moral dilemma has been defined as a situation where an individual's obligations require two or more possible pathways or alternatives, but only one is possible (Hamric, Spross, and Hanson, 2009). Ethical dilemmas (or conflicts) occur in health care environments on a daily basis. The ability to recognize a potential conflict with possible intervention to prevent the conflict from advancing to a dilemma is a valuable skill for the health care manager's professional toolkit. Table 14.3 contains examples of possible health-related ethical conflicts or dilemmas. See which ones you can identify with and what strategies you could use to intervene or prevent the situation from advancing into a more serious situation.

Table 14.3 Health Care Conflicts and Ethical Principles

Ethical Principle	Definition	Ethical Issue for Consideration
Autonomy	Duty to respect individual rights of "personal liberty, values, beliefs and choices"	Shirley's daughter tells you that her father is "old and doesn't know what he is doing." She will be making his decisions for him and is taking him off of two of his medications.
Nonmaleficence	"Duty not to inflict harm"	Joe Smith increases Jerome Terrell's pain medication because he can't stand to see the child suffer due to a sickle cell crisis. Jerome becomes unconscious and lapses into a coma.
Beneficence	"Duty to do good and prevent/remove harm"	Sue Jacobson, a 34-year-old woman with metastatic breast cancer, has a hip fracture and is waiting in the emergency room to be seen. You are walking through the ER on your way to a meeting when you see Sue reaching for her purse on a bedside stand just out of her reach. She is about to roll onto the floor.
Formal Justice	"Duty to treat equals equally"	Miguel and Roxanne are patients of yours with the same diagnosis of multiple sclerosis (MS). There is an experimental drug that proposes to reverse signs and symptoms and reduce pain in MS patients. Both Miguel and Lin are moaning in pain, the same age, and at the same stage of MS. You have only enough of the drug for one person.
Veracity	"Duty to tell the truth"	Dr. Fred has just diagnosed Mrs. Olsen with advanced ovarian cancer. Her prognosis is four months at the most. Since Dr. Fred likes this patient and she is old (89 years old), he decides to not "upset her" and keeps her diagnosis to himself.
Fidelity	"Duty to honor commitments"	Roger is a health care provider who is employed under an integrated health care system. The organization has told him not to continue treating Baby X because the insurance carrier has denied the last two months' worth of claims. Baby X is four months old, and you have been his only health care provider since birth. You promised his mother that you would look after him just before she died in childbirth. While you are committed to the health care organization that employs you, you made this promise to Baby X's mother.

DEBATE TIME: Ethical Dilemmas for Health Care Managers *(Continued)*		
Confidentiality	"Duty not to disclose information shared in a trusted manner"	"She told me not to tell anyone, but I know I can trust you"—conversation overheard in the elevator at a large metropolitan medical center between two nurses you know. The person they are discussing turns out to be your boss's wife. What do you do?
Privacy	"Duty to respect limited access to individuals"	Sarah works in medical records. She learns that her son's girlfriend, Raquel, is an inpatient on the psychiatric floor. She decides to "sneak a peek" at Raquel's medical records to see why she is there; after all, her son's welfare may be at stake!

SOURCE: Adapted from Beauchamp and Childress (2009).

SUMMARY AND MANAGERIAL GUIDELINES

1. Technological advances, changes in societal communication, and access to information have contributed to the consumer-driven health care movement. Consumers expect different modes of health care delivery, access to understandable information, involvement in their health care decisions, and high quality and satisfaction with health services and health providers.

2. Consumer-driven health care has contributed to increased individual expectations and has fueled new markets and applications, such as retail medicine, EMRs and PHRs, and personalized health reimbursement and insurance models.

3. Personal health information is protected by HIPAA regulations, but this applies only to "covered entities" (e.g., health care providers, health plans, and health care clearinghouses). It is important for health care managers and leaders to keep in mind that not all health information is covered under the HIPAA regulations, such as health networking sites (e.g., PatientsLikeMe, CureTogether) or PHRs (e.g., Google Health or Microsoft's HealthVault).

4. Health plans and employer-sponsored health care reimbursement have moved toward a consumer-driven model that encourages the use of HDHPs. These plans generally have optional health accounts for noncovered health expenses that participants have the option to participate in. While many of these plans are still considered part of the managed care model, health care managers need to be aware of the criteria of these health plans from the standpoint of the limitations and extent of reimbursement coverage for organizations, health providers, and employees.

5. Ethical behavior and standards are vital components of effective high-quality health care organizations. Awareness of key ethical principles, common occurrences of specific ethical conflicts, and how their organization regulates compliance with ethical standards are vital aspects of the health care manager's professional role. Important ethical principles to understand include autonomy, privacy, confidentiality, fidelity, veracity, nonmaleficence, beneficence, and justice.

6. Bioethical considerations in clinical and behavioral research impact the success and quality of an organization and are a reflection of the leadership staff. Adherence to human subjects protections standards and ethical behavior in research and organizational activities are required and monitored by Institutional Review Boards (IRBs) and federal agencies, such as the Office of Human Research Protections (OHRP), the National Institute of Health (NIH), and U.S. Department of Health and Human Services (HHS).

DISCUSSION QUESTIONS

1. How has the consumer-driven health movement impacted health care service delivery?

2. What is the impact of Bachman's "five building blocks of health care consumerism" for health care managers?

3. How do HIPAA regulations protect the public's privacy in regards to electronic medical records (EMRs), personal health records (PHRs), and health information used in social health networking groups (e.g., PatientsLikeMe)?

4. How have consumer-directed health plans (CDHPs) and high-deductible health plans (HDHPs) changed health care service reimbursement and health insurance expectations?

5. What is the difference between health savings accounts (HSAs), medical savings accounts (MSAs), flexible spending arrangements (FSAs), and health reimbursement arrangements (HRAs)?

6. What is retail medicine, and should it be of concern to health care managers and leaders in for-profit and not-for-profit environments?

7. Why has retail medicine become popular with consumers? How can health care managers and organizations leverage retail medicine concepts to enhance current service delivery practices in nonretail environments?

8. How do electronic medical records (EMRs) and personal health records (PHRs) differ? How are they similar?

9. Consider Google (Google Health) and Microsoft's (HealthVault) impact on the consumer-driven health movement and the public's need to participate in their own health care. What are the pros and cons of this type of consumer health application? What barriers to expansion of this concept do you foresee in the near future?

10. How can consumers become more involved in their own health care? What products and resources are available for people who wish to take control of their health or monitor chronic disease states from home?

11. Name five key ethical principles that impact the health care environment. What examples of each are commonly seen in health care and why?

12. How do nonmaleficence and beneficence differ, and why are they important in health care?

13. Why do IRBs exist, and how do they impact biomedical, behavioral, and clinical research activities?

14. Do all health care organizations and providers need to comply with the Patient's Bill of Rights? Why or why not?

15. Should health care providers always tell the truth to their patients, even if the truth may cause pain or distress?

CASE

Consumer-Driven Changes for the ABC Health Options Clinic

Robert has been made the new director of the ABC Health Care Options Clinic in Phoenix, Arizona. The clinic is a large, freestanding, multispecialty clinic providing general and specialty health services to the southeastern Phoenix area. It has been in existence since 1963, with 53 physicians and 10 multiphysician groups. The Internal Medicine (IMP), Family Practice (FMP) and OB-GYN (OGP) groups are the largest and have a history of exerting the most control in the clinic's affairs.

Before he took early retirement, the previous director began a plan to make the clinic more "consumer-friendly," incorporating new additions, such as mandatory electronic medical records based on a tethered system, Saturday office hours, and two freestanding satellite minor emergency and primary care clinics in southeastern Phoenix to assist with the uninsured and underinsured population groups. In the last meeting, the chiefs of staff for each of the three primary physician groups expressed their opinions regarding some of the new changes, particularly the satellite clinics for the uninsured and underinsured populations. Dr. Smee, chief of staff for IMP, was concerned that this would bring in "an unfavorable sort into our clinic," decrease their fiscal solvency, and increase the liability. Whereas Dr. Loo, chief of staff for FMP, felt that this was a good way that the clinic can impact the issue of lack of access to care and would increase its ability to provide quality health care to all but was wary of how the clinics would be staffed particularly over the weekends.

Dr. Rodriguez, an endocrinologist specializing in diabetes care, stated concern about the tethered electronic medical record system, which is proposed to be linked with Google Health and HealthVault. Her primary concern was the safety of the information and presumed privacy of health information in personal health records that would be linked to the clinics records. Drs. Blue and Green from rheumatology and orthopedics felt that this push to increase the clinic's public image and consumer appeal is a good strategy and one which could increase the clinic's ability to remain competitive. Mary Johnson, the lead nurse practitioner (NP) from the family practice group, felt that the move toward a more consumer-friendly system and increasing access to care for all was a good move and stated that she and six other NPs were willing to staff the satellite clinics on Saturdays on a rotating basis.

For the last two weeks, Robert has been reviewing all the meeting notes and interviewing representatives from the physicians in each clinic. While the majority of the physicians and groups were in favor of the changes, the Internal Medicine group (IMP) was opposed to the changes and felt threatened by any new change to its accustomed routines.

Robert has called an all-clinic meeting on Friday to discuss these changes and how they will impact the routine of the clinic or if they should be done at all. As he ponders his situation, he has to decide what the best choices are.

Questions

1. What are the key problems?
2. How will these consumer-driven changes affect the clinic overall? Per physician group?
3. Are the tethered medical records a good idea?
4. What ethical concerns have been expressed by the physicians that could impact the success (or failure) of these new changes?
5. Are the satellite clinics such a good idea? What will their impact be on the clinic financially? Will one group bear the majority of the financial obligation and liabilities for this population?

REFERENCES

Agency for Healthcare Research and Quality. (2018). Multiple chronic conditions. Retrieved October 18, 2018 from https://www.ahrq.gov/professionals/systems/long-term-care/resources/multichronic/mcc.html

Agrawal, A. J. (2016). It's not all bad: The social good of social media. *Forbes*. Retrieved October 17, 2018, from https://www.forbes.com/sites/ajagrawal/2016/03/18/its-not-all-bad-the-social-good-of-social-media/#214eeaf7756f.

Allan, J., & Englebright, J. (2000). Patient-centered documentation: An effective and efficient use of clinical information systems. *Journal of Nursing Administration, 30*(2), 90–95.

Americas Health Insurance Plans (AHIP). (2017). 2016 survey of health savings account – high deductive health plans. Retrieved October 18, 2018, from https://www.ahip.org/wp-content/uploads/2017/02/2016_HSASurvey_Draft_2.14.17.pdf.

American Hospital Association. (1992–1998). *AHA—Patient bill of rights. American Hospital Association Mandatory Advisory.* Retrieved January 19, 2010, from http://www.patienttalk.info/AHA-Patient_Bill_of_Rights.htm.

American Hospital Association. (2003). *Understanding expectations, rights, and responsibilities.* Retrieved January 19, 2010, from http://www.aha.org/aha/content/2003/pdf/pcp_english_030730.pdf.

American Hospital Association. (2018). About History: Jan 1, 1973 patient's bill of rights. Retrieved October 18, 2018, from https://www.aha.org/about/history.

Association of American Physicians and Surgeons, Inc. (AAPS). (n.d.). Physician oaths. Retrieved October 18, 2018, from http://www.aapsonline.org/ethics/oaths.htm.

Anonymous. (2008). Microsoft offers online health records. *Information Management Journal, 42*(1), 19.

Bachman, R. E. (2006). *Healthcare consumerism: The basis of a 21st century intelligent health system.* Retrieved November 30, 2009, from http://www.healthtransformation.net/galleries/wp-consumerism/Healthcare%20Consumerism%20-%20The%20Basis%20of%20a%2021st%20Century%20Intelligent%20Health%20System.pdf.

Balasubramani, V. (2014). Nurse properly fired and denied unemployment due to Facebook rant. *Technology and Marketing Law Blog.* Retrieved October 18, 2018, from http://blog.ericgoldman.org/archives/2014/01/nurse-properly-fired-and-denied-unemployment-due-to-facebook-rant.htm.

Barnett, H. (2007). Complementary and alternative medicine and patient choice in primary care. *Quality in Primary Care, 15*, 207–212.

Beauchamp, T. L., & Childress, J. F. (2009). *Principles of biomedical ethics* (6th ed.). Oxford: Oxford University Press.

Becker's Hospital Review. (2016). From the Hippocratic oath to HIPAA: A history of patient privacy. Retrieved October 18, 2018, from https://www.beckershospitalreview.com/healthcare-information-technology/from-the-hippocratic-oath-to-hipaa-a-history-of-patient-privacy.html.

Berkman, N. D., Sheridan, S. L., Donahue, K. E., et al. (2011). Low health literacy and health outcomes: An updated systematic review. *Annals of Internal Medicine, 155*(2), 97–107.

Blais, K. & Bollinger, N. (2014). Chapter 5: Teaching older adults and their families. In K. L. Mauk (Ed.), *Gerontological nursing: Competencies for care* (3rd ed.) (pp. 133–135). Burlington, MA: Jones & Bartlett Learning.

Boyd, D. M., & Ellison, N. B. (2007). Social network sites: Definition, history, and scholarship. *Journal of Computer-Mediated Communication, 13*(1), article 11.

Burke, T. (2014). Federally funded insurance exchanges under the Affordable Care Act: Implications for public health policy and practice. *Public Health Reports, 129*(1), 94–96. doi:10.1177/003335491412900114.

Cahin, V., & Lancashire, J. (2008, March 27). *Older Americans 2008: Key indicators of well-being, press notes.* Retrieved November 12, 2009, from http://www.agingstats.gov/agingstatsdotnet/main_site/default.aspx.

Ciampa, M. (2015). *CompTIA security + guide to network security fundamentals* (5th ed.). Boston, MA: Cengage Learning.

Cohen, R. A., & Stussman, B. (2010, February). Health information technology use among men and women aged 18–64: Early release of estimates from the National Health Interview Survey, January–June 2009. Retrieved February 2, 2010, from http://www.cdc.gov/nchs/data/hestat/healthinfo2009/healthinfo2009.htm.

Collaborative Institutional Training Initiative (CITI). (n.d.). About the Collaborative Institutional Training Initiative. Retrieved January 19, 2010, from http://www.citiprogram.org/aboutus.asp?language=english.

Colon, A. (2018). The best fitness trackers of 2018. *PC Magazine.* Retrieved October 18, 2018 from https://www.pcmag.com/article2/0,2817,2404445,00.asp

Congress.gov. (2018). H.R. 4872—Health Care and Education Reconciliation Act of 2010. 111th Congress (2009–2010). Retrieved October 17, 2018, from https://www.congress.gov/bill/111th-congress/house-bill/4872/text.

Convenient Care Association. (2018). About CCA. Convenient Care Association, Retrieved October 18, 2018 from https://www.ccaclinics.org/about-us/about-cca

Cordina, J., Kumar, R., & Moss, C. (2015). Debunking common myths about healthcare consumerism. *McKinsey & Company.* Retrieved October 18, 2018, from https://www.mckinsey.com/industries/healthcare-systems-and-services/our-insights/debunking-common-myths-about-healthcare-consumerism.

Department of the Treasury, Internal Revenue Service. (2008, November 25). *Health savings accounts and other tax-favored health plans.* Retrieved December 30, 2009, from http://www.irs.gov/pub/irs-pdf/p969.pdf

DesRoches, C. M., Painter, M. W., & Jha, A. K. (2015). Health information technology in the United States 2015. *Robert Wood Johnson Foundation.* Retrieved October 18, 2018, from https://www.rwjf.org/en/library/research/2015/09/health-information-technology-in-the-united-states-2015.html.

Dissent. (2008, April 2). UCLA staffer looked through Farrah Fawcett's medical records. Retrieved May 31, 2010, from: http://www.phiprivacy.net/?p=189.

Ethics & Compliance Initiative (ECI). (2018). Business ethics and compliance timeline. Retrieved October 18, 2018, from https://www.ethics.org/resources/free-toolkit/ethics-timeline/.

Federal Interagency Forum on Aging-Related Statistics. (2008, March). *Older Americans 2008: Key indicators of well-being.* Retrieved November 22, 2009, from http://www.agingstats.gov/agingstatsdotnet/Main_Site/Data/2008_Documents/OA_2008.pdf.

Frakt, A. (2015). Why consumers often err in choosing health plans. *New York Times.* Retrieved October 18, 2018, from https://www.nytimes.com/2015/11/02/upshot/why-consumers-often-err-in-choosing-health-plans.html.

Fronstin, P., & Elmlinger, A. (2017). Consumer engagement in health care: Findings from the 2016 EBRI/ Greenwald & Associates consumer engagement in health care survey. *Employee Benefit Research Institute (EBRI.org).* Retrieved October 18, 2018, from https://www.ebri.org/pdf/briefspdf/EBRI_IB_433_CEHCS.25May17.pdf.

Froomkin, A. M. (2008). *The new health information architecture: Coping with privacy implications of the personal health records revolution.* Retrieved January 19, 2010, from http://www.projecthealthdesign.org/media/file/social-life-info-15.pdf.

Gardner, A. (2010). *Patient's bill of rights too tough to read.* Retrieved January 19, 2010, from http://www.healthfinder.gov/news/newsstory.aspx?docID=624592.

Garnett, C. (2018). AI workshop surveys landscape, assess big ideas. NIH Record, LXX (18). Retrieved October 18, 2018, from https://nihrecord.nih.gov/newsletters/2018/09_07_2018/story1.htm.

Goodman, J. C. (2006, March 29). *Transparency in health care.* Retrieved December 30, 2009, from http://www.ncpa.org/pub/ba548.

Guzys, D., Kenny, A., Dickson-Swift, V., et al. (2015). A critical review of population health literacy assessment. *BMC Public Health, 15*(1), 1–7. doi:10.1186/s12889-015-1551-6.

Hajat, C. & Kishore, S. P. (2018). The case for a global focus on multiple chronic conditions. *BMJ Global Health,* 3(3), 2000874 doi:10.1136/bmjgh-2018-000874.

Hamric, A. B., Spross, J. A., & Hanson, C. M. (2009). *Advanced nursing practice* (4th ed.). St. Louis, MO: Saunders Elsevier.

Havlin, L. J., McAllister, M. F., & Slavney, D. H. (2003, September). How to inject consumerism into your existing health plans. *Employee Benefits Journal, 28*(3), 7–14.

He, W., Goodkind, D., & Kowal, O. (2016). An aging world: 2015. Report No. P95-16-1. United States Census Bureau. Retrieved October 18, 2018, from https://www.census.gov/content/dam/Census/library/publications/2016/demo/p95-16-1.pdf.

HealthCare.gov. (2017a). 3 things to know before you pick a health insurance plan. Retrieved October 18, 2018, from https://www.healthcare.gov/choose-a-plan/comparing-plans/.

HealthCare.gov. (2017b). Affordable Care Act (ACA). Retrieved October 18, 2018, from https://www.healthcare.gov/glossary/affordable-care-act/.

HealthIT.gov. (2016). Are there different types of personal health records (PHRs)? Retrieved October 18, 2018, from https://www.healthit.gov/providers-professionals/faqs/are-there-different-types-personal-health-records-phrs.

Healthy People 2020. (2014). National plan to improve health literacy. *Office of Disease Prevention and Health Promotion.* Retrieved October 18, 2018, from https://www.healthypeople.gov/2020/tools-resources/evidence-based-resource/national-action-plan-improve-health-literacy.

Healthy People 2010. (n.d.). *What are the leading health indicators?* Retrieved January 19, 2010, from http://www.healthypeople.gov/LHI/lhiwhat.htm.

Hilgers, D. W. (2005). The rise of retail medicine: Adding new complexity to the practice of health care law. *National CLE conference.* Snowmass: Law Education Institute.

History of Medicine Division. (2012). Greek medicine: Hippocratic Oath. *National Library of Medicine, National Institutes of Health.* Retrieved October 18, 2018, from https://www.nlm.nih.gov/hmd/greek/greek_oath.html.

Hofmann, P. B., & Nelson, W. A. (2001). *Managing ethically: An executive's guide.* Chicago, IL: Health Administration Press.

Internal Revenue Service. (2017). Publication 969, health savings accounts and other tax-favored health plans. Retrieved October 18, 2018 from https://www.irs.gov/publications/p969.

Internal Revenue Service. (2018). Publication no. 969: Health savings accounts and other tax-favored health plan. IRS tax map—IRS.gov. Retrieved October 14, 2018, from https://taxmap.irs.gov/taxmap/pubs/p969toc.htm.

Jarousse, L. A. (2015). Population health and the rise of consumerism. Hospitals & Health Networks. Retrieved from https://www.hhnmag.com/articles/3220-population-health-and-the-rise-of-consumerism

Leonard, J., & Rosenbaum, S. (2011). Health insurance exchanges: Implications for public health policy and practice. *Public Health Reports, 126*(4), 597–600. doi:10.1177/003335491112600417.

Marjoua, Y., & Bozic, K. J. (2015). Brief history of quality movement in US healthcare. *Current Review Musculoskeletal Medicine, 5*(4), 265–272. doi:10.1007/s12178-012-9137-8.

Maryland Department of Mental Health and Hygiene. (2007, June 13). *What is HIPAA?* Retrieved December 30, 2009, from http://www.dhmh.state.md.us/hipaa/whatishipaa.html.

McBride, M. (2008). Google Health: Birth of a giant. *Health Information Technology, 29*(5), 8–9.

MD Anderson Cancer Center, University of Texas. (2009). *About complementary/integrative medicine.* Retrieved December 29, 2009, from http://www.mdanderson.org/education-and-research/resources-for-professionals/clinical-tools-and-resources/cimer/about-complementary-integrative-medicine/index.html.

Medline Plus. (2009, December 30). *Complementary and alternative medicine.* Retrieved December 31, 2009, from http://www.nlm.nih.gov/medlineplus/complementaryandalternativemedicine.html.

Merriam-Webster. (2017). Social networking. Retrieved October 18, 2018, from https://www.merriam-webster.com/dictionary/social%20networking.

Milani, R. V., & Franklin, N. C. (2017). The role of technology in healthy living medicine. *Progress in Cardiovascular Diseases, 59*(5), 487–491. https://doi.org/10.1016/j.pcad.2017.02.001.

Moffett, P., & Moore, G. (2011). The standard of care: Legal history and definitions: The bad and good news. *Western Journal of Emergency Medicine, 12*(1), 109–112. Retrieved October 18, 2018, from https://www.ncbi.nlm.nih.gov/pmc/articles/PMC3088386/pdf/wjem12_1p0109.pdf.

Moscovitch, B. (2018). How the increased use of electronic health records intersects with patient safety. The Pew Charitable Trusts. Retrieved October 17, 2018, from https://www.pewtrusts.org/en/research-and-analysis/articles/2018/06/04/how-the-increased-use-of-electronic-health-records-intersects-with-patient-safety.

Musgrave, C. (2018). EHR, telemedicine, and E-risk. The Doctors Company. Retrieved October 17, 2018, from https://www.thedoctors.com/articles/ehr-telemedicine-and-e-risk/.

Nash, D. B., Jacoby, R., & Murtha, M. (2008, July 14). *Retail medicine and the quality of care.* Retrieved December 31, 2009, from http://www.medpagetoday.com/Columns/10113.

National Center for Healthcare Leadership. (2010). Health leadership competency summary. Retrieved from http://nchl.org/Documents/NavLink/Competency_Model-summary_uid31020101024281.pdf.

National Center for Healthcare Leadership (2012). National healthcare leadership competency model. (v2.1). Retrieved from http://www.nchl.org/Documents/NavLink/NCHL_Competency_Model-full_uid892012226572.pdf.

National Institutes of Health. (n.d.). *Bioethics.* Retrieved January 19, 2010, from http://www.bioethics.nih.gov/home/index.shtml.

National Network of Libraries of Medicine (NNLM). (2017). Health literacy. Retrieved from https://nnlm.gov/professional-development/topics/health-literacy.

NCSBNInteract. (2011). Social media guidelines for nurses. Retrieved from https://www.youtube.com/watch?v=i9FBEiZRnmo.

NCSBN (2011). White paper: A nurse's guide to the use of social media. Retrieved from www.ncsbn.org/Social_Media.pdf.

Office of Civil Rights. (2018). Personal health records and the HIPAA privacy rule. U.S. Department of Health & Human Services. Retrieved October 18, 2018, from https://www.hhs.gov/sites/default/files/ocr/privacy/hipaa/understanding/special/healthit/phrs.pdf.

Office of History and Stetten Museum. (2018). Timeline of laws related to the protection of human subjects. Office of History and Stetten Museum, National Institutes of Health. Retrieved October 18, 2018, from https://history.nih.gov/about/timelines_laws_human.html.

Office of Human Research Protections (OHRP). (2005, September). *Office of human research protections, fact sheet.* Retrieved January 19, 2010, from Office of Human Research Protections, U.S. Department of Health & Human Services: http://www.hhs.gov/ohrp/about/ohrpfactsheet.htm.

Office of Human Research Protections (OHRP). (2008, November 13). *The Belmont report.* Retrieved January 19, 2010, from http://www.hhs.gov/ohrp/belmontArchive.html.

Office of Human Research Protections (OHRP). (n.d. a). *History of human subjects protection system.* Retrieved January 19, 2010, from http://www.hhs.gov/ohrp/irb/irb_introduction.htm.

Office of Human Research Protections (OHRP). (n.d. b). *Jurisdiction of the Institutional Review Board. In the Institutional Review Board guidebook.* Retrieved January 19, 2010, from http://www.hhs.gov/ohrp/irb/irb_chapter1.htm.

Olen, H. (2017). Choosing a health insurance plan is not "shopping." *New York Times.* Retrieved October 18, 2018, from https://www.nytimes.com/2017/11/02/opinion/health-insurance-shopping-obamacare.html.

Oxford English Dictionary. (1989a). *Autonomy.* Retrieved January 19, 2010, from http://www.oed.com/cgi/entry/50015226?single=1&query_type=word&queryword=autonomy&first=1&max_to_show=10.

Oxford English Dictionary. (1989b). *Beneficence.* Retrieved January 19, 2010, from http://www

.oed.com/cgi/entry/50020270?single=1&query_type=word&queryword=beneficence&first=1&max_to_show=10.

Oxford English Dictionary. (1989c). *Bioethics.* Retrieved January 19, 2010, from http://www.oed.com/cgi/entry/50022316?single=1&query_type=word&queryword=bioethics&first=1&max_to_show=10.

Oxford English Dictionary. (1989d). *Confidential.* Retrieved January 19, 2010, from http://www.oed.com/cgi/entry/50046956?single=1&query_type=word&queryword=confidentiality&first=1&max_to_show=10.

Oxford English Dictionary. (1989e). *Fidelity.* Retrieved January 19, 2010, from http://www.oed.com/cgi/entry/50084378?single=1&query_type=word&queryword=fidelity&first=1&max_to_show=10.

Oxford English Dictionary. (1989f). *Hippocratic oath.* Retrieved January 19, 2010, from http://dictionary.oed.com/cgi/entry/50106410/single=1&query_type=word&queryword=hippocratic&firts=1&max_to_show=10.

Oxford English Dictionary. (1989g). *Justice.* Retrieved January 19, 2010, from http/www.oed.com/cgi/entry/50124865/query_type=word7queryword=justice&first=1&max_to_show=10&sort_type=alpha&result_place=1&research_id=eUe9-9fXtzj-8471&hilite=50124865.

Oxford English Dictionary. (1989h). *Oxford English Dictionary Online* (2nd ed.). Oxford, UK: Oxford University Press.

Oxford English Dictionary. (1989i). *Privacy.* Retrieved January 19, 2010, from http://www.oed.com/cgi/entry/50188914/signle=1&query_type=word&queryword=privacy&first=1&max_to_show=10.

Oxford English Dictionary. (1989j). *Veracity.* Retrieved January 19, 2010, from http://www.oed.com/cgi/entry/50276176?single=1&query_type=word&queryword=veracity&first=1&max_to_show=10.

Patientslikeme.com (2018). About us. Patienstlikeme.com Retrieved October 18, 2018, from https://www.patientslikeme.com/about.

Patterson, M. P. (2004). Defined contribution health plan to consumer driven health benefits: Evolution and experience. *Benefits Quarterly, 20*(2), 49–59.

Piscotty, R., Martindell, E., & Karim, M. (2016). Nurses' self-reported social media and mobile device use in the work setting. *Online Journal of Nursing Informatics, 20*(1), 9–11. Retrieved from http://www.himss.org/nurses-self-reported-use-social-media-and-mobile-devices-work-setting.

Potter, J. (1988). Consumerism and the public sector: How well does the coat fit? *Public Administration, 66*(2), 149–164.

Ransom, E. R., Joshi, M. S., Nash, D. B., et al. (Eds.). (2008). *The healthcare quality book: Vision, strategy, and tools* (2nd ed.). Chicago, IL: Health Administration Press.

Robert Wood Johnson Foundation. (2008, June). *Health information technology in the United States.* Retrieved January 19, 2010, from http://www.rwjf.org/pr/product.jsp?id=31831.

Robert Wood Johnson Foundation. (2010). *Feature: The power and potential of personal health records.* Retrieved January 19, 2010, from http://www.rwjf.org/pioneer/product.jsp?id=49988.

Robinson, J. C., & Ginsburg, P. B. (2009). Consumer-driven health care: Promise and performance. *Health Affairs, 28*(2), w272–w281.

Roland, J. (2015). The pros and cons of Obamacare: The Affordable Care Act. *Healthline.* Retrieved October 18, 2018, from https://www.healthline.com/health/consumer-healthcare-guide/pros-and-cons-obamacare.

Rosenbaum, S. (2011). The patient protection and affordable care act: Implications for public health policy and practice. *Public Health Reports, 126*(1), 130–135. doi:10.1177/00333549112600118.

Ryan, C. (2018). Computer and internet use in the United States. Census.gov. U.S. Department of Commerce. Retrieved October 18, 2018, from https://www.census.gov/content/dam/Census/library/publications/2018/acs/ACS-39.pdf.

Saver, C. (2006). Nursing—today and beyond. *American Nurse Today, 1*(1), 18–25.

Shane, S. (2017). The fake Americans Russia created to influence the election. *New York Times.* Retrieved October 18, 2018, from https://www.nytimes.com/2017/09/07/us/politics/russia-facebook-twitter-election.html.

Shane, S., & Goel, V. (2017). Fake Russian Facebook accounts brought $100,000 in political ads. *New York Times.* Retrieved from https://www.nytimes.com/2017/09/06/technology/facebook-russian-political-ads.html.

Silverman, S. M. (2009, May 11). Farrah Fawcett breaks her silence. *People* magazine; Time, Inc. Retrieved May 31, 2010, from http://www.people.com/people/article/0,,20278026,00.html.

Stewart, D. (2009). Socialized medicine: How personal health records and social networks are changing healthcare. *EContent, 32*(7), 30–35.

The Jellyvision Lab, Inc. (2016). What your employees think about your benefits communication: New research from Jellyvision conducted by Harris Poll. Retrieved October 14, 2018 from https://www.nytimes.com/2017/11/02/opinion/health-insurance-shopping-obamacare.html

The Joint Commission. (2015). Health literacy and palliative care. Retrieved October 18, 2018, from https://www.jointcommission.org/health_literacy_and_palliative_care/.

The Joint Commission. (2017). Facts about patient-centered communications. Retrieved October 18, 2018, from https://www.jointcommission.org/facts_about_patient-centered_communications/.

Thompson Reuters. (2017). IRS announces 2018 HSA contribution limits, HDHP minimum deductibles, and HDHP out-of-pocket maximums. Retrieved October 18, 2018, from https://tax.thomsonreuters.com/checkpoint-ebia-newsletter/irs-announces-2018-hsa-contribution-limits-hdhp-minimum-deductibles-and-hdhp-out-of-pocket-maximums/.

Total Administrative Services Corporation (TASC). (2008a). *What is a health reimbursement arrangement (HRA)?* Retrieved December 30, 2009, from http://www.tasconline.com/businessresourcecenter/hra.html.

Total Administrative Services Corporation (TASC). (2008b). *What is a health savings account?* Retrieved December 30, 2009, from http://www.tasconline.com/businessresourcecenter/hsa/index.html.

Treasury, U.S. (2004, March 30). *Treasury issues additional guidance on health savings accounts (HSAS).* Retrieved December 29, 2009, from http://www.treas.gov/press/releases/js1278.htm.

Treasury, U.S. (2008, November 19). *HSA frequently asked questions: The basics of HSAs.* Retrieved December 29, 2009, from http://www.ustreas.gov/offices/public-affairs/hsa/faq_basics.shtml.

UCLA Media Relations. (2008, April 2). UCLA health system statement on report about Farrah Fawcett's medical records. *UC Regents.* Retrieved May 31, 2010, from http://newsroom. ucla.edu/portal/ucla/fawcett-48120.aspx?id=.

United States Census Bureau. (2018). Older people projected to outnumber children for the first time in U.S. history. Retrieved October 18, 2018, from https://www.census. gov/newsroom/press-releases/2018/cb18-41-population-projections.html.

United States Department of Labor (n.d.). COBRA continuation health coverage FAQs. United States Department of Labor. Employee Benefits Security Administration. Retrieved October 18, 2018, from https://www.dol.gov/agencies/ ebsa/about-ebsa/our-activities/resource-center/faqs/ cobra-continuation-health-coverage-compliance.

U.S. Department of Health and Human Services. (2009, December). *Health information privacy: HIPAA administrative simplification statute and rules.* Retrieved December 31, 2009, from http://www.hhs.gov/ocr/privacy/hipaa/ administrative/index.html.

U.S. Department of Health and Human Services (2012). About health literacy, p. 1. Retrieved from http://hrsa.gov/ publichealth/healthliteracy/healthlitabout.html.

U.S. Department of Health and Human Services. (n.d. a). *Patient Safety and Quality Improvement Act of 2005 statute and rule.* Retrieved December 30, 2009, from http://www.hhs .gov/ocr/privacy/psa/regulation/index.html

U.S. Department of Health and Human Services. (n.d. b). *Summary of the HIPAA privacy rule.* Retrieved December 20, 2009, from http://www.hhs.gov/ocr/privacy/hipaa/ understanding/summary/index.html.

Vert, G., Claesson-Vert, A. L., Roberts, J., et al. (2017). Chapter 3: Model for detection of advanced persistent threat in networks and systems using a finite angular state velocity machine (FAST-VM). In Daimi, K. (Ed.), *Computer and network systems essentials.* New York: Springer. doi:10.1007/978-3-319-58424-9.

Weaver, J. (2013). More people search for health online. Telemedicine. *NBC News.* Retrieved October 18, 2018, from http://www.nbcnews.com/id/3077086/t/more-people-search-health-online/#.WgoTM03ruM8.

Wolsko, P., Ware, L., Kutner, J., et al. (2000). Alternative/ complementary medicine: Wider usage than generally appreciated. *Journal of Alternative and Complementary Medicine, 6*(4), 321–326.

Chapter 15

The Globalization of Health Care Delivery Systems

Jon Chilingerian, John R. Kimberly, and Eilish McAuliffe

CHAPTER OUTLINE

- Introduction
- The Flow of Clinical Information and the Emergence of Online Patient Communities
- The Flow of Patients across International Borders
- The Flow of Health Workers across Borders

LEARNING OBJECTIVES

After completing this chapter, the reader should be able to:

1. Explain how this increasing global interconnectedness is playing out in the world of health and health care
2. Discuss the managerial challenges of a health care system locating in another country
3. Describe global online patient communities
4. Define medical tourism and how flows across national borders have changed
5. Describe the evolution and effect of patient flows on comparative advantage
6. Describe the effect of health worker mobility on health systems
7. Describe the flow of policy instruments and managerial practices across borders
8. Discuss the managerial and policy implications of health care globalization

KEY TERMS

Brain Drain

Comparative Advantage

Diagnosis-Related Groups (DRGs)

Focused Clinics

General Agreement on Trade in Services (GATS)

Global Health Workforce Alliance (GHWA)

Globalization

Infant Mortality Rates

Joint Commission International (JCI)

Kohl and Dekker Cases

Managed Migration

Medical Innovation

Medical Tourism

Migrant Remittances

Millennium Development Goals (MDGs)

Patient Communities

Patient-Driven Health Care

Patient Classification System

Prospective Payment

Retrospective Reimbursement

Reverse Innovation

Technological Innovation

• • • IN PRACTICE: A Country Case Study on the Partnership between Abu Dhabi and the Cleveland Clinic in the United States[1]

The subject of health care globalization often focuses on the migration of medical workers. Especially troubling is the flow of physicians and other clinical professionals from the developing to the developed world. This problem has been labeled a "brain drain." There are, however, some examples of developed countries bringing advanced medical services closer to the developing countries in Africa, Asia, and the Middle East. Cleveland Clinic in Abu Dhabi is a case in practice.

Abu Dhabi is the capital of the United Arab Emirates, a federation of seven Emirates. A modern city set on the Arabian Gulf, it is hydrocarbon-based—with 8.5 percent of the world's oil reserves and 3.3 percent of the world's natural gas. With a population of 2.784 million, of which 536,741 are nationals, the majority of the other 120 nationalities are expatriates, and 98 percent are younger than 65. All UAE nationals have a government-funded, mandatory health insurance provided by a public or private option. In the Emirates, 21 percent of the population suffers from diabetes, and 85 percent of breast cancer cases are diagnosed late. The leading causes of death are cardiovascular disease (25 percent) and motor vehicle accidents (10.4 percent).

In 2015, according to the Abu Dhabi Health Authority, the top four outpatient and inpatient episodes by diagnosis were (1) respiratory infections and disease (11.8 percent outpatient, 11.6 percent inpatient), (2) cardiovascular disease (7.5 percent/11.7 percent), (3) diabetes mellitus (7.5 percent/2.6 percent), and (4) musculoskeletal disease (7.4 percent/4.7 percent). Although 39 of the 104 hospitals in the UAE are in Abu Dhabi, 2,100 acute beds will be needed by 2025—an annual growth rate of 3.8 percent. Many of the acute care services are oversubscribed; historically, cardiology, oncology, psychiatry, urology, cardiac surgery, neurosurgery, orthopedic surgery, and thoracic surgery have had long waits. Consequently, many Emiratis travel overseas to obtain access to world-class health care; each year the government spends 25 percent of its health budget in sending patients to other countries to obtain medical care. To stem the flow of patients abroad, one of the government's global targets is to create health care services that meet and exceed international standards.

In 2006, Mubadala,[2] a pioneering investor working with the local government of Abu Dhabi, invited and challenged the Cleveland Clinic to not only build a 490-bed hospital but also to transplant its clinical know-how, culture, people, and quality standards to Abu Dhabi (Erhart, 2008; Fares, 2009). When design and planning began in 2006, Cleveland Clinic Abu Dhabi (CCAD) was to be 4 million square feet with expandable capacity to 490 beds, 7,500 rooms, 72 ICUs, 25 operating rooms, and 200+ patient visit spaces. Complicated questions had to be answered, such as if you open 200 beds, how many services can you offer? Can you offer 1 clinical service, 5 services, or 50? Arguably, this was the largest global health care project ever undertaken.[3]

In 2015, construction was completed on CCAD, a state-of-the-art 364-bed multispecialty hospital. Under the executive leadership of CEO Dr. Tomislav Mihaljevic, MD, CCAD began booking appointments in March 2015 and opened its doors to patients in May 2015.

Dr. Mihaljevic seeks to replicate the culture and best practices of the Cleveland Clinic 7,000 miles away from Cleveland. The Cleveland Clinic's organizational model is based on Cleveland's physician-led multispecialty approach with a shared vision of achieving "outstanding patient experiences," "superior clinical outcomes," and "improved quality of life for the people." The hospital in Abu Dhabi is a spectacular glass-enclosed state-of-the-art facility. The patient rooms are not cold and sterile; the rooms are beautiful, with comfortable modern couches for family and guests. The majority of patients (70 percent) are coming from Abu Dhabi, 20 percent from the other Emirates, and 10 percent from other countries, beyond the surrounding countries—Saudi Arabia, Kuwait, Oman, Bahrain, and Qatar. Given the population, 55 percent will be UAE national citizens and 45 percent will be expatriates and medical tourists.

The CCAD hospital is not a "general hospital"; it will not offer pediatrics, obstetrics, or gynecology and will not take people under the age of 14 years old. CCAD will be highly focused on more complex adult diagnoses and procedures. They will be organized by service lines, divided into five specialty institutes and seven subspecialty institutes. The concept of an institute was pioneered by Cleveland Clinic and can be best illustrated by Heart and Vascular institute. To break down the usual silos, cardiology, vascular medicine and vascular surgery, and cardiac surgery will be physically located and formally arranged in one unit. The five institutes are the following: (1) Digestive Disease (colorectal and gastroenterology), (2) Heart and Vascular, (3) Neurosciences (neuroscience and neurosurgery), (4) Ophthalmology, and (5) Respiratory and Critical Care. The seven subspecialty institutes

• • • IN PRACTICE: A Country Case Study on the Partnership between Abu Dhabi and the Cleveland Clinic in the United States *(Continued)*

are the following: (1) Anesthesiology, (2) Pathology & Laboratory Medicine, (3) Imaging, (4) Emergency Medicine, (5) Medical Subspecialties, (6) Surgical Subspecialties, and (7) Quality & Patient Safety. Each institute has a detailed operating manual (see "In Practice: Cleveland Clinic Abu Dhabi: The Future of Health Care Globalization Is Already Here").

At CCAD, patient care is managed by salaried, Western-trained, U.S. board-certified or equivalent specialists called "the responsible physician" and assisted by physicians without admission or operating theatre privileges. They have developed well-integrated information technology (IT) platforms and electronic medical records (EMR) aligned with state-of-the-art clinical support services and a delivery system built on a patient-centered model. All physicians, clinicians, and other employees are called "caregivers." Each caregiver received six months of training on care pathways, process work flows, order entry, and EMR, including practicing in their state-of-the-art simulation center. All caregivers receive annual employee reviews, and they will get ongoing training and development. Cleveland clinic's goal is to bring world-class medical care to the people of the world wherever possible.

Discussion Questions

1. Diagnose the health care problems that countries like UAE are facing.
2. What is the strategic opportunity for Abu Dhabi?
3. Why would the U.S.-based Cleveland Clinic want to set up another clinic in Abu Dhabi?
4. What are the risks and uncertainties for Abu Dhabi and Cleveland Clinic?

CHAPTER PURPOSE

Health care has been globalizing. But what does this mean? A hallmark of globalization is the increasing openness of national borders to flows of goods and services, financial and human capital, information, and expertise (Friedman, 2005). In the domain of health care, we would point specifically to flows of investment capital; of patients; of physicians, nurses, and other health workers; of medical technology; of pharmaceutical products; of policy tools and initiatives; of a variety of types of information and expertise; and of diseases, such as H1N1, HIV/AIDS, etc., across national borders as indicators to use in examining how health care is globalizing. To the extent that these flows are increasingly common and increasingly significant as measured by their frequency and volume, we can conclude that the process of globalization is accelerating. Accelerating globalization is, of course, a mixed blessing. Flows that are welfareenhancing in some countries have the opposite effect in other countries. Some flows are mutually beneficial, and as we will argue later, some are of dubious legal and ethical value.

In this chapter, we will present four illustrations of how increasing flows of various kinds across national borders are changing the landscape of health care. The first example focuses on flows of information and shows how the ability to access and share patient knowledge and experience globally is empowering patients, creating online communities, and paving a new road for **patient-driven health care**. The second illustration focuses on flows of patients and explores the concept and implications of **medical tourism**, when patients travel out of their local region or country to obtain health care services. The third illustration focuses on flows of health workers and

---

[1] Note: Information for this case study was based on interviews conducted by Jon Chilingerian in Abu Dhabi between 2008 and 2016. The information was also sourced on March 10, 2017, from the Cleveland Clinic Abu Dhabi's website, retrieved from https://www .clevelandclinicabudhabi.ae/en/pages/default.aspx?gclid=CKneoain99MCFZ5KDQodMx4Gbw.

[2] One of the catalysts for change in Abu Dhabi is Mubadala Development Company PJSC (Mubadala). Established and owned by the government, the company's strategy is built on the management of long-term, capital-intensive investments that deliver strong financial returns and tangible social benefits for the Emirate. They partner with "best-of-breed" international organizations, attracting world-class experts to help diversify the economy in several business units, such as aerospace, infrastructure, real estate and hospitality, and health care. Mubadala has formed alliances with leading international health care organizations including Cleveland Clinic and Johns Hopkins Medicine International of the United States and Imperial College London. (See http://www.mubadala.com/ for a complete list).

[3] In 2007, Cleveland Clinic took over Sheik Khalifa Medical Center in Abu Dhabi, a 570-bed hospital. Their team of Cleveland physicians and managers brought very high standards of care into an environment that had not supported those standards. They learned how to work in the region and how to deliver on their promise of excellence.

investigates issues related to the global distribution of health care professionals, with attention to the impact on middle- and low-income health systems. The fourth and final example focuses on flows of policy instruments and managerial practices and describes the spread of various reimbursement systems that require patient classification (e.g., Diagnosis-Related Groupings) to countries around the globe. The chapter will conclude with a discussion of the implications of these and other examples of globalization for future health care managers.

INTRODUCTION

When *The Borderless World* was published in 1990, Kenichi Ohmae's groundbreaking book changed the mindsets of business leaders (Ohmae, 1990). Ohmae foreshadowed how the flow of financial and industrial activity was growing evidence that future growth opportunity and threats were becoming global. Thinking beyond corporate strategy, a global strategy, required a relentless focus on customer needs and business system requirements in every potential geographic market. To succeed, global companies had the dual challenge of identifying "universal" service and product designs for large core markets and supplemental product and services designs for local preferences.

Over the next 20 years, as global competition became a reality, other observers referred to head-to-head competition in *known market space* as becoming a "bloody red ocean" where overcrowded industries saw major global brands becoming more similar, differentiation strategies more difficult, and profits harder to sustain (Kim and Mauborgne, 2015). The future no longer meant merely beating the competition but required making them irrelevant by discovering a vast "blue ocean" of unknown and untapped market space. Creating a blue ocean meant the reconstruction of market boundaries, the discovery and targeting of noncustomers, and breaking the trade-off between cost and quality (Kim and Mauborgne, 2015).

New digital platforms and social media (Amazon, Facebook, YouTube, etc.) began to accelerate globalization in the twenty-first century, connecting people to knowledge intensive flows of data, information, and ideas (McKinsey Global Institute, March 2016). Digitalization manifested a new world in which information on products, services, and prices is instantly available on a global basis. People increasingly could make choices based on price and value.[4] With the emergence of digital commerce, collaborative initiatives, and the information and attention economy, some

organizations quickly adopted new practices, such as idea and crowd sourcing, cloud computing, and the arbitrage of excess capacity. With simple devices, such as an app from a cell phone, brands and expertise could be accessed. Upstart newcomers, such as Alibaba, Airbnb, Amazon, BlaBlaCar, Uber, and Victors & Spoils created seismic upheavals in the retail, hotel, transportation, and advertising industries by improving productivity, plummeting the marginal costs of managing a business, and offering customers lower prices (Rifkin, 2015).

We have been seeing very similar global trends in health care. Over the last 10 years, we have seen an acceleration of global investments in health care. While the vast majority of health organizations remain local and provincial, other organizations like Apollo Hospitals of India, Cleveland Clinic, Houston Methodist, Imperial College Diabetes Center, Johns Hopkins International, and MD Anderson have become insiders in key global health markets. They have been able to reconstruct the market boundaries and customers from local to global. Some health care organizations are sending their best physicians to global destinations. They are demonstrating that if they can drive costs down while driving value up they can achieve global success. Somehow, these organizations have overcome the cognitive problem of inattentional global blindness in health care—the unconscious lack of attention to growing global opportunities and threats (Chilingerian and Savage, 2005). (See "In Practice: Cleveland Clinic Abu Dhabi: The Future of Health Care Globalization Is Already Here.")

Globalization has both admirers and critics (Ghemawat, 2007). Pankaj Ghemawat (2017), for example, argues that digitalization exaggerates the importance of globalization and underestimates how national borders, off-shoring jobs, and populist backlash will stem globalization. He points out that much of the world of commerce involves transactions that are essentially local and the rest is "globaloney." Whether one agrees or disagrees, our question is, "Will these trends affect the management of health care organizations and where will medical practice be in 10 years?"[5]

How is this increasing interconnectedness playing out in the world of health and health care? Globalization includes a wide range of activities and interactions. For example, to succeed in a world economy, we must ensure and promote healthy lives throughout the world. The "Global Goals" for health care are simple and clear—ensuring healthy lives and the promotion of well-being

---

[4] The new global era is evolving unevenly for institutions and organizations. Each institution (such as banks, communities, families, fashion, governments, hospitals, news media, universities, and the like) appear to be cognitively locked into different time and geographic horizons.

[5] For example, among the top pharmaceutical and biotechnology companies, irrespective of countries and borders, the processes, technologies, and tools for drug discovery, development, and clinical trials are very similar, thus enabling scientists to easily move from one R&D facility to another. That same "easy" mobility across borders is true for hospitals and clinicians as well.

for people of all ages.[6] All health care delivery systems can contribute to this goal.

Health care managers must learn to think globally and learn to work collaboratively with governments and other institutions to develop effective global strategies. To improve *health for all*, for example, will require collaborative global partnerships and evidence that they can offer excellent medical outcomes, outstanding patient experiences, and efficient, low-cost care.

While the technical challenges of bringing health care to people in other countries or recruiting health care professionals are daunting, the more significant issues are adapting to local cultures and understanding their political systems. Globalization requires throwing money, reputation, and talent into uncertainty. Moreover, global strategies expose health care organizations to risk—the chance of small or large losses, depending on the investment. For the remainder of this chapter, we illustrate globalization trends in health care with four examples.

The first example focuses on flows of clinical information. The second analyzes medical tourists flows across national borders. The third example looks at health worker flows across borders. The fourth and final example traces the flow of policy instruments across borders. In each case, we present evidence that these flows are increasing, which is a testimony to some of the ways in which globalization in health and health care is taking place. We conclude with some examples of cross-border flows that are cause for concern and that illustrate a dark side to globalization. The next section involves the flow of clinical information. Owing to the Internet, clinical information flows have been globalizing faster than anyone expected. An even more surprising development has been the emergence of online patient support networks.

• • • IN PRACTICE: Cleveland Clinic Abu Dhabi: The Future of Health Care Globalization Is Already Here[7]

Dr. Tomislav Mihaljevic, MD, landed in Abu Dhabi following a meeting with the CEO of the Cleveland Clinic in Cleveland, Ohio. Though it was late in the evening, he went straight from the airport to the newly opened hospital facility. At the hospital, he managed a few items, checked-in with some clinical staff, and reviewed the charts of some patients. While returning to his apartment to get some rest, he reflected on his career in medicine and management and, at age 51, becoming the CEO of Cleveland Abu Dhabi (CCAD).

Dr. Mihaljevic had obtained his medical education in native country, Croatia, and did his cardiac surgery training in Switzerland. He took a job as a cardiothoracic surgeon at the Brigham and Woman's Hospital and Harvard Medical School in the United States and after a few years joined the Cleveland Clinic in the United States. He moved to Abu Dhabi in 2011, when he was asked to be chief of staff at CCAD, and in 2015 he was appointed chief executive officer of CCAD.

When Dr. Mihaljevic woke at 5:00 a.m. the next day, he felt the usual pressures of the day—multiple formal and informal meetings with clinical and nonclinical executives, 30-minute huddles with the clinical staff, rounds in the hospital, surgeries in the operating theater, meeting VIPs giving hospital tours, checking messages, returning phone calls, check-ins and follow-ups with the board, and being on call in the hospital that evening.

When he arrived at the hospital, he was informed of an urgent meeting with Mubadala, the visionary partners with Cleveland Clinic in the United States and a global network of other world-class health care facilities. He took care of a few items and went back in his car and drove to that meeting. Driving back to the hospital, he remembered that he was scheduled for a trip to London later that week. This was just a typical day for this global health leader.

As a global hospital CEO, Dr. Mihaljevic was prepared to go between Abu Dhabi and London; Cleveland, Ohio; the Gulf Region and Africa; and many other destinations. Being an MD-CEO required being both a team player and a coach taking multiple roles—clinical leader, cardiothoracic surgeon, chief strategist, visionary, and figurehead. While being CEO and a physician is daunting, he would not have it any other way. Dr. Mihaljevic explained,

If I can borrow a metaphor from the military, I say that medicine ought to be led at the level of the Corporal and not the General (as long as each Corporal is not only qualified but also is the best soldier). A hospital CEO ensconced in meetings in the C-suite and meeting with VIPS, is like a General who is 5 miles away, they

---

[6] We have outlined global health goals and the policymaking institutions and organizations comprising the global health system in an Appendix.

[7] This case is a short version of a longer case written by Jon Chilingerian, PhD. It is intended to be used as a basis for class discussion rather than to illustrate either effective or ineffective handling of an administrative situation.

• • • IN PRACTICE: Cleveland Clinic Abu Dhabi: The Future of Health Care Globalization Is Already Here (Continued)

can get out-of-touch. So, for me it would be difficult to envision that I could run a hospital effectively without knowing what hospital life is really like.

He went on to say:

I am a thoracic surgeon and I am a CEO. As a surgeon when I perform a minimally invasive robotic heart surgery I must be available for that patient 24-7; as the responsible physician working with the most qualified workforce as a team, I can make decisions that put the patient first; in addition, I understand intimately our internal problems . . . As the hospital CEO, I have morning huddles, administrative meetings and rounds, and other duties. Playing both roles enables me and every other physician leader here at CCAD to understand the clinical, managerial and policy worlds we deal with every day.

Today CCAD is a 364-bed hospital with expandable capacity, offering 55 medical and surgical specialties. The breathtakingly beautiful facility has 5 clinical floors, 3 diagnostic and treatment levels, and 13 floors of acute and critical beds. In 2017, there were 3,500 employees from 62 countries and a multispecialty group with 325 physicians.

This bold experiment in globalization opened one of the largest health care organizations with a brand-new team that had never worked together before. The investors not only wanted access to the most innovative, most advanced care, and technology, they also wanted CCAD to transplant the "exact" culture and care processes from Cleveland in the United States to Abu Dhabi. That experiment had never been attempted.

For an idea like this to become reality, there are at least four organizational design challenges:

Challenge (1) Selecting, training, and retaining the best people, able to perform the most advanced clinical and nonclinical tasks in a multispecialty, team-based, collaborative group setting. People who not only thrive on hard work but are also able to work at a faster pace

Challenge (2) Organizing the care structure into clinical institutes based on the Cleveland multispecialty group practice model

Challenge (3) Performing clinical tasks and making clinical decisions that adhere to scientific evidence, care pathways, online order entry steps, and algorithms supported by a single electronic health record

Challenge (4) Establishing a culture and professional work environment for people who not only thrive on hard work but are also able to work at a faster pace, offering an outstanding patient experience while obtaining the best results observed in practice

When Dr. Mihaljevic and his team thought about those four challenges, people, formal architecture, culture, and work tasks, they felt that the first major responsibility was recruitment of *the most qualified clinical workforce*. This was challenge number one.

Thirty physicians applied for every opening. Over 9,000 applications were reviewed, and the finalists went through 20 interviews at Cleveland Clinical in the United States and 20 interviews at Cleveland in Abu Dhabi. When asked why he required 40 interviews for each physician, Mihaljevic said,

You can fool 20 people but not 40. We wanted to recruit for attitude and select the most qualified and most responsible physicians to care for our patients in Abu Dhabi.

By 2017, CCAD hired 325 physicians, 80 percent were trained in the United States and 20 percent were trained in Europe. They also hired some 3,500 employees they called "caregivers." The second set of challenges are directly connected to recruiting the right staff—how do we "onboard" organize and align 3,500 caregivers effectively?

To improve communication, teamwork, and coordination of patient care, CCAD designed clinical, *educational, and support institutes* rather than traditional departments. The CCAD hospital developed highly focused service lines organized into five clinical institutes and seven support institutes.[8] Mihaljevic and his team explained that

---

[8] The concept of an Institute was pioneered by Cleveland Clinic. The five institutes are (1) Digestive Disease (colorectal and gastroenterology), (2) Heart and Vascular, (3) Neurosciences (neuroscience and neurosurgery), (4) Ophthalmology, and (5) Respiratory and Critical Care. The seven subspecialty institutes are (1) Anesthesiology, (2) Pathology & Laboratory Medicine, (3) Imaging, (4) Emergency Medicine, (5) Medical Subspecialties, (6) Surgical Subspecialties, and (7) Quality & Patient Safety.

• • • IN PRACTICE: Cleveland Clinic Abu Dhabi: The Future of Health Care Globalization Is Already Here (Continued)

by clustering cardiology, cardiac surgery, and thoracic surgery into the heart and vascular institute, there is one physical space for all intermediate services, such as echocardiograms and EKGs. If a patient needs to see a heart surgeon, have a CT scan, and do some respiratory function tests, all of this is done in one site on two floors. The physical colocation formalizes the authority structure and leadership into one unit; silos among those subspecialties begin to break down. Each institute has a chair and every member of the institute reports to the chair.

The institute chair reports to CCAD chief of staff who reports to the CCAD CEO. A CCAD chair is an exceptional physician, admired and respected for clinical skills and with responsibility for operations, quality, and finance of their institute. The chair of an institute hires, fires strategizes, and manages the budget and smaller capital items with the team. If nurses, surgeons, or even intensivists in the ICU are managed by different people, the architecture will fail. Having one chair for each institute creates a structure of accountability and of unity.

Having organized 3,500 people into these institutes, the third challenge became how to coordinate all critical tasks and work processes into a seamless service process? How to schedule appointments and how to deal with no-shows? In the operating room, for example, who should do what and with whom? What if the patient does not arrive on time? How to handoff one step to how perform the next step in the care process?

At CCAD, there are 3,500 employees from 72 countries. That means that every "caregiver" will have his or her own ideas about how to do every task, such as booking a patient for a clinical appointment, putting a cast on a broken leg, or doing coronary bypass grafting. To coordinate work flows and tasks the Cleveland way (Cosgrove, 2014) requires an operating manual that gives step-by-step detail. An operating manual introduces predictability, accountability, transferability of Cleveland quality and cost, and reflective improvability (learning) within each institute and across each institute to share best practices.

To manage every one of these service processes, CCAD has developed an original *operating manual* for every single institute for every care and support process.[9] They accounted for task interdependences, handoffs, and uncertainties. They developed operating procedures for both routine and nonroutine tasks and jokingly call it a *Wikipedia cookbook for clinical medicine.*

Since 80 percent of the institute chairs are leaders from Cleveland, they knew how things worked at Cleveland. Guided by their cognitive knowledge and combing the literature for evidence and best practices, they translated clinical algorithms into decision rules and procedures.

The operating manuals depicted a mission and vision statement, an organizational chart, staffing formulas and hiring practices, scope of services, physical plant, patients' journey, standard operating procedures for most commonly performed operations, and all other procedures for the institute and its entities. Once the manuals were completed, the clinical and nonclinical leaders engaged the new hires in thousands of hours of onboarding, training, and mock operations.

Dr. Mihaljevic said,

I am a member of the heart and vascular institute. We developed a manual that guides each cardiac surgeon so a coronary by-pass grafting will be done identically, regardless of the name of surgeon. We are all using the same surgical instruments, the same suture, the same valves, same coronary by-pass set up . . . We trained everyone and hold them accountable for their actions. Adherence to the protocols and procedures should reduce performance variations . . . To my knowledge, no other hospital in the world has such a manual that holds people accountable for every support and every care process they provide. At CCAD, we do!

Having developed operating manuals for every piece of clinical and nonclinical work in every institute, the final challenge was bringing Cleveland's culture to Abu Dhabi.

Mihaljevic and his team believed that structure not only generates behavior, it is also the most powerful way to reduce human variation and performance differences. They had to embed the right values and work ethic in the work environment; ultimately, CCAD has transferred the Cleveland, Ohio culture (7,000 miles away) to Abu Dhabi.

---

[9] In general, while most hospitals have some procedures and documentation, few have highly comprehensive operating manuals. When new technology requires new care processes and skill sets, collective memory and organizational culture guide the implementation. They reinforce doing a task based on how people work together and how they take decisions in that hospital's culture.

• • • IN PRACTICE: Cleveland Clinic Abu Dhabi: The Future of Health Care Globalization Is Already Here *(Continued)*

Through formal and informal conversations and discussion, Mihaljevic and the team embedded and reinforced three underling values of the Cleveland culture. The primary value is that "the patient comes first," and this value necessitates relentless communication and deep leadership throughout the organization. Every clinical leader in every situation must continually communicate this value.

A second value that must be built into the architecture, operating manuals, and culture is "to always view care from the patient's point-of-view." For example, since patients reside in their rooms, they should be taken care of in their rooms because patients desire convenience. Patients expect competence and commitment, so *the most qualified workforce* should always be available in the hospital to guide and make decisions and to always bring care to the patients. The third core value is that every person in a leadership position must be an exceptionally good physician. That value has to be built into the human resource practices and aligned with the critical tasks.

Physicians working in other hospitals in the Emirates offered other insights about the CCAD experiment. While Cleveland could try to export their quality standards and metrics to Abu Dhabi, they would have to adapt to the local culture in the Middle East. As one Western-trained physician working in another Abu Dhabi hospital observed,

> When CCAD opened in 2015, there was pent up demand. Patients saw this beautiful facility and they wanted to come in for an appointment within one or two days. To accommodate the patients, CCAD began booking thousands of appointments. Soon, each of these highly-skilled physicians were seeing 25–30 patients a day. However, some patients only speak Arabic and not every Cleveland physician speaks Arabic. If a physician is waiting for translators and has 25 other patients coming in, it will mean long, hard days for clinicians and staff.

Once caregivers are seeing patients, the subtle cross-cultural issues begin to manifest. One cross-cultural issue is how people experience and manage time. In the United States and parts of Europe (such as Germany or England), time is money and most patients expect clinical events to happen in a sequential order—they value punctuality and staying on schedule. By and large, patients are more likely to be on time and keep surgical appointments.

Another Western-trained physician working in another Abu Dhabi hospital explained,

> In parts of the Middle East, the past, present and future are interwoven and time is very flexible. In Western hospitals if visiting hours end at 9 PM, families obey the rules. Here they like to stay with a family member till 3 AM. Since time is more flexible, it doesn't matter whether a patient appointment is at 3:00 PM or 8:00 AM, many patients will come in at 10:00 AM and say—Please, where is my doctor? When time is more flexible, people believe they can cancel a surgery that morning—they know that they can call any other hospital in Abu Dhabi, my hospital, and they will be accommodated for a surgery tomorrow or the next day . . . On the other hand, if a patient is told the wait is 2–3 months, they will become impatient. Some of them will call the owners and complain. The CEO will get many, many of these calls. That will be how he spends some of his time.

Another cross-cultural issue is about the amount of time it takes to build a patient–physician relationship and the initial distrust of the health system. In Western cultures, a patient may see a physician and get a second opinion. In the Emirates, some patients have already seen five or more cardiologists and cardiac surgeons. While there is pent-up demand, a lot of that demand is "regurgitated" patients. As one physician from a competing hospital said,

> In the Emirates patients perhaps rightly so, do not automatically trust the health care system. So, they will see every doctor in town until they find one who connects with them, and they can trust. Some have already been to physicians in Germany and England. But they do not tell you. When they get to see a sub-specialist at CCAD, they will be thinking, "I want you to impress me, doctor from Cleveland." So, CCAD will have to learn how to accommodate the clash of cultures so that their staff does not get demoralized.

Despite the cynics and nay-sayers, in May 2015, CCAD began to treat patients. By December 2015, they had done 30,000 patient visits and performed 1,600 surgical procedures. By March 2016, they performed complex surgeries never provided in Abu Dhabi, such as robotic cardiac surgery, percutaneous treatment for structural

• • • IN PRACTICE: Cleveland Clinic Abu Dhabi: The Future of Health Care Globalization Is Already Here (Continued)

heart disease, percutaneous valve replacement, endoscopic resections of colon cancer, innovative treatments for refractive issues with eyes, and endoscopic treatment for chronic obstructive pulmonary lung disease.

In March 2016, Dr. Mihaljevic added,

> Everything is working better than anticipated. Our entire focus has been to perfect the delivery of care informed by science. Our team has created effective processes that are standardized and documented. We have designed a continuous improvement model associated with this effort to deliver the best possible care to every single individual under our roof.

> The leadership challenges are internal. We continually are steering a multicultural, diverse workforce to re-energize, re-commit themselves to Cleveland Clinic standard. Ask any caregiver here and they will say that they are part of a hard-working clinical organization.

> One year after opening its doors, patients from 42 countries were traveling to Cleveland Clinic in Abu Dhabi to obtain a level of care they could not access in their native countries. Patients came from Canada, England, Europe, Mexico, and even the United States. So far, this experiment and partnership with the Cleveland Clinic has been a watershed. The government of Abu Dhabi is fulfilling its mission to provide "world-class healthcare in the Emirates." Although this represents just one case example, there are lessons and implications for the globalization of health care management.

Questions

1. What were the four organizational design challenges facing CCAD and what results have CCAD achieved to date?
2. What is the role of Dr. Mihaljevic, MD, CEO of CCAD? Where does the CEO spend his time? Is this a good model for health care?
3. How must a health care organization like Cleveland Clinic adapt to become a patient-centered health organization in the Middle East?
4. What are the lessons for managing health care organizations?

THE FLOW OF CLINICAL INFORMATION AND THE EMERGENCE OF ONLINE PATIENT COMMUNITIES

Facilitating globalization has been the presence of the Internet and the emergence of online **patient communities**. Several powerful innovations have led to the development of these communities and health data–sharing platforms.[10] A few patients started googling their symptoms, researching and networking with other patients to understand their diagnosis and treatments. Physicians jokingly referred to the Internet as "Dr. Google." But this was not a fad or a joke, as other patients also began demanding better clinical experiences, better quality, shorter waiting periods, and less costly drugs. Motivated patients began traveling to destinations around the world for health care.

As the Internet enabled patients to share symptoms, diagnoses, and treatments, and to collaborate with clinicians, something else blossomed. Now patients could join virtual support groups. There were patient-initiated websites, social networks, and health data platforms that opened new health care opportunities on a truly global scale. These trends enabled patients, clinics, and countries to participate in the self-care movement. The ability of online

---

[10] The emergence and the confluence of four innovations have influenced our mindsets and changed our behaviors. The first innovation was the ability to digitize text (health records), images (X-ray), voice (recognition), videos, and sounds into a single binary code that could be both stored or sent anywhere. The second was the broadening of access to the Internet and the gradual integration of digital technologies. A third influence is the explosion of information availability enabled by the development of powerful search engines, such as Google. The fourth major influence is the commercialization of a variety of personal digital devices that enable access to information by anyone at any time and any place in the world. Together, these forces have reinforced one another and have transformed the traditional doctor–patient relationship from one dominated by authoritative professionals to what is now called patient-centered and patient-driven health care.

patient communities to source new knowledge globally changed the balance of power from the medical authorities to the patients. Examples of new sites founded by patients and families include Organization for Autism Research, QuitNet, Association of Cancer On-Line Resources (ACOR), and PatientsLikeMe. The remainder of this section will focus on one online community—PatientsLikeMe—as an example of new information flows. And will consider its managerial implications.

Organic Growth of PatientsLikeMe (PLM)

PatientsLikeMe (PLM) labels itself the "world's leading health data sharing platform" (Aggarwal and Chick, 2017). PLM was launched in 2004 when the brother of one of the founders was diagnosed with amyotrophic lateral sclerosis (ALS), a deadly neurodegenerative disorder without any effective therapy. What began as a social network of patients with ALS has grown steadily. Following requests from patients, PLM takes about one year to understand illness condition, design a platform, and to recruit patients. Today, PLM is an online global community of over 500,000 people living with 2,700 conditions that aim to "put patients first" (see www.patientslikeme .com/about).

People with new diagnoses can share their personal information, exchange ideas, and learn from others. Patients are invited to report symptoms (ranging from difficulties speaking and swallowing to walking or sleeping), test results, treatments with start and stop dates, and demographic information. For some diseases, access to a global online population can generate a large-enough data sets to conduct observational studies that can contribute to clinical and patient discovery. This enabled PLM to shift from only being a social network patient platform to becoming a research platform. How this evolved will be explained in the next section.

Clinical Discovery Using Data from PLM's Online Community

Worldwide, the total number of patients with ALS is approximately 450,000. Patients with serious and deadly neurodegenerative diseases like ALS often experiment with vitamins and unproven treatments that do not have regulatory approval and they are left to running their own experiments. In 2008, lithium carbonate therapy was reported to slow the progression of ALS. In 2011, PLM did a global clinical study to explore whether lithium could slow the progression of ALS.

PLM had 3,674 members with ALS and 9 percent had reported taking lithium. Consequently, they could conduct a patient-initiated observational study with self-reported outcomes. PLM developed an algorithm to match 149 treated patients to multiple controls using their patient members. By leveraging their database, PLM refuted the potential efficacy of that therapy with its finding that lithium had no effect on the progression of the horrific disease. PLM staff published their findings in *Nature Biotechnology* (Wicks et al., 2011), demonstrating how globalization of patients can contribute to clinical research and the practice of medicine.

Implications for Health Care Management

The PLM community is an example of how a patient-centric approach coupled with global patient sourcing and a global health data–sharing platform could lead to faster clinical insights in advance of clinical trials. The collective intelligence of an online patient group that can source global knowledge may equal or perhaps surpass the knowledge of a single general practitioner or even some medical specialists. Whether clinics and physicians respect and legitimize online groups is irrelevant. These empowered patients will fact-check, challenge medical experts, and legitimize themselves.

Patient-driven health care will continue to be supported and enabled by the Internet and by mobile technology. Some 260,000 health apps help patients throughout the world manage their conditions, share information, and gather and analyze data. As big data analytics learns how to separate important clinical signals from noise, wearables and dazzling digital health tools will monitor and transmit fast-moving streams of information on patients from hundreds or thousands of miles away (Rifkin, 2015).

The next section will focus on the second example of globalization, the flow of patients across international borders. We explore the size, scope, and reasons that patients travel from their home country to an international destination for the sole purpose of obtaining access to health services. The legal, ethical, and managerial issues will come into sharper relief.

THE FLOW OF PATIENTS ACROSS INTERNATIONAL BORDERS

Although health care delivery is usually done locally, some patients are increasingly willing to travel to other countries to obtain health care services (Chilingerian and Savage, 2005; Cohen, 2015; Cortez, 2008; Francis, 2008; Schroth and Khawaja, 2007; Woodman, 2015). Patients who require advanced surgical procedures can go to the Internet and search by country or medical specialty and find an international smorgasbord of "best care" accredited hospitals and world-class physicians

(Cote, 2014; Woodman, 2015). In addition to sophisticated medical services at international destinations, medical travelers may also find "white glove" concierge services, patient ambassadors, luxury hotels, lake and seaside resorts, as well as big cost savings (see Woodman Medical Tourism Association, 2017, http://www.medical-tourismassociation.com/en/index.html). In this section, we examine the flow of patients around the globe—a trend that has been called *medical tourism.*

For purposes of this chapter, we define a medical tourist as a patient seeking value in any or all of the following six ways: (1) more comprehensive care, (2) more advanced care, (3) more specialized care, (4) less costly care, (5) improved quality, and (6) better access and better patient experiences. Porter (1987, p. 45) argues that "the global competitor can locate activities wherever comparative advantage lies, decoupling comparative advantage from the firm's home base or country of ownership." Comparative advantage, when applied to health care, refers to the discovery and deployment of significant differences in a nation's cost, quality, or access such that a medical or surgical procedure, health activity, or service creates patient value. Consequently, a highly rated care program for lung cancer or organ transplantation with excellent technical outcomes, outstanding patient experience, and lower costs could become a "power offering" to anyone, anywhere in the world.

Travel in search of medical services is not a new phenomenon. The royals, retirees, rich, and famous have done this for generations. What is new, however, is the realization that both low and high GDP countries that have efficient, high-quality, technologically advanced health care organizations can attract medical tourists and not only achieve a comparative advantage but also make the competition *temporarily* irrelevant. Conversely, both low and high GDP countries also have inefficient, low-quality, technologically weak health care organizations with long waits or poor service attitudes, and these countries will therefore lose some of their patients to other countries.

In 2008, one study found that the average weighted price of a procedure in the United States was $10,629 versus $1,410 for other accredited international destinations (Keckley and Underwood, 2008). One 53-year-old American traveled to India to replace both hips and one knee for a total out-of-pocket cost less than $30,000 (Comarow, 2008). This price included all hospital charges, physician fees, ancillary services airfare, visas, and other miscellaneous expenses—easily a price that is substantially below what he would have paid out of pocket in the United States (see Crooks et al., 2011).

When one marketing director for an American business coalition heard about American patients going abroad, he organized a due diligence mission, investigating both quality and prices from U.S. facilities and abroad. His leadership team reached a dramatic conclusion:

> We came to believe that quality of care in facilities credentialed by the Joint Commission International (JCI) in foreign countries, and in India in particular, is as good as or better than that in the United States, and offers a 70–80 percent cost differential in many cases. (Douglas, 2007, p. 36)

Some third-party payors in the United States reached similar conclusions. For example, Blue Cross and Blue Shield of Wisconsin, Florida, California, and South Carolina launched pilot programs to send patients to India, Mexico, and Thailand (Keckley and Underwood, 2009). If hospitals or physicians refuse to negotiate their prices for patients, insurance companies, or sick funds, some patients will cross borders.

The following section explores the size of the market for inbound and outbound patients and considers the reasons patients are willing to travel for their health care. Among the patients traveling abroad for health care are those in need of organ transplants, which raises many ethical issues. Perceived demand for medical treatments abroad has spawned rivalry among nations whose delivery systems target medical tourists; consequently, it is becoming a more competitive market. The section concludes with specific implications for health care managers and leaders as they develop global health care strategies that require excellent patient experiences, outstanding technical outcomes, and efficient, low-cost care.

How can the number of patients actually crossing national borders to obtain health care be estimated? We will explore this question by examining the size of the global market for inbound and outbound patients.

Size of the Global Market: The Myths and Half-Truths of Medical Tourism

A literature review reveals that there are neither definitive studies nor very accurate estimates of the size of the global market for medical travelers. The data on medical travelers often come from tourism boards, newspaper accounts, and government estimates of hospital claims, social media, stakeholder media, or hospital websites. Estimates often include expatriates obtaining acute and primary care in their current locations, outpatient visits, visitor emergency cases, and tourists obtaining alternative medical care, such as acupuncture (see Cohen, 2015).

A study by Ehrbeck, Guevara, and Mango (2008) that excluded expatriates, emergencies, traumas, cosmetic surgeries, and outpatient visits estimated the size of the global acute market to be quite small—between 60,000 and 85,000 people (see Francis, 2008). More recent studies that include cosmetics, dentistry, weight loss, scans, and tests with acute care estimated some 14 million cross-border patients worldwide in 2015 (Woodman, 2015). In 2015, some 100,000 Russians patients traveled to Turkey, Israel, or the United States for their medical treatment; another 600,000 Indonesian patients went to Singapore and Malaysia for both routine and more complex treatment unavailable locally (Woodman, 2015). Governments in the UAE, Mexico, and India have been investing billions of dollars to improve health care and attract the global health patients.

Despite the seemingly exaggerated size of the market for medical tourists by ad agencies and medical tourist boards, people do travel to other countries for the sole purpose of obtaining health care. Why is this the case, and what are the implications?

Understanding the Reasons for Outbound Patient Flows

Why do people go abroad for medical care? The Ehrbeck, Guevara, and Mango (2008) acute care study found five reasons for medical travel to an international destination: (1) better quality and patient experiences (40 percent), (2) the most advanced technology (32 percent), (3) quicker access (15 percent), (4) lower costs for medically necessary procedures (9 percent), and (5) lower costs for discretionary procedures (4 percent). What becomes clear is that 87 percent of acute medical travelers want good quality and fast service rather than low costs. An obvious conclusion is that a key factor for global competition is a provider's clinical reputation,

defined in terms of (1) outcomes, (2) technological backup, and (3) use of the most advanced medical procedures. In many countries, health insurance excludes cosmetic, weight loss, infertility, behavioral health, and other procedures and treatments, which is another reason to travel.

Table 15.1 helps us to visualize the global flow of acute patients around the world (Ehrbeck, Guevara, and Mango, 2008). Patients who travel can come from countries with high per capita gross domestic product (GDP) or low per capita GDP. Latin American countries (87 percent) and the Middle Eastern countries (58 percent) favor travel to North America. North America favors travel to Latin America (26 percent) and Asia (45 percent). Oceana (99 percent), African (95 percent), and Asian countries (93 percent) favor travel to Asia. Finally, European travelers are divided between North American (33 percent) and Asian countries (39 percent). Thus, a strong health care infrastructure with excess capacity gives some countries a disproportionate share of the patient flow and consequently a comparative global advantage.

Marketing studies have also found that patients who travel to India, Singapore, and Thailand have been mostly satisfied with the care (Cohen, 2015; Ehrbeck, Guevara, and Mango, 2008; Woodman, 2015). Several factors may affect a patient's willingness to travel across national borders to seek heath care: clinical reputation of the local and national providers, an individual's ability to afford the total cost of care abroad, and the value to the patient when the perceived sacrifices are considered in relation to the perceived benefits. We will segment medical tourists into the three significant patient groups for reasons of better quality, lower cost, and improved access (Alsagoff, 2005; Chilingerian and Savage, 2005).

Table 15.1 Global Trade Routes for Acute Patients by Point of Origin and Destination*

	From Africa	From Asia	From Europe	From Latin America	From Middle East	From North America	From Oceana
To Africa	0%	0%	0%	0%	0%	0%	0%
To Asia	95%	93%	39%	1%	32%	45%	>99%
To Europe	4%	1%	10%	0%	8%	0%	0%
To Latin America	1%	0%	5%	12%	0%	26%	<1%
To Middle East	0%	0%	13%	0%	2%	2%	0 percent
To North America	0%	6%	33%	87%	58%	27%	0%
To Oceana	0%	0%	0%	0%	0%	0%	0%
Total Value	100%	100%	100%	100%	100%	100%	100%

*SOURCE: Adapted from Ehrbeck, Guevara, and Mango (2008).

Wealthy Patients from High GDP Countries That Lack Advanced or Comprehensive Health Services

According to Alsagoff (2005), the number of infant deaths per 1,000 live births is highly associated with degree of local health care infrastructure. In general, countries with high per capita GDP have lower infant mortality rates (Alsagoff, 2005). There are also outlier countries. For example, Qatar, Bahrain, and United Arab Emirates have a higher per capita GDP and higher infant mortality rates—14 infant deaths per 1,000 live births (Alsagoff, 2005). Although the problems may be more complex, the presence of a rich population and the absence of adequate health care facilities may lead to medical travel. Some countries, like Abu Dhabi, are taking this very seriously (see "In Practice: A Country Case Study on the Partnership between Abu Dhabi and the Cleveland Clinic in the United States" and "In Practice: Cleveland Clinic Abu Dhabi: The Future of Health Care Globalization Is Already Here"). Studies have identified countries, such as Turkmenistan, Jordan, Malaysia, Vietnam, the Philippines, Pakistan, Indonesia, India, and China as countries whose wealthy patients are willing to travel for medical care if they cannot get an advanced surgical procedure or comprehensive care within their own country.

Patients from High GDP Countries with Relatively Expensive Health Care Services

The United States and Japan have excellent and comprehensive health care systems; however, they are very expensive. Apollo Hospitals of India offer very low cost and immediate access for people who want to avoid the lengthy waits that often accompany the higher-cost alternatives. Table 15.2 displays the cost advantages of traveling to other countries for health care.

A patient from the United States can fly to India and have a coronary artery bypass graft for 16 percent of the average U.S. price—paying only $14,400 versus $88,000 for the procedure. Medical travelers who go to Mexico pay $11,500 for a hip replacement versus $33,000 in the United States.

Patients Seeking Better Access, Shorter Wait Times and Less Time in Pain

From time to time, patients living in high GDP countries with government-sponsored national health systems can have trouble getting access to all medical services across the continuum of patient care. As health care expenditures keep rising, governments try to limit spending. When services are underfunded and patient demand exceeds the capacity constraint, the result is overutilization, bottlenecks, and longer wait times for all services.

Lengthy waits can be psychologically and physically damaging to older patients. For example, a study of older people in Scotland needing hip and knee replacements found that patients with urgent cases were waiting as long as 30 months and nonurgent cases waited as long as 78 months (Roy and Hunter, 1996). These patients experienced great pain, mobility restrictions, an inability to go out or climb stairs, and one-fourth had been forced to retire. A Canadian study of patients waiting for hip and knee replacements found that some patients had been waiting up to three years (36 months) (Williams et al., 1997). In another study, cataract patients from Canada, Denmark, and Spain were asked if they would be willing to pay out of pocket to shorten their wait times (Anderson, Modrow, and Tan, 1992). Approximately 38 percent of the Canadians, 17 percent of the Danes, and 29 percent of the Spanish were willing to pay $500 for a shorter wait.

In July 2002, the British Medical Association conducted a survey of 2,000 adults in the United Kingdom. These citizens, entitled to free care from the National Health Service (NHS), were asked how far they would be willing to travel if they faced a lengthy wait for health

Table 15.2 Cost Comparison of Selected Procedures

Procedure	United States	India	Malaysia	Mexico	Singapore	Thailand
Heart Bypass (CABG)	$88,000	$14,400	$20,800	$37,800	$54,500	$23,000
Hip Replacement	$33,000	$8,000	$12,500	$11,500	$21,400	$16,500
Knee Replacement	$34,000	$7,500	$12,500	$12,800	$19,200	$11,500
Gastric Bypass	$18,000	$6,800	$8,200	$13,800	$13,500	$12,000
Rhinoplasty	$6,200	$2,800	$3,600	$2,800	$4,740	$4,300
IVF Cycle (Not Including Medication)	$15,000	$3,300	$7,200	$7,800	$9,450	$6,500

SOURCE: Adapted from Woodman (2015) and Cohen (2015).

care services. More than 40 percent were willing to travel outside the United Kingdom, 15 percent would travel anywhere in Europe, and 26 percent would travel anywhere in the world (Beecham, 2002).

A 2016 study in Canada found an average of a 20-week wait for "medically necessary" procedures and treatments and for some specialties like neurosurgery up to 47-week waits (Barua and Ren, 2016). One patient from Canada facing a lengthy one-year wait for a hip replacement went to India, was treated immediately, and paid a total of $4,500 for the entire procedure versus an average price of $15,000 or more in Western Europe or the United States.

In 2016, the average wait time for hip and knee replacements, hernias, and other routine surgeries in the England was more than 100 days. Some people from England, Canada, and other parts of the world are willing to become medical tourists because their perception of value includes such factors as spending less time in pain and the high quality of life that results, in relation to the perceived sacrifice of leaving home and paying out of pocket. Patients dissatisfied with the quality of the health care services offered by their country, but unable to pay any out-of-pocket costs, had to accept the inconveniences rather than fight.

In Europe, a 1988 ruling by the European Court of Justice gave citizens of Europe the right to travel abroad to receive health care. The now famous **Kohl and Dekker cases** established that health care resources should be treated as any other part of the European Union economy with regard to the free movement of goods and services. Patients can seek treatment across borders unless the same treatment can be provided more conveniently within their own country. European patients are no longer held hostage by their local providers.

We have focused on three reasons for outbound patient flows: (1) better quality, (2) improved access, and (3) lower costs. Next, we explore patients who require a treatment that may be unavailable or subject to long waits in their native country—that is, patients who need organ transplants. Organ transplantation raises ethical issues.

Ethical Challenges to Outbound Patient Flows

There is an ethical challenge to medical tourism when patients need an organ transplant. Transplant tourists are residents of one country who travel to a medical destination in another country to obtain a readily available organ, such as a kidney that is temporarily or permanently unavailable in their resident country. These organs often come from the poor in the destination country who have sold them in an effort to alleviate their poverty. Alternatively, they may have been harvested from

executed prisoners in countries where tuberculosis and hepatitis are more prevalent. Profound ethical questions are raised in either case and lead to the question of how transplant tourism should be regulated.

According to the U.S. Department of Health and Human Services, in 2017 there were 118,003 U.S. patients on a wait list for organ transplants of which nearly 100,000 are waiting for a kidney (see https://optn.transplant.hrsa.gov). Twenty-two people die each day waiting for an organ transplant and 13 of the 22 die each day waiting for a kidney (see https://optn.transplant.hrsa.gov). Liver candidates are triaged based on a Model for End-Stage Liver Disease (or MELD) scoring system that ranges from a score of 6 for the earliest stages of their liver disease to 40 for the most critically ill. One study estimated that some 400 Americans jump their queue and travel out of the United States to avoid the wait (Schiano and Rhodes, 2010). Often, they come back home for follow-up care, which requires expensive immunosuppressant drugs.

The risks involved in obtaining a transplant in another country are alarming. One study reported by Delmonico (2009) followed 33 transplant tourists from the United States. Nine required hospitalization upon return and 17 had infections. The one-year graft survival of the 33 patients was 89 percent versus 98 percent for a matched cohort (Delmonico, 2009).

A study carried out by two physicians reported that their patient, HQ, was on the list for one year. During that time, his MELD score went from 18 to 21 (see Schiano and Rhodes, 2010). HQ visited the People's Republic of China and received a transplant two weeks after arriving. In China, the organs of executed prisoners are used for transplantation. HQ came back to the United States and checked in to a U.S. hospital for follow-up care. On the one hand, the America Society of Transplantation has a policy that optimal care will be provided to patients, even if they sought their transplant abroad. On the other hand, should the U.S. government take a position against the exploitation of donors and the practice of taking organs from executed prisoners or paid living donors?

Medical tourism raises ethical issues and can even involve false advertising or fraud. Some treatments are experimental, offering large risks and only modest benefits. For example, in the United States, some stem cell treatments are only available in clinical trials, and some patients may not be eligible. Heart failure patients can travel to Bangkok, Thailand, for stem cell heart therapy, an unproven treatment (Cohen, 2013; Vastag, 2008). Ethical issues will intensify as the demand for treatments increases.

We discussed the view that medical tourism has been increasing as patients seek better outcomes, better access, better patient experiences, and/or lower costs. Does this lead to competition for medical tourists?

The Growing Rivalry for Inbound International Patients

By 2017 at least 50 countries with hospitals and clinics not only targeted medical tourists but also claimed that they were able to outperform North American or Western European hospitals and doctors. In 2014 alone, 1 million Americans left the United States to get affordable, world-class medical treatment in other countries and that number will increase by 40 percent (Woodman, 2015). There is evidence that medical tourism is growing into a multi-billion-dollar global health industry, and with growing demand comes growing competitive rivalry.

Although these temporal changes in patient flows have not received much attention because they have been difficult to track, global rivalry for patients appears to be heating up. In 2017, 950 hospitals have been accredited by the **Joint Commission International (JCI)** worldwide—with 161 hospitals and clinics receiving JCI accreditation in the United Arab Emirates alone. Countries like UAE, Belgium, Costa Rica, Cuba, India, Israel, Mexico, Poland, Singapore, South Korea, Taiwan, Thailand, and Malaysia are becoming major players (Al-Hammouri, 2008; Benveniste, 2008; Fleni, 2008; Heyman, 2008; Keckley and Underwood, 2009; Woodman, 2015). Not unlike the Olympics, the health care playing field is leveling, allowing both high- and low-GDP countries to compete for each other's patients.

Many Asian countries report large numbers of inbound medical tourists. Malaysia, for example, claimed to have more than 600,000 tourists annually, India 250,000, Singapore 550,000, and Thailand 1.2 million (Woodman, 2015). The best of breed in medical tourism is Thailand's Bumrungrad Hospital in Bangkok. Each year this hospital treats 550,000 international patients from 200 countries and reports that 55,000 of the inbound patients are from the United States (for their latest statistics, see www.bumrungrad.com).

There are many reasons why medical tourism accounts for a high proportion of Bumrungrad's patient revenues. With more than 200 U.S.-trained, board-certified physicians, Bumrungrad Hospital is fully accredited by the Joint Commission for International Accreditation. They offer five-star hotel services with deluxe rooms, VIP and royal suites, laptop computers, a swimming pool, and a fitness center, and the hospital is within walking distance of Bangkok's most prestigious restaurants, shopping, and entertainment venues. Patients' families or significant others are able to enjoy the exotic beaches, while the patient undergoes a procedure.

The difference between inbound and outbound medical tourism not only has an effect on a hospital but can also have a significant effect a nation's health care system (Chilingerian and Savage, 2005; Fried and Harris, 2007). In 2007, 750,000 outbound American medical tourists spent $2.1 billion, whereas 400,000 inbound international patients spent $5.0 billion for care in the United States (Keckley and Underwood, 2009). If these estimates are correct, the United States came out ahead by almost $3.0 billion.

Nevertheless, outbound patients represent losses in revenue. Conservative estimates of the revenue that would have been generated if the 750,000 patients had received care in the United States were $15.6 billion versus the $5 billion from the inbound patients (Keckley and Underwood, 2008).

International inbound patients (flowing to the United States) were projected to grow to only 500,000 by 2017; on the other hand, U.S. outbound patients are projected to be 1.4 million. The projected increase in the number of outbound American medical tourists represents a potential $30.3–$79.5 billion spent oversees for medical care, resulting in a revenue loss of anywhere between $228.5 and $599.5 billion for the United States. What we learn by observing inbound patient flows around the world is that medical tourism is not only competitive but also a "disruptive innovation" that deserves more clinical and managerial attention (see Cohen, 2015). What are the implications for managers?

Managerial Implications of Medical Tourism

We have shown that many patient-centered, integrated health care organizations are attracting patients across national borders because they offer high quality and high efficiency. Hospitals and clinics that focus on a small set of diagnoses or diseases, such as cataract procedures or hip replacements, have chosen a strategy of being a "focused clinic." **Focused clinics** can deliver better results at lower costs and often outperform general hospitals that offer a wider range of clinical services.

Two examples of focused clinics offering excellent outcomes, low cost, and superb patient experiences are the Coxa clinic, which specializes in joint replacements and performs 3,000 procedures annually in Finland, and the Canadian hernia hospital, Shouldice, which performs 7,000 simple inguinal hernia repairs annually. Both Coxa and Shouldice attracted medical tourists and Table 15.3 explains why a hernia hospital attract medical tourists. (To learn what it takes to organize and manage a clinical service that can offer outstanding patient experiences and superior technical outcomes at a low cost, see "In Practice:. Case Study: Canada's High-Quality, Low-Cost Hernia Hospital.")

• • • IN PRACTICE: Case Study: Canada's High-Quality, Low-Cost Hernia Hospital[11]

Shouldice hospital in Ontario, Canada, is an 89-bed hospital with five operating theaters. Founded in 1945, the hospital focuses on the surgical repair of simple inguinal hernias. It is not only efficient but also offers high-quality care and, over many decades, has attracted medical tourists.

The Shouldice hernia repair almost never uses general anesthesia; in well over 95 percent of the cases, operations are performed under local infiltration and a light sedative (Glassow, 1973, 1986). The avoidance of general anesthesia significantly reduces the risk of harm to patients. Moreover, Shouldice surgeons are carefully selected and trained over four months before they are allowed to operate. Whereas a general surgeon may perform 50 hernia repairs a year, each Shouldice surgeon performs over 600 per year. Additionally, the surgery is not done on an outpatient basis; each patient stays for a minimum of three days. What makes the clinical work challenging and rewarding for a Shouldice surgeon is repairing a hernia that another surgeon was unable to repair.

Every day at noon, the surgeons operate on patients with a hernia recurrence. These patients may have already had one or two hernia procedures, but the hernia returned because it was not properly repaired. Performing a procedure over old scar tissue is tricky work for any surgeon. Nevertheless, these are the cases that motivate Shouldice surgeons, because they provide clinical evidence of the superiority of the Shouldice technique with its specialized incision, suturing, and early ambulation. Shouldice surgeons can guarantee their patients (and themselves) that they are the best hernia surgeons in the world (Odell, 2000).

Shouldice is not just a hernia repair technique; it is a well-designed service proposition that has clinical value for specific group of patients (Urquhart and O'Dell, 2004). The care process includes a stay in a pleasant and relaxed environment, continuity of relationships, low prices, and high quality. The physician–patient interaction differs from most surgical encounters; when patients are admitted, the first person they see is their surgeon who confirms their diagnosis, explains the procedure, and what to expect.

Once selected for Shouldice, patients are educated to become partners and co-producers in every aspect of the care process, which builds both trust and self-confidence. For example, they walk into the operating room, they are awake and can talk with the surgeons during the surgery, and they are invited to get off the operating table and walk (with the help of the surgeon) to the postoperative room because early ambulation is part of the recovery process.

Recovery is completely programmed to include wake-up, medication, breakfast, exercise classes, rest periods, lunch in the dining room, more exercise, dinner, and more activity. To encourage mobility and interaction, there are no televisions or telephones in the rooms. Meals must be eaten in a dining room, and patients must take themselves to the toilets. The facility has stairs with low risers, putting greens, exercise cycles, walking paths, and other activities aimed at a speedy recovery.[12]

Every patient, physician, nurse, and employee at Shouldice is an alumnus. Patients, providers, and staff are fully engaged, understand their roles and responsibilities, and share an attitude and a mindset. Through mutual interaction, learning, and understanding, they are committed to the mission and goals of the clinical care process and adopt a Shouldice identity. The nurses know that their job is not to perform menial tasks but to educate patients, help them to exercise, and relieve physicians of simple nonclinical tasks. These are powerful lessons in the repositioning of the primary clinical activities and the role of management in the formulation of care practices into a care process. Value is created for patients, value is created for clinicians, and value is created for the organization (see Table 15.3).

Case Questions

1. From a medical tourist perspective, compare Shouldice with the traditional hospital in terms of the key factors of competition.

2. Using Table 15.3, would Shouldice attract patients from outside the local province? Why?

3. How is value created for patients, for clinical and nonclinical professionals, and for the Shouldice Hospital as an organization?

4. Which segment or type of medical travelers would Shouldice attract?

---

[11] Information for this case study is based on several days of observations and interviews at Shouldice Hospital with Dr. Shouldice and staff members in October 1985 and March 2016. It also draws on a paper by Chilingerian and Savage (2005) and on an interview in October 2000 with Mr. Alan Odell.

[12] Every patient who had experienced Shouldice Hospital would be invited to annual reunions. This practice ended a few years ago. Nevertheless, every patient is a member of the Shouldice patient network.

Table 15.3 Key Factors for Competition for Shouldice Hospital

Excellent outcomes/Strong Clinical Reputation

- Low Recurrence rates: less than 1% over last 10 years
- Complications rates less than 0.5%
- On average patients go back to work sooner

Extremely high patient satisfaction—exceeding patient expectations

- 98% are extremely satisfied with the care and 2% "merely" satisfied
- Excellent Pain Management
- 100% willing to recommend the service again

Low Cost

- High degree of coordination of patient care across operating units
- Average cost per case is less than the average local community hospital

Efficient decision making

- Quick diagnosis to treatment
- Optimal involvement of the patient in the care process

Some amenities, one standardized care process

- Short waits once admitted
- Excellent dining services and food

Excellent relationships, psychological support and information

- High degree of trust and confidence
- Nurses and physicians spend time answering questions
- Annual patient reunions/long term relationship

SOURCE: Adapted from Chilingerian (2004).

Depending on patients from abroad may not be a sustainable strategy, however. It is difficult to make global competition irrelevant by merely outperforming a rival on hotel and food, hygiene, safety and outcomes, friendly services, JCI, U.S. and European board certifications, robotic technology, and the like, as these resources and capabilities can be easily replicated by most competitors. So, investing millions to become a "most-traveled" destination for medical tourists is a temporary designation at best. Moreover, geography, global economics, and politics expose health care management to risks and uncertainties.

In the year 2000, patients from the Gulf states reportedly spent approximately $27 billion to obtain care abroad and the United States received 44 percent of all acute patients from Middle Eastern countries (Alsagoff, 2005). Following the events in New York on September 11, 2001, entry to the United States from the Gulf region became very difficult and time-consuming. Subsequently, U.S. hospitals lost between $750 million and $1.25 billion in international patient revenues from just two

countries, Saudi Arabia and the United Arab Emirates (Landers, 2002). In 2002, the U.S. share of Middle East patients dropped from 44 percent to 16 percent, and in 2003 and 2004 it dropped further, from 16 percent to only 8 percent. International patients who formerly went to U.S. destinations like the Mayo Clinic or John Hopkins discovered health care in Thailand, Malaysia, and India (Chilingerian and Savage, 2005). Accreditation from the JCI can quickly bring legitimacy to a provider (Ehrbeck, Guevara, and Mango, 2008). If patients want to find JCI-accredited health care organizations, they can go online to sites, such as Health Travel Media.

The decision to go out of one's country to obtain care depends on the perceived value of medical travel in relation to the perceived sacrifices. The perception of sacrifice can be driven by local and global events that influence perceptions of air safety, transportation costs, national rivalry for patients, the global economy, national moods, and health policies and politics that influence barriers to entry. Many of these factors are out of the control of hospital managers.

Some health care organizations are shifting their international strategy from attracting medical tourists to "exporting its know-how" to other countries. In the mid-1980s, Shouldice, the Canadian hernia clinic, reported more than 40 percent of their patients were medical tourists; today, that is no longer the case. Coxa, the joint replacement clinic in Finland, has also seen a significant decline in international patients over the last 10 years. In fact, Coxa is no longer depending on medical tourists. Coxa's CEO, Tarmo Martikainen, said,

> We believe it is far better to transfer our knowledge help countries develop the ability to perform a procedure with our outcomes, patient experience, and efficiency rather than attracting patients to fly thousands of kilometers for surgery in another country. (Martikainen, 2016)

In 2015, Coxa developed a partnership with Nairi Medical Center in Armenia. It sent orthopedic surgeons, nurses, and physiotherapists to Armenia to transfer Coxa's unique care processes; knowledge of best practices for hygiene, medications, pain relief, operating room technology; and supply-chain advantages. From a global strategy standpoint, they are trying to achieve a better local–global balance by moving away from medical tourism and moving toward transferring their advanced surgical knowledge for hip and knee replacements and their managerial skills and operating strategies to other countries (see Chilingerian and Savage, 2005).

In summary, there are bright and dark sides to medical tourism. If health care systems can give international patients better care at a lower cost, there is an argument that medical tourism can advance social justice. For example, if the outbound flow of patients motivates a country to improve its health care system, as in the case of Abu Dhabi, that advances the well-being of people (see "In Practice: A Country Case Study on the Partnership between Abu Dhabi and the Cleveland Clinic in the United States" and "In Practice: Cleveland Clinic Abu Dhabi: The Future of Health Care Globalization Is Already Here"). On the other hand, if medical tourists are patients desperately seeking an organ transplant, or an unproven experimental therapy unavailable in their homeland, we have legitimate concerns. Medical tourism has an added challenge since it can also be associated with the flow of the health workers across borders. To attract international patients requires a substantial investment in facilities, equipment, service processes, and service-minded people who can "delight" patients. Hospitals and clinics that want to serve medical tourists must recruit "world-class" clinical talent at a time when there is a global shortage of skilled professionals such as nurses, physicians, therapists, pharmacists, and others. Medical worker migration may be one of most serious global health care issues and is addressed in the next section.

THE FLOW OF HEALTH WORKERS ACROSS BORDERS

Technological and **medical innovation** coupled with an ageing population has increased the demand for health care worldwide. Countries are finding it difficult to keep pace with these changes, and many countries are experiencing shortages of health human resources. The 10 percent of nurses and 20 percent of physicians from Africa who work in other continents create a severe shortfall of clinicians and contribute to public health problems (Bradby, 2014). Rwanda is a case in point.

Between 1990 and 2014, Rwanda made dramatic improvements in population health. Maternal mortality rates have decreased 77 percent, deaths for children under 5 per 100,000 live births have 71 percent, and by 2013, Rwanda achieved an average life expectancy of 64 years of age.[13] Despite these improvements, between 1990 and 2013, deaths attributable to cardiovascular disease went from 7 percent to 15 percent. The number of acute myocardial infarctions is estimated to be about 5,000, with 25,000 reported cases of rheumatic heart disease. Although the number of physicians is directly related to positive outcomes in cardiovascular disease (Bradby, 2014), in 2016 there were no cardiac surgeons and only four cardiologists in Rwanda (Bowser et al., 2016).

As the labor market became more globalized and health professionals become more mobile, countries looked beyond their national boundaries to recruit the skills and expertise to meet their health care delivery needs (Chen and Wilson, 2013). From the 1950s until today, physicians and eventually nurses from low-income countries have served as a buffer or "reserve army of labor" when demand for health care increases (Bradby, 2014). There has always been an imbalance in the distribution of health workers (akin to the broad imbalance in resource availability). The increasing demand for health workers and the ability of high-income countries to offer more attractive remuneration packages have exacerbated this maldistribution—a phenomenon known as the "brain drain."

In this section of the chapter, we explore the extent of this maldistribution of health professionals, the financial implications, and its impact on middle- and low-income health systems. We explore the variety of coping mechanisms put in place to reduce the impact of the shortages,

---

[13] This is still significantly lower than China, Mexico, Malaysia, or India.

giving examples of human resources initiatives from several countries. We also consider the broader implications for how we should staff our health systems of the future. The section concludes with specific implications that managers and leaders in health care need to consider as they face the challenge of staffing their health delivery system in an ethical, cost-effective, and efficient manner.

Health Worker Mobility

Somewhere between 23 percent and 34 percent of physicians practicing in Australia, Canada, New Zealand, the United Kingdom, and the United States have trained elsewhere (Bradby, 2014).[14] In an increasingly globalized labor market, national health systems can no longer rely on the commitment of graduates to work within their own country and so must look to the international labor market to meet their demands for health professionals. It has therefore become common for high-income countries to recruit portions of their health labor force from middle- and low-income countries.

This health worker migration first became an issue for African countries in the postcolonial period, when developing countries were starting to expand their health services and to train their own nationals to deliver these services. These developments coincided with the rapid expansion of health systems in high-income countries and a shortage of health professionals to meet service requirements. Thus, opportunities opened up for health care workers in search of better pay and enhanced career opportunities to work in these countries, and the term "brain drain" was coined to describe the large-scale movement of health professionals from low-income to high-income countries (Bach, 2004). This process has been facilitated by the growth of free trade blocks, reinforced by service sector liberalization that arose from the General Agreement on Trade in Services (GATS) (OECD, 2002). For example, the European Union has established an inclusive model of mutual recognition of qualifications in which registered nurses or midwives are free to work in any member state. Bach claims that the migration of health workers is distinctive because it is strongly influenced by the regulatory frameworks of individual governments that control the training, recruitment, and deployment of health professionals; such frameworks giving rise to particular national patterns of migration. (2003, p. 3). However, this centrality of government regulation also provides greater scope for policy interventions that address migration of health workers, as we discuss later in this chapter.

The Scale of the Flow

The establishment of accurate data on the flows of health workers presents a challenge, given the different classification, regulation, and registration systems for health professionals in every country. As Clemens and Pettersson (2007) point out, no comprehensive and systematic bilateral database of the international flows of people for all countries exists. All high-income countries collect occupation-specific data on people who arrive in the country but most do not do so for people who depart the country, making high-frequency occupation-specific data on bilateral gross migration flows impossible to compile (2007, p. 15). However, identifying the stock of health workers in different regions of the world gives us some sense of the inequities that exist in the distribution of health workers. The sub-Saharan average was 15.5 physicians for 100,000 people, 73.4 nurses per 100,000 people, 30.9 midwives per 100,000 people, and 1.1 pharmacists per 100,000 people in 2002. In contrast, the average among the Organization for Economic Co-operation and Development (OECD) countries was approximately 311 physicians and 737.5 nurses per 100,000 people in 2002. On average, African countries have about 20 times fewer physicians and 10 times fewer nurses than high-income countries. Even compared to other emerging countries, SSA numbers are strikingly low. For India, Korea, Singapore, and Vietnam, in the early years of the last decade the average number of physicians per 100,000 people was estimated at 106.3; for nurses it was 220.4 (Liese Blanchet, and Dussault, 2003).

Clemens and Pettersson (2007) estimate that approximately 65,000 African-born physicians and 70,000 African-born professional nurses were working overseas in a high-income country in the year 2000. This represents about one-fifth of African-born physicians in the world and about one-tenth of African-born professional nurses. The fraction of health professionals abroad varies enormously across African countries, from 1 percent to over 70 percent according to the occupation and country.

In 2014, almost one-quarter of U.S.-based physicians were foreign-trained (OECD Health Data, 2016). The corresponding percentage was as low as 10 percent for France and Germany and as high as 42 percent in New Zealand. The majority of these doctors originated from India, Pakistan, and Dominica. In 2014, the United States imported 2,659 nurses from the Philippines alone.

---

[14] In the United States, for example, 25.8 percent of the physician workforce are foreign-born or-educated, 5.4 percent of registered nurses were foreign born and educated abroad, and 20.9 percent of direct care workers were born outside the United States (Chen et al. 2013).

Impact on Health Systems of Low- and Middle-Income Countries

The global shortage of health professionals is having an impact on all countries; however, a disproportionately large amount of this burden falls on countries with the greatest health needs. Africa carries 25 percent of the world's disease burden, yet has only 1.3 percent of the world's health workers (Commission for Africa, 2005). The health personnel to population ratio in Africa has always lagged behind the rest of the world, falling far short of the WHO (World Health Organization) minimum standard of 2.3 trained health workers per 1,000 population (230 per 100,000).

The latest available WHO statistics show the scale of this inequity with number of physicians per 1,000 population ranging from 2.544 in the United States (2013) to 767 in South Africa (2015), 0.725 in India (2015), and 0.03 in Tanzania (2012), for example. The ratios of practicing nurses and midwives show similar patterns with 9.884 in the United States (2005), 5.113 in South Africa (2015), 2.049 in India (2013), and 0.428 in Tanzania (2012).

The Joint Learning Initiative (JLI), a network of global health leaders, launched by the Rockefeller Foundation, suggested that on average countries with fewer than 2.5 health care professionals (counting only doctors, nurses, and midwives) per 1,000 population failed to achieve an 80 percent coverage rate for deliveries by skilled birth attendants or for measles immunization (Chen et al., 2004). The World Health Organization has highlighted the alarming global shortage of approximately 4.3 million doctors and nurses, which constitutes a shortfall of 15 percent of the total number of doctors and nurses worldwide. It is estimated that 57 poor countries are facing a severe crisis in that they have insufficient human resources to meet minimum needs (WHO, 2006). Liese, Blanchet, and Dussault (2003) argue that the proportion of health personnel to population has stagnated or declined in nearly every African country since 1960. Among the countries that attract African health workers in relatively large numbers are the United States, the United Kingdom, Canada, Australia, France, Spain, Portugal, Belgium, and South Africa (attracting workers from other African countries). It is clear that these nine countries play a significant role in depleting the resources of struggling health systems. The European Commission estimated that without further measures to meet the challenge of health personnel shortages, a potential shortfall of around 1 million health care workers will take place by 2020, rising up to 2 million if long-term care and ancillary professions are taken into account (European Commission, 2010). This means that around 15 percent of total care will not be covered compared to 2010. Although there is no consensus on the subject, some researchers in the United States are projecting shortages of 85,000 doctors by 2020 and 260,000 nurses by 2025 (Crisp and Chen, 2014). Countries with fast-growing economies, such as India, China, Brazil, and South Africa, want more trained health workers, and critical shortages remain in the world's poorest countries.

Kapur and McHale (2005a, b) point out that those with tertiary education are the most likely to emigrate, and "the dilemma is that those most likely to be institution-builders are those most likely to emigrate" (2005, p. 4). This results not only in gaps in the delivery of care but also in the development of services. Active recruitment by high-income countries tends to focus on attracting the most experienced health professionals. McAuliffe et al. (2010) argue that the gap in experienced health workers, coupled with the increased output of newly graduated health professionals, is creating its own difficulties for health systems. The shortage of experienced health professionals raises concerns about training, clinical supervision and ultimately the quality of care (McAuliffe et al., 2010). WHO makes the link between supervision and performance: "If supervisory visits become sterile administrative events, or are seen as fault-finding and punitive, they have little positive effect and may have negative effects. In contrast, supervision that is supportive, educational and consistent and helps to solve specific problems, can improve performance, job satisfaction and motivation" (WHO, 2006, p. 76). Good supervision made a difference in staff motivation and performance between public hospitals and autonomous quasi-government hospitals in Ghana (Dovlo et al., 1998). An additional impact identified in a study by Troy, Wyness, and McAuliffe (2007) is that the health workers who remain in low- and middle-income countries are faced with increased workloads and rising stress levels because of the depleted numbers. This has led to increased sick leave and absenteeism, further demotivating the remaining staff. In addition, a high prevalence of burnout has been reported in health professionals in many of the countries experiencing brain drain (Biksegn et al., 2016; Khamisa, Peltzer, and Oldenburg, 2013; Okwaraji and Aguwa, 2014).

Financial Implications

The exodus of health workers from low- and middle-income countries continues to maintain and increase the dependence of those countries on more developed nations, ironically the nations to which health personnel migrate. The recruitment of the best-qualified health personnel from low-income countries, at no training cost to the recipient countries, is increasingly being recognized as unethical. Almost 50 percent of doctors trained to work in Africa leave to work abroad (see Liese, Blanchet, and Dussault, 2003). With an estimated cost of $60,000 for training a general medical practitioner in the Southern African Development Cooperation (SADC) region, outflows from the region to more "developed" countries amount to a $500 million reverse subsidy per annum. Martin, Abella, and Kuptsch (2006) assert that South Africa is "suffering" from a "brain drain" of doctors and nurses with a financial loss of over $1 billion. UNCTAD has estimated that the United States has saved $3.86 billion as a consequence of importing 21,000 doctors from Nigeria alone.

Clemens and Petersson (2007) suggest a relationship between the loss of professionals and economic and political stability. Angola, Congo-Brazzaville, Guinea-Bissau, Liberia, Mozambique, Rwanda, and Sierra Leone all experienced civil war in the 1990s and they found that all had lost more than 40 percent of their physicians by 2000. Kenya, Tanzania, and Zimbabwe all experienced decades of economic stagnation in the late twentieth century and, by its end, each had lost more than half of its physicians. By contrast, countries with greater stability and prosperity—Botswana, South Africa, and pre-collapse Côte d'Ivoire—managed to retain their doctors (2007, p. 14).

However, some argue that the movement of workers from low-income to high-income countries is positive for the source countries as well as the host countries. Pritchett (2006) *argues that* "the gains to people in poor countries from labor mobility are enormous compared to everything else on the development agenda." Pritchett cites estimates that if rich countries were to permit a mere 3 percent increase in the size of their labor force by easing restrictions on labor mobility, the benefits to citizens of poor countries would be $305 billion a year—almost twice the combined annual benefits of full trade liberalization ($86 billion), foreign aid ($70 billion), and debt relief (about $3 billion in annual debt service savings). Pritchett argues that demographic forces for greater international labor mobility are being slowed by immovable anti-immigration ideas of rich-country citizens. He highlights the difficult political and ethical issues that the movement of people across national borders presents to the current system and proposes breaking the gridlock through policies that support development while also being politically acceptable in rich countries. These include greater use of temporary worker permits, permit rationing, reliance on bilateral rather than multilateral agreements, and protection of migrants' fundamental human rights.

One of the positive financial implications of labor migration from low-income to high-income countries is the value of remittances to families in low-income countries. **Migrant remittances**, defined as the transfer of funds from migrants to relatives or friends in their country of origin, have become an increasingly important feature of modern economic life. Indeed, remittances are now recognized as an important source of global development finance (Department for International Development, 2006). They not only supplement the incomes of families but also provide a much needed source of foreign exchange to these countries. The report of a study of UK migrants undertaken by DFID in 2006 states that "international remittance flows by migrant workers are huge and growing, with remittance flows perhaps exceeding development aid and without doubt playing a substantial role in alleviating poverty in recipient countries" (2006, p. 6) The report cites three factors to explain this trend:

- Remittance flows are now the second largest source of external funding for development countries (foreign direct investment being the largest)
- Remittances are one of the least volatile sources of foreign exchange for developing countries
- Remittances are expected to rise significantly in the long term. (Department for International Development, 2006, p. 6)

The recognition that remittances are playing an important role in supporting families in low-income countries has resulted in international organizations, bilateral donors, and nongovernment organizations taking initiatives to better understand the nature and scope of migrant remittances and to identify ways of maximizing their development impact in countries of origin.

In addition, international migration has been used to stimulate economies in some low-income countries. The export of contract labor as a strategy for stimulating domestic market conditions is a primary feature of Philippine economic policy (Matejowsky, 2006). Since the 1970s, millions of Filipinos have responded to slow economic growth at home by taking advantage of nonpermanent job opportunities abroad. There are also considerable benefits to be gained, should the migrants return to their home countries. They usually return having improved their education and expanded their skills sets and bring with them an international network that they can tap into for ongoing support and development.

International Response[15]

Increased awareness of the scale of health worker migration and the belief that migrant health worker flows will continue have shifted the attention of governments

---

[15] See the Appendix for a description of the complex policymaking institutions, organizations, and agencies that comprise the global health care landscape and the health care targets for 2030.

toward the concept of "managed migration"—a term that signals attempts to link international migration to the health policy goals of individual states and to regulate the flows of health workers in a way that is beneficial to both source and destination countries (Bach, 2003). The practice of recruitment agencies in high-income countries actively encouraging migration has been heavily criticized because of its impact on low-income countries. These countries are effectively utilizing scarce resources of low-income countries to educate health professionals, only for high-income country health systems to reap the benefits. There have been calls for a tax or compensation payment by countries that recruit large numbers of health workers from countries that can ill afford to lose them. Attempts have been made to develop international recruitment guidelines, but these have been fraught with difficulty and have had little impact on the management of international migration of overseas nurses (Buchan and Perfilieva, 2006). The Commonwealth Code of Practice has a strong emphasis on mutuality of benefits for both countries.

> Many developing Commonwealth countries have expressed the view that recruiting developed countries should in some way compensate source countries for the loss of personnel trained at great expense. Compensation may be in a variety of ways such as building capacity in training institutions. (2003, p. 7)

According to Bach (2003), this was "a step too far" for Australia, Canada, and the United Kingdom, and they declined to sign the code because of the statements on compensation. As such codes and guidelines are not mandatory, many countries have chosen not to follow them and therefore, at best, they serve to highlight good employment practices when adhered to.

Bilateral agreements between countries, such as policies on return, the incorporation of ethical codes of practice into national recruitment practice, and measures to cap the numbers of internationally recruited health workers entering countries have met with limited success. The UK National Health Service ended its active recruitment of staff from Sub-Saharan Africa in 2001. However, this has not entirely stemmed the flow, and some writers are calling for more radical measures to address the problem. Alkire and Chen (2004) urge that high-income countries' migration policy "should adopt 'medical exceptionalism' based on moral and ethical grounds". Kapur and McHale caution against "poaching" health workers from developing countries and claim that the case is "obvious" for "restraint" in the recruitment of doctors and nurses. Labonte, Packer, and Klassen (2006) in a study of Canadian policy makers found that reducing pull factors by increasing domestic self-sufficiency and reducing push factors by strengthening source country health systems have the greatest policy traction in Canada.

The Global Health Workforce Alliance (GHWA) partnership was established in 2006 to identify and implement solutions to the global health workforce crisis. It assists countries with their efforts to develop and implement plans for scaling up the health workforce. It brings together a variety of actors, including national governments, civil society, finance institutions, workers, international agencies, academic institutions, and professional associations in addressing the crisis. The 2010 WHO Global Code of Practice on the International Recruitment of Health Personnel aimed to bring awareness to richer countries of the importance of reducing recruitment from poorer nations that have health worker shortages (WHO, 2010). However, wider measures, including increased investment, improved training, and better human-resources management are needed to address the shortfalls in both rich and poor countries (Chen and Boufford, 2005). Despite widespread assertions of the right to health, it is estimated that at least 1 billion people do not have access to a trained health worker (Crisp and Chen, 2014).

National Level Responses

Individual countries, alarmed by the scale of emigration from their health systems and the devastating impact this has had, have begun to take serious measures to address their human resources crisis. Dovlo and Martineau (2004) identify the role that countries need to play to stem the flow of health workers, stating that "the critical issue is that countries need to improve their workforce planning and monitoring, assess incentive packages and how well these work; improve human resources and personnel administration systems as well as better planning; new flexible pay systems and more accessible and shorter specialist training" (2004).

The prospect of financial gain is believed to be a pivotal factor in the decision to migrate. In order to counteract this, many African countries have introduced top-up salaries and other kinds of benefits and allowances for some cadres of health workers. Namibia is reported to be offering generous end of service payments and subsidized house-owning schemes and car ownership. In Ghana, the government has increased incomes, especially for physicians. Nigeria also introduced a separate duty allowance structure for physicians. Botswana introduced 30 percent overtime allowance for nurses and 15 percent for physicians. Other countries, such as Kenya, South Africa, Zambia, Malawi, Tanzania, and Mozambique have increased salaries of various cadres of health workers in an effort to retain them. While countries, such as Thailand and Ireland have had some degree of success in persuading physicians who have migrated abroad to return home by providing monetary incentives and research funds, as well as services and assistants (Pang, Lansang, and Haines, 2002), it has been argued that providing monetary incentives alone will not alter migration significantly, considering the enormous wage differentials in the source and recipient countries (Vujicic et al., 2004). Most SSA countries cannot compete with the financial incentives of overseas countries, but it has been argued that nonfinancial incentives, which have been found to be important in motivating health workers, can be used to supplement these financial incentives. Indeed, there is growing evidence that other factors in the work environment may also be acting as strong push factors. Workload and staff shortages are contributing to burnout, high absenteeism, stress, depression, low morale, and demotivation, and these factors are responsible for driving workers out of the public sector (McAuliffe et al. 2010; Sanders and Lloyd, 2005). Poor working conditions are reported to seriously undermine health system performance by thwarting staff morale and motivation and directly contributing to problems in recruitment and retention (Troy, Wyness, and McAuliffe, 2007; WHO, 1996). Financial incentives are only one part of a much more complex picture of motivational factors and perceived fairness and management support in particular are important motivators (Madede et al., 2017; McAuliffe et al., 2009, 2016).

One strategy being used to alleviate health worker shortages and to improve access and quality of health services is task shifting or the delegation of tasks that would traditionally fall within the scope of practice of doctors or nurse to other health workers who have undergone shorter periods of training (see "In Practice: A Country Case Study on Ethiopia's Flooding and Retention Strategy"). These cadres have different titles in different countries but are commonly referred to as mid-level workers or nonphysician clinicians. Mid-level workers are health care providers who have received less training and have a more restricted scope of practice than professionals. These workers, in contrast to community or lay health workers, however, do have a formal certificate and accreditation through their countries' licensing bodies (Lehman, 2008, p. iv). Mullan and Frehywot (2007)

identified nonphysician clinicians (NPCs) in 25 of 47 countries in sub-Saharan Africa, although their roles varied widely between countries. In nine countries, numbers of NPCs equaled or exceeded numbers of physicians. In general, NPCs' training costs less than a physician's and lasted for an average period of three to four years postsecondary school. All NPCs do basic diagnosis and medical treatment, but some were trained in specialty activities, such as caesarean section, ophthalmology, and anesthesia. Many NPCs were recruited from rural and poor areas and worked in these same regions (Mullan and Frehywot, 2007). NPCs deliver health services in low-, middle-, and high-income countries. For example, more than 300,000 NPCs practice alongside physicians in the United States (Cooper, Laud, and Dietrich, 1998). Much innovation in such roles is taking place in low-income and middle-income countries in which the scarcity of resources has prompted this diversification of roles. In Mozambique, técnicos do cirurgia—mainly nurses with extra training—perform nearly all cesarean sections, with outcomes that are as good as those observed when the procedure is performed by physicians, and at a much lower cost (Chilopora et al., 2007; Kruk et al., 2007; Pereira et al., 2007). In Pakistan "Lady Health Workers" have shown the ability to influence health promotion and treatment in villages (Oxford Policy Management, 2002). Community health workers, such as those in Bangladesh, are contributing to better child survival in many countries (Haines et al., 2007). One particularly interesting case study is the use of the mid-level cadres in Ethiopia (see "In Practice: A Country Case Study on Ethiopia's Flooding and Retention Strategy"). This initiative, although progressing well, is not sufficiently advanced to assess the true impact on the availability of health services or on the country's health indicators. If successful, however, it will raise interesting questions about the wisdom of attempting to populate low-income countries with Western-trained, expensively produced doctors.

• • • IN PRACTICE: A Country Case Study on Ethiopia's Flooding and Retention Strategy[16]

Ethiopia is a federal government, comprising 9 regional states, 2 city administrations, 624 districts, and 15,000 villages. Federal Ministry of Health data from 2006 showed that 85 percent of the population, or 77.3 million persons, lived in rural areas. It is estimated that 60 percent to 80 percent of the country's health problems are due to largely preventable communicable diseases, such as malaria, pneumonia, and TB. HIV/AIDS is also a growing problem. Ethiopia suffers from an acute shortage of health workers at every level, and rural areas have been particularly chronically underserved. The government's Health Sector Development Program, which began to be implemented in 1997, is focused on achieving the health-related **Millennium Development Goals (MDGs)** and

---

[16] Information for this case study was sourced from the Ethiopia's Ministry of Health website, Carter Center, and WHO GHWA's Country Case Study: Ethiopia's Human Resources for Health Programme retrieved from www.who.int/workforcealliance.

• • • IN PRACTICE: A Country Case Study on Ethiopia's Flooding and Retention Strategy (Continued)

on providing comprehensive and integrated primary care services, mainly at community-based health facilities. One of the program's eight components is to expand the supply and productivity of health personnel. The initial focus was on community-level provision, with the initiation of the Health Extension Program (HEW) in 2004. This program aims to improve primary health services in rural areas through an innovative community-based approach that focuses on prevention, healthy living, and basic curative care. It introduced a new cadre of health worker, health extension workers (HEWs), and defined a package of essential interventions for them to deliver from village health posts. Female high school graduates are recruited and trained for one year (candidates must have completed grade 10 in school, need to be from the local community, and speak the local language). They are trained to deliver a package of 16 preventive and basic curative services that comprise four main components: hygiene and environmental sanitation, family health services, disease prevention and control, and health education and communication. The program aims to train 30,000 new HEWs to work at local health posts and is well advanced in achieving this.

A second initiative is the Ethiopia Public Health Training Initiative (EPHTI)—a partnership between the Ethiopian government ministries of Health and Education, The Carter Center, seven Ethiopian universities, and other nongovernmental organizations—aims to improve the quality of preservice training to health science professionals within Ethiopia. Because the biggest hurdle to better health in Ethiopia is the lack of access to health personnel, the mission of EPHTI is to build a team of qualified health care workers across the country, especially in underserved rural populations. EPHTI has three primary goals:

• Assist Ethiopians in developing their own training and educational health learning materials
• Strengthen the teaching capacity of Ethiopian university faculty members
• Improve the campus teaching and learning environments of Ethiopian health sciences universities

In 2005, EPHTI began to implement the Accelerated Health Officer Training Program in Ethiopia. The health officer is the leader of the community-based health center professional staff, and the program's objective is to train 5,000 health officers by 2010. Health officers provide clinical services at health centers and manage both the health center and world health offices. Five universities and 20 hospitals are involved in the training program. The majority of students in the training program were practicing nurses who received basic science education in the first year, followed by two years of tailored instruction at a training hospital. By mid-2008, more than 900 had graduated, and 3,168 were under training.

The Ethiopian government is to be commended for its novel approach to addressing the health worker shortage. In 2014, the Ethiopia government announced that the country had achieved the 4th Millennium Development Goal of reducing child mortality by two-thirds from 1990 levels. In a review of the progress of Ethiopia's Health Financing Strategy by Harvard School of Public Health, Alebachew et al. (2015) report that more than 35,000 health extension workers on government salary provide services in rural and urban kebeles throughout the country. Significant scale-up in training physicians and other health workers was underway and preparations were advanced to launch social health insurance and expand community-based health insurance. However, despite this impressive level of progress, there remains considerable inequity in service provision, as the following extract from the above-mentioned report demonstrates:

> Overall, despite the marked achievement on the supply side toward enhancing the Primary Health Care through accelerated expansion of Primary Health Care Units, given the poverty level in the country and the limited coverage and implementation of the fee-waiver and health insurance scheme; the equity objective of the HCF reform is far from met as households still finance 34 percent of total health expenditure (as per NHA) and this puts a great burden of ill health in poor households. Hence, major work is required on the demand side to make health care to provide equitable and acceptable standards of service for all segments of the population. On the supply side, in addition to improving access it is also important to review the service availability and functionality of the Primary Healthcare Units. (2015, p. 84)

Some countries have continued to produce highly trained doctors and nurses but have adopted a strategy of over-production. The Philippines has, for more than a decade, been exporting its degree-level nurses to many countries throughout the world. The government has deliberately adopted this strategy of overproduction in the belief that the country would benefit both from remittances of their emigrants and from the additional expertise and knowledge of returning migrants. This strategy has certainly been welcomed by countries who have benefited from this large pool of nursing staff, for example, Canada, United States, Ireland, and United Kingdom. However, interviews with directors of nursing in the Philippines showed that, while acknowledging these benefits to the emigrant nurses, their concerns on the detrimental effect on nursing and the health systems in their own country were noticeable; "the nurses that migrate from low and middle income countries tend to be experienced and highly skilled" (Troy, Wyness, and McAuliffe, 2007, p. 3). Castro-Palaganas et al. (2017) summarizes the impact this strategy of overproduction for migration has had on the Philippines Health System. "The migration of health workers has both negative and positive consequences for the Philippine health system and its health workers . . . migration has resulted in the loss of investment in human capital. The gap in the supply of health workers has affected the quality of care delivered, especially in rural areas. The opening of overseas opportunities has commercialized health education, compromised its quality, and stripped the country of skilled learning facilitators. The social cost of migration has affected émigrés and their families. At the household level, migration has engendered increased consumerism and materialism and fostered dependency on overseas remittances" (2017, p. 25).

Cuba also presents an interesting case (see "In Practice: A Country Case Study on Cuba's Internationalist Principle and the Latin American Medical School Program"). When faced with a critical shortage of doctors following the revolution, it began to not only overproduce but also to change the very nature and structure of medical training in an attempt to engender values of solidarity and loyalty to local communities in its new medical graduates. Health indicators in this country have shown huge improvements and Cuban doctors have assisted many low-income countries to build their supply of medical manpower. Again this could be seen as a challenge to the traditional model of training and deployment of health professionals to staff our health systems.

• • • IN PRACTICE: A Country Case Study on Cuba's Internationalist Principle and the Latin American Medical School Program[17]

The devastation caused in Central America and the Caribbean in 1998 by hurricanes George and Mitch prompted Cuba to send 1,000 Cuban doctors to volunteer in the disaster areas. The scale of the disaster and the impact for populations without health care led the Cuban government to a decision to offer Cuban medical teams for longer-term assistance to strengthen local health systems and to open a medical school in Cuba offering 10,000 scholarships to students from those countries. This became the Comprehensive Health Program (CHP).

By 2007, over 3,000 foreign doctors had graduated from this school. Government-to-government agreements have expanded the program to 27 countries, and in the case of the United States, attracted students even in the absence of a bilateral agreement. The program is distinctive in its underlying mission to train doctors to serve local communities by combining population-based public health principles and prevention with clinical medicine. Students are placed in polyclinics (the basic unit of the system, which serves a population of 25,000 to 30,000) to work with local Cuban communities even in their basic science years. The focus of the training is biopsychosocial—individual, family, and community. This prepares students well for working in resource poor settings where the close association between poverty and ill health means that health professionals must have a good understanding to the economic, social, cultural, and environmental determinants of health in order to be effective. The Cuban principle is that "medicine as merchandise has not—and will not—guarantee health for the world's poor majorities" (Frank and Read, 2008, p. 3). Health professionals must believe in health as a human right and must be prepared to make sacrifices to deliver on this right.

As well as this large-scale training of doctors, Cuba also trained auxiliary personnel, such as nursing auxiliaries and health technicians, to serve in the rural areas and to meet the changing needs of the health system.

---

[17] Materials for this case study were sourced from: Presentations at the Global Forum for Health Research, Havana, November 2009. Marquez, M. (2009). Health-workforce development in the Cuban health system. *The Lancet, 374*(9701), 1574–1575. Frank, M., & Reed, G. (2008). Doctors for the (developing) world, training physicians for global health, MEDICC Review. Retrieved from www.medicc.org/publications/medicc_review/0805/spotlight.html.

• • • IN PRACTICE: A Country Case Study on Cuba's Internationalist Principle and the Latin American Medical School Program (Continued)

Marquez (2009) writing in *The Lancet* claims that "the development of a diversified workforce has been crucial for the provision of free-of-charge services along the continuum of care, particularly ambulatory services in polyclinics . . .The system's community healthcare approach has allowed the placement of a doctor trained in primary care and a nurse in every neighborhood (serving about 150 families)."

Cuba now has one of the best doctor-to-population ratios in the world with 61 percent female. It has better health indicators than countries that have substantially higher per capita spending on health. It has been ranked by Save the Children as the number one country in Latin America to be a mother. One hundred percent of pregnant women have more than four prenatal visits, compared with 97 percent in the United States. Cuba's infant mortality rate in 2013 was 4.70 per 1,000, compared with 6.17 for the United States (Erwin and Bialek, 2015). These achievements are considerable in the context where according to World Bank Statistics (accessed June 26, 2017), Cuba's health expenditure per capita (PPP) in 2014 was 2.475, while the United States spent almost four times this amount at 9.403 per capita.

The Implications for Health Care Managers

As we have shown above, migration of health workers has increased over the past several decades and there are many indications that it will continue to be a feature of the landscape for the foreseeable future—the world is indeed flattening for health workers. Some of these migration flows are predictable, others less so. An example that serves to highlight this is the case of nurses migrating from the Philippines to Ireland. Earlier we described the strategy of overproduction that was adopted by this country in the 1990s. In the late 1990s, Ireland had a critical shortage of nurses and began to recruit hundreds of Filipino nurses to fill gaps in the services. They came, they settled, and their families followed them. Ireland considered its problem solved until it was discovered that those who had been in the country for four to five years were moving on to the United States or Canada in search of higher salaries and greater opportunities for skill development. South Africa experiences similar problems with unpredictable migration flows. At the service delivery level, coping with this unpredictability requires careful manpower planning, matching supply with current and predicated future demand. It is no longer sufficient to expect domestic labor markets to fulfil the needs of service delivery. Recruiting beyond one's own national boundaries is inevitable (and desirable from the perspective of the health professional who wishes to travel and broaden his or her clinical expertise).

In an era of ever-increasing health care demands, all health systems need to be strengthened and further developed. However, such development needs to be conducted with due recognition of health as a basic human right—entitling everyone to affordable health care regardless of their means or their address. If the international mobility of highly skilled workers is likely to increase, what of the future of developing countries already experiencing substantial losses and struggling to provide basic health care for their populations? Lowell and Findley (2001) in a report synthesizing the International Labor Office's research advise that immigration policies of developed countries should facilitate movement; yet, they should incorporate mechanisms that encourage developing country economic growth.

> Developed countries might: encourage temporary and return migration; restrict recruitment from at risk countries; establish best practices; regulate recruitment agencies; establish bilateral agreements; and standardize GATS commitments. (2001, p. ii)

As discussed earlier, there are many ways in which high-income countries can help strengthen low-income country health systems, from monetary (recruitment tax paid to source country) to capacity building (contributing to source country training, exchange of staff and expertise, etc.) methods. The migration of health workers has also led to questions about how health workers can be retained; happy health workers tend to stay in jobs longer. Understanding and improving the motivation of health workers is a key task for any health care manager, regardless of context or scarcity of resources. Creating an environment that attracts and retains health professionals has become a focus of many low-income countries' attempts to stem the brain drain.

However, the hard reality is that, at the global level, there is an insufficient supply of health professionals to meet current service demands. It is this reality that prompted Ethiopia and several other African countries to adopt alternative methods of staffing their health systems. Shorter training, more specialized training, task shifting to lower cadres, etc., are all features of these environments.

This formula seems to be working. Does this suggest that it might be time to change how we staff our health systems in high-income countries? Are some professionals overtrained for the work that they do? Can we afford to continue training health professionals for periods of 5 to 10 years or is this now a luxury we can no longer afford? With increasingly sophisticated technological and medical diagnostic aids, how important is the human element in the process? These questions about health care worker mobility will be debated as health care demand continues to grow.

We have focused on the flow of clinical information, the flow of patients across borders, and the flow of health care workers as three examples of how interconnectedness is playing out in the world of health and health. Turning now to our fourth and final illustration, we describe new policy instruments and management practices that are spreading from country to country.

The Flow of Policy Instruments and Management Practices across Borders

Two key ingredients of an effective health care system are the health policy instruments and the quality of management. Health policy defines a service vision with care priorities and specific goals and targets for society, such as paying for performance and reducing social injustices. Management quality defines the general ability of health managers to coordinate care, uncover low performers, manage inefficient utilization of health services, and adopt best practices (Bradley, Taylor, and Cuellar, 2015; Chilingerian, 2008). To manage effectively, it is essential to understand the connection between care production, the resources used, and the results achieved. But how is this understanding achieved?

To advance the science of medicine and management, the "products" of health care had to be defined, measured, and differentiated. Gradually a consensus emerged in the 1950s and 1960s that the utilization of clinical resources during treatment should be measured on a per-case or episode basis, and that meant every patient illness had to be classified. Health care management came of age with the realization that a meaningful patient classification was needed to enable health care managers to track patterns of resource consumption with respect to episodes of care.

On April 1, 1983, the first patient classification system (PCS) used for paying hospitals for services they provided was adopted by the U.S. Congress. As Kimberly, Pouvourville, and D'Aunno (2008) state, "For the first time a payer—in this case Medicare—had a way of comparing the outputs of one hospital with those of another as a basis for paying hospitals in a standardized, consistent fashion for the 'products' they produced. This system is a policy instrument whose impact on management practices in hospitals and other health care facilities has been profound."

What Is the Policy Instrument in Question?

The patient classification system that was adopted by the U.S. Congress, known as diagnosis-related groups, or DRGs, was developed by a team of researchers at Yale University in the late 1970s. DRGs have been called the single most significant innovation in medical financing and perhaps the most influential health care management research project ever undertaken (Chilingerian, 2008). Worldwide adoption followed in the wake of this American experiment.

The lead researcher, Robert Fetter, was trained as an industrial engineer and brought an industrial engineer's mindset to the analysis of hospital performance—a mindset that placed a premium on standardizing production processes and applying basic cost accounting principles to those processes. If you didn't know how much it cost to produce whatever product(s) you were producing, how could you ever know how to price them in a way that insured that your revenues would exceed your costs? This logic was completely foreign to the world of health care management in a time when hospitals would justify higher costs by asserting that their patients were sicker and therefore cost more to treat. Fetter and his team reasoned that case mix differences from one hospital to the next were important in determining costs. Patients with similar illnesses should incur similar costs for treatment, and if patients were classified correctly by diagnosis (and if the resources necessary to treat them were correctly specified), it would be possible to determine what a treatment cost is and then pay hospitals accordingly. Furthermore, hospitals could be paid prospectively rather than being reimbursed retrospectively on the basis of what they charged. This would lead to significant improvements in efficiency at the hospital level and result in significant cost savings at the national level. Retrospective reimbursement is a payment method where the amount paid depends on the volume and the type and intensity of the services (i.e., lab tests, medications, amount of time in the operating rooms, etc) that the health care organization provided. Prospective payment is a payment method in which the health care organization will know in advance what the payment will be for a procedure or diagnosis, irrespective of the volume or intensity of the services.

The logic underlying the development of DRGs was truly revolutionary at the time, and, once the system was adopted by the U.S. Congress, it forced hospitals to adopt management practices that would allow them to understand their costs; it put incentives in place for hospitals to manage themselves more efficiently than they ever had in the past. They knew in advance what they would be paid for a whole range of procedures. If they were able to deliver a given procedure for less than they would be paid, they would realize a profit; if not, they would experience a loss. The result, it was hoped, would, at the very least, be a slowing of the rate of increase in health costs.

Nearly 40 years later we find that various versions of this system are being used in as many as 37 countries around the globe. We see this as a good illustration of the flow of policy instruments across national borders. Some version of the DRG patient classification system is being used in countries as diverse as Sweden, Hungary, Singapore, Italy, and Japan. This is another indicator of the globalization of health care—similar policy instruments are being adopted by countries in very different parts of the world with very different health systems and are influencing management practice as a consequence. The emergence of online patient communities, patients seeking care across national borders, health professionals finding jobs across national borders, and similar policy instruments being used across national borders are all examples of globalization.

The Drivers of Cross-Border Flow

Why have DRG-based patient classification systems spread so widely around the globe? Perhaps the most obvious reason is that this particular policy instrument is seen at the macro level as having the potential to help countries contain, if not control, the cost of health care—a problem that nearly every country has been facing for decades and that only seems to be growing in significance with the passage of time. Additionally, at the micro or provider level, it encourages investment in capabilities that allow a given provider to understand its cost structure in a more detailed fashion and to make certain operational and investment decisions with a greater degree of managerial sophistication. Finally, it allows clinicians and managers to engage in dialogue around questions of resource consumption and performance in a data-driven, as opposed to a more rhetorical and intuitive, fashion.

While the cost-containing potential of DRG-based patient classification systems may help to explain their spread across national borders, other factors have played and continue to play an important role as well. If we think of the business aspects of health care, and if we consider the kinds of opportunities that lie behind the flow of policy instruments across national borders, we are led to examine how the development and spread of these systems was motivated by market forces and opportunities to benefit as perceived by a variety of interested parties—researchers, policy makers, consultants, and software developers, to name only the most obvious. Individual members in each of these groups saw opportunities for gain, and a few invested time, effort, and, in many cases, money very early in the process to explore the potential further. The research group at Yale, for example, became actively involved in helping to develop awareness of the instrument's potential by holding seminars on campus and in a number of locations around the globe, including France, England,

Australia, and New Zealand. Once the system had been adopted by the federal government in the United States, policy makers were invited to speak about its structure and advantages in other countries. A number of consulting firms began offering advice on the design and implementation of patient classification systems both in the United States and in other countries. 3M began actively marketing the grouper software it had developed to providers and national systems both at home and abroad.

In 1987, as awareness of the instrument and its potential spread across national borders, a group of researchers and policy makers interested in sharing experiences and in defining "best practices" formed PCS Europe, which later, as interest in patient classification systems grew further, became PCS International. The organization they founded played an important role both as a focal point for information about patient classification systems and as a catalyst for further dissemination. It is difficult to determine exactly when, what Malcolm Gladwell (2002) has called a "tipping point" was reached, but the formation and growth of PCS International is a key indicator of the extent to which the DRG-based policy instrument has been adopted globally.

Barriers to Cross-Border Flow

Resources and ideas do not cross national borders seamlessly. A host of possible barriers exists, including regulatory, political, economic, and cultural barriers. As any company doing business in more than one county knows, differences in labor laws, product safety codes, political priorities, economic vibrancy, and underlying values and habits all influence the character and outcomes of multi-country business ventures. One size does not necessarily fit all, and it is always a challenge to balance the advantages of standardization with the need for sensitivity to local customs and preferences. Nowhere is this more true than in health care, where local practices, medical knowledge, and available resources vary widely, not only from one country to the next but also from one region to another within any particular country.

In the case of health workers, one barrier could be the exporting of Western-style medical training to many developing countries. Cuba's "training for context" serves to highlight the potential that can be realized with the removal of such a barrier. In the case of DRG-based patient classification systems, a significant potential barrier is the fact that the original system was developed in the United States. Although the United States is widely recognized as a leader in medical research and education, it is also widely criticized for its lack of universal access to care. It may also be a matter of national pride in some cases to avoid adopting a policy instrument that was developed elsewhere. Known as the "not-invented-here" syndrome, this simply refers to the well-known skepticism about the appropriateness and/or relevance of something not invented at home for the home. The Japanese, for example, might question the relevance for their country of a system developed in a country with different medical practices and different epidemiological characteristics.

In point of fact, different countries have used the system in quite different ways to meet idiosyncratic situations and particular needs (Kimberly, Pouvourville, and D'Aunno, 2008). The flexibility and adaptability of the system have allowed it to be adopted for multiple uses in a variety of contexts. Thus, the potential impact of the NIH syndrome has been mitigated to a certain extent.

The Situation Today

Two conclusions and one lesson can be drawn clearly from the history of cross-border flow of patient classification systems in general and the DRG-based systems in particular. First, the flow has been substantial. The number of countries using some version of the DRG-based system continues to grow and, perhaps most important, the operations management mindset as applied to the management of hospitals and other health care facilities continues to spread and change profoundly the way policy makers and managers think about the intersection of clinical and managerial practice. In this sense, we have seen a globalizing of managerial practice in health care. Second, and just as important, the search for improved instruments, tools, and practices that will help to contain costs in health care continues. The DRG-based PCS may have been the first of its kind to have had a certain degree of global uptake, but it has also spawned a host of initiatives intended to replace it. This pattern is just what we would expect in a robust, globalizing industry that is ripe for innovation.

VI. Additional Considerations

So far, we have made the case that flows of a variety of types across national borders are increasing in the world of health care and health care management, and that these increases indicate that the business of health care is globalizing. To illustrate, we have presented concrete examples of how this process is unfolding: one dealing with online communities, another with the flows of patients across national borders, a third focusing on flows of health workers across national borders, and a fourth describing the spread of a policy instrument across national borders that enables better health care management.

We turn now to three additional considerations. First, the directionality of flows is important. We should not assume that what the developed countries have should flow to the less developed countries nor should we assume that increased flows are necessarily beneficial to all concerned.

As we saw with patient flows, in some cases, wealthy patients from less developed countries seek care in more developed ones, the assumption being that care will be "better" in the latter. But we also see patients from developed countries seeking care in less developed countries because that care is less expensive and is of comparable quality. We also see health workers from less developed countries migrating to more developed countries, a pattern that further exacerbates shortages of qualified health workers in the countries they leave behind and which can hardly be viewed as beneficial to those countries. And yet, if you ask any U.S. health professionals who have worked in a low-income country about their experience, they will invariability refer to it as a life-changing experience and enthuse about how much they have learned. As Immelt, Govindarajan, and Trimble (2009) contend, the developed countries have a lot to learn from others if they will only be open to the possibility. They make the case for what they call "**reverse innovation**," by which they mean that rather than modifying products and services developed in the West for emerging markets, innovation should be sourced in smaller, less developed markets and then introduced in to larger, more developed markets. For example, the innovations in skill mix and task shifting adopted by many African countries may have lessons for the West. This argument turns the generally accepted thought process upside down and encourages us to ask what might be learned about health maintenance, health promotion, health care delivery, and health care management through careful observation and analysis of practices used in less developed settings. The point we are making is simple but not simplistic. Flows are multidirectional, and we must be careful not to overlook unexpected value-creating possibilities.

Second, we should be mindful of how **technological innovation** can change the landscape of health care across national borders. A particularly vivid example is teleradiology, the ability to read and interpret images taken in one place and sent digitally to another. Effectively, this means that the reading and interpretation of radiological images is "borderless," and consequently that it depends only on the expertise of the reader, no matter where he or she may be located. The technology enables virtually instantaneous transmission of the images, making "place" irrelevant. Another example is robotic surgery, a technology that permits a surgeon located in one part of the world to operate on a patient located elsewhere. Again, this technology makes traditional borders irrelevant and hinges primarily on the availability of the technology and the surgical and support capabilities.

And finally, we must remember that that not all cross-border flows in health care are positive. The enhanced frequency and volume of cross-border flows has a dark side as well. We have already discussed the problem that the movement of health workers from less to more developed countries poses for source countries. There are more sinister examples as well. Global trafficking in human organs is a case in point, as are global markets for blood supplies. In both cases, cross-border flows are enabled by a combination of sophisticated communication and logistical technologies, and in both cases, we see systematic exploitation of the underprivileged for the benefit of the wealthier.

CONCLUSION

Health care is global. Online patient communities are sourcing and sharing information across national and regional borders, patients are seeking care outside their home countries, health workers are relocating to new countries, and new policy instruments and management

practices are spreading from country to country. Although health care is still primarily a "local" business—local practice patterns and health-seeking behavior vary considerably, both within and across national borders—there are signs that at least some aspects of the business are becoming more global as awareness of opportunities increases and as enabling technologies to become available.

The challenge is to encourage the spread of those technologies and managerial practices that are welfare-enhancing and to discourage the spread of those that are not. History tells us that this challenge is daunting. Globalization is not, in and of itself, a force for good or a force for evil. Ultimately, the challenge is to maintain equity through a sense of global responsibility, while capitalizing on the potential benefits globalization affords to health care.

SUMMARY AND MANAGERIAL GUIDELINES

1. The fundamental question that must be addressed in examining globalization in any domain, including health care, is how flows of various kinds—both legal and illegal—across national borders have changed.

2. Comparative advantage, when applied to health care, refers to the discovery and deployment of significant differences in a nation's cost, quality, or access such that a medical or surgical procedure, health activity, or service creates patient value. Care program for lung cancer or organ transplantation could become a "power offering" to anyone, anywhere in the world. The difference between inbound and outbound medical tourism can have a significant effect an economy.

3. The rapid growth of the Internet has facilitated the flow of clinical information to patients worldwide trying to manage their health issues. The development of global online patient communities, like PatientsLikeMe (PLM), create value in two fundamental ways. First, they facilitate the development of social networking among patients with particular diseases and diagnoses. The patients get information, emotional support, and relationships with other patients to help them manage their health problems. The second way they create value is by sharing deidentified patient-level data to understand disease progression and palliative treatments. Using patient-generated data, PLM was able to conduct a small observational study that showed that a potential treatment for ALS had no effect on disease progression.

4. Medical tourism may be a "disruptive innovation" that deserves more clinical and managerial attention. Studies predict that in the coming years, patients traveling across country borders for the sole purpose of obtaining acute health services will grow into a multi-billion-dollar global industry. The key factors for global competition will be a provider's clinical reputation, defined in terms of (1) outcomes, (2) technological back-up, and (3) use of the most advanced medical procedures.

5. The number of infant deaths per 1,000 live births is highly associated with degree of local health care infrastructure. In general, countries with high per capita GDP have low infant mortality rates. Health care managers should pay attention to these numbers.

6. Enhancing the patient experience can bring a great return to a hospital. For example, Bumrungrad Hospital in Bangkok, with five-star hotel services and accreditation from the Joint Commission for International Accreditation, receives 37 percent of its patient revenues from international patients from 154 countries. They offer deluxe rooms, VIP and royal suites, laptop computers, a swimming pool, fitness center, and are walking distance to Bangkok's most prestigious restaurants, shopping, and entertainment venues. To attract loyal international patients requires substantial investments in buildings, equipment, service processes, and people who can "delight" patients. There is growing rivalry among nations to attract medical tourists with no guarantee of permanent patient loyalty.

7. The market for international patients has many risks and uncertainties—for example, of air safety, transportation costs, national rivalry for patients, the global economy, national moods, global economics, and politics. The flow of patients abroad depends on perceived value of medical travel in relation to the perceived sacrifices.

8. Africa carries 25 percent of the world's disease burden, yet has only 1.3 percent of the world's health workers. Approximately 37 of the 47 sub-Saharan African countries (SSA) have less than 20 doctors per 100,000 people; the sub-Saharan average was 15.5 physicians for 100,000 people and 73.4 nurses per 100,000 people. In contrast, the average among the Organization for Economic Co-operation and Development (OECD) countries was approximately 311 physicians and 737.5 nurses per 100,000 people in 2002. On average, African countries have about 20 times fewer physicians and 10 times fewer nurses than high-income countries.

9. Countries like Angola, Congo-Brazzaville, and Sierra Leone all experienced civil war in the 1990s and they found that all had lost more than 40 percent of their physicians by 2000. Kenya, Tanzania, and Zimbabwe all experienced decades of economic stagnation in the late twentieth century and, by its end, each had lost more than half of its physicians. Countries with greater stability and prosperity—Botswana, South Africa, and pre-collapse Côte d'Ivoire—managed to retain their doctors.

10. Migrant remittances, defined as the transfer of funds from migrants to relatives or friends in their country of origin, have become an increasingly important feature of modern economic life. Indeed, remittances are now recognized as an important source of global development finance. One report stated that international remittance flows by migrant health workers play a substantial role in alleviating poverty in recipient countries.

11. Countries need to improve their workforce planning and monitoring to assess incentives for retaining their health workers. By developing flexible pay systems, shorter specialist training, and improving human resources and personnel administration systems, countries can change the scale of emigration. Delegation of tasks that would traditionally fall within the scope of practice of doctors or nurse to other health workers who have undergone shorter periods of training is another effective strategy to alleviate health worker shortages.

12. Nonphysician clinicians (NPCs) are trained with less cost than physicians for an average period of three to four years postsecondary school. In sub-Saharan Africa, 25 countries use NPCs, and, in nine of these countries, NPCs equaled or exceeded numbers of physicians. NPCs do basic diagnosis and medical treatment, but some are trained in specialty activities, such as caesarean section, ophthalmology, and anesthesia.

13. Countries that attract health workers may do so for short time periods. Ireland had a critical shortage of nurses and began to recruit hundreds of Filipino nurses to fill gaps in the services. However, the nurses who had been in the country for four to five years and who therefore had gained excellent experience were now moving on to the United States or Canada in search of higher salaries and greater opportunities for skill development. Retaining health workers is as important as recruiting them.

14. DRGs were developed in the United States in the late 1960s. They were adopted in the United States in 1983. In 2010, various versions of this system are being used in at least 36 countries around the globe, and we see this as a good illustration of how the flow of policy instruments across national borders is indicative of "flattening" in the sense Friedman intended. Some version of the diagnosis-related group (DRG) patient classification system is being used in countries as diverse as Sweden, Hungary, Singapore, Italy, and Japan.

15. DRGs have the potential to help countries contain, if not control, the cost of health care. Additionally, DRGs encourage investment in capabilities that allow a given provider to understand its cost structure. Finally, DRGs allow clinicians and managers to engage in dialogue around questions of resource consumption and performance in a data-driven, as opposed to a more rhetorical and intuitive, fashion.

16. Although health care is still primarily a "local" business—local practice patterns and health-seeking behavior vary considerably, both within and across national borders—there are signs that at least some aspects of the business are becoming more global as awareness of opportunities increases and as enabling technologies become available.

DISCUSSION QUESTIONS

1. What factors contribute to the directionality of flows in health care? Patients, health workers, managerial practices?

2. What results has Cleveland Clinic in Abu Dhabi achieved to date and what lessons have been learned about globalizing a health care clinic?

3. What value do online patient communities, like PatientsLikeMe, bring to patients and clinicians?

4. Discuss the implications of the following statement: "We came to believe that quality of care in facilities credentialed by the Joint Commission International (JCI) in foreign countries, and in India in particular, is as good as or better than that in the United States, and offers a 70–80 percent cost differential in many cases."

5. What are the five segments of patients who are willing to travel across borders to obtain health care? Are there other patient segments beside these five that explain why patients are willing to travel to a foreign destination for health care?

6. What explains the global price differential among hospitals? Why would countries like the United States have 4×s the charges for procedures like hip replacements?

7. Why is there growing rivalry for inbound international patients? Under what conditions should a hospital invest in hospitals, clinics, VIP facilities, and special equipment to attract international patients? What are the risks and uncertainties?

8. Cleveland clinic's goal is to bring world-class medical care to the people of the world wherever possible. Is it working? Are they attracting medical tourists?

9. From a medical tourist perspective, compare Shouldice with the traditional hospital in terms of the key factors of competition. Using Table 15.3, why would Shouldice attract patients from outside the local province? Which segment or type of medical travelers would Shouldice attract?

10. What is the scale of the outflow of health workers? What are the financial implications of health worker flows from low- and middle-income countries?

11. With respect to worker flows, what international and national responses have been effective?

12. Is there a "brain drain" in health care? How does it affect countries?

13. The Ethiopian government has a novel approach to addressing the health worker shortage. How might it retain these newly trained professionals and achieve an equitable distribution of health care workers?

14. What lessons does Cuba have for training health professionals? Is training for context one way to address the migration problem?

15. Why is there an insufficient supply of health professionals to meet current service demands? Should higher-income countries follow Ethiopia and adopt shorter training, more specialized training, and task shifting to allied health professionals?

16. How many countries have adopted DRGs? Why? Have DRGs reduced health care costs or improved quality? Are there policy instruments and/or management practices that can reduce the outflow of health workers and related inequity in access to health care?

DEBATE TIME

1. Make a convincing set of arguments in favor of the hypothesis that the world of health care is globalizing. What are the counterarguments?

2. Why are most medical travelers from nearly every continent choosing Asia for their health care? Under what conditions would you consider going to another country to receive health care?

3. When people get transplants abroad, should they expect to get follow-up care in their home country? And should their insurance or governments pay for that follow-up care? More importantly, should governments take a position against the exploitation of organ donors, in particular, taking organs from prisoners or paid living donors?

4. What international agency regulates unproven and/or experimental treatments? Who will ensure that evidence-based methods are used and comparative effectiveness studies are being conducted? Finally, do these providers who serve medical tourists have an institutional review board that oversees its medical ethics?

5. Is health care worker migration a problem or benefit for source countries? For receiving countries? For the workers themselves? Should global entities try to regulate the flow of health care workers across countries? How so?

6. Do you agree that migrant remittances to their homeland make the flow of health workers less of an ethical issue?

7. Should Cuba and/or Ethiopia's model be considered by high-income countries? What are the advantages? Are there any disadvantages?

REFERENCES

Aggarwal, R., & Chick, S. (2017). *PatientsLikeMe: Using social network health data to improve patient care.* Fontainebleau: INSEAD. Case No. 6248.

Alebachew, A., Yusaf, Y., Mann, C., et al. (2015). Ethiopia's progress in health financing and the contribution of the 1998 HCFS in Ethiopia. Resource Tracking and Management Project, Harvard T. H. Chan School of Public Health & Breakthrough International Consultancy PLC, March 2015, Harvard, Boston.

Al-Hammouri, F. (2008). Jordan as medical destination: A spotlight on Middle East. *World Medical Tourism & Global Health Congress*, San Francisco.

Alkire, S., & Chen, L. (2004). "Medical exceptionalism" in international migration: Should doctors and nurses be treated differently?, JLI Working Paper 7-3, Global Health Trust. Retrieved January 26, 2007, from http://www .globalhealthtrust.org/doc/abstracts/WG7/Alkirepaper.pdf.

Alsagoff, F. (2005). Singapore General Hospital: On local shores and beyond. Unpublished master's thesis. INSEAD, Fontainebleau, France.

Anderson, D. H. A., Modrow, R. E., & Tan, J. K. H. (1992). Surgical waiting lists: Definition, desired characteristics, and uses. *Healthcare Management FORUM, 5*(2), 17–22.

Bach, S. (2003). International migration of health workers: Labour and social issues. Sectoral Activities Programme, Working Paper. Geneva: International Labour Office.

Bach, S. (2004). Migration patterns of physicians and nurses: Still the same story? *Bulletin of the World Health Organisation, 82*(8), 624–625.

Barua, B., & Ren, F. (2016). *Waiting your turn.* Retrieved December 2016 from Fraser Institute website: https://www.fraserinstitute.org/studies /waiting-your-turn-wait-times-for-health-care-in-canada-2016.

Beecham, L. (2002). British patients willing to travel abroad for treatment. *British Medical Journal, 325*, 10.

Benveniste, I. (2008). High quality of care available in the Middle East: Is developing countries' trend for getting treatment in the USA now reversed? Medical Tourism Association Conference. Acibadem Healthcare Group, Turkey.

Biksegn, A., Kenfe, T., Matiwos, S., et al. (2016, March). Burnout status at work among health care professionals in a tertiary hospital. *Ethiopian Journal of Health Science, 26*(2), 101–108.

Bowser, D., Bigiimana, N., Patton-Bolman, C., et al. (2016, March). *Health system strengthening for cardiovascular disease in Rwanda.* Unpublished Report, Brandeis University, MA.

Bradby, H. (2014). International medical migration: A critical conceptual review of the global movements of doctors and nurses. *Health, 18*(6), 580–596. doi:10.1177/1363459314524803.

Bradley, E. H., Taylor, L. A., & Cuellar, C. J. (2015). Management matters: A leverage point for health systems strengthening in global health. *International Journal of Health Policy and Management, 4*(7), 411–415.

Buchan J., & Perfilieva, G. (2006). *Health worker migration in the European region: Country case studies and policy implications.* Copenhagen: WHO Regional Office for Europe.

Castro-Palaganas, E., Spitzer, D. L., Midea, M., et al. (2017). An examination of the causes, consequences, and policy responses to the migration of highly trained health personnel from the Philippines: The high cost of living/leaving—a mixed method study. *Human Resources for Health, 15*, 25. doi:10.1186/s12960-017-0198-z.

Chen, L., Evans, T., Anand, S., et al. (2004) Human resources for health: Overcoming the crisis. *Lancet, 364*, 1984–1990.

Chen, L. C., & Boufford, J. I. (2005). Fatal flows—doctors on the move. *New England Journal of Medicine, 353*, 1850–1852.

Chen, L. H., & Wilson, M. E. (2013). The globalization of healthcare: Implications of medical tourism for the infectious disease clinician. *Clinical Infectious Diseases: An Official Publication of the Infectious Diseases Society of America, 57*(12), 1752. doi:10.1093/cid/cit540.

Chen, P. G., Auerbach, D. I., Muench, U., et al. (2013). Policy Solutions To Address The Foreign-Educated And Foreign-Born Health Care Workforce In The United States, HEALTH AFFAIRSVOL. 32, NO. 11: REDESIGNING THE HEALTH CARE WORKFORCE. Accessed on July 3, 2017, https://doi. org/10.1377/hlthaff.2013.0576

Chilingerian, J. (2008). Origins of DRGS in the United States: A technical, political and cultural story. In J. Kimberly, G. de Pouvourville, & T. D'Auno (Eds.), *The globalization of managerial innovation* (pp. 1–33). Cambridge: Cambridge University Press

Chilingerian, J. A. (2004). Who has star quality? In R. E. Herzlinger (Ed.), *Consumer-driven health care: Implications for providers, payers, and policy-makers* (pp. 443–453). San Francisco, CA: Jossey-Bass.

Chilingerian, J. A., & Savage, G. T. (2005). The emerging field of international health care management. In G. T. Savage, J. A. Chilingerian, & M. Powell (Eds.), *Advances in health care management* (Vol. 5). Boston, MA: Elsevier JAI.

Chilopora, G., Pereira, C., Kamwendo, F., et al. (2007). Postoperative outcome of caesarean sections and other major emergency obstetric surgery by clinical officers and medical officers in Malawi. *Human Resources for Health, 5*, 17.

Clemens, M. A. & Pettersson, G. (2007). New data on African health professionals abroad. Working Paper Number 95, Centre for Global Development, February.

Cleveland Clinic Abu Dhabi to be operational in 2011. (2008). *Arab Health Online*, April 20.

Cohen, G. I. (2013). Introduction. In I. G. Cohen (Ed.), *The globalization of healthcare*. New York: Oxford University Press.

Cohen, G. I. (2015). *Patients with passports: Medical tourism, law and ethics*. New York: Oxford University Press.

Comarow, A. (2008). Saving on surgery by going abroad. *U.S. News & World Report*, May 1 (pp. 42–50). *USNews.com*, September 16. Retrieved October 10, 2009, from http://health.usnews.com/articles/health/special-reports/2008/05/01/saving-on-surgery-by-going-abroad.html.

Commission for Africa. (2005). Our common interest. Retrieved July 4, 2017, from http://www.commissionforafrica.info/wp-content/uploads/2005-report/11-03-05_cr_report.pdf.

Cooper, R. A., Laud, P., & Dietrich, C. L. (1998). Current and projected workforce of non-physician clinicians. *Journal of American Medical Association, 280*, 788–794.

Cortez, N. (2008). Patients without borders: The emerging global market for patients and the evolution of modern health care. *Indiana Law Journal, 83*(71), 71–132.

Cosgrove, T. (2014). The *Cleveland way*. New York: McGraw Hill Education.

Cote, J. (2014). *HealthCare Elsewhere: Inspiring medical tourism stories*. Huntsville: Vipernet, Inc.

Crisp, N., & Chen, L. (2014). Global supply of health professionals. *New England Journal of Medicine, 370*, 950–957. doi:10.1056/NEJMra1111610.

Crooks, V. A., Turner, L., Snyder, J., et al. (2011). Promoting medical tourism to India: Messages, images, and the marketing of international patient travel. *Social Science & Medicine, 72*(5), 726–732. doi: http://dx.doi.org/10.1016/j.socscimed.2010.12.022.

Delmonico, F. L. (2009, February). The hazards of transplant tourism. *Clinical Journal of American Society of Nephrology, 4*(2), 249–250.

Department for International Development. (July 27, 2006). *BME remittance survey—research report*, UK.

Douglas, D. E. (2007). Is medical tourism the answer? *Frontiers of Health Services Management, 24*(2), 35–40.

Dovlo, D., & Martineau, T, (2004). A review of the migration of Africa's health professionals. A Joint Learning Initiative: Human Resources for Health and Development Working Paper.

Dovlo, D., Sagoe, K., Ntow, S., et al. (1998). Ghana case study: Staff performance management. In *Reforming health systems* (research report). Retrieved February 17, 2006, from http://www.liv.ac.uk/lstm/research/documents/ghana.pdf.

Ehrbeck, T., Guevara, C., & Mango, P. D. (2008). Mapping the market for medical travel. *McKinsey & Company Quarterly Report*. McKinsey & Company.

Erhart, M. (2008, February 10). Unpublished interview with Jon Chilingerian. Abu Dhabi, UAE.

Erwin P. C., & Bialek, R. (2015, August). A matter of perspective: Seeing Cuban and United States health systems through a cultural lens. *American Journal of Public Health, 105*(8), 1509–1511.

European Commission. (2010). An agenda for new skills and jobs: A European contribution towards full employment. COM, 682 final.

Fares, Z. (2009, February 13). Unpublished interview with Jon Chilingerian. Abu Dhabi, UAE.

Fleni. (2008). Fundacion de Lucha contra las Enfermedadaes Neurologicas de la Infancia. World Medical Tourism & Global Health Congress. San Francisco.

Francis, T. (2008). Medical tourism is still small. Getting care abroad may be less usual than once thought. May 8, 2008. *Wall Street Journal Online.* Retrieved October 10, 2009, from http://online.wsj.com/public/article_print/SB121004330575669909.html.

Friedman, T. (2005). *The world is flat: A brief history of the twenty first century*. New York: Farrar, Straus and Giroux.

Frank, M., & Reed, G. (2008) Doctors for the (developing) world, training physicians for global health. *MEDICC Review*. Retrieved July 5, 2017, from www.medicc.org/publications/medicc_review/0805/spotlight.html

Fried, B. J., & Harris, D. M. (2007). Managing healthcare services in the global marketplace. *Frontiers of Health Services Management, 24*(2), 3–17.

Ghemawat, P. (2007). Businesses beware: The world is not flat. Interview, Harvard Business School Working Knowledge, October 15.

Ghemawat, P. (February 2017). Even with digitalization, globalization is not inevitable. *Harvard Business Review*. Retrieved March 10, 2017, from https://hbr.org/2017/02/even-in-a-digital-world-globalization-is-not-inevitable.

Gladwell, M. (2002). *The tipping point: How little things can make a big difference*. New York: Little, Brown & Company.

Glassow, F. (1973). The surgical repair of inguinal and femoral hernias. *Canadian Medical Association Journal, 108*(3), 308–313.

Glassow, F. (1986, July–September). The Shouldice Hospital technique. *International Surgery, 71*(3), 148–153.

Haines A., Sanders D., Lehmann U., et al. (2007). Achieving child survival goals: Potential contribution of community health workers. *Lancet, 369*, 2121-2131

Heyman, J. (2008). AMA perspective on globalization. World Medical Toursim & Global Health Congress. San Francisco.

Immelt, J., Govindarajan, V., & Trimble, C. (2009). How GE is disrupting itself. *Harvard Business Review*. October.

Kapur D., & McHale J. (2005a). Policy options. In *Give us your best and brightest: The global hunt for talent and its impact on the developing world*. Washington, DC: Center for Global Development.

Kapur, D., & McHale, J. (2005b) The global migration of talent: What does it mean for developing countries? Centre for Global Development Brief. Retrieved August 6, 2010, from www.cgdev.org.

Keckley, P. H., & Underwood, H. R. (2008). *Medical tourism: Consumers in search of value*. Washington, DC: Deloitte Center for Health Solutions.

Keckley, P. H., & Underwood, H. R. (2009). *Medical tourism: An update*. Washington, DC: Deloitte Center for Health Solutions.

Khamisa N., Peltzer, K., & Oldenburg, B. (2013, June). Burnout in relation to specific contributing factors and health outcomes among nurses: A systematic review. *International Journal of Environmental Research and Public Health, 10*(6), 2214–2240. doi:10.3390/ijerph10062214.

Kim, W. C., & Mauborgne, R. (2015). *Blue ocean strategy: How to create uncontested market space and make the competition irrelevant*. Boston, MA: Harvard Business Review Press.

Kim, J. Y., Farmer, P., & Porter, M. E. (2013, September). Re-defining global health delivery. *The Lancet, 382*(9897), 21–27; 1060–1069

Kimberly, J. R., Pouvourville, G., & D'Aunno, T. (2008). *The globalization of managerial innovation in health care*. London: Cambridge University Press.

Kruk, M. E., Pereira, C., Vaz, F., et al. (2007). Economic evaluation of surgically trained assistant medical officers in performing major obstetric surgery in Mozambique. *BJOG, 114*, 1253–1260.

Labonte, R., Packer, C. & Klassen, N. (2006). Managing health professional migration from sub-Saharan Africa to Canada: A stakeholder inquiry into policy options. *Human Resources for Health, 4*, 22.

Landers, S. J. (2002). Heightened security keeping international patients away: U.S. hospitals with substantial international programs see a decline in revenue; doctors see a boost in telemedicine consults. Retrieved March 20, 2005, from http://www.ama-assn.org/amednews/2002/09/16/hlsc0916.htm.

Lehman, U. (2008). Mid-level health workers: The state of the evidence on programmes, activities, costs and impact on health outcomes, a literature review. World Health Organization, Department of Human Resources for Health. Geneva, July 2008.

Liese, B., Blanchet, N., & Dussault. G. (September 15, 2003). The human resource crisis in health services in sub-Saharan Africa. The World Bank. Retrieved July 4, 2017, from http://documents.worldbank.org/curated/en/146661468767966818/310436360_20050276022409/additional/269620The0Human0Resource0Crisis.pdf.

Lowell, B. L., & Findlay, A. M. (2001). Migration of highly skilled persons from developing countries: Impact and policy responses. Synthesis Report, International Labor Office, Geneva.

Madede, T., Sidat, M., McAuliffe, E., et al. (2017). The impact of a supportive supervision intervention on health workers in Niassa, Mozambique: A cluster-controlled trial. Human Resources for Health HRHE-D-16-00101R1.

Marquez, M. (2009). Health-workforce development in the Cuban health system. *The Lancet, 374*(9701), 1574–1575.

Martikainen, T. (2016). Personal communication, January 9.

Martin, P., Abella, M., & Kuptsch, C. (2006). *Managing labor migration in the twenty-first century*. New Haven, CT: Yale University Press.

Matejowsky, T. S. (2006). Overseas contract labor, remittances, and household consumption: A case study from San Fernando City, the Philippines. *Research in Economic Anthropology, 24*, 11–36.

McAuliffe, E., Manafa, O., Maseko, F., et al. (2009). Understanding job satisfaction amongst mid-level cadres in Malawi: The contribution of organisational justice. *Reproductive Health Matters, 17*(33), 80–90.

McAuliffe, E., Manafa, O., Bowie, C., et al. (2010). Managing and motivating: Pragmatic solutions to the brain drain. In S. Kebane (ed.), *Human resources in healthcare, health informatics and health systems*. Hersey, PA: IGI Global.

McAuliffe, E., Galligan, M., Revill, P., et al. (2016). Factors influencing job preferences of health workers providing obstetric care: Results from discrete choice experiments in Malawi, Mozambique and Tanzania. *Globalization and Health, 12*(86), 1–19.

McKinsey Global Institute. (2016, March). Digital globalization: The new era of global flows. Retrieved March 16, 2017, from https://www.mckinsey.com/business-functions/digital-mckinsey/our-insights/digital-globalization-the-new-era-of-global-flows.

Mullan, F., & Frehywot, S. (2007). Non-physician clinicians in 47 African countries. *Lancet, 370*, 2158–2163.

Odell, A. (2000, October). Unpublished interview with Jon Chilingerian. Harvard Business School, Cambridge, MA.

OECD. (2002). GATS: The case for open services markets. Paris.

OECD Health Data. (2016, October). 2014 figures. Paris: Organisation for Economic Co-operation and Development.

Ohmae, K. (1990). *The borderless world: Power and strategy in the interlinked economy*. New York: Harper Collins.

Okwaraji, F. E. & Aguwa, E. N. (2014, March). Burnout and psychological distress among nurses in a Nigerian tertiary health institution. *African Health Sciences, 14*(1), 237–245. doi: 10.4314/ahs.v14i1.37.

Oxford Policy Management. (2002). External evaluation of the National Programme for Family Planning and Primary Health Care: Quantitative survey report. Lady Health Workers Programme, Pakistan. Oxford, England: PatientsLikeMe. Retrieved from https://www.patientslikeme.com/.

Pang, T, Lansang, M. A., & Haines, A. (2002). Brain drain and Health professionals. *BMJ, 324*, 499–500.

Pereira C., Cumbi, A., Malalane, R., et al. (2007). Meeting the need for emergency obstetric care in Mozambique: Work performance and histories of medical doctors and assistant medical officers trained for surgery. *BJOG, 114*(12), 530–1533.

Porter, M. (1987). Changing patterns of international competition. In D. J. Teece (Ed.), *The competitive challenge*. Cambridge: Ballinger Publishing Company.

Pritchett, L. (2006). Let their people come. Washington, DC: Center for Global Development.

Rifkin, J. (2015). *The zero marginal cost society*. New York: Palgrave Macmillan.

Roy, C. W., & Hunter, J. (1996). What happens to patients awaiting arthritis surgery? *Disability and Rehabilitation, 18*(2), 101–105.

Sanders, D., & Lloyd, B. (2005). South African health review 2005. In P. Ijumba & P. Barron (Eds.), *Human resources:*

*International context (pp. 76–87). Durban (South Africa): Health Systems Trust.

Schiano, T. D., & Rhodes, R. (2010). The dilemma and reality of transplant tourism: An ethical perspective for liver transplant programs. *Liver Transplantation, 16*, 113–117.

Schroth, L., & Khawaja, R. (2007). Globalization of healthcare. *Frontiers of Health Services Management, 24*(2), 19–30.

Troy, P., Wyness, L., & McAuliffe, E. (2007). Nurses' experiences of recruitment and migration from developing countries: A phenomenological approach. *Human Resources for Health, 5*,15.

Urquhart, D. J. B., & O'Dell, A. (2004). A model of focused health care delivery. In R. E. Herzlinger (Ed.), *Consumer-driven health care: Implications for providers, payers, and policy-makers* (pp. 627–634). San Francisco, CA: Jossey-Bass.

Vastag, B. (2008). Unproven treatments. U.S. News & World Report. May 1, 2008. *USNews.com*. September 16, 2008, p. 50. Retrieved October 10, 2009, from https://www.ncbi.nlm.nih.gov/pubmed/18655696 US News World Rep. 2008 May 12;*144*(13):50.

Vujicic, M., Zurn, P., Diallo, K., et al. (2004). The role of wages in slowing the migration of health care professionals from developing countries. Department of Health Services Provision, World Health Organization, Geneva, Switzerland.

Wicks, P., Vaughan, T. E., Massagli, M. P., et al. (2011) Accelerated clinical discovery using self-reported patient data collected online and a patient-matching algorithm. *Nature Biotechnology, 29*, 411–414. doi:10.1038/nbt.1837.

Williams, J. I., Llewellyn, T. H., Arshinoff, R., et al. (1997). The burden of waiting for hip and knee replacements in Ontario. *Journal of Evaluation in Clinical Practice, 3*(1), 59–68.

Woodman, J. (2015). *Patients without borders: Everybody's guide to affordable world-class medical travel* (3rd ed.). Chapel Hill, NJ: Health Travel Media.

Woodman Medical Tourism Association (2017). Retrieved on July 6, 2017, from http://www.medicaltourismassociation.com/en/index.html.

World Bank. (2017). Health expenditure per capita (PPP). Retrieved June 26, 2017, from www.data.worldbank.org.

World Health Organisation. (1996). Strengthening nursing and midwifery: Progress and future directions, 1996–2000. Geneva, WHO.

World Health Organisation. (2006). *Working together for health*. World Health Report 2006, Geneva, WHO.

World Health Organisation. (2010). The WHO global code of practice on the international recruitment of health personnel http://www.who.int/hrh/migration/code/WHO_global_code_of_practice_EN.pdf.

APPENDIX
Global Health Architecture

The global health landscape is a complex array of actors and policy makers. A large and ever-expanding number of organizations and partnerships contribute toward the common goal of improving health for all. We will briefly outline the functions of the more established and recognized of these in relation to global health. Such international health organizations are usually divided into three groups: multilateral organizations, bilateral organizations, and nongovernmental organizations (NGOs). The term "multilateral" means that funding comes from multiple governments (as well as from nongovernmental sources) and is distributed to many different countries. The major multilateral organizations are all part of the United Nations (UN). The UN came into being in 1945, following the devastation of World War II, with one central mission: the maintenance of international peace and security. It has 193 member states. A key purpose or guiding principle of the UN is the promotion and protection of human rights. One of the purposes of the UN, as stated in its Charter, is "to achieve international co-operation in solving international problems of an economic, social, cultural, or humanitarian character." Improving people's well-being continues to be one of the main focuses of the UN. The global understanding of development has changed over the years, and countries now have agreed that sustainable development—development that promotes prosperity and economic opportunity, greater social well-being, and protection of the environment—offers the best approach to improving the lives of the world's population. The World Health Organization (WHO) is the primary international health organization. Technically it is an "intergovernmental agency related to the United Nations." WHO and other such intergovernmental agencies are separate, autonomous organizations that, by special agreements, work with the UN and each other through the coordinating machinery of the Economic and Social Council. WHO has three main divisions. The governing body, the World Health Assembly, meets once a year to approve the budget and decide on major matters of health policy. All the 190 or so member nations send delegations. The main function of WHO is directing and coordinating international health activities and supplying technical assistance to countries. It develops norms and standards, disseminates health information, promotes research, provides training in international health, collects and analyzes epidemiologic data, and develops systems for monitoring and evaluating health programs. The Pan American Health Organization (PAHO) serves as the regional field office for WHO in the Americas. The World Bank is the other major intergovernmental agency that plays a key role in global health. The World Bank loans money to poor countries on advantageous terms not available in commercial markets.

Three subsidiary agencies of the UN Economic and Social Council are heavily committed to international health programs. The United Nations Children's Fund (UNICEF) spends the majority of its program budget on health care. UNICEF's work focused on the world's most vulnerable children, devoting most of its resources to the poorest countries and to children under five years old. In 1994, UNICEF received about $1 billion in contributions, all voluntary—70 percent from governments and 30 percent from private sources. The U.S. government is the largest single donor to UNICEF. The United Nations Population Fund (UNFPA) supports reproductive health care for women and youth in more than 150 countries and aims to achieve "a world where every pregnancy is wanted, every childbirth is safe and every young person's potential is fulfilled." The United Nations Development Programme (UNDP) contributes a sizable portion of its budget to health and focuses primarily on HIV/AIDS, maternal and child nutrition, and maternal mortality. In conjunction with WHO and the World Bank, it sponsors the Special Programme for Research and Training in Tropical Diseases (TDR).

Bilateral Agencies

Bilateral agencies are governmental agencies in a single country, which provide aid to low- and middle-income countries. The largest of these is the United States Agency for International Development (USAID). Most industrialized nations have a similar governmental agency. Many of these agencies prioritize particular countries or causes, based on political and historical reasons ranging from former colonies to religious order ties, but some prioritize on grounds of greatest need or high mortality and morbidity rates. USAID channels most of this aid through "cooperating agencies"—private international health agencies that contract with USAID.

Nongovernmental Organizations

Nongovernmental organizations (NGOs) play an important role in the delivery of health care services in many low- and middle-income countries. Most of these organizations are small- or medium-sized operations involved in the direct provision of care through hospitals and clinics and often filling the gaps that are left by inadequate or patchy government provision of health care. One of the major challenges for governments is influencing what or how these organizations provide in terms of health care. In many countries, they operate independently of the government health infrastructure and follow procedures and guidelines set by their parent organizations, with no obligation to comply with the national guidelines of the country they are operating in. Recently, there has been a more concerted attempt by some countries to implement guidelines for NGO activities, as their noncompliance with national salary scales for health professionals has resulted in may health care professionals moving from government-run health facilities to better remunerated posts in NGO-run clinics.

Philanthropic Organizations and Foundations

Philanthropy has always provided some funding for health care through wealthy individuals' and corporations' desire to help the less fortunate in poorer countries. As international rich lists have expanded and the asset portfolios of the richest have increased and diversified, so too have the size and scale of philanthropic organizations. One of the most prominent examples in the health care landscape is the Bill and Melinda Gates Foundation. It has contributed approximately $40 billion since its inception both in the United States and to over 100 countries worldwide, much of it targeted toward improving health. In addition to the substantial financial and personal contribution of Bill and Melinda Gates, the foundation has also benefited from Warren Buffett (a U.S. multibillionaire) who pledged most of his fortune to the Gates Foundation in 2006 allowing it to expand in size and scope. It currently employs over 1,400 people. The Clinton Health Access Initiative (CHAI) is a similarly large organization with 1,500 employees focused mainly on improving the lives of those living with HIV/AIDS but more recently partnering with the American Cancer Society and pharmaceutical companies to provide access to life-saving cancer treatments for people in poorer countries.

Humanitarian Assistance and Health

In addition to the range of agencies described above, there are a multitude of international, national, and local governmental and nongovernmental organizations working to provide disaster relief and humanitarian aid to refugees and other populations in crisis due to natural and man-made disasters, for example, floods, drought, war, etc. Many of these agencies play a strong role in the provision of health care. Two examples are the International Red Cross and Red Crescent Movement (ICRC) and Medicine Sans Frontiers (MSF). ICRC is the largest and most prestigious of the world's humanitarian NGOs, founded in 1863 and mandated by the Geneva Conventions to protect and assist prisoners of war and civilians in international armed conflicts. Its functions include setting up surgical hospitals or providing expatriate teams to work in existing hospitals; providing other types of medical assistance and relief, especially rehabilitation of war-disabled patients; development and dissemination of educational materials concerning health care of prisoners and victims of war. MSF provides health aid to victims of war and natural disasters. In addition to aiding in acute disasters, MSF also provides aid in "chronic emergencies" (e.g., Somalia, Sudan), is involved in several long-term health projects, and publishes a series of field manuals/texts on disaster medicine.

Global Health Policy

At the Millennium Summit in September 2000, the largest gathering of world leaders in history adopted the UN Millennium Declaration, committing their nations to a new global partnership to reduce extreme poverty and setting out a series of targets, with a deadline of 2015, that became known as the Millennium Development Goals.

The Millennium Development Goals (MDGs) served as the world's time-bound and quantified targets for addressing extreme poverty in its many dimensions—income, poverty, hunger, disease, lack of adequate shelter, and exclusion—while promoting gender equality, education, and environmental sustainability.

For 15 years, the MDGs drove progress in reducing poverty, providing much needed access to water and sanitation, driving down child mortality, and drastically improving maternal health. They also spawned a global movement for free primary education, inspiring countries to invest in their future generations. Most significantly, the MDGs made huge strides in combating HIV/AIDS and other treatable diseases, such as malaria and tuberculosis. UNDP list the following as the key achievements of the MDGs:

- More than 1 billion people have been lifted out of extreme poverty (since 1990).
- Child mortality dropped by more than half (since 1990).
- The number of out-of-school children has dropped by more than half (since 1990).
- HIV/AIDS infections fell by almost 40 percent (since 2000).

Significant strides have been made in increasing life expectancy and reducing some of the common killers associated with child and maternal mortality, and major progress has been made on increasing access to clean water and sanitation, reducing malaria, tuberculosis, polio, and the spread of HIV/AIDS. However, only half of women in developing countries have received the health care they need, and the need for family planning is increasing exponentially, with more than 225 million women having an unmet need for contraception.

The Sustainable Development Goals (SDGs) were born at the United Nations Conference on Sustainable Development in Rio de Janeiro in 2012. The objective was to produce a set of universal goals that meet the urgent environmental, political, and economic challenges facing our world.

The SDGs, also termed the Global Goals, replace the Millennium Development Goals (MDGs). The SDGs, officially known as "Transforming Our World: The 2030 Agenda for Sustainable Development," are a set of 17 "Global Goals" with 169 targets covering a broad range of sustainable development issues. Goal Number 3 is Good Health and Well-being Table 15.4 sets out the detailed elements of Goal 3, which will provide the health agenda up to 2030.

Goal 3: Good Health and Well-Being
Good Health and Well-Being—Ensure healthy lives and promote well-being for all at all ages

Global Health Delivery Systems

The funding mechanisms and delivery models for health services provision vary substantially across countries. Comprehensive coverage to address the population health needs is an elusive goal that many countries are far from reaching. Even in the most advanced countries' health systems, there are pockets on inequity and gaps in provision. The myriad of actors involved in global health delivery makes for a highly fragmented system characterized by inequities, duplication, and inefficiencies and problems in accessibility, availability, and quality. Kim, Farmer, and Porter (2013) writing in the *Lancet*, highlight the consequences of fragmented delivery: "The current, fragmented approach is costing us dearly in terms of duplication, inefficiency, poor use of human resources, and high procurement costs. It is costing patients most of all: they are dying of preventable diseases and suffering without therapies readily available elsewhere" (2013, p. 1061). They argue for a more strategic approach to global health delivery and stress the importance of knowledge sharing and learning across actors and settings. They suggest the need for clearinghouse for information about program design, best practices, lessons learned, synergies, policy constraints, environmental determinants, and other elements of global health care delivery.

Table 15.4 Time-Bound Targets for Goal 3

- By 2030, reduce the global maternal mortality ratio to less than 70 per 100,000 live births
- By 2030, end preventable deaths of newborns and children under 5 years of age, with all countries aiming to reduce neonatal mortality to at least as low as 12 per 1,000 live births and under-5 mortality to at least as low as 25 per 1,000 live births
- By 2030, end the epidemics of AIDS, tuberculosis, malaria and neglected tropical diseases and combat hepatitis, water-borne diseases and other communicable diseases
- By 2030, reduce by one third premature mortality from non-communicable diseases through prevention and treatment and promote mental health and well-being
- Strengthen the prevention and treatment of substance abuse, including narcotic drug abuse and harmful use of alcohol
- By 2020, halve the number of global deaths and injuries from road traffic accidents 3.7
- By 2030, ensure universal access to sexual and reproductive health-care services, including for family planning, information and education, and the integration of reproductive health into national strategies and programmes
- Achieve universal health coverage, including financial risk protection, access to quality essential health-care services and access to safe, effective, quality and affordable essential medicines and vaccines for all
- By 2030, substantially reduce the number of deaths and illnesses from hazardous chemicals and air, water and soil pollution and contamination
- Strengthen the implementation of the World Health Organization Framework Convention on Tobacco Control in all countries, as appropriate
- Support the research and development of vaccines and medicines for the communicable and noncommunicable diseases that primarily affect developing countries, provide access to affordable essential medicines and vaccines, in accordance with the Doha Declaration on the TRIPS Agreement and Public Health, which affirms the right of developing countries to use to the full the provisions in the Agreement on Trade Related Aspects of Intellectual Property Rights regarding flexibilities to protect public health, and, in particular, provide access to medicines for all
- Substantially increase health financing and the recruitment, development, training and retention of the health workforce in developing countries, especially in least developed countries and small island developing States
- Strengthen the capacity of all countries, in particular developing countries, for early warning, risk reduction and management of national and global health risks

SOURCE: www.globalgoals.org.

The push for better integration of health services delivery can also be seen in the policy prominence afforded to health system strengthening in donor governments and recipient country governments over the past decade. Health Systems Global is an international membership organization that was established in 2012 to convene researchers, policy makers, and implementers from around the world to develop the field of health systems research and use their collective capacity to create, share, and apply knowledge to strengthen health systems.

Appendix

Acronyms

ACF	Agency for Children and Families	CIO	Chief information officer
ACHE	American College of Healthcare Executives	CITI	Collaborative Institutional Training Initiative
ACO	Accountable care organization		
ACTION	Accelerating Change in Transforming Networks	CMS	Centers for Medicare and Medicaid Services
AFDC	Aid to Families with Dependent Children	COGME	Committee on Graduate Medical Education
AHA	American Hospital Association		
AHIP	America's Health Insurance Plans	CON	Certificate of need
AHRQ	Agency for Healthcare Research and Quality	COO	Chief operating officer
		COSTAR	Computer stored ambulatory record
AIDET	Acknowledge, Introduce, Duration, Explanation, Thank You	CPOE	Computerized physician order entry
		CPR	Computer-based patient records
AIDS	Acquired immune deficiency syndrome	CQI	Continuous quality improvement
AKS	Anti-Kickback Statute	CRM	Crew resource management
AMA	American Medical Association	CSHSC	Center for Studying Health System Change
ANA	American Nursing Association	DHCP	Decentralized hospital computer system
AoA	Administration on Aging	DMAIC	Define, Measure, Analyze, Improve, Control
ARRA	American Recovery and Reinvestment Act		
ART	Antiretroviral therapy	DO	Doctor of osteopathy
ASQ	American Society for Quality	DOJ	Department of Justice
ATSDR	Agency for Toxic Substances and Disease Registry	DOL	Department of Labor
		DRAM	Dynamic random access memory
BATNA	Best Alternative to a Negotiated Agreement	DRG	Diagnosis-related group
		DTC	Direct-to-consumer advertising
BCG	Boston Consulting Group	EHR	Electronic health record
BIDMC	Beth Israel Deaconess Medical Center	EI	Emotional intelligence
BPR	Business process reengineering	EMR	Electronic medical record
CAHME	Commission on the Accreditation of Healthcare Management	EMTALA	Emergency Medical Treatment and Labor Act
CAM	Complementary and alternative medicine	EPHTI	Ethiopia Public Health Training Initiative
CBO	Congressional Budget Office	ERISA	Employee Retirement Income Security Act
CCAD	Cleveland Clinic Abu Dhabi	FCA	False Claims Act
CCC	Convenient care clinic	FDA	Food and Drug Administration
CCCA	Convenient Care Clinic Association	FSA	Flexible spending accounts
CCR	Continuity of care	FTC	Federal Trade Commission
CDC	Centers for Disease Control and Prevention	GAO	Government Accountability Office (formerly General Accounting Office)
CDHP	Consumer-directed health plan		
CEO	Chief executive officer	GATS	General Agreement on Trade in Services
CER	Comparative clinical effectiveness research	GAVI	Global Alliance for Vaccines and Immunization
CFO	Chief financial officer	GDP	Gross domestic product
CHCS	Composite health care system	GE	General Electric
CHIP	Children's Health Insurance Program	GHWA	Global Health Workforce Alliance
CHP	Comprehensive health program	GPO	Group Purchasing Organization
CIA	Corporate integrity agreement	HCA	Hospital Corporation of America

HCO	Health care organization	MSA	Medical savings account
HCQIA	Health Care Quality Improvement Act	MSO	Management services organization
HDHP	High-deductible health plan	NCHL	National Center for Healthcare Leadership
HELP	Health, Education, Labor, and Pensions Committee (U.S. Senate)	NCI	National Cancer Institute
HELP	Health Evaluation through Logical Processing	NCQA	National Committee for Quality Assurance
		NCSL	National Conference of State Legislatures
HEWs	Health extension workers	NEJM	New England Journal of Medicine
HHS	Department of Health and Human Services	NHE	National health expenditures
HIE	Health information exchange	NHS	National Health Service
HIMSS	Health Information and Management Systems Society	NIH	National Institutes of Health
		NIHS	Not-invented-here syndrome
HIPAA	Health Insurance Portability and Accountability Act	NPCs	Non-physician clinicians
		NPDB	National Practitioner Data Bank
HIT	Health information technology	NQF	National Quality Forum
HIV	Human immunodeficiency virus	NRH	Norman Regional Hospital
HLA	Health Leadership Alliance	OHRP	Office for Human Research Protections
HMO	Health maintenance organization	OIG	Office of the Inspector General
HPR	Hospital-physician relationships	P4P	Pay-for-performance
HPWP	High-performance work practices	PA	Physician's assistant
HR	Human resources	PBRN	Provider base research network
HRA	Health Reimbursement Accounts	PCS	Patient classification system
HRO	High-reliability organization	PDA	Personal Digital Assistant
HRSA	Health Resources and Services Administration	PHI	Protected health information
		PHO	Physician-hospital organization
HSA	Health Savings Account	PHQID	Premier Hospital Quality Incentive Demonstration
IBM	International Business Machines		
ICU	Intensive care unit	PHR	Personal health record
IDN	Integrated delivery network	PPO	Preferred Provider Organization
IDS	Integrated delivery system	PPP	Public-private partnership
IHS	Indian Health Service	PPS	Prospective Payment System
IOM	Institute of Medicine	ProPAC	Prospective Payment Assessment Commission
IOR	Interorganizational relationship		
IPA	Independent Practitioner Association	PSQIA	Patient Safety and Privacy Act
IPP	Implementation policies and practices	PVC	Preventative Services Chart
IRB	Institutional Review Board	QI	Quality improvement
IRS	Internal Revenue Service	QIO	Quality Improvement Organization
IS	Information systems	QM	Quality management
ISM	Integrated salary model	QUERI	Quality Enhancement Research Initiative
IT	Information technology	R&D	Research and development
JAMA	Journal of the American Medical Association	RAC	Recovery audit contractor
		RBRVS	Resource Based Relative Value System
JCI	Joint Commission International	RD Teams	Research and development teams
JLI	Joint Learning Initiative	RFID	Radio frequency identification
LMX theory	Leader-member exchange theory	RFP	Request for proposal
M&A	Merger and acquisition	RHIOs	Regional Health Information Organizations
M&M	Morbidity and Mortality	ROI	Return on investment
MBO	Management by objectives	SADC	Southern African Development Cooperation
MCO	Managed-care organization		
MDGs	Millennium Development Goals	SAMHSA	Substance Abuse and Mental Health Services Administration
MedPAC	Medicare Payment Advisory Commission		
MELD	Model for end-stage liver disease	SBU	Strategic business unit
MHA	Master's in Health Administration	SDLC	Systems development life cycle
MRI	Magnetic resonance imaging	SEPT	South Essex Partnership University NHS Foundation Trust

SMART	Specific, Measurable, Achievable, Realistic and Time Bound	UNCTAD	United Nations Conference on Trade and Development
SNA	Social network analysis	UNOS	United Network of Organ Sharing
SNS	Social network sites	USD	United States dollars
SOP	Standard operating procedure	VA	Veterans Administration (Department of Veterans Affairs)
SSA	Sub-Saharan Africa		
SSI	Supplemental Security Income	VBP	Value-based purchasing
SWOT	Strengths, weaknesses, opportunities, threats	VHA	Veterans Health Administration
		VIP Model	Virtual integrated practice model
TQM	Total quality management	VISN	Veterans Integrated Service Network
TVA	Tennessee Valley Authority	VP	Vice president
UBIT	Unrelated business income tax	WHO	World Health Organization

Glossary

ACA (Patient Protection and Affordable Care Act): The comprehensive health care reform law enacted in March 2010 (sometimes known as ACA, PPACA, or "Obamacare") which had three primary goals: (1) make affordable health insurance available to more people, (2) expand the Medicaid program to cover all adults with income below 138 percent of the federal poverty level, and (3) support innovative medical care delivery methods designed to lower the costs of health care generally.

Accountable Care Organization: A group of health care providers who give coordinated care, and chronic disease management, and thereby improve the quality of care patients get. The organization's payment is tied to achieving health care quality goals and outcomes that result in cost savings.

Accountability in Teams: The entities to which teams are formally accountable, which may be internal to the team as well as external to the team and organization.

Accreditation: An entity receives accreditation when it meets the quality standards defined by the accrediting organization.

Adaptive Leadership: A prominent model within the contingency theory of leadership, which describes how effective leadership techniques vary according to the amount of uncertainty in the environment.

Adaptive Learning: A form of learning in which problem solvers adjust their behavior and work processes in response to changing events or trends. Adaptive learning is similar to single-loop learning.

Administrative Leadership: The instrumental and interpersonal support provided by those who hold senior positions in the organization such as chief executive officer, chief operating officer, and vice president for performance improvement.

Alliance Objectives: The goals pursued by the parties in a strategic alliance that serve as the stated purpose of the alliance.

Alliance Problems: This distinction highlights that there is often disagreement as to why alliances fail, and that this disagreement is often rooted in mistaking a root cause for a mere symptom.

Alliance Process: The flow of activities in the life cycle of a strategic alliance.

Alliance Risk: The risk that a strategic alliance will fail. This risk must be balanced against the expected rewards.

Alliance Symptom: The easily observable problems that develop in a troubled strategic alliance as opposed to the root causes (i.e., alliance problems).

Ambassador Activities: Activities carried out by team members involving communication with those above them in the organizational hierarchy, often carried out to protect the team from outside pressures, to persuade others to support the team, and to lobby for resources.

Ambidexterity: An important attribute of high-performing organizations, which is based on the ability to conduct two seemingly opposed sets of activities.

Anchoring Bias: A psychological effect whereby an initial offer in negotiation tends to influence subsequent thinking.

Anti-Kickback Statute (AKS): Prohibits the knowing and willful solicitation or receipt of remuneration by any person in connection with items or services for which payment could be made by Medicare or Medicaid.

Antitrust Law: The body of law intended to promote competition.

Autonomy: Relates to the freedom to follow or act according to one's own will.

Balancing Feedback Loops: Feedback loops that counteract or oppose whatever is happening in a system.

Barriers to Communication: The psychological factors that distort the substance of a message, such as credibility, relationships, beliefs, interests, and communication styles.

BATNA: This stands for "Best Alternative to a Negotiated Agreement" and represents the best option left with if the current negotiations fail and an agreement cannot be reached.

Behavioral Norms: Rules that standardize how people act at work on a day-to-day basis, while performance norms are rules that standardize employee output.

Behavioral Theories: Leadership theories that examine how those in leadership roles act toward those they are influencing.

Belmont Report: A result of work by the National Commission for the Protection of Human Subjects of Biomedical and Behavioral Research in the 1970s with revisions by the Department of Health and Human Services (HHS) in the late 1970s and early 1980s for the protection of human subjects.

Benchmarking: A key feature of many QI approaches, benchmarking is the process of comparing an organization's performance metrics (e.g., quality, cost, operational efficiency) to those of other "best practice" or peer organizations.

Bending the Cost Curve: This refers to reducing health spending relative to projected trends in spending.

Beneficence: The obligation to do good, prevent or remove harm, and to act in a kind or benevolent manner.

Bioethics: The discipline concerned with ethical questions and actions in medicine and biology.

Boundary Permeability: The fluidity of team membership, whereby members may enter or exit according to the team's needs.

Boundary-Spanning Roles: Individuals who help enhance communication and coordination with other organizations or teams.

Bounded Rationality: This refers to the limits on the correctness of managerial decisions due to limits on managers' cognition of all variables and forces in the environment.

Brain Drain: An imbalance in the distribution of health workers, due to increasing demand for health workers and the ability of high-income countries to offer more attractive remuneration packages.

Bureaucracy: Literally, this means government by bureaus or offices. More generally, it refers to an organization structured on bureaucratic principles with clear roles, lines of authority and accountability, procedures, and rules.

Business Models: The core elements of a firm and how it is organized to deliver value to its customers and generate revenues.

Centers for Medicare and Medicaid Services (CMS): One of the largest programs in HHS, which manages the Medicare and Medicaid programs.

Centralization: The concentration of responsibilities and authority vertically at higher levels or horizontally within one or only a few people or organizational units.

Certificate of Need: A form of approval that is sometimes legally required for the creation of a health care organization, purchase of equipment, or provision of a service. State agencies grant this approval based on their determination of community need.

Charismatic Power: Power gained by a leader through the use of strong personal communication and social skills as opposed to power gained by respect for observable and concrete achievements.

Classical School of Administration: The management school that emphasized general principles and the best way to structure organizations.

Clayton Act: Prohibits mergers, acquisitions, and joint ventures that threaten to substantially lessen competition or are likely to create a monopoly.

Clinical Leadership: Instrumental and interpersonal support provided by those who hold clinical positions, such as physicians and nurses.

Clinical Practice Guidelines: Typically developed by expert panels, clinical practice guidelines synthesize evidence from the literature and make recommendations regarding treatment for specific clinical conditions. The National Guideline Clearinghouse (http://www.guideline.gov) is a publicly available resource for evidence-based guidelines covering a full range of clinical conditions.

Coalition: A limited-term alliance among individuals or groups that is formed in order to increase power and further the respective interests.

Coercion: The use of subtle influence dynamics to achieve desired goals.

Cognitively Active: Constantly and intentionally focusing on all parties instead of only focusing on oneself.

Collaborating: A negotiation strategy where parties try to help each other get what they want and in the process maximize the value created in the negotiation.

Combinatorial complexity: Also known as "detail" complexity, this arises from the number of constituent elements of a system or the number of interrelationships that might exist among them.

Communication: The exchange of information among individuals. Especially important, in the context of achieving coordination in an organization, are the frequency, timeliness, accuracy, and focus on problem solving in information exchange.

Communication Networks and Structure: The manner and patterns through which communication is disseminated in an organization; these include both formal and informal modes of communication.

Communication Technology: The variety of methods used for communication within an organization or team.

Community Benefit Standard: To maintain tax-exempt status as charitable organizations under Section 501(c)(3) of the federal Internal Revenue Code, nonprofit health care providers must meet a community benefit standard. Examples of relevant factors under this standard include the presence of a community board, the operation of an emergency room open to all, and the provision of charity care.

Comparative Advantage: The discovery and deployment of significant differences in a nation's cost, quality, or access such that a medical or surgical procedure, health activity, or service creates patient value.

Comparative Clinical Effectiveness: A type of research that involves a systematic comparison of the impact of drugs, devices, procedures, or services on patient health outcomes.

Competencies: The knowledge, skills, and abilities needed to be an effective leader of an organization.

Contingency Theories: Leadership theories that argue that no singular set of traits and behaviors is adequate for explaining who will be effective in leadership roles, but rather that the needed behaviors depend on the circumstance or environment in which one is leading.

Competing: A negotiation strategy where one party tries to get as much value for themselves as possible, with little, if any, concern for the other party.

Competitive Advantage: The long-term market position and uniqueness that is not easily duplicable by rivals, that enables a firm to outperform its rivals. It could also be called "key success factors."

Complex Adaptive System: A system that is comprised of people and activities that mutually influence each other in complex ways with often unpredictable outcomes. Elements of the system co-evolve as people and activities move forward together and interact over time.

Complex Systems: A management theory that reflects developments in biology, ecology, and evolutionary theory that believes that organizations are richly interconnected, dynamic, nonlinear systems that are constantly changing and do not settle into predictable patterns but still display complex forms of order.

Compliance: An organization's compliance program consists of the steps it takes to ensure that it follows applicable statutes, regulations, and rules.

Compromising: A negotiation strategy where the parties in the negotiation divide value and find a solution that partially satisfies everyone.

Confidential: An expectation of a certain privacy and nondisclosure regarding information relayed to another person.

Confidentiality: The nature of a confidence or confiding of secrets or private information from one to another.

Confirming Evidence Bias: The tendency for people to seek out and pay attention only to information that confirms prior beliefs.

Consumer-Driven Health Care: A strategy that encourages and enables people to take charge of their personal health through: (1) knowledge of their current status and needs, (2) informed decision making, (3) wise use of health care dollars, and (4) confident and active participation in their own health care decisions and treatment choices.

Consumer-Driven Health Plan (CDHP): A health plan designed to allow the employees greater choice in their health care, thus enabling them to be wise consumers.

Consumer: A person who uses up a commodity. Also known as a purchaser of goods or services, or customer.

Consumerism: A movement that advocates that patients be active participants in their own healthcare decisions, acting like consumers who choose the healthcare options that they believe are best for them. This is a change from the traditional relationship between patients and healthcare professionals in which patients followed the advice given to them without playing an active part in decision making.

Contingency Theory: This theory posits that the selection of the most appropriate form of organization is dependent upon the particular circumstances of the environment in which the organization operates. Contingency theory does not advocate an either/or approach but rather views the process as a continuum from mechanistic/bureaucratic to organic forms.

Continuous Quality Improvement (CQI): A participative, systematic approach to planning and implementing a continuous organizational improvement process.

Control: Control indicates influence, and an influence can come from many sources, of which ownership is only one.

Convenient Care Clinic (CCC): Walk-in services for a limited scope of medical conditions, usually staffed by advanced practice health professionals such as nurse practitioners (NPs) or physician assistants (PAs).

Convenient Care Clinic Association: An organization of health care systems and companies that offer accessible, cost-effective, quality health services located in retail-based environments.

Coordination: Achievement of synchronized action among individuals and work units so that their work is mutually reinforcing and contributing to organizational goals.

Corporate Integrity Agreement: An agreement imposed by the HHS Office of the Inspector General on a health care provider in the aftermath of a health care fraud investigation. It is intended to promote adherence to health care laws and regulations by imposing specific compliance obligations on a health care provider.

Cost Reduction: This distinction highlights that the strategic intent behind alliances may differ on fundamental dimensions, such as cost versus value, and that such differences imply different bases for evaluating the success of an alliance.

Culturally Derived Power: Power that derives from the informal aspects of organization, such as norms, values, beliefs, and assumptions.

Curse of Knowledge: The problem of imagining another person's state of mind when you have a piece of knowledge that they lack.

Decentralization: The delegation of responsibilities and authority vertically to lower levels or horizontally among many people or organizational units. (*See also* centralization.)

Decisional Authority: The continuum of roles that teams may play in decision making from no decision authority to being able to make all decisions.

Decision-Making School: The management school that emphasized how decisions are made and how goals are set within the firm, with a view towards controlling managerial behavior.

Deeming Authority: Authority granted to an accreditation organization such that a provider meeting accreditation requirements is deemed to also meet certain Medicare requirements.

Delphi Technique: An approach to decision making in which a panel of experts is asked for their views on an issue followed up by controlled feedback and repeated until consensus is reached. This technique encourages member participation.

Department of Health and Human Services (HHS): The principal federal government agency for health care under which the Public Health Service and 11 other public health agencies are governed.

Department of Justice (DOJ): The DOJ, along with the Federal Trade Commission (FTC), is responsible for federal enforcement of the antitrust laws. These federal agencies coordinate their efforts in investigating and prosecuting antitrust cases.

Detail Complexity: Another name for combinatorial complexity.

Diagnosis-Related Groups (DRGs): The patient classification system adopted by Congress and developed by a team of researchers at Yale University in the late 1970s.

Differentiation: The segmentation of an organization into units together with the structuring of those units and development of organizational practices and systems and employees' cognitive and emotional orientations that are suited to each unit's unique tasks and sub-environment.

Direct Contact: A structural alternative for coordination in which individuals in different functional departments coordinate efforts through direct interaction with each other. Direct contact is a weak structural alternative to coordination.

Discovery: A form of learning in which innovators learn about possible action alternatives, outcome preferences, and contextual factors. Discovery is similar to double-loop or generative learning in that it opens up and investigates possibilities.

Distortion: Factors that affect how a listener understands a message. These factors include the content of the message, the medium of the message (face-to-face, written, or electronic communication), and the listeners themselves.

Diversity and Inclusion: Diversity often refers to differences in professional background, age and generation, gender, hierarchical level, demographic and cultural background, as well as in consumer versus professional status. Inclusion is an organizational environment that accepts and promotes diversity.

Donors: Individuals or groups that provide funds or resources to a nonprofit organization who are not immersed in the daily activities of the organization but can have substantial influence on its mission and activities.

Double-Loop Learning: A form of learning in which problem solvers attempt to close the gap between desired and actual states of affairs by questioning and modifying those organization's policies, plans, values, and rules that frame organizational problems and guide organizational action. Double-loop learning is similar to generative learning.

Dynamic complexity: A form of complexity that arises from the operation of feedback loops.

Electronic Health Record (EHR): An electronic record of health-related information on an individual that conforms to nationally recognized interoperability standards and that can be created, managed, and consulted by authorized clinicians and staff across more than one health care organization.

Electronic Medical Record (EMR): An electronic record of health-related information on an individual that can be created, gathered, managed, and consulted by authorized clinicians and staff in one health care organization.

Emergence: New ideas, products, practices, and relationships that arise spontaneously and are neither predicted nor anticipated by participants or observers.

Emotional Contagion: When emotions are transmitted from one party to another.

Empowerment: A strategy in which employees are given information, knowledge, and power to make decisions when the traditional hierarchical management structure and the command-and-control management techniques are no longer viable. Teams, when used as an extension of the general employee empowerment strategy, occur along four dimensions: potency, meaningfulness, autonomy, and consequences.

EMTALA (Emergency Medical Treatment and Labor Act): Established in 1986, the EMTALA is designed to prevent institutions from denying care to anyone seeking emergency medical treatment, regardless of citizenship, insurance status, or ability to pay.

Entry and Exit Barriers: Entry barriers are obstacles that make it difficult for a new firm to enter a market and are not borne by companies that are already part of the market. Exit barriers are obstacles that make it difficult or prohibit a firm from leaving a market.

Environmental Context: The mix of external factors that significantly affect or may affect the team or organization.

Equity-Based Alliances: Non-contractual alliances where the alliance partners invest equity capital in the alliance's formation and thus have ownership stakes tied to such investments.

ERISA (Employee Retirement Income Security Act): A statute which imposes minimum requirements on retirement and health benefit plans.

Ethos, Pathos, Logos: Aristotle's terms for "character," "emotion," and "logic," the three modes of communicating one's message.

Evidence-Based Medicine: The systematic identification and application of available scientific information for clinical decision making by health care professionals. Scientific information includes findings related to process and outcome-based measures of quality, as well as findings related to cost and cost-effectiveness.

Expectancy: The perceived link between effort and performance (e.g., the relationship between how hard an employee tries and how well he or she does in terms of job performance).

External Environment: The conditions, entities, and factors surrounding an organization that influences its activities and choices.

Fairness: An incentive for work motivation where individuals perceive a balance between their work effort and their treatment by managers relative to coworkers.

FCA (False Claims Act): A law that prohibits knowingly submitting or causing to be submitted a false claim to the government, such as a Medicare claim for a service different from the one that was actually provided.

Feedback: Feedback approaches to coordination entail the exchange of information among staff usually while work is being carried out. Feedback approaches permit staff to change or modify work activities in response to unexpected requirements. Feedback also refers to the part of the communication process through which the sender and receiver engage in a two-way process of communication. It reverses the sender and receiver roles so that information can be shared, recycled, and fine-tuned to achieve unambiguous and mutual understanding in the communication process.

Federal Trade Commission: An independent agency of the U.S. government whose mission is to protect consumers and prevent anticompetitive, deceptive, and unfair business practices.

Fidelity: The obligation to honor commitments.

First Mover Advantage: The advantage an organization attains by being the first competitor to pursue a particular source of competitive advantage.

Fixed-Pie Bias: An erroneous assumption made in conflict management that concludes that the benefits gained by one side in an agreement equal the costs paid by the opposing side and that the outcome of the negotiation sums to zero.

Flexible Spending Account or Arrangement (FSA): A blanket term for financial accounts where pretax monies are held to be used for reimbursement for noncovered medical expenses.

Focused Clinics: Clinics that specialize in specific diseases or surgical procedures.

Followership: Those who share a common purpose with the leader, believe in what the organization is trying to accomplish, and want both the leader and the organization to succeed.

Formal Leadership: Leadership based on formal authority conferred by the organization to an individual.

Fractioning: A negotiation tactic that involves separating out the various components of a specific issue.

Free Rider Syndrome: A situation where a team member obtains the benefits of group membership but does not accept a proportional share of the costs of membership.

Front-Line Managers: Those who provide supervision directly to care providers.

Functional Fixedness: When a negotiator bases his or her strategy on familiar, rather than the most effective, methods.

Functional Organization Structure: The organizational form that is based on segmentation, at the highest level of an organization structure, of responsibilities and authority for achievement of an organization's primary task, into units that represent different functions. In industrial firms, these functions are typically research, engineering, manufacturing, marketing, and sales. In health care organizations, the functions are typically professions and disciplines directly involved in delivery of services to patients, such as medical specialties and subspecialties, nursing, social work, therapies, and transportation.

General Agreement on Trade in Services (GATS): A 1995 treaty of the World Trade Organization (WTO) created to extend the multilateral trading system to the service sector, in the same way that the General Agreement on Tariffs and Trade (GATT) provides such a system for merchandise trade.

Generative Learning: A form of learning in which problem solvers attempt to eliminate problems by changing the underlying structure of the system. This underlying structure includes the "operating policies" of the decision makers and actors in the system (e.g., their values and assumptions). Generative learning is similar to double-loop learning.

Generic Strategies: The label Michael Porter gave to two prominent position strategies: low-cost and high differentiation. He argued that most firms naturally gravitate to one or the other, and thus he called these "generic" positions.

Global Health Workforce Alliance (GHWA): An international partnership established in 2006 to identify and implement solutions to the global health workforce crisis.

Globalization: A process by which regional economies, societies, and cultures have become integrated through a global network of communication, transportation, and trade.

Goals: The larger aspirations of the organization.

Goal Setting: A motivational technique based on the concept that the practice of setting specific goals enhances performance, and that setting difficult goals results in higher performance than setting easier goals.

Governance: The activities and decisions that focus on the determination of mission, strategy, and goals of an organization, as well as its broad policies. In addition, it is the governance structure that holds the organization's leadership accountable for their actions and performance. Typically, the board of trustees performs the governance functions in a health care organization, and a collective body representing the medical staff performs its governance activities, such as determining its policies and regulations.

Governing Board: A board of directors, managers, or trustees elected or appointed to direct and supervise an institution's policies.

Groupthink: A team decision-making phenomenon in which a desire for consensus overrides the full exploration of alternative courses of action.

HCQIA (Health Care Quality Improvement Act): At the time of its enactment in 1986, HCQIA reflected two primary concerns, one relating to weaknesses in existing peer-review processes, and the other to the ease with which incompetent physicians were able to move between states without a record of their malpractice experience or professional disciplinary action. HCQIA is designed to address these issues by encouraging physicians to identify and discipline fellow physicians who are incompetent or who engage in unprofessional behavior, so as to improve the quality of care.

Health Information Technology: A general term used to describe a broad range of technologies for transmitting and managing health information for use by consumers, providers, payers, insurers, and others interested in health care.

Health Insurance Portability and Accountability Act (HIPAA): Federal legislation that specifies regulations for the privacy of personal health information, portability of health insurance, and the organization of the interchange of electronic data for certain financial and administrative operations.

Health Reimbursement Account (HRA): A financial arrangement that is used for reimbursement of substantiated medical expenses.

Health Savings Account (HSA): A tax-exempt financial account used to reimburse medical expenses not covered under existing health plans.

Health Systems: Arrangements among hospitals, physicians, and other provider organizations that involve direct ownership of assets on the part of the parent system.

Hierarchy of Authority: The arrangement of responsibilities and authority for actions and decisions such that successively higher levels in the organization have authority over units below them. The hierarchy of authority is used specifically in this book as a macro-level approach to coordination.

High-Deductible Health Plan (HDHP): A type of consumer-driven health plan that offers a broad provider network, limited involvement with medical management, higher deductibles, and lower premiums.

High-Performance Work Practices (HPWPs): Workforce or human resource practices that have been shown to improve an organization's capacity to effectively attract, select, hire, develop, and retain high-performing employees.

Horizontal Integration: An expansion strategy that occurs when organizations producing similar products merge or are acquired.

Hospital–Physician Relationships: The array of economic, noneconomic, and clinical integration mechanisms designed to link hospitals more closely with their medical staffs and community-based physicians.

Human Relations School: The management school that focuses on the individual and the group, and the importance of their participation in organizational decision making.

Human Subjects: In the context of research, human subjects are living individual(s) who provide data or other material with which researchers conduct studies.

Hybrid Organization: An organization that maintains its traditional functional structure and creates program structures for just one or two programs.

Hygiene Factors: Factors related to the work environment (such as extrinsic factors) whose presence prevents dissatisfaction but does not lead to satisfaction or motivation.

Implementation: The processes involved and occurring between the decision to adopt the QI innovation and the routine use of the QI innovation, or the integration of a new idea or practice into the operating system of the organization.

Inclusive Leadership: A leadership style that invites and appreciates others' words and deeds, collaborates with others across the professional hierarchy, shares power with others, frames tasks as a team effort, and facilitates a positive work climate for all staff members, regardless of profession and position.

Individually Derived Power: A source of power rooted in an individual's legitimate authority, ability to reward another, knowledge or expertise, charisma, coercive ability, and informational centrality.

Infant Mortality Rates: An often-used health statistic measured in the number of infant deaths per 1,000 live births; shown to be highly associated with the degree of local health care infrastructure.

Informal Leadership: Leadership that is not formally established or sanctioned by the organization, but develops as a result of other sources of power and authority.

Innovation: An idea, practice, or object that is perceived as new by an individual or other unit adopting it. Innovation also refers to the act (or process) of introducing something new into an environment or setting.

Institutional Review Boards: Administrative entities established by institutions to protect the ethical rights of human subjects who participate in research conducted under their supervision.

Institutional Theory: The management school that emphasizes that organizations face environments characterized by external norms, rules, and requirements to which they must conform in order to receive support and legitimacy.

Instrumental Support: Various forms of tangible assistance such as providing resources, removing organizational barriers, developing structures to facilitate change efforts, and information sharing.

Integrated Delivery System Network: An organization consisting of subunits that provide different types of care across the continuum. Integrated delivery systems typically include hospitals, long-term care facilities, rehabilitation facilities, ambulatory care facilities, and home health agencies, and structurally they vertically integrate these different suborganizations. They may provide services in one or several geographic regions.

Integration: Coordination of activities among organizational units, including the management of conflict among the units, to achieve synchronized actions and decisions.

Integrators: Individuals whose primary responsibility is coordination. Care managers are a prime example of integrators in health care. (*See also* Lateral Relations.)

Interconnectedness of Work: The property of work itself that inherently requires different parts or elements to fit together to be performed well. For example, the decisions and actions performed in the care of an individual patient are interconnected elements of work.

Interdependence: The nature and degree to which the performance of work (taking actions and making decisions) by an individual or organization unit is dependent upon or is (potentially) affected by the performance of work by other individuals or organization units.

Intergroup Relationships and Conflict: Patterns and types of interactions and interdependence among groups in an organization, including conflicts among groups.

Interpersonal Support: Intangible actions that often contribute to individuals' feeling valued and appreciated, such as providing encouragement, offering feedback, and being inclusive.

Internal Environment: The conditions and elements within an organization, including employees, management, and culture, that affect the firm's choices and activities.

Intrinsic Motivation: Intrinsic motivation exists when employees complete tasks because they are meaningful, interesting, and enjoyable—as compared to situations in which motivation derives from extrinsic rewards such as money or status.

Iron Triangle: Refers to the difficulty of seeking to improve quality of care, improve access to care, and reduce the cost of care simultaneously.

Job Redesign: Altering certain aspects of the job to better satisfy an employee's psychological needs. Examples include task identity, skill variety, task significance, knowledge of results, and feedback.

Joint Commission International (JCI): A private sector, U.S.-based, not-for-profit organization focused on improving the safety of patient care through the provision of accreditation and certification services.

Joint Venture: A legal entity formed between two or more parties to undertake an economic activity together.

Justice: The quality of being (morally) just or righteous, including just conduct, integrity, and conformity to a moral right or reason.

Knowledge-Based Sources of Power: Power that derives from a group's control over the expertise needed to make key decisions and organize production.

Kohll and Decker Cases: Two cases by the European Court of Justice in 1998, which established that health care resources should be treated as any other part of the European Union economy with regard to the free movement of goods and services.

Leader-Member Exchange (LMX): A contingency theory leadership model that recognizes distinctive relationships between people in leadership roles and specific staff in followership roles.

Leadership: The process in which one engages others to set and achieve a common goal, often an organizationally defined goal.

Lean: A management and operations improvement approach, often described as a "transformation" that focuses on eliminating waste across "value streams" that flow horizontally across technologies, assets, and departments (as opposed to improving within each). The intent of a Lean approach is cost-effectiveness, error reduction, and improved service to customers. The term "Lean" was originally coined by Jim Womack to describe innovations in Toyota's manufacturing process (http://www.lean.org).

Learning: The acquisition of knowledge or skills through study, instruction, or experience. Learning is essentially a feedback process.

Learning Organization: An organization skilled at creating, acquiring, and transferring knowledge, and at modifying its behavior to reflect new knowledge and insights.

Liaison Roles: A boundary-spanning role within a unit or department whose responsibilities are to serve as a point of contact and coordination with other units or departments.

Licensure: State agency—granted authority to practice a profession or operate a facility.

Logrolling: A negotiation tactic that involves trading off on issues of different value to each party.

Macro Perspective: The unit of analysis in organizational theory and research that focuses on the organization as a social system in the context of other organizations.

Managed Migration: The linkage of international migration to the health policy goals of individual states; the regulation of the flows of health workers in a way that benefits both source and destination countries.

Management: The process of accomplishing predetermined objectives through the effective use of human, financial, and technical resources.

Management Teams: Teams that coordinate and provide direction to the subunits under their jurisdiction; such subunits may exist at multiple organizational levels.

Market Niche Strategy: A strategy in which a competitive organization seeks advantage by focusing on a single or small number of product lines or population segments.

Matrix Organization: The organization form in which responsibilities and authority are allocated between two equally powerful hierarchies, one representing functions and the other representing programs, overlaid on each other. The "matrixed" individuals have two supervisors—a functional supervisor, and a program supervisor.

Medical Innovation: A new development that improves patient care (e.g., new medications), helps doctors care for patients (e.g., electronic medical records), or lowers the cost of delivery.

Medical Savings Account: A type of tax-exempt financial account created to offset non-covered medical expenses for self-employed individuals or employees of small businesses (fewer than 50 workers).

Medical Tourism: The practice of traveling across international borders to obtain health care.

Medicare Payment Advisory Commission (MedPAC): An independent congressional agency, MedPAC has played a significant role in shaping a variety of Medicare reform initiatives. MedPAC advises Congress on a broad range of issues and is also tasked with analyzing access to care, quality of care, and other issues affecting Medicare.

Membership Fluidity: The extent to which, and the frequency with which, team membership changes; this is related in part to boundary permeability, or the extent to which a team's core membership is maintained over time and the ease with which new members can enter and current members exit the team.

Mental Models: The discipline of constantly surfacing, testing, and improving our assumptions about how the world works.

Message: Communication that is delivered using one or more of the three persuasive means of conveying a message—ethos (character), pathos (emotion), and logos (logic).

Micro Perspective: The unit of analysis in organizational theory and research that focuses on the individual, group, and departments within the organization.

Middle Managers: Those who have responsibility for entire units within a health care organization.

Migrant Remittances: The transfer of funds from migrants to relatives or friends in their country of origin. Migrant remittances have become an increasingly important feature of modern economic life.

Millennium Development Goals (MDGs): Eight time-bound goals, agreed upon by world leaders in 2000, that provide a framework for the entire international community to work together towards a common end of global development.

Mission: The foundation for strategic direction. A mission provides the reason for the company's existence and forms the basis for strategy. It should guide the firm to focus its energies and frame its choices of strategy and commitments of resources.

Model for End- Stage Liver Disease (MELD): A scoring system for assessing the severity of chronic liver disease that later was adopted for determining prognosis and prioritizing for receipt of a liver transplant.

Monopoly: A market when there is only one provider of a supply or service.

Moral Hazard: Moral hazard arises when people covered by health insurance utilize more health care than they would if they paid for services out of pocket (i.e., from their own resources without insurance).

Motivators: Factors related to the work content (i.e., intrinsic factors) whose presence increases job satisfaction and motivation but whose absence does not lead to job dissatisfaction. Motivators include achievements, recognition, the work itself, responsibility, and advancement.

Mutual Adjustment: The direct communication between two individuals who are not in a hierarchical relationship for the purpose of coordinating their interdependent activities. It is one of three types of feedback approaches to coordination.

National Practitioner Data Bank: A federal repository of data on medical malpractice payments and adverse actions taken against health care practitioners (such as license terminations or hospital privileges revocations). A federal statute specifies what information state licensing boards, hospitals, insurers, and others are required to report and how often they are expected to report.

Network Centrality: A situation within an organization where one work group or unit lies at the intersection of other work groups or units, as a result becoming a repository of knowledge about how the entire organization works.

Nominal Group Technique: A model of team decision making in which members pool their individual judgments in a guided systematic manner. This technique encourages member participation.

Non-malfeasance: The obligation to do no harm upheld by physicians by virtue of their Hippocratic Oath.

Nonspecific Compensation: A negotiation tactic that involves adding issues that are not tied to money or compensation.

Non-Physician Clinician (NPC): Health care professionals trained with less cost than physicians for an average period of three to four years post secondary school.

Notice of proposed rulemaking: A precursor to the creation of a new federal regulation. Agencies' notices of proposed rule-making describe the rules they intend to enact and then solicit public comments; the agencies may subsequently revise initially proposed rules in light of comments received.

Not-Invented-Here Syndrome (NIHS): The well-known skepticism about the appropriateness or relevance of something not invented in one's homeland.

Objectives: Subordinate goals that must be achieved to accomplish the overall organizational goal.

Office for Human Research Protections: A branch of the U.S. Department of Health and Human Services that provides leadership regarding protection of human subjects involved in research activities.

Office of the Inspector General: With the cooperation of the Department of Justice, the Office of the Inspector General dedicates considerable resources to enforcing federal fraud and abuse laws.

Oligopoly: A market in which there are a small number of firms, and the competitors believe that their rivals have sufficient market power to influence their long-term survival. They therefore consciously adapt their strategies in response to their assessments of rival competitive advantages and expected strategic maneuvers.

Open Systems Theory: The management school that emphasizes that organizations are part of the external environment and, as such, must continually change and adapt to meet the challenges posed by the environment. The need for openness, adaptability, and innovation are consistent with the open system view.

Organization Design: The arrangement of authority, responsibilities, and flow of information by segmentation into organizational subunits, designation of scopes of authority and responsibility vertically and horizontally, and creation of structures to facilitate coordination among those subunits. A broader view of organization design also includes development of policies and design of control, reward, evaluation, and information systems.

Organization Structure: The graphical representation of segmentation of authority and responsibility into organization units and their interrelationships, resulting from organization design. Also called "table of organization."

Organizational Culture: The deepest level of beliefs, values, and norms that are shared by members of the organization. These beliefs, values, and norms represent the unique character of the organization and provide the context for action and behavior.

Organizational Learning: An organization-wide process that involves the systematic integration and collective interpretation of new knowledge.

Organizational Politics: The ongoing interplay of interests and power among people and groups in an organization. Different coalitions of interest or influence vie for the opportunity to achieve their desired goals.

Outcome Measures of Performance: Metrics based on the results of work performed. Examples include health status, patient satisfaction, and mortality.

Ownership: Ownership stakes in an alliance do not necessarily result in greater control of an alliance. Control indicates influence, and an influence can come from many sources, of which ownership is only one.

Parallel Organization: An organization structure that operates "parallel" to the primary structure. Parallel organizations are often used for large-scale change programs. Parallel structures also refer to integrating mechanisms that are used for managing programs that cross a functional structure.

Parallel Teams: Teams typically composed of people from different work units or jobs who carry out functions not regularly performed in the organization.

Partner Orientation: A summary characterization of the degree to which an alliance partner is interested in working cooperatively with his or her partner.

Path-Goal Model: A leadership contingency theory that argues that effective leadership requires a supervisor who provides the information, support, and resources that staff need to achieve the objectives in a particular situation.

Patient Classification System: A policy instrument that allows for output comparisons to be made across hospitals and provides a basis on which hospitals can be paid in a standardized, consistent fashion for the products they produce.

Patient-Centered Communication: A model of communication designed to maximize the effectiveness of communication between health care providers and patients.

Pay-for-Performance (P4P): Reimbursement for health care services that is designed to link payment incentives to quality and performance outcomes. Demonstration programs to test various approaches have been under way through the Centers for Medicare and Medicaid Services.

Performance Norms: Formal or informal rules that standardize employee output in a team.

Performance Outcomes: A management tool used to clarify goals and document progress toward achieving those goals.

Personal health record (PHR): An electronic record of health-related information on an individual that conforms to nationally recognized interoperability standards and that can be drawn from multiple sources while being managed, shared, and controlled by the individual.

Personal Mastery: The discipline of individual learning, without which organizational learning cannot occur. Personal mastery involves continuously clarifying our individual sense of purpose and vision, and continuously learning how to see the world as it is without distortion.

Performance Measures: Metrics and measurements used to determine the level of quality achieved by organizations.

Planning and Goal Setting: Global-level approaches to coordination that are used in addition to hierarchy of authority when an organization faces relatively low levels of uncertainty.

Policy Resistance: The tendency for interventions to be delayed, diluted, or defeated by the response of the system to the intervention itself.

Pooled Interdependence: A type of interdependence among team members in which each member makes a contribution to group output without the need for interaction among members. (*See also* Reciprocal Interdependence, Sequential Interdependence, and Simultaneous Interdependence.)

Pooling Alliances: Pooling alliances reflect two or more organizations contributing similar resources for mutual gain.

Population Ecology: The management school that emphasizes the environment's "selecting out" of certain organizations for survival. Organizational success is more dependent upon environmental selection than managerial decision making and implementation.

Porter's Five Forces Framework: A framework developed by Michael Porter of Harvard University to analyze the five main forces that affect competition in a market.

Portfolio Analysis: A method that compares the value of the strategic business units (SBUs) of firms. Components of companies are categorized by their competitive market position and their environmental attractiveness.

Power: The ability to exert influence or control over others.

Power Abuse: Situations where one or more organizational stakeholders uses power in ways that are generally not acceptable, often involve self-interest, and can inflict negative outcomes on the organization.

Power Stratification: When different stakeholders have unique opportunities to access power based upon their particular characteristics or circumstances.

Preemption: The displacement of one law by another, rendering the displaced law ineffective. When federal and state statutes conflict, the federal statute preempts the state statute.

Privacy: The right or choice to be alone, undisturbed, or free from public attention or intrusion.

Process Measures of Performance: Refer to indicators of the activities involved in carrying out work in an organization. Activities such as reviewing medical records to ensure completion of patient education, monitoring physician and nurse compliance with organizational standards for cleanliness, or evaluating the use of central lines are examples of process metrics.

Programming: Approaches to workplace coordination that include standardization of work, skills, and output.

Project Teams: Teams that are typically time limited, producing one-time outputs such as a new product, service, or support function (e.g., a new information system) in the organization.

Psychological Safety: An individual's perceptions about the consequences of taking interpersonal risks in the work environment. It is a largely taken-for-granted belief about how others will respond when one puts oneself on the line, such as by asking a question, seeking feedback, reporting a mistake, or proposing a new idea.

Quality Improvement (QI): An organized approach to planning and implementing continuous improvement in performance. QI emphasizes continuous examination and improvement of work processes by teams of organizational members trained in basic statistical techniques and problem-solving tools, and empowered to make decisions based on their analysis of the data.

Quality Improvement (QI) Interventions: Interventions designed to decrease medical errors and enhance patient safety.

Receiver: The person for whom a message is intended in the communication process.

Reciprocal Interdependence: A type of interdependence among team members in which the outputs of each member become inputs for the others. (*See also* Pooled Interdependence, Sequential Interdependence, and Simultaneous Interdependence.)

Reciprocity: The tendency for others to exchange equal levels of goods and services.

Recovery Audit Contractor: Entity under contract with Medicare to review claims for the purpose of identifying payment errors and fraud.

Regulation: Governmental oversight of the private marketplace.

Reinforcing Feedback Loops: Feedback loops that amplify or intensify whatever is happening in a system.

Relational Coordination: A relational process involving a network of communication and relationship ties among people whose tasks are interdependent to achieve coordination.

Relational Theories: Leadership theories that emphasize the relationship between people in leadership and followership roles.

Relationship Conflict: Conflict regarding some inherent characteristic of the other party.

Relationships: One of the two interacting components of relational coordination, relationships can be seen as consisting of shared goals, shared knowledge, and mutual respect.

Research: A systematic investigation, including research development, testing, and evaluation, designed to develop or contribute to generalizable knowledge.

Resource Dependence Theory: The management school that emphasizes the importance of the organization's abilities to secure needed resources from its environment in order to survive.

Retail Medicine: Health care services that are provided in "retail settings" or nonhospital, nontraditional medical environments.

Retrospective Reimbursement: A payment method in which rates are set on the basis of costs already incurred.

Revenue Enhancement: One of the two main outcome goals of organizational alliances, revenue enhancement refers to the decision to form an alliance with the goal of increasing revenue rather than cutting costs.

Reverse Innovation: An innovation either seen first or used first, in small or less developed markets before spreading to the larger, more developed markets.

Rules and Procedures: Approaches to coordination specifying how work is to be done and providing guidance to behavior. Rules and procedures augment use of an organization's hierarchy in coordinating work that is programmable.

Safety Zones: In antitrust guidelines, safety zones are outlines of the factual elements of business arrangements viewed as acceptable by the Department of Justice and the Federal Trade Commission. Such arrangements will generally not be prosecuted for antitrust violations, barring extraordinary circumstances.

Scaffolding: A method of team goal setting that utilizes a light organizational structure that does not require consistent individual members but rather assigns collective responsibility for a defined set of tasks.

Scientific Management School: The management school that emphasizes the application of scientific methods (e.g., time-motion studies) to maximize worker productivity and conformance to the one best way of production.

Scout Activities: Activities carried out by team members involving general scanning for ideas and information about the external environment.

Self-Fulfilling Prophecy: The process by which one party's beliefs cause another party to behave in such a way that supports that belief.

Sender: The person who is delivering a message in the communication process.

Senior Management: A team member who holds a leadership role in a health care organization, such as the CEO. According to the IOM, all individuals in leadership roles must develop, implement, and sustain systems that improve the safety, timeliness, efficiency, cost-effectiveness, equity, and patient-centeredness of care delivered in their organizations.

Sequential Interdependence: A type of interdependence in which one group member must act or produce an output before another one can begin or complete a task. (*See also* Pooled Interdependence, Reciprocal Interdependence, and Simultaneous Interdependence.)

Service Line: An organizational arrangement designed to coordinate the work of people from multiple professions and disciplines for a specific service in a health care organization. A service line is a health care variant of the general program organization. There are several variations of service line structures, characterized by the degree to which they facilitate integration. Service lines in health care can focus on diseases, patient populations, or technologies.

Shared Vision: The discipline of generating a common answer to the question, "What do we want to create?"

Sherman Act: Section 1 of this antitrust law prohibits contracts and other agreements that unreasonably restrain trade. This provision applies to situations where individuals or organizations that are in a competitive situation with one another also collaborate to achieve common business objectives. Section 2 prohibits activities that are undertaken to obtain or achieve a monopoly. This section is aimed at the conduct of a single entity that undertakes anticompetitive activities to strengthen its competitive position.

Simultaneous Interdependence (Team Interdependence): A situation in which team members diagnose, solve problems, and collaborate as a group while performing work or work-related activities.

Single-Loop Learning: A relatively simple error-and-correction process whereby problem solvers look for solutions within an organization's policies, plans, values, and rules. Single-loop learning is similar to adaptive learning.

Six Sigma: A data-driven methodology for eliminating defects in any process by applying a consistent framework of DMAIC (define, measure, analyze, improve, control) to minimize variation and improve processes. Six Sigma was started at Motorola and has been widely adopted at other companies, including GE. (http://www.isixsigma.com).

Skill- and Knowledge-Based Pay: A type of reward system in which employees are rewarded for acquiring new value-added skills, knowledge, or competencies.

SMART: An acronym that means specific, measurable, achievable, realistic, and time-bound. It is commonly used to describe the types of objectives that are most effective in strategic problem solving.

Social Capital: In health and human service systems, the web of cooperative relationships between providers that involve interpersonal trust, norms of reciprocity, and mutual aid.

Social Loafing: In teams, behaviors associated with obtaining the benefits of group membership without accepting a proportional share of the costs of membership (synonymous with Free Rider).

Social Media: Web 2.0 interactive communication technology.

Social Network Approach: The management school that emphasizes the role of social relationships among individuals and groups in explaining organizational behavior.

Social Networks: The connections among a group of people and the broader environment in which they live and work.

Speaker–Listener Model: A model of communication in which the speaker sends a message directly to the listener.

Specialization: The process of focusing on a narrow field of work to develop a depth of expertise. In organization design, specialization means developing different work units so that each unit can perform work that differs from that in other units in terms of its character, content, and information requirements (e.g., medical specialties). Specialization is one component of differentiation.

Stages of Team Development: A relatively predictable series of developmental stages experienced by teams. A team's stage of development may be related to team functioning and effectiveness.

Stakeholder: A person or group of people who are affected by an idea or message.

Stakeholder Analysis: The mapping of stakeholders according to power and interests.

Standardization of Output: The specification of goals or of characteristics of a product or service for the purpose of coordinating the interdependent activities of two or more people or organizational units. It is one of three types of programming approaches to coordination.

Standardization of Skills: The specification of specific training or skills required for people in different jobs, for the purpose of coordinating the interdependent activities of people in those jobs or the organizational units in which those jobs reside. Often, this is achieved through specification of minimum levels and types of education, certification as evidence of meeting minimum qualifications, or on-the-job training. It is one of three types of programming approaches to coordination.

Standardization of Work: The use of rules, regulations, schedules, plans, procedures, policies, and protocols to specify activities to be performed. It is one of three types of programming approaches to coordination.

Stark Physician Self-Referral Law (Stark): A federal fraud and abuse law that prohibits physicians from referring patients to certain health services providers with which the physicians have a financial relationship.

Status Differences: A characteristic of a team defined by the extent of variation in the status of each team member.

Strategic Alliance: Any formal agreement between two or more organizations for purposes of ongoing cooperation and mutual gain.

Strategic Management: The creation, implementation, and overall direction for a firm. As such, it requires both internal and external management functions to facilitate the development, implementation, and monitoring of strategy within an organization.

Strategic Management Perspective: The strategic management perspective emphasizes the importance of positioning the organization relative to its environment and competitors in order to achieve its objectives and assure its survival.

Strategic Problem Solving: An eight-step approach to integrating the strategic functions of leadership involving goal and objective setting, with the subsequent organizational action required to achieve the set objectives.

Strategy: The development of a broad formula prescribing a way in which a business competes and collaborates, sets goals, and establishes policies to carry out those goals in order to achieve the organizational mission.

Structural Measures of Performance Quality: Measures based on aspects of an organization or an individual's actions that could impact overall quality or organizational performance. Examples include indicators such as the number and type of beds in a given organization, the presence of shared governance structures, and the existence of a computerized provider order entry (CPOE) system with decision support features.

Structurally Derived Power: Power that is derived from the formal or bureaucratic aspects of an organization.

Study of Conflict Management: The study of conflict management concerns how parties approach, deal with, and resolve conflict and which personal, social, and environmental factors affect that process.

Supervision: The exchange of information among two or more people, one of whom is responsible for the work of the others. It reflects the use of an organization's hierarchy for the purpose of coordinating interdependent activities of people or organizational units. It is one of three types of feedback approaches to coordination.

Support Teams: Teams that enable others in the organization to do their work, serving such functions as quality improvement, strategic planning, and search committees.

Switching Cost: The cost incurred when a customer changes from one supplier or product to another.

SWOT Analysis: A simple analytical framework that includes assessments of strategically important factors both internal (strengths and weaknesses) and external (opportunities and threats) to organizations.

System Perspectives: A set of new perspectives on individual and organizational behavior, emphasizing the wider social and societal systems that condition this behavior.

Systems Thinking: The discipline of seeing wholes, perceiving the structures that underlie dynamically complex systems, and identifying high-leverage change opportunities.

Task Conflict: Conflict regarding differences among the parties in understanding and carrying out tasks.

Task Coordinator Activities: Activities carried out by team members involving communication and coordination with other groups and persons at lateral levels in the organization. These activities include discussing problems with others, obtaining feedback, and coordinating and negotiating with outsiders.

Task Force: A temporary, interdisciplinary group formed to coordinate work of different departments, usually for a specific objective, such as planning a new service. Task forces are one of several types of lateral relations, or structural mechanisms, to achieve coordination across specialized departments. (*See also* Integrators, Team.)

Task Interdependence: The level and manner in which information or resources are exchanged in carrying out team tasks; this often refers to the degree in which sub-tasks in a team are related to each other in carrying out the work of a team.

Task Uncertainty: A characteristic of work reflecting lack of knowledge of cause-and-effect relationships and/or predictability of events affecting task performance. Task uncertainty is a central factor in design of organizational units (*see also* differentiation) and in interdependence, which directly affects the need for coordination.

Tax Exemption: Freedom from an obligation to pay taxes, such as income or property taxes. Nonprofit health care providers seeking to maintain tax- exempt status are subject to a number of legal obligations not shared by for-profit entities.

Team: In the context of coordination, an enduring interdisciplinary group of people working together to achieve one or more common goals. Teams are one of several types of *lateral relations*, or structural mechanisms to facilitate coordination across specialized departments. (*See also* Integrators, Task Force.)

Team-Based Rewards: Financial or non-financial rewards given to team members for the accomplishment of team goals. This sometimes refers to rewarding team members for their contributions to the work of the team.

Team Cohesiveness: The extent to which members are committed to each other, often related to trust, emotional support, and ability to mutually adjust to changes in the behavior of others.

Team Composition: Membership on a team, which may be defined in aggregate numbers or according to another characteristic, such as professional status or gender.

Team Goals: The formal purposes of a team, which may vary by goal clarity, complexity of goals, and diversity of goals. This should be distinguished from informal team goals, which may or may not be related to the formal purposes of a team.

Team Interdependence: A situation in which team members diagnose, solve problems, and collaborate as a group while performing work or work-related activities. Team interdependence requires a workflow that is simultaneous and multidirectional.

Team Leadership: Team members who are formally assigned leadership roles, or who informally assume such roles.

Team Learning: Activities carried out by team members through which a team obtains and processes data that allows it to adapt and improve.

Team Norms: Standards that are shared by team members and regulate member behavior.

Team Performance: Formal measures of the effectiveness of a team in achieving its goals.

Team Processes: Methods of interacting and performing work by team members alone and in interaction with each other.

Team Size: A measure of team membership, often related to a variety of measures of team performance, member satisfaction, and other team processes.

Teaming: The ability to actively build and develop teams even as a project is in process.

Technical Leadership: A contingency theory of leadership that is appropriate for situations with little uncertainty and involves motivating the execution of established problem-solving processes.

Temporal Nature of Teams: A measure of the permanence of a team over time.

Tenure Diversity: The length of time during which members have been on a team.

Testing: A form of learning in which innovators learn about action—outcome relationships. In particular, through successive experimentation, they learn which actions sreliably produce desired outcomes. Testing is similar to single-loop or adaptive learning.

Threat Rigidity Effect: When individuals feel threatened, their thinking becomes rigid or inflexible.

Trading Alliances: Trading alliances are based on the notion of combining dissimilar—but complementary—resources for mutual gain.

Trait Theories: Theories of leadership that examine personality traits associated with leadership success.

Transactional Leadership: A leadership theory composed of these four behavioral elements: (1) making rewards contingent on performance, (2) correcting problems actively when performance goes wrong, (3) refraining from interruptions of performance if it meets standards (i.e., passive management of exceptions), and (4) a laissez-faire approach to organizational change.

Transformational Leadership: An influential model of leadership style in contemporary theories that includes four key behaviors: (1) influence through a vision, (2) motivating through inspiration, (3) stimulating the intellect of subordinates, and (4) individualized consideration.

Transparency: Proponents of transparency in the health care setting advocate wide dissemination of information about health care providers and their services, including information about service quality and prices.

Triple Aim: The attempt to improve the experience of care, improve the health of populations, and reduce per capita costs of health care.

Turbulence: The external circumstances that create an uncertain environment for an organization.

Turbulent Environment: This refers to the situation whereby an organization is facing rapidly changing external circumstances and greater interconnectedness and interdependence between itself and other organizations.

Uncertainty Reduction: An important benefit of strategic alliances, when compared with alternative approaches to growth, given the exit options typically found in alliance agreements.

Value: In economics, value is the quotient of quality divided by cost, the combined benefits among all the parties in the negotiated agreement.

Value-Based Payment: A payment structure used as a strategy for improving the performance of health care organizations that entails linking financial incentives to the accomplishment of assigned performance goals related to efficiency, productivity, or quality.

Value Chain: This refers to the interlinked activities among a set of organizations whereby suppliers provide raw material inputs to manufacturers who process them and produce outputs for downstream markets.

Value in Negotiation: The combined benefits among all the parties in a negotiated agreement drafted as a strategy to solve a conflict.

Values: The expression of the ethics that guide employees' actions. They should constrain how the mission and vision is accomplished.

Vertical Information Systems: Approaches to coordination based on increasing the information-processing capacity of the hierarchy by facilitating information flow up and down the hierarchy and by increasing the capabilities of various managers to handle more information.

Vertical Integration: An expansion strategy that occurs when an organization acquires a business in its value chain that is a supplier (backward expansion) or a buyer of the organization's products (forward expansion).

Vision: A statement about what the organization wants to become. It focuses on the future.

Winner's Curse: The feeling of unhappiness after a reached settlement where one side feels that it should have asked for more.

Work Teams: Groups of people responsible for producing goods or providing services.

Author Index

Blanchet, N., 397, 398, 399
Blau, P. M., 168
Blayney, K. D., 91
Blegen, M. A., 230
Block, P., 142
Blumenthal, D. M., 6, 326, 327, 333, 334, 335
Boards of Trustees, 308
Bobbio, A., 47
Bodnar, W., 263
Bogardus, S. T., 43
Bogue, R., 21
Bohmer, R. M., 74, 124, 196
Bollinger, N., 352
Bonabeau, E., 22
Bonache, J., 118
Bonacum, D., 224
Bono, J. E., 35, 36
Boothman, R. C., 323
Borah, A., 279
Bornstein, R., 136
Boufford, J. I., 400
Boulton, J. G., 188, 189
Bourgeois, L. J., 165, 263
Bowditch, J. L., 195
Bowman, C., 188, 189
Bowser, D., 396
Boyd, D. M., 359
Bozic, K. J., 365
Bradby, H., 396, 397
Bradley, E. H., 13, 38, 40, 43, 47, 48, 49, 405
Brandenburger, A., 253
Brass, D. J., 168
Braverman, H., 15, 16
Bray, N., 22
Breland, J., 121
Brimhall, K. C., 48
Britten, N., 136
Brockner, J., 86
Brook, R. H., 7
Brown, B., 117
Brown, G. D., 217
Brown, S. L., 205
Buchan J., 400
Buntin, M. B., 325
Buono, A. F., 195
Burawoy, M., 168
Burgess, J. F., 326
Burke, C. S., 119
Burke, T., 357
Burkhardt, M. E., 168
Burnes, B., 188
Burns, L. R., 5, 9, 10, 12, 14, 15, 17, 19, 20, 22, 24, 243, 244, 256, 260, 278, 279, 280, 281, 283, 288, 289, 293, 298, 299

Burns, T., 19, 60, 62
Burnum, J. F., 334
Burt, R. S., 21, 143
Business Dictionary, 249
Business Insights, 299
Byrne, D. S., 188, 189
Byrne, M., 65, 69

C

Cahin, V., 350
Caldararo, K. L., 254
Caldwell, D. F., 111, 121
Calhoun, J. G., 49
Callaghan, G., 188, 189
Calloway, M., 119
Cameron, K. S., 124
Campbell, J. P., 86
Campion, M. A., 111
Cannon-Bowers, J. A., 119
Cappelli, P., 25
Carayon, P., 106
Cardinal, L., 15
Carey, K., 326
Carli, L. L., 35
Carman, J. M., 226, 228
Carnevale, P. J., 172
Carpenter, G., 265
Cartwright, D., 122
Casalino, L. P., 23, 280, 289
Castro-Palaganas, E., 403
Caumont, A., 245
Center for Studying Health System Change (CSHSC), 324
Centers for Disease Control and Prevention (CDC), 271, 272
Centers for Medicare and Medicaid Services (CMS), 11, 40, 89, 157, 165, 309, 325
Cerasoli, C. P., 86
Chaiken, S., 174
Chaliand, G., 249
Chan, C., 18
Chandler, A. D., 17
Chang, C.-H., 83, 86
Charns, M. P., 65, 67, 69, 70, 71, 72, 73, 74, 89
Chassin, M. R., 218, 325
Chen, G., 83, 86, 118
Chen, L. C., 5, 397, 398, 400
Chen, L. H., 396
Chick, S., 388
Childress, J. F., 365, 366, 367, 368, 372
Chilingerian, J. A., 382, 388, 390, 393, 394, 395, 396, 405
Chilopora, G., 401
Chimonas, S., 327
Chiquan, G., 252

Choi, C., 204
Chou, A. F., 271
Christakis, N., 143
Christianson, J. C., 20
Christianson, M., 20
Chuang, Y. T., 192
Chukmaitov, A. S., 254
Chullen, C. L., 47
Cialdini, R. B., 175
Ciampa, M., 362
Clancy, C. M., 230
Clark, J. R., 48
Clegg, S. R., 167, 205
Clemens, M. A., 397, 399
CMS, 245, 254
CMS Quality Strategy, 255
Cobb, J. A., 19
Coffey, J., 135
Cohen, G. I., 388, 389, 390, 391, 392, 393
Cohen, R. A., 358
Cohen, S. G., 102, 109, 118
Cohn, D., 245
Collins, J. C., 19, 139, 200
Collis, D., 247, 249
Colon, A., 360
Colquitt, J. A., 109
Colwell, J., 269
Comarow, A., 389
Commission for Africa, 398
Commission on Accreditation of Healthcare Management Education (CAHME), 49
Commonwealth Fund, 5, 6, 253
CompareMaine, 324
Congressional Budget Office, 6
Conley, S., 15
Conner, M., 88
Conover, C. J., 321
Conrad, D., 187
Conte, J. M., 35
Convenient Care Association, 364
Coons, A., 36
Cooper, R. A., 7, 401
Coopman, S. J., 121
Cordina, J., 350, 351, 359, 362, 363, 364
Corrigan, J. M., 230
Cortez, N., 388
Cosby K. S., 112
Cosgrove, T., 385
Cosier, R. A., 114
Cote, J., 389
Covey, S., 137
Cowden, T., 47
Coye, M. J., 341
Cramton, C. D., 178
Crean, K., 254
Cresswell, K. M., 341

Subject Index